Contemporary Issues in the Treatment of Schizophrenia

Contemporary Issues in the Treatment of Schizophrenia

Edited by

Christian L. Shriqui, M.D.
Henry A. Nasrallah, M.D.

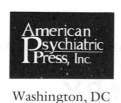

American Psychiatric Press, Inc.

Washington, DC
London, England

Copyright © 1995 American Psychiatric Press, Inc.
ALL RIGHTS RESERVED
Manufactured in the United States of America on acid-free paper
98 97 96 95   4 3 2 1
First Edition

American Psychiatric Press, Inc.
1400 K Street, N.W., Washington, DC   20005

Library of Congress Cataloging-in-Publication Data
Contemporary issues in the treatment of schizophrenia / edited by Christian L. Shriqui, Henry A. Nasrallah.
    p.   cm.
  Includes bibliographical references and index.
  ISBN 0-88048-681-3 (alk. paper)
    1. Schizophrenia. 2. Schizophrenia—Treatment.   I. Shriqui, Christian L, 1961- . II. Nasrallah, Henry A.
  [DNLM: 1. Schizophrenia—therapy.   WM 203 C762 1995]
  RC514.C617 1995
  616.89'8206—dc20
  DNLM/DLC   95-2032
  for Library of Congress   CIP

British Library Cataloguing in Publication Data
A CIP record is available from the British Library.

Dedication

To our wives,
Carol Ann and Amelia,
without whose personal support and understanding
this book would not have been possible.

Contents

Section I

Biochemistry, Neuropathology, and Genetics of Schizophrenia

Section II

Clinical and Diagnostic Issues in Schizophrenia

Section III

Pharmacological Treatments

Contributors

Gerard Addonizio, M.D.
Associate Professor of Clinical Psychiatry, New York Hospital–Westchester Division, Cornell University Medical Center, White Plains, New York

Lawrence Annable, B.Sc., Dip. Stat.
Associate Professor, Department of Psychiatry, McGill University; Medical Scientist, Allan Memorial Institute, Montreal, Québec, Canada

A. George Awad, M.B., B.Ch., Ph.D., F.R.C.P.C.
Professor of Psychiatry and Director of Psychopharmacology Program, University of Toronto; Psychiatrist-in-Chief, Wellesley Hospital, Toronto, Ontario, Canada

Bernhard Bogerts, M.D.
Professor, Department of Psychiatry, University of Magdeburg, Magdeburg, Germany

Richard L. Borison, M.D., Ph.D.
Professor and Chairman, Department of Psychiatry, Medical College of Georgia and Augusta Veterans Administration Medical Center, Augusta, Georgia

Walter A. Brown, M.D.
Professor, Department of Psychiatry and Human Behavior, Brown University School of Medicine and Veterans Administration Medical Center, Providence, Rhode Island

Daniel E. Casey, M.D.
Chief, Psychiatry Research and Psychopharmacology, Department of Veterans Affairs Medical Center, Portland Division; Professor of Psychiatry and Neurology, Oregon Health Sciences University, Portland, Oregon

Evan J. Collins, M.D., F.R.C.P.C.
Head, Clinical Research Section, Schizophrenia Research Program, Queen Street Mental Health Centre; Assistant Professor, Department of Psychiatry, University of Toronto, Ontario, Canada

Nancy Curcio, Psy.D.
Research Associate, Department of Psychiatry, Schizophrenia Research Program, St. Luke's–Roosevelt Hospital Center, New York, New York

John R. DeQuardo, M.D.
Assistant Professor of Psychiatry, University of Michigan Medical Center, Ann Arbor, Michigan

Bruce I. Diamond, Ph.D.
Professor, Department of Psychiatry, Medical College of Georgia and Augusta Veterans Administration Medical Center, Augusta, Georgia

Lisa Dixon, M.D.
Assistant Professor, Department of Psychiatry, University of Maryland School of Medicine; Medical Director, Assertive Community Treatment Team, University of Maryland Medical Center, Baltimore, Maryland

Ahmed M. Elkashef, M.D.
Senior Staff Research Fellow, Department of Health and Human Services, National Institute of Mental Health, Neuropsychiatry Research Hospital, Washington, D.C.

Peter Falkai, M.D.
Senior Physician, Department of Psychiatry, University of Düsseldorf, Düsseldorf, Germany

Michael Flaum, M.D.
Assistant Professor, Mental Health Clinical Research Center, University of Iowa Hospitals and Clinics and Department of Psychiatry, University of Iowa College of Medicine, Iowa City, Iowa

Sridhar Gowda, M.D.
Fellow, Department of Psychiatry, Medical College of Georgia and Augusta Veterans Administration Medical Center, Augusta, Georgia

Hans Häfner, M.D., Ph.D., Drs.h.c.
Professor and Head, Central Institute of Mental Health, Mannheim, Germany

Courtenay M. Harding, Ph.D.
Assistant Professor, Department of Psychiatry, and Associate Director, Program for Public Psychiatry, University of Colorado School of Medicine, Denver, Colorado

Susan Haverstock, M.D.
Assistant Professor, Department of Psychiatry, Medical College of Georgia and Augusta Veterans Administration Medical Center, Augusta, Georgia

Marvin I. Herz, M.D.
Professor, Department of Psychiatry, University of Rochester Medical Center, Strong Memorial Hospital, Rochester, New York

Steven R. Hirsch, M.D., F.R.C.Psych.
Professor and Chairman, Academic Department of Psychiatry, Charing Cross Hospital, London, England

Anne L. Hoff, Ph.D.
Lecturer, Department of Psychiatry, Stanford University, Stanford, California; Adjunct Assistant Professor, State University of New York at Stony Brook; Research Coordinator, Biological Psychiatry Treatment and Research Center, Napa State Hospital, Napa, California

Fuad Issa, M.D.
Senior Staff Research Fellow, Department of Health and Human Services, National Institute of Mental Health, Neuropsychiatry Research Hospital, Washington, D.C.

Michael D. Jibson, M.D., Ph.D.
Assistant Professor of Psychiatry, University of Michigan Medical Center, Ann Arbor, Michigan

Barry D. Jones, M.D., F.R.C.P.C.
Professor of Psychiatry, McMaster University; Director of Postgraduate Education, Hamilton Psychiatric Hospital, Hamilton, Ontario, Canada

John M. Kane, M.D.
Professor of Psychiatry, Albert Einstein College of Medicine, New York City; Chairman of Psychiatry, Hillside Hospital (Division of Long Island Jewish Medical Center), Glen Oaks, New York

Bruce J. Kinon, M.D.
Assistant Professor of Psychiatry, Albert Einstein College of Medicine, New York City; Director of Psychopharmacology, Hillside Hospital (Division of Long Island Jewish Medical Center), Glen Oaks, New York

Dora Kohen, M.D., M.R.C.Psych.
Senior Lecturer and Honorary Consultant, Academic Department of Psychiatry, Charing Cross Hospital, London, England

Pierre Lalonde, M.D., F.R.C.P.C.
Professor, Department of Psychiatry, University of Montreal; Director, Young Adult Schizophrenia Program, Hôpital Louis-H. Lafontaine, Montreal, Québec, Canada

J. Steven Lamberti, M.D.
Assistant Professor of Psychiatry, University of Rochester Medical Center; Director, Strong Ties Clinic, Strong Memorial Hospital, Rochester, New York

Yvon D. Lapierre, M.D., F.R.C.P.C.
Professor and Chairman, Department of Psychiatry, University of Ottawa; Psychiatrist-in-Chief, Royal Ottawa Hospital, Ottawa, Ontario, Canada

Julian Leff, M.D.
Professor and Director, Medical Research Council Social and Community Psychiatry Unit, London, England

Ira M. Lesser, M.D.
Professor of Psychiatry and Director of Residency Training, Department of Psychiatry, Harbor University of California at Los Angeles Medical Center, Torrance, California

Jeffrey A. Lieberman, M.D.
Associate Professor of Psychiatry, Albert Einstein College of Medicine, New York City; Director of Psychiatric Research, Hillside Hospital (Division of Long Island Jewish Medical Center), Glen Oaks, New York

Pierre-Michel Llorca, M.D.
Assistant des Hôpitaux, Chef de Clinique Universitaire, Service de Psychiatrie, Hôpital Ste. Marguerite, Marseille, France

Stephen R. Marder, M.D.
Professor of Psychiatry, University of California at Los Angeles; Staff Psychiatrist, Veterans Affairs Medical Center, Los Angeles, California

Kurt Maurer, Ph.D.
Psychologist and Senior Scientist, Schizophrenia Research Unit, Central Institute of Mental Health, Mannheim, Germany

Michel Maziade, M.D., F.R.C.P.C.
Associate Professor of Psychiatry, Laval University; Scientific Director, Centre de Recherche Université Laval Robert-Giffard, Beauport, Québec, Canada

Tasha Mott, M.A.
Research Associate, Department of Psychiatry, Schizophrenia Research Program, St. Luke's–Roosevelt Hospital Center, New York, New York

Heather Munroe-Blum, M.S.W., Ph.D.
Vice President–Research, and Professor, Departments of Social Work and of Psychiatry, University of Toronto; Professor, Departments of Psychiatry and of Clinical Epidemiology and Biostatistics, McMaster University, Hamilton, Ontario, Canada

Henry A. Nasrallah, M.D.
Chairman, Department of Psychiatry, and Professor of Psychiatry and Neurology, Ohio State University College of Medicine, Columbus, Ohio

Luc Nicole, M.D., F.R.C.P.C.
Lecturer, Department of Psychiatry, Laval University; Director, Residency Training, Centre Hospitalier Robert-Giffard, Beauport, Québec, Canada

Ananda Pathiraja, M.D.
Assistant Professor, Department of Psychiatry, Medical College of Georgia and Augusta Veterans Administration Medical Center, Augusta, Georgia

Peter J. Prendergast, M.B., M.R.C.Psych., F.R.C.P.C.
Psychiatrist-in-Chief, Whitby Psychiatric Hospital, Whitby, Ontario; Director of Continuing Medical Education, Department of Psychiatry, University of Toronto, Ontario, Canada

Vincent Raymond, M.D., Ph.D.
Senior Scientist, Molecular Endocrinology Laboratory, Centre de Recherche du Centre Hospitalier de l'Université Laval, Sainte-Foy, Québec; Assistant Professor, Department of Psychiatry, Laval University, Beauport, Québec, Canada

Thomas A. Rebori, M.D.
Addictions Psychiatry Fellow, Department of Psychiatry, University of Maryland School of Medicine; Assertive Community Treatment Team, University of Maryland Medical Center, Baltimore, Maryland

Gary J. Remington, M.D., Ph.D., F.R.C.P.C.
Assistant Professor, Department of Psychiatry, University of Toronto, Neuropsychopharmacology Research Unit and Schizophrenia Research Program, Clarke Institute of Psychiatry, Toronto, Ontario, Canada

S. Craig Risch, M.D.
Professor of Psychiatry, and Director, Schizophrenia Research and Treatment Program, Medical University of South Carolina, Institute of Psychiatry, Charleston, South Carolina

Allan Z. Safferman, M.D.
Associate Medical Director–Clinical and Scientific Affairs, Clinical Research Division, Pfizer, Inc., New York, New York

Christian L. Shriqui, M.D., M.Sc., F.R.C.P.C.
Assistant Professor of Psychiatry, Laval University, Centre Hospitalier Robert-Giffard and Centre de Recherche Université Laval Robert-Giffard, Beauport, Québec, Canada

Samuel G. Siris, M.D.
Professor of Psychiatry, Albert Einstein College of Medicine, New York City; Director, Psychiatric Day Programs, Hillside Hospital (Division of Long Island Jewish Medical Center), Glen Oaks, New York

Virginia L. Susman, M.D.
Associate Professor of Clinical Psychiatry, New York Hospital–Westchester Division, Cornell University Medical Center, White Plains, New York

J. Randolph Swartz, M.D.
Assistant Professor, Department of Psychiatry, Harbor University of California at Los Angeles Medical Center, Torrance, California

Sally R. Szymanski, D.O.
Assistant Professor, Neuropsychiatry Program, Department of Psychiatry, University of Pennsylvania, Philadelphia, Pennsylvania

Rajiv Tandon, M.D.
Associate Professor of Psychiatry, and Director, Schizophrenia Program, University of Michigan Medical Center, Ann Arbor, Michigan

Stephan F. Taylor, M.D.
Lecturer in Psychiatry, University of Michigan Medical Center, Ann Arbor, Michigan

Theodore Van Putten, M.D.[†]
Professor of Psychiatry, University of California at Los Angeles; Staff Psychiatrist, Veterans Affairs Medical Center, Los Angeles, California

---

[†]Deceased.

Peter J. Weiden, M.D.
Associate Professor, Department of Psychiatry, and Director, Schizophrenia Research Program, St. Luke's–Roosevelt Hospital Center, New York, New York

Scott A. West, M.D.
Fellow, Biological Psychiatry Program, Department of Psychiatry, University of Cincinnati College of Medicine, Cincinnati, Ohio

Marc-Alain Wolf, M.D.
Assistant Professor of Psychiatry, McGill University, Douglas Hospital Centre, Verdun, Québec, Canada

Richard Jed Wyatt, M.D.
Chief, Neuropsychiatry Branch, Department of Health and Human Services, National Institute of Mental Health, Neuropsychiatry Research Hospital, Washington, D.C.

Preface

The objective of this book is to provide a clinical, state-of-the-art overview of treatment-related topics in schizophrenia. The book is primarily targeted for psychiatrists and psychiatric residents, but can be useful to neurologists, psychologists, nurses, and other mental health professionals. In addition to pharmacotherapy and psychosocial treatments, we have attempted to integrate a wide range of issues relating to the biochemistry, neuropathology, genetics, brain imaging, cognitive functioning, and neuroleptic side effects of schizophrenia, as well as several clinical and diagnostic aspects of the illness.

The history behind the cover illustration of this book is a moving and inspiring story. In 1985, one of us (C.L.S.) attended a posthumous exhibition of the works of Martin Ramirez at the Goldie Paley Gallery in Philadelphia. Martin Ramirez suffered from paranoid schizophrenia and rarely communicated verbally. He spent most of his adult life institutionalized in a state psychiatric hospital in Auburn, California, where he died in 1963. Mr. Ramirez, a man of Mexican origin, had received no previous art training and began to develop a passion for his art after 20 years in the hospital. When suitable paper was not available to him, he would frequently gather scraps of paper and glue them together with mashed potatoes and saliva. To protect his works from hospital staff, who were instructed to confiscate and burn the works of patients, Mr. Ramirez would often hide them under his mattress bed. Although trapped in a mute state, Ramirez somehow managed to express himself in a brilliant and unique art form. His story is a compelling testimony to the power of human creativity. We are delighted to have this particular Ramirez work on the book cover. In its own right, the Ramirez story is a triumph of the human spirit and provides hope for all concerned about schizophrenia: physicians, mental health professionals, families, advocates, and of course, our patients. For permission to use this work, we express our gratitude to Gladys Nilsson, Jim Nutt, Elsa Weiner Longhauser, and Phyllis Kind.

We believe we have gathered an outstanding group of chapter authors, composed of both senior and junior investigators. **To each contributor in this book, we express our heartfelt appreciation.** We were saddened to learn of the death of Theodore Van Putten, M.D., who coauthored the chapter on the clinical use of neuroleptic plasma levels. Dr. Van Putten helped characterize the art of pharmacotherapy for psychosis, and his studies of antipsychotic side effects have made clinicians more sensitive to the feelings of their patients.

We would like to thank several organizations and individuals who either encouraged or assisted us in the publication of this book: the Fonds de la Recherche en Santé du Québec (FRSQ); the Centre de recherche université Laval Robert-Giffard and Centre hospitalier Robert-Giffard, Beauport, Quebec; the late Ramzy Yassa, M.D.; Serge Champetier; Nicole Brunet; Myriam de Courval; Beth Deley; Marjolaine Roy; and Josée Plamondon.

We are also grateful to Claire Reinburg, Editorial Director; Carol C. Nadelson, M.D., Editor in Chief; Pamela Harley, Managing Editor, Books; Rebecca Richters, Project Editor, Books; and other editorial staff members at American Psychiatric Press, Inc., for their valuable assistance.

We sincerely hope that this book will be a useful addition to the library of clinicians involved in the treatment and care of individuals with schizophrenia.

Christian L. Shriqui, M.D.
Henry A. Nasrallah, M.D.

Introduction

O f all the existing mental disorders, schizophrenia is the most devastating biopsychosocial illness. With an estimated lifetime prevalence of 1%, schizophrenia is probably the most frequently occurring of all psychotic disorders. For several decades, the prognosis for schizophrenic patients was generally considered to be poor with a progressive deteriorating course. However, recent long-term prospective studies on the course and outcome of schizophrenia have confirmed that such an outcome is no longer true for many individuals with this illness.

This book is divided into five major sections. In Section I, the chapter authors focus on the biochemical basis, neuropathology, and genetics of schizophrenia and their relationship to its etiology and treatment.

In Section II, clinical and diagnostic issues in schizophrenia (i.e., diagnostic classification [including DSM-IV criteria]; the epidemiology, pathophysiology, and treatment implications of positive and negative symptoms; depression in schizophrenia; diagnostic and treatment issues in late-onset schizophrenia; neuropsychological function; the relationship of structural brain changes to antipsychotic drug response; and gender differences) are discussed.

In Section III, the chapter authors concentrate on pharmacological treatments and cover standard and novel antipsychotic drugs and their potential mechanisms of action. Also included are specific chapters on drug treatment of negative symptoms, drug treatment implications on the long-term course of schizophrenia, neuroleptic noncompliance issues, clinical use of neuroleptic plasma levels, whether neuroleptic-responsive and neuroleptic-resistant patients have different illnesses, neuroleptic maintenance strategies, and use of non-neuroleptic adjunctive agents in treatment-refractory schizophrenic patients.

In Section IV, the broad spectrum of neuroleptic-induced side effects, including acute extrapyramidal side effects (EPS), neuroleptic malignant syndrome, non-EPS symptoms, tardive dyskinesia, and the clinical evidence supporting the concept of tardive psychosis are covered.

In Section V, the multifaceted psychosocial treatment dimensions of schizophrenia are addressed. Biopsychosocial factors affecting the course of schizophrenia are presented as well as chapters on family management of the illness; psychiatric and vocational rehabilitation; psychotherapeutic interventions, social skills training, and various case management approaches; quality of life issues; psychosocial treatment of the substance-abusing schizophrenic patient; the need for better integration of pharmacological and psychosocial treatments; and the relevance of individualizing treatment needs.

Some of chapters presented in this book (e.g., Chapters 16, 19, and 26) express some highly interesting, although speculative, viewpoints; the reader is advised to keep the recommendations in these chapters in perspective.

We are currently witnessing a surge of new knowledge and technological breakthroughs in the field of brain imaging and molecular biology, as well as the development of several novel antipsychotic agents that, when used appropriately with psychosocial treatments, are likely to confer greater therapeutic benefit and improved quality of life to patients. In an era of shrinking health care budgets, one of the many challenges ahead will be how to give schizophrenic patients greater access to novel antipsychotic drugs.

SECTION I

Biochemistry, Neuropathology, and Genetics of Schizophrenia

CHAPTER 1

The Biochemical Basis of Schizophrenia

Ahmed M. Elkashef, M.D.,
Fuad Issa, M.D., and Richard Jed Wyatt, M.D.

Ever since schizophrenia was described almost 100 years ago by Kraepelin (1919), researchers have sought a biochemical abnormality that could be fingered as a cause of this disorder. This has triggered a search for what has proven to be a very elusive chemical in the body fluids and tissues of schizophrenic patients. As measuring techniques have grown more sophisticated and new brain chemicals have been discovered, many hypotheses and ideas involving various neurotransmitters and neuromodulators have been advanced, and some have been discarded only to be reintroduced.

In this chapter, we review several of the biochemical hypotheses of schizophrenia and focus on some of the current issues involving each. Because space is limited, this chapter is not a comprehensive review of the literature, but rather a selective overview that we hope will introduce readers to this extremely complex topic.

The authors are grateful to Ioline de Saint Ghislain for her editorial assistance.

The Monoamines

Dopamine

The most promising biochemical theory, and the one that has generated the most studies, is the *dopamine hypothesis*. Advanced in the 1960s and early 1970s, the dopamine hypothesis posits, in its simplest form, that schizophrenia is caused by hyperactivity of dopamine (DA) in the brain. Support for this theory was derived mostly in an indirect manner through the then newly discovered action of antipsychotic medications and psychotogenic drugs.

For example, indirect DA agonists like amphetamine and L-dopa, which act to increase DA in the synapse, can induce a schizophrenia-like psychosis in healthy subjects and worsen the psychotic symptoms of schizophrenic patients (Angrist et al. 1973; Connell 1958; Janowsky et al. 1973; Meltzer and Stahl 1976; Tatetsu 1976). In addition, antipsychotic medications, including chlorpromazine and haloperidol, increase the DA metabolite, 3-methoxytyramine (Carlsson and Lindquist 1963), suggesting that antipsychotic medications are involved in increasing the turnover of DA through a feedback loop after blocking DA receptors. Finally, there is a strong correlation between the relative clinical potencies of antipsychotic medications and their ability to bind to DA receptors in vitro (Creese et al. 1976).

Since the dopamine hypothesis was first advanced, it has stimulated extensive work in the search for direct evidence of "hyperdopaminergia," and has been subjected to many challenges and revisions along the way. In the following sections we review some of this work and present several current views on the hypothesis. (See Figure 1–1 for an overview of dopamine synthesis and metabolism; see Figure 1–2 for the major dopaminergic tracts in the brain.)

Postmortem Studies

A number of studies have focused on the concentration of DA and its metabolites—especially homovanillic acid (HVA)—and DA receptor density in the brains of schizophrenic individuals. The findings of these studies have varied depending on the antipsychotic medication

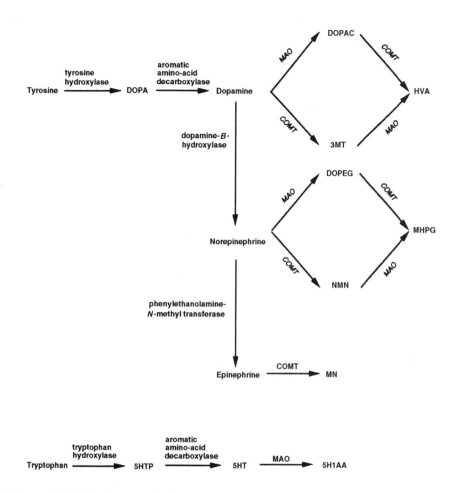

Figure 1–1. The basic catecholamine metabolic pathways. DOPA = dihydroxyphenylalanine; DOPAC = dihydroxyphenylacetic acid; DOPEG = dihydroxyphenylethyleneglycol; 5-HIAA = 5-hydroxyindoleacetic acid; 5-HT = 5-hydroxytryptamine (serotonin); 5-HTP = 5-hydroxytryptophan; HVA = homovanillic acid; MHPG = 3-methoxy-4-hydroxyphenylglycol; MN = meta-nephrine; 3-MT = 3-methoxytyramine; NMN = normetanephrine; COMT = catechol-O-methyl transferase; MAO = monoamine oxidase.

status of the patients, the brain region studied, and methodological issues (e.g., agonal and postmortem changes, assay techniques employed, number of cases reported). Overall, these studies have provided only limited support for the dopamine hypothesis.

Dopamine and homovanillic acid concentration studies.   In their study, Owen et al. (1978) found increased DA in the caudate nucleus, but not in the nucleus accumbens, of 15 schizophrenic patients. Mackay et al. (1982) found increased DA in the nucleus accumbens, but not in the caudate, of 34 schizophrenic patients compared with 34 normal control subjects. Crow et al. (1979) noted increased DA in the caudate and putamen of 9 schizophrenic patients who were taking

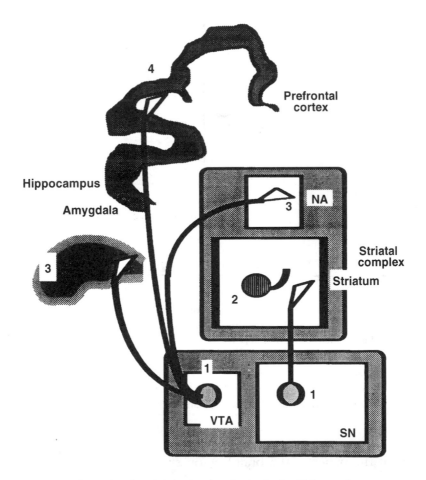

Figure 1–2. The major dopaminergic tracts in the brain. NA = nucleus accumbens; SN = substantia nigra; VTA = ventral tegmental area. 1–2 = nigrostriatal tract; 1–3 = mesolimbic tract; 1–4 = mesocortical tract.

antipsychotic medications. In another study (Toru et al. 1988), elevated HVA was reported in the nucleus accumbens of 5 schizophrenic patients who were not taking antipsychotic medications compared with another 5 schizophrenic patients who were taking those medications, whereas no change was detected in the DA concentration of either group. In another study of 13 schizophrenic patients (Bridge et al. 1985), no difference in DA concentration was found when patients were compared with normal control subjects. However, when the researchers compared schizophrenic patients who had dementia with those who did not, a significant increase in DA concentration was found in the nucleus accumbens of the latter group.

DA and HVA levels in various cortical regions have been investigated in two studies. In one, Bacopoulos et al. (1979) reported increased HVA in the temporal, cingulate, and frontal cortices of schizophrenic patients taking antipsychotic medications compared with those who were not and with normal control subjects. Authors of a second study (Reynolds et al. 1983) reported an increase of DA in the amygdala of schizophrenic patients, but not in normal control subjects, with concentrations being higher in the left amygdala.

Dopamine receptor density (B_{max}) studies.　　There are at least five types of central nervous system DA receptors—D_1 through D_5—identified on the basis of their DNA sequence. Of these, the D_1 and D_2 receptors are the most well studied. D_1 and D_2 can be differentiated by selective agonists and antagonists that bind specifically to each. For example, SKF 82526 is a selective D_1 agonist, whereas SCH 23390 is a selective D_1 antagonist. Sulpiride is a selective D_2 antagonist. D_1 receptors stimulate, and D_2 receptors inhibit, adenylate cyclase activity. Both receptors can exist in either a high- or a low-affinity state, and are found predominately in areas receiving dopaminergic projections, such as the prefrontal cortex and the striatum and limbic structures. D_2 receptors are also located presynaptically, where they regulate DA synthesis and release. Most antipsychotic medications bind to both D_1 and D_2 receptors.

Most studies of DA receptor density have used [^{3}H]spiperone to measure D_2 receptors. In the majority of studies (Cross et al. 1981; Crow et al. 1978; Hess et al. 1987; Mackay et al. 1982; Seeman et al.

1987), increased D_2 receptor densities in the striatum of schizophrenic patients have been reported. These results were confounded by the fact that most of the schizophrenic patients had received antipsychotic medications prior to their death. However, in the majority of studies where schizophrenic patients free of antipsychotic medications for at least a few weeks were compared with normal control subjects, an increase in D_2 receptors in the schizophrenic patients was found (Joyce et al. 1988; Mita et al. 1986; Seeman et al. 1984; Toru et al. 1988). In one study in which patients were free of antipsychotic medication for a few days before their death (Kornhuber et al. 1989b), no increase in D_2 receptor density was found. This finding raises some doubt about the interaction between antipsychotic treatment and the increase in D_2 receptor density.

Although most studies of D_1 receptor density have indicated no difference between schizophrenic patients and normal control subjects (Seeman and Niznik 1990), authors in two studies (Carenzi et al. 1975; Memo et al. 1983) did report elevated D_1 receptor density in schizophrenic patients.

Positron-Emission Tomography and Single Photon Emission Computed Tomography Studies

In vivo studies of D_2 receptor densities in schizophrenic patients have had mixed results. Five positron-emission tomography (PET) studies have been conducted with either neuroleptic-naive or unmedicated schizophrenic patients. In the first of these studies, Wong et al. (1986) used [^{11}C]methylspiperone with 10 neuroleptic-naive schizophrenic patients; these researchers reported robust increases of about 250% in the D_2 receptors of schizophrenic patients compared with those of normal control subjects. Farde et al. (1990) studied D_2 receptor densities in 18 drug-naive schizophrenic patients using [^{11}C]raclopride and reported no significant differences between the schizophrenic patients and the normal control subjects; however, in the schizophrenic patients, the elevation of D_2 receptors was significantly higher in the left putamen compared with the right. Using the same ligand ([^{11}C]raclopride), Hietala et al. (1991) found no differences between 11 neuroleptic-naive schizophrenic patients and matched normal control subjects, although 4 of the schizophrenic patients had D_2 densities that were highly elevated compared with those of the control subjects. Similarly negative findings were reported in two studies by Martinot et al. (1990, 1991). In the 1990 study, 12 schizophrenic patients (9 of whom were neuroleptic naive and 3 of whom had not received antipsychotic medications for at least 1 year prior to the study) and 12 normal control subjects were observed using [^{76}Br]bromospiperone. In Martinot et al.'s replication study (1991), a different ligand, [^{76}Br]bromolisuride, was used to measure D_2 receptor densities in 19 schizophrenic patients (10 of whom were neuroleptic naive and 9 of whom had not received antipsychotic medications for at least 6 months prior to the study) and 14 normal control subjects.

In another PET study, Crawley et al. (1986) used [^{77}Br]bromospiperone to study 12 schizophrenic patients, 4 of whom were neuroleptic naive and 8 of whom had not received antipsychotic medications for 6 months prior to the study. The authors reported a modest but statistically significant increase of 11% in the striatum-cerebellum ratios in schizophrenic patients compared with normal control subjects. Researchers in one single photon emission computed tomography (SPECT) study (Konig et al. 1991) used [^{123}I]pyrrolidinemethylbenzamide (IBZM) to measure D_2 receptor density in 27 schizophrenic patients, 8 of whom were unmedicated. No significant differences were reported between the unmedicated schizophrenic patients and the normal control subjects. Significant increases in D_2 receptor density were found in the schizophrenic patients treated with antipsychotic medications in comparison with those in the unmedicated group, suggesting, as in the postmortem studies, that chronic treatment with antipsychotic medications can increase D_2 receptor density (B_{max}).

The conflicting results of the above-described tests have stimulated further analyses (Buchsbaum 1992; Seeman 1992a) in an attempt to understand the discrepancies that appear to permeate these studies.

Cerebrospinal Fluid and Plasma Homovanillic Acid Studies

The dopamine hypothesis of schizophrenia has motivated efforts to find peripheral measurements that reflect central dopaminergic activity. Cerebrospinal fluid (CSF) HVA and plasma HVA, DA's major metabolite (see Figure 1–1), have been most widely measured. There are, however, several confounding factors that affect CSF HVA levels that must be kept in mind (Issa et al. 1994a), including patients' height and weight and circadian and seasonal variations. Also, the validity of such measurements relies on several assumptions (Kahn and Davidson 1993), including that DA turnover is a reflection of neuro-transmission, and that what is present in the CSF and plasma is representative of what is taking place in the brain.

Conflicting results have been obtained when CSF HVA and plasma HVA measurements are used as an indicator of baseline central DA function. In 11 studies that compared CSF HVA levels between a medication-free patient group and healthy control subjects (reviewed in Issa et al. 1994a), authors in the majority of studies did not find any difference between the two groups, whereas authors of 2 studies found a decrease in the HVA of the patient group (Bjerkenstedt et al. 1985; Lindström 1985). Attempts to correlate CSF HVA with psy-chopathological ratings have yielded equally conflicting results. Post et al. (1975) reported a significant negative correlation between CSF HVA and Schneiderian first-rank symptoms. Lindström (1985) re-ported a significant negative correlation between CSF HVA and lassi-tude and slowness of movement. Pickar et al. (1990) found that the levels of CSF HVA of unmedicated schizophrenic patients correlated negatively with the patients' Brief Psychiatric Rating Scale (BPRS; Overall and Gorham 1962) total score and BPRS positive symptom score. A negative correlation between CSF HVA levels and BPRS total score in unmedicated schizophrenic patients was similarly noted by Hsiao et al. (1993). Issa et al. (1994b) did not find any correlation between CSF HVA levels and Psychiatric Symptom Assessment Scale (Bigelow and Berthot 1989) mean item score or any of its subscales. Furthermore, plasma HVA levels provided a basis for differentiating between the patient and control groups in some, but not all, of the studies (Davis et al. 1991). Similarly, contradictory results were found when plasma HVA was correlated with psychopathology.

More consistent results, however, were obtained when change in central DA activity was studied using CSF and plasma HVA. Initial reports on CSF HVA (Bowers 1975; Fyrö et al. 1974; Gerlach et al.

1975; Sedvall et al. 1974) indicated an acute rise shortly after initiation of treatment with antipsychotic medications. In addition, plasma HVA has mostly been found to decrease after treatment with antipsychotic medications (Bowers et al. 1984; Chang et al. 1990; Davidson et al. 1991; Pickar et al. 1986; Sharma et al. 1989; Wolkowitz et al. 1988), with this decrease being associated with clinical response. Pickar et al. (1990) found that, in a stepwise multiple regression model, CSF and plasma HVA were the only two variables that made a statistically significant contribution to the variance of the BPRS total score. They proposed that plasma HVA reflects subcortical DA activity, while CSF HVA reflects cortical DA activity. This argument was used to support the dysregulation hypothesis (see below).

The Dopamine Hypothesis 20 Years Later

Two decades after the dopamine hypothesis was first advanced, there is still no direct evidence of increased DA in the brains of schizophrenic patients. Although authors of some studies have shown some indirect evidence of increased DA, its metabolite HVA, or D_2 receptors, that evidence is subtle and inconclusive.

Clinical evidence suggests that at least 30% of schizophrenic patients do not respond to traditional treatment with antipsychotic medications, implying that D_2 blockade, and presumably DA hyperactivity, are not the major pathophysiologic processes involved in these patients. Furthermore, PET data have shown that some schizophrenic patients continue to have active symptoms despite the fact that D_2 receptors in the striatum are markedly blocked.

The similarities noted by Mesulam (1986) between deficit symptoms in schizophrenic patients, deficit symptoms in patients with frontal lobe lesions, and the behavior observed in primates with frontal lobe lesions aroused the notion that the deficit state in schizophrenic patients could be an expression of frontal lobe hypofunction. PET blood flow and metabolic studies have shown that schizophrenic patients are unable to activate their prefrontal cortex, specifically the dorsolateral prefrontal region, when challenged with tasks that would normally activate this area (Andreasen et al. 1992; Buchsbaum et al. 1992; Weinberger et al. 1988). These findings have led to the emergence of new theories and variations on the original dopamine hypothesis in an attempt to explain the various symptoms and phenotypes of schizophrenia, including deficit symptoms, cognitive impairments, and positive symptoms.

A theory concerning dysregulation of the mesocortical and mesolimbic DA tracts was recently advanced (Davis et al. 1991; Heritch 1990; Weinberger 1987). It has been proposed that a lesion involving the dorsolateral prefrontal region renders the mesocortical dopaminergic tract hypoactive. This would explain the deficit symptoms and the impairment in cognitive functioning found in schizophrenic patients. The lesion would also remove the inhibitory cortical regulation on mesolimbic dopaminergic systems that become hyperactive; this would be responsible for the production of positive symptoms. The evidence that best supports this theory is the PET data of hypofrontality and the data from other PET studies that have shown increased blood flow in the frontal region of schizophrenic patients after the administration of the DA agonists, amphetamine and apomorphine (Daniel et al. 1989, 1991). In these studies, hypofrontality was indirectly linked to DA. Finally, some CSF and plasma HVA studies have shown an inverse correlation between HVA levels and deficit symptoms or HVA levels and poor response to medication (Davidson and Davis 1988; Widerlöv 1988).

Another variant of the dopamine hypothesis is that an underlying decrease in dopaminergic function in the prefrontal cortex is responsible for some of the prodromal symptoms seen in schizophrenic patients prior to the first acute phase as well as for the deficit symptoms seen later in the illness (Wyatt 1986). This decrease, associated with deficit symptoms, is attributed to stress, which is part of psychotic relapse. Stress has been shown to increase DA turnover (Breier et al. 1991; Roth et al. 1988), which could have a damaging neurotoxic effect on the catecholaminergic systems in the frontal cortex and in other regions.

New Frontiers

DA remains the core of both the older and the more recent revisions of the original dopamine hypothesis; therefore, much research still emphasizes an understanding of the role of DA in schizophrenia. As mentioned previously, the revolution in molecular biology has enabled five DA receptor subtypes—which are G protein–coupled receptors—to be cloned. The first receptor to be cloned was the D_2 receptor (Bunzow et al. 1988), followed by the D_3 receptor, which appears to be a D_2 isoprotein in terms of binding characteristics. The D_4 receptor, which behaves pharmacologically like a D_2 receptor, has also been cloned. Another D_2 type receptor, differing by virtue of its calcium channel gating, has also been described. (The nomenclature of these receptors is still undergoing refinement, as are the defining characteristics of each.) Furthermore, the D_2 receptor gene itself was found to be subject to alternative splicing, leading to the D_{2A} and D_{2B} isoforms. It is not yet clear if these isoforms correspond to the high- and low-affinity states of the receptor. The D_1 receptor has also been cloned (Dearry et al. 1990), and two more D_1-type receptors, possibly isomers, have been identified. One of these closely resembles the original D_1 receptor, whereas the other has a significantly higher dopaminergic affinity. In addition, still another D_1 receptor with different pharmacological characteristics has been designated as D_5. It is very likely that more DA subtype receptors-isomers will be identified in the near future (Niznik and Van Tol 1992).

Rapid advances in the cloning of DA receptors and the availability of specific probes could lead to a better definition of specific alterations in the gene expression of various DA receptors in postmortem tissue, and to a better understanding of their biochemical and pharmacological characteristics (Seeman 1992b). Such cloning has also enabled scientists to look for genetic linkages between chromosomal regions containing the genetic information for the receptors within schizophrenic families, efforts that so far have been unsuccessful (Moises et al. 1991).

The imaging techniques of PET and SPECT methodology continue to be refined and could offer a direct window into brain DA. PET studies to look at presynaptic DA using ligands like 6-^{18}F-dopa are already under way. The controversial issue of D_2 receptor density can be further investigated using SPECT. SPECT offers an advantage over PET because it can be used to perform multiple studies of the same subject; ideally, it could be used to study the effect of antipsychotic medications on DA receptors.

Norepinephrine

In noradrenergic neurons, the cell bodies of which are primarily in the locus coeruleus, norepinephrine (NE) is produced from DA by the enzyme dopamine-β-hydroxylase (DBH). (See Figure 1–1 for NE synthesis and metabolism.) Stein and Wise (1971) hypothesized that there is a loss of noradrenergic neurons secondary to neurotoxic accumulation. The hypothesis was based on preclinical observations of loss of drive and decreased reward-seeking behavior in animals with lesions in noradrenergic pathways. Stein and Wise also speculated that such a loss of noradrenergic neurons would lead to chronic deterioration and the negative symptoms of schizophrenia. The hypothesis was later supported by their finding of decreased DBH activity in schizophrenic patients. Other studies, however, could not replicate this finding (Crow et al. 1979; Wyatt et al. 1975). More recently (van Kammen et al. 1983), decreased DBH was reported in the CSF of schizophrenic patients, which correlated with both negative symptoms and increased ventricle-to-brain ratio (VBR) on computed tomography scans. This finding revitalized interest in the role of NE in schizophrenia.

Noradrenergic receptors are subdivided into two types: α-receptors, found in cortical and limbic structures, and β-receptors, found in cortical projections and the cerebellum. α-noradrenergic receptors have been further subdivided into α_1- and α_2-receptors, and β-noradrenergic receptors have similarly been subdivided into β_1- and β_2-receptors. Presynaptic receptors are α_2, whereas postsynaptic neurons contain α_1-receptors. Antipsychotics have potent α_1- and α_2-receptor–binding capacities, a property that has been reported to correlate with their relative clinical efficacy (R. M. Cohen et al. 1988).

Increased NE has been reported in the CSF (Beckmann et al. 1983; Gomes et al. 1980; Kemali et al. 1982; Lake et al. 1980), plasma (Albus et al. 1982; Bogerts et al. 1983; Naber et al. 1985), and postmortem brains of schizophrenic patients (Bridge et al. 1985; Carlsson 1978; Crow et al. 1979; Farley et al. 1978). CSF, NE, and 3-methoxy-4-hydroxyphenylglycol (MHPG) levels have been reported to be state dependent in schizophrenia; an increase has been reported with relapse and a decrease has been associated with remission or a stable condition (Linnoila 1983; van Kammen et al. 1985,

1989a, 1990). Ko et al. (1985) reported an increase in α_2-receptor binding in one postmortem study, and researchers in two other studies (Kafka and van Kammen 1983; Sternberg et al. 1982) reported a decrease. These findings seem to mirror the changes in DA and its metabolites. Similar changes in the noradrenergic system and its metabolites were also reported in anxiety disorders and mania (Post et al. 1981).

In one study, R. Freedman et al. (1982) found that, when the α_2-receptor agonist clonidine was used as the sole treatment for schizophrenia, it had a transient therapeutic effect. Authors of another study (van Kammen et al. 1989b) reported an antipsychotic effect of clonidine comparable to that of antipsychotic medications in 13 acutely psychotic patients. However, no other studies have reported beneficial effects of clonidine on psychotic symptoms, and some have reported a worsening of symptoms (Fields et al. 1988; Jimerson et al. 1980; Simpson et al. 1967).

In conclusion, there is no strong evidence for direct involvement of NE in schizophrenia. The data, however, seem to suggest a role for NE in the stress and anxiety associated with schizophrenia. It is possible that changes in NE could be early predictors of relapse in schizophrenia.

Serotonin

The idea that serotonin (5-HT) may play a role in schizophrenia was proposed in the 1950s (Gaddum and Hameed 1954; Woolley and Shaw 1952), based on the finding that the hallucinogen lysergic acid diethylamide (LSD), a 5-HT antagonist, could cause a psychosis similar to that observed in schizophrenia. That idea was later formulated into a hypothesis when LSD was found to be both a 5-HT agonist and antagonist. The hypothesis suggested that, in schizophrenic patients, there is a disturbance in 5-HT production that leads to both increased and decreased periods of production and, in turn, to a cyclic pattern of psychosis (Woolley 1957). At the time, the hypothesis was not heavily investigated, mainly because of the concurrent introduction of antipsychotic medications and the emergence of the dopamine hypothesis. Currently, four classes of 5-HT receptors have been characterized:

5-HT$_1$ through 5-HT$_4$ (see Figure 1–1 for synthesis and metabolism). More recently, the introduction of the atypical antipsychotic medication clozapine, which blocks 5-HT$_2$ receptors, has revived interest in the role of 5-HT in schizophrenia.

Postmortem Studies

Crow et al. (1979) reported increases in 5-HT in the putamen of 9 schizophrenic patients. In another study, Farley et al. (1980) found that levels of 5-HT and its metabolite, 5-hydroxyindoleacetic acid (5-HIAA), were also increased in the globus pallidus and nucleus accumbens of schizophrenic patients compared with normal control subjects. Similarly, significant increases in 5-HT were reported in the basal ganglia of 30 schizophrenic patients; increases of 5-HIAA in the occipital cortex were also found (Korpi et al. 1986). Winblad et al. (1979) reported decreased 5-HT in the hypothalamus, medulla oblongata, and hippocampus of 12 schizophrenic patients. Joseph et al. (1979) reported no differences in 5-HT or 5-HIAA in the putamen or temporal cortex of 15 schizophrenic patients.

Other postmortem studies assessed 5-HT$_2$ receptor density. Bennett et al. (1979) reported decreased binding of [^{3}H]LSD in 21 schizophrenic patients, whereas Whitaker et al. (1981) reported no change in 5-HT$_2$ in the frontal cortex of 13 schizophrenic patients in comparison with normal control subjects. Decreased binding of [^{3}H]ketanserin, a 5-HT$_2$–specific ligand, was reported in the prefrontal cortex of 9 schizophrenic patients investigated (Bennett et al. 1979), although this finding was not replicated in another study (Reynolds et al. 1983).

More recently, Joyce et al. (1993) reported an increase of 5-HT reuptake sites in the striatum, as measured with [^{3}H]CN-IMI, and a marked reduction of such sites in the anterior cingulate and frontal and temporal cortices of schizophrenic patients. Similarly, Laruelle et al. (1993) found decreased uptake sites in the frontal and anterior cingulate.

Cerebrospinal Fluid Studies

5-HIAA levels in the CSF were measured following the administration of probenecid, a drug that blocks amino acid transporter systems, in several studies of unmedicated schizophrenic patients. Decreased 5-HIAA was reported in three of these studies (Ashcroft et al. 1966; Bowers 1970; Gattaz et al. 1982b), but most researchers (Bowers et al. 1969; Nyback et al. 1983; Post et al. 1975; Potkin et al. 1983; Rimon et al. 1971) reported no significant differences in unmedicated schizophrenic patients compared with control subjects. An interesting correlation between decreased 5-HIAA, cortical atrophy, and increased VBR was reported by Losonczy et al. (1986), Nyback et al. (1983), and Potkin et al. (1983). Authors of three other studies (Banki et al. 1984; Ninan et al. 1984; van Praag 1983) reported a correlation between decreased 5-HIAA and suicidal behavior in schizophrenic patients.

Platelet Studies

Platelet 5-HT and monoamine oxidase (MAO) activity have been studied in schizophrenic patients as a model of brain 5-HT. Increased platelet or whole blood 5-HT has been reported in most studies of both medicated and unmedicated schizophrenic patients (DeLisi et al. 1981; D. X. Freedman et al. 1981; Garelis et al. 1975; Jackman et al. 1983; King et al. 1985; Stahl et al. 1985; Todrick et al. 1960). Some investigators (e.g., DeLisi et al. 1981) have also reported a strong correlation between increased platelet 5-HT and structural brain abnormalities in either schizophrenic patients or a specific subtype of schizophrenic patients.

MAO is the enzyme that metabolizes 5-HT into 5-HIAA. MAO activity was studied because it was thought that decreased MAO might represent a genetic predisposition for schizophrenia and might therefore explain the increased 5-HT reported in platelet studies (Wyatt et al. 1973). Studies have reported decreased MAO activity in schizophrenic patients with auditory hallucinations (Casacchia et al. 1975; DeLisi et al. 1981; Meltzer and Aurora 1980). In general, the decrease in platelet MAO in such patients is probably attributable to the presence of antipsychotic medications.

Treatment Trials

Clinical studies attempting to manipulate brain 5-HT have focused on two opposing strategies. In some studies (Bigelow et al. 1979; Wyatt et al. 1972), 5-hydroxytryptophan was used in combination with carbidopa in an attempt to increase brain 5-HT, with mixed results. In another study (DeLisi et al. 1982), para-chlorophenylalanine, an inhibitor of tryptophan hydroxylase, was used in an attempt to decrease brain 5-HT; in this study, negative results were reported except for some decrease in withdrawal behavior and social isolation.

Fenfluramine, a 5-HT uptake inhibitor and 5-HT$_2$ agonist, was tried in schizophrenic patients with no significant effect in one study (Shore et al. 1985) and with some improvement of negative symptoms in another study (Stahl et al. 1985).

Ritanserin, a potent 5-HT$_2$ antagonist, has been shown to be effective in improving negative symptoms when used as an adjunct to standard antipsychotic medication (Gelders et al. 1985a). In two other studies, Ceulemans et al. (1985) and Gelders et al. (1985b) compared ritanserin as a sole treatment with haloperidol in a double-blind design, finding that the ritanserin caused an overall improvement of psychotic symptoms.

Recently, challenge studies using the 5-HT selective agonist *m*-chlorophenylpiperazine (MCPP), an active metabolite of trazodone, were conducted to test the hypothesis that this agent would worsen psychosis in schizophrenic patients. When MCPP was administered intravenously, exacerbation of psychotic symptoms was reported in two studies (Iqbal et al. 1991; Seibyl et al. 1989). In another study (Kahn et al. 1992), a decrease in the BPRS (Overall and Gorham 1962) psychosis subscore was reported after oral administration of MCPP in a randomized double-blind fashion.

In conclusion, these studies seem to suggest that there is a relationship between central 5-HT dysfunction and negative symptoms, suicidal behavior, and, to a lesser extent, positive symptoms in schizophrenia.

Serotonin-Dopamine Interaction and Future Research

Serotonergic neurons, originating mainly from the medial and dorsal raphe nuclei, directly innervate the dopaminergic neurons in the striatum and the substantia nigra, where they exert an inhibitory modulating effect (Jenner et al. 1983). Manipulation of the 5-HT system could therefore be of great value in secondarily regulating the DA system. It is highly plausible that the observed therapeutic effects of 5-HT antagonists on negative symptoms are attributable to the fact that the DA neurons of the mesocortical tract are no longer inhibited.

The atypical antipsychotic medication clozapine, which binds to both $5\text{-}HT_2$ and $D_1\text{-}D_2$ receptors, has proven remarkably effective in treating those schizophrenic patients who have shown a poor response to typical antipsychotic medications. Efforts at producing medications similar to clozapine are therefore ongoing. Setoperone and risperidone are two such medications that have proven to be effective in poorly responsive schizophrenic patients (Ceulemans et al. 1985; Chouinard et al. 1993). In addition, such medications produce few, if any, motoric side effects (i.e., dystonia and parkinsonism). Their development not only will enhance our understanding of 5-HT and DA interaction, but will also offer better treatment for patients.

The Amino Acid Neurotransmitters

Glutamate

The N-Methyl-D-Aspartate Receptor Complex

The N-methyl-D-aspartate (NMDA) receptor, one of the five excitatory amino acid receptors, is an ion-gated channel receptor complex. The complex has many recognition sites that regulate the Ca^{++} channel. The identified sites include glutamate, glycine, Zn^{++}, spermidine, Mg^{++}, and phencyclidine (PCP). The PCP site is located inside the ion channel and leads to an antagonism of the glutamate effect (Javitt and Zukin 1990).

The Glutamate Hypothesis of Schizophrenia

In the glutamate hypothesis, which was advanced by Kim et al. (1980), it is suggested that an impairment of glutamatergic neurons might be related to schizophrenia. The basis for the hypothesis dates back to the 1950s, when Luby et al. (1959) proposed a model for schizophrenia based on the psychotomimetic effects of PCP. PCP psychosis resembles schizophrenia not only in the positive symptoms of agitation, catatonia, hallucinations, and delusions, but also in the deficit symptoms and the cognitive impairment.

Administration of PCP to schizophrenic patients has led to the exacerbation of psychotic symptoms (Davies and Beech 1960; Domino and Luby 1981; Luby et al. 1959). Low CSF glutamate levels have been reported in schizophrenic patients (Kim et al. 1980), a finding that was not replicated in two other studies (Gattaz et al. 1982a; T. L. Perry 1982). In their postmortem studies of the brains of schizophrenic patients using [^{3}H]kainic acid (which labels the non-NMDA site) and [^{3}H]MK-801 (which binds to the NMDA site), both Deakin et al. (1989) and Kornhuber et al. (1989a) reported increased densities in the temporal as well as the parietal cortex.

Evidence of a glutamatergic deficiency in schizophrenia has been reported in synaptosomes that were prepared with frozen sections taken from the brains of schizophrenic patients (frontal and temporal areas) and normal control subjects and then subjected to veratridine, a substance that induces release of excitatory amino acids and gamma-aminobutyric acid (GABA) (Sherman et al. 1991). Both glutamate and GABA release were reduced in the schizophrenic patients compared with the normal control subjects.

Serine hydroxymethyltransferase (SHMT), the enzyme responsible for converting serine to glycine, was found to be deficient in the temporal lobes of brains of schizophrenic patients (Waziri et al. 1990). Glycine is essential for the facilitation of the glutamate effect on the NMDA site. Glycine, which does not cross the blood-brain barrier readily, has been used in high dosages as an adjunct to antipsychotic medications, and was reported to be effective in improving the deficit symptoms of schizophrenic patients (Rosse et al. 1989; Waziri 1988; Zukin et al. 1992).

Overall, various studies have provided sufficient evidence that glutamate could play a role in schizophrenia. Given that the glutamate hypothesis is still in its infancy, future studies will involve more work at the molecular level in order to better understand the very complicated and rapidly changing knowledge about the NMDA receptor complex. On a pharmacological level, glycine-like agents are being developed that can potentiate the action of glutamate at the NMDA receptor and cross the blood-brain barrier more readily than glycine. Studies are currently under way with two such medications: milacemide and cycloserine.

Recently, water-suppressed proton magnetic resonance ([^{1}H]MR) spectroscopy was used to investigate in vivo [^{1}H]MR spectra in schizophrenic patients. This technique allows for quantification of certain excitatory amino acids and their metabolites in a certain volume of the brain. These include *N*-acetyl aspartate (NAA), glutamate, glutamine, aspartate, creatine, choline, and inositol. In one study (Stanley 1992), 6 neuroleptic-naive schizophrenic patients were found to have lower levels of prefrontal glutamate and aspartate compared with normal control subjects. In another study (Moore et al. 1992), NAA levels were lower in both the frontal and the temporal lobes of schizophrenic patients (25 of whom were taking antipsychotic medications and 5 of whom were neuroleptic naive) compared with normal control subjects. Nasrallah (1992) reported decreased mean NAA levels in the right hippocampus in 11 schizophrenic patients compared with 11 normal control subjects. This promising new technique will definitely add to the understanding of the role excitatory amino acids may have in schizophrenia.

Dopamine-Glutamate Interaction

DA and glutamate terminals converge on the same neurons in those subcortical structures that are of relevance to schizophrenia. The corticostriatal fibers and the dopaminergic nigrostriatal fibers both converge on GABA neurons in the striatum. DA acting at D_2 receptors inhibits GABA release, and glutamate acting on NMDA receptors stimulates GABA release (Carlsson and Carlsson 1989). Thus, corticostriatal glutamate could be viewed as an antagonist to the nigrostriatal DA system. An increase in dopaminergic activity (as is proposed by the DA hypothesis) could have the same effect as a decrease in glutamatergic transmission (as is postulated in the glutamate hypothesis).

Other sites of interaction occur in the striatum and nucleus accumbens, where DA release is regulated by intermediate cholinergic neurons, which are in turn regulated by cortical glutamate fibers. Decreased glutamate will remove the inhibitory effect on these cholinergic fibers and subsequently increase DA release (Scatton et al. 1982). In the cingulate cortex, the presynaptic DA terminals possess NMDA receptors (Javitt 1987). Glutamate can thus directly increase DA release. Likewise, a postulated decrease in glutamate in this region could decrease DA release.

It is obvious that glutamate-dopamine interactions are complex and occur at multiple levels. More work needs to be done in this area to better understand their involvement in schizophrenia in a unified way.

Gamma-Aminobutyric Acid

GABA is produced from glutamate by the enzyme glutamic acid decarboxylase (GAD). There are two major types of GABA receptors—$GABA_A$ and $GABA_B$—and their subdivision is based on their location, pharmacological properties, and effect on second messengers. GABA neurons directly inhibit the dopaminergic neurons in the basal ganglia. In 1972, Roberts proposed that reduced GABA inhibition could be responsible for the hypothesized hyperactive DA system in schizophrenia.

Measurements of CSF and plasma GABA levels have been widely inconsistent (Garbutt and van Kammen 1983; van Kammen and Gelernter 1987; van Kammen et al. 1982). Reynolds et al. (1990) reported a reduction of GABA uptake sites in the hippocampus that was associated with increased DA in the amygdala of schizophrenic patients.

When benzodiazepines, which are GABA agonists, have been used in clinical trials as the sole treatment for schizophrenic patients, their effects have been largely negative (Wolkowitz and Pickar 1991); however, when benzodiazepines have been used as an adjunct to antipsychotic medications, a mild to moderate therapeutic effect has been reported (Wolkowitz and Pickar 1991). Benzodiazepines have also proven beneficial when administered at early signs of relapse, as they appear to decrease the stress-induced symptoms that may precipitate a relapse (Kirkpatrick et al. 1989).

Overall, studies have not demonstrated strong evidence for GABA involvement in schizophrenia, but GABA agonists may be of some benefit when used as an adjunctive treatment, as they alleviate the stress and anxiety associated with psychosis.

The Neuropeptides

Several neuropeptides have recently been identified in the brain. Studies have been conducted in an attempt to identify the role of these agents in the central nervous system (CNS) in general and in schizophrenia in particular. The most commonly studied neuropeptides in schizophrenia are β-endorphin, cholecystokinin (CCK), and neurotensin. The study of most of these peptides arose from the observation that all three exhibit antipsychotic medication–like effects.

β-Endorphin

β-Endorphin is the most potent of the natural opioids and one of the proopiomelanocortin (POMC)-derived peptides. Because it was found that an injection of β-endorphin in rats precipitated a catatonic state (Bloom et al. 1976), this neuropeptide has received wide attention. It was later discovered that β-endorphin is the parent peptide for two smaller fragments: α- and γ-endorphin. γ-Endorphin has been reported to have an antipsychotic effect in preclinical studies, and was found to antagonize the behavioral effects induced by injection of DA agonists (van Ree et al. 1982a, 1982b). This discovery led to the formulation of a hypothesis by de Wied in 1978 that endorphins may be endogenous antipsychotic agents whose deficiency could be related to schizophrenia.

In the rat brain, γ-endorphin binding sites have been identified in the orbital cortex, cingulate cortex, entorhinal cortex, amygdala, and nucleus accumbens (Ronken et al. 1989). Chronic treatment with γ-endorphins in rats has resulted in decreased DA release and decreased HVA and dihydroxyphenylacetic acid (DOPAC) in the nucleus accumbens (Radhakishun et al. 1988; van Ree et al. 1982c).

The effects of γ-endorphin as an antipsychotic medication were compared with those of haloperidol in 30 schizophrenic patients in a double-blind design by Kissling et al. (1984). After 2 weeks of treatment, it was reported that γ-endorphin was as effective as haloperidol and had no adverse effects. Azorin et al. (1986) compared γ-endorphin with placebo as an adjunct to antipsychotic medication. A significant effect was reported in patients' psychotic symptoms after 4 weeks of treatment. Other studies have reported less encouraging results (Manchanda et al. 1988; van Ree et al. 1986). In general, these studies support the idea that γ-endorphin could be of help as an adjunctive treatment to standard antipsychotic medications. Benefits might include long-term improvement in social functioning and a decreased relapse rate.

Postmortem studies of β-endorphin in schizophrenic patients have provided inconsistent data, further compounded by the fact that most patients had been treated with antipsychotic medications, which are known to influence the POMC system.

Cholecystokinins

The cholecystokinins (CCKs) are straight-chain amino acids that are widely distributed in the CNS (Vanderhaeghen et al. 1981). They exist in several molecular forms based on the length and derivation of amino acid residues. In the human brain, CCK-8 and CCK-33 are the most abundant. CCK binding sites have been identified in the brain, mostly in the cerebral cortex, basal ganglia, and hypothalamus (Geola et al. 1981). CCK was found to colocalize in the DA neurons of the ventral tegmental area (VTA) and the substantia nigra (Hokfelt et al. 1980). This finding triggered the search for the CCKs' role in interactions with DA. Similar to γ-endorphin, CCK-8 has been reported to have an antipsychotic effect in animal studies and to counteract the behavioral effects of DA and DA agonists (S. L. Cohen et al. 1982; Schneider et al. 1983; van Ree et al. 1983). However, this effect was not replicated in two other studies (Kovacs et al. 1981; Widerlöv et al. 1983). Fuxe et al. (1983), Mashal et al. (1983), and Wang and White (1983), in their studies of CCK-8 interactions with DA, all reported inhibition of DA release, turnover, and binding.

In schizophrenic patients, CCK was measured both in the CSF

and in the brain. Two studies measured CCK in the CSF of unmedicated schizophrenic patients: Gerner and Yamada (1982) reported no significant differences in 13 schizophrenic patients who had been off antipsychotic medications for 2 weeks, whereas Verbanck et al. (1984) reported a significant reduction in CCK in 9 schizophrenic patients following a 6-week drug-free period. Three postmortem studies in schizophrenic patients reported inconsistent results: Kleinman et al. (1982) reported a marked increase in CCK in the amygdala; Ferrier et al. (1983) reported significant reductions in CCK in the temporal cortex; and no differences in CCK were found in the entorhinal cortex by R. H. Perry et al. (1981).

Multiple clinical trials have been conducted with schizophrenic patients using CCK or the chemically related decapeptide cerulein as an adjunct to antipsychotic medications. In 8 of the 11 studies reviewed by Nair et al. (1986), some improvement was reported, although only 5 of these 11 studies were double-blind, placebo-controlled ones.

Neurotensin

Neurotensin (NT), a tridecapeptide isolated in 1973 (Carraway and Leeman 1973), has been found to exist in high concentrations in the CNS (Uhl and Snyder 1977), especially in the substantia nigra, nucleus accumbens, and caudate (Griffiths et al. 1984). Anatomically, the interaction between NT and DA has been described at different levels. Like CCK, NT has been found to colocalize within the DA neurons of the mesocortical tract (Bean et al. 1990), and NT receptors were identified on DA neurons in the nigrostriatal tract (Quirion et al. 1982). In the frontal cortex, the distribution of the NT receptors was analogous to that of the D_1 receptors (Tassin et al. 1988). In preclinical studies, centrally administered NT exhibited antipsychotic characteristics in blocking the action of DA, similar to the action of β-endorphin and CCK (Kilts et al. 1986; Quirion 1983).

Clinically, NT is the least studied peptide of the three described here. Lindström et al. (1988) and Widerlöv et al. (1982), in their CSF studies, reported a decrease of NT levels, in schizophrenic patients free of antipsychotic medications, that normalizes following treatment

(Widerlöv et al. 1982), suggesting that NT-CSF levels could be a state marker in schizophrenia. In one postmortem brain study, Nemeroff et al. (1983) found an increase in NT in the nucleus accumbens, amygdala, and striatum of schizophrenic patients who had received antipsychotic medications prior to death. No clinical trials of NT have been conducted, as it does not cross the blood-brain barrier.

Future research in the area of neuropeptides should involve the development of chemical analogues that have receptor-binding qualities similar to the naturally existing ones but that also have the ability to cross the blood-brain barrier. Another promising avenue of research is the ability to measure these peptides in peripheral blood. Like platelets for 5-HT and MAO, neuropeptide concentrations can be measured in peripheral blood mononuclear cells (PBMC). Panza et al. (1992) reported β-endorphin and CCK levels in the PBMC of schizophrenic patients consistent with data from CSF and autopsy studies.

Conclusion

In this chapter we have presented an overview of some of the most widely studied biochemical hypotheses in schizophrenia. We did not cover some areas (e.g., metabolism, prostaglandins), although these have extensive hypotheses associated with them.

Of the brain chemicals reviewed here, DA is still viewed as the core neurotransmitter involved in schizophrenia and is still the focus of considerable research. Our emphasis on the interactions between different neurotransmitters and DA reflects the increased frequency of such studies in the literature. If an aberrant DA system is found to be at the core of the schizophrenic disorder, it could be either a primary cause or a downstream effect.

More importantly, we believe the focus should be on studying the interactions of these different chemical systems in an integrative way. Likewise, their relationship to different aspects of schizophrenia (e.g., symptom profile, neuroanatomical data, treatment response) should be viewed in a similar manner. These studies can naturally be conducted in a number of ways. CSF and plasma neurotransmitters and metabolites should be studied in a multidimensional neurochemical and multivariate statistical manner. The study of second-messenger systems (e.g., G proteins), on which the first-messenger neurotransmitters converge and compete to exert their effects, can also be explored. With the development of new radiotracers, imaging studies of such interactions are being conducted in primates, and as the methods are refined, they will be applied to humans. The study of regional brain metabolism with PET or nuclear magnetic resonance spectroscopy, coupled with the activation or challenge by various agonists or antagonists of a specific neurotransmitter system, is another way of understanding these interactions at a metabolic level.

References

Albus M, Ackenheil M, Engel RR, et al: Situational reactivity of autonomic functions in schizophrenic patients. Psychiatry Res 6:361–370, 1982

Andreasen NC, Rezai K, Alliger R, et al: Hypofrontality in neuroleptic-naive patients and in patients with chronic schizophrenia. Arch Gen Psychiatry 49:943–958, 1992

Angrist BM, Dathananthan G, Wilk S, et al: Behavioural and biochemical effects of L-dopa in psychiatric patients, in Frontiers in Catecholamine Research. Edited by Usdin E, Kopin IJ, Barchas J. Oxford, UK, Pergamon, 1973, pp 991–994

Ashcroft GW, Crawford TTB, Eccleston D, et al: 5-Hydroxyindole compounds in the cerebrospinal fluid of patients with psychiatric or neurologic disease. Lancet 2:1049–1052, 1966

Azorin JM, Charbaut J, Granier F, et al: Des-enkephalin-gamma-endorphin in exacerbation of chronic schizophrenia: a double blind, placebo controlled study. Paper presented at the Symposium on Neuropeptides and Brain Function, Utrecht, Netherlands, 1986

Bacopoulos NG, Spokes EG, Bird ED, et al: Antipsychotic drug action in schizophrenic patients: effect on cortical dopamine metabolism after long-term treatment. Science 205:1405–1407, 1979

Banki CM, Arato M, Papp Z, et al: Cerebrospinal fluid amine metabolites and neuroendocrine changes in psychoses and suicide, in Catecholamines: Neuropharmacology and Central System—Therapeutic Aspects. Edited by Usdin E, Carlsson A, Dahlstrom A. New York, Alan R Liss, 1984, pp 153–159

Bean AJ, During MJ, Roth RH: Effects of dopamine autoreceptor stimulation on the release of colocalized transmitters: in vivo release of dopamine and neurotensin from rat prefrontal cortex. Neurosci Lett 1089:143–148, 1990

Beckmann H, Waldmeier P, Lauber J, et al: Phenylethylamine and monoamine metabolites in CSF of schizophrenics: effects of neuroleptic treatment. J Neural Transm 57:103–110, 1983

Bennett JP, Enna SJ, Bylund D, et al: Neurotransmitter receptors in frontal cortex of schizophrenics. Arch Gen Psychiatry 36:927–934, 1979

Bigelow LB, Berthot BD: The Psychiatric Symptom Assessment Scale (PSAS). Psychopharmacol Bull 25:168–179, 1989

Bigelow LB, Walls P, Gillin JC, et al: Clinical effects of L-5-hydroxytryptophan administration in chronic schizophrenic patients. Biol Psychiatry 14:53–67, 1979

Bjerkenstedt L, Edman G, Hagenfeldt L, et al: Plasma amino acids in relation to cerebrospinal fluid monoamine metabolites in schizophrenic patients and healthy controls. Br J Psychiatry 147:276–282, 1985

Bloom F, Segal D, Ling N, et al: Endorphins: profound behavioral effects in rats suggest new etiological factors in mental illness. Science 194:630–632, 1976

Bogerts B, Häntsch J, Herzer M: A morphometric study of the dopamine-containing cell groups in the mesencephalon of normals, Parkinson patients, and schizophrenics. Biol Psychiatry 18:951–969, 1983

Bowers MB Jr: Cerebrospinal fluid 5-hydroxyindoles and behavior after L-tryptophan and pyridoxine administration to psychiatric patients. Neuropharmacology 9:599–604, 1970

Bowers MB Jr: Thioridazine: central dopamine turnover and clinical effects of antipsychotic drugs. Clin Pharmacol Ther 17:73–78, 1975

Bowers MB Jr, Heninger GR, Gerbode FA: Cerebrospinal fluid, 5-hydroxyindoleacetic acid and homovanillic acid in psychiatric patients. International Journal of Neuropharmacology 8:255–262, 1969

Bowers MB Jr, Swigar ME, Jatlow PI, et al: Plasma catecholamine metabolites and early response to haloperidol. J Clin Psychiatry 45:248–251, 1984

Breier A, Wolkowitz OM, Pickar D: Stress and schizophrenia, in Schizophrenia Research. Edited by Schulz SC, Tamminga CA. New York, Raven, 1991, pp 141–152

Bridge TP, Kleinman JE, Karoum F, et al: Postmortem central catecholamines and antemortem cognitive impairment in elderly schizophrenics and controls. Neuropsychobiology 14:57–61, 1985

Buchsbaum MS: Commentary on "The current status of PET scanning with respect to schizophrenia." Neuropsychopharmacology 7:67–68, 1992

Buchsbaum MS, Haier RJ, Potkin SG, et al: Frontostriatal disorder of cerebral metabolism in never-medicated schizophrenics. Arch Gen Psychiatry 49:935–942, 1992

Bunzow JR, Van Tol HHM, Grandy DK, et al: Cloning and expression of a rat D_2 dopamine receptor cDNA. Nature 336:783–787, 1988

Carenzi A, Gillin JG, Guidotti A, et al: Dopamine-sensitive adenylyl cyclase in human caudate nucleus. Arch Gen Psychiatry 32:1056–1059, 1975

Carlsson A: Antipsychotic drugs, neurotransmitters and schizophrenia. Am J Psychiatry 135:164–173, 1978

Carlsson M, Carlsson A: The NMDA antagonist MK-801 causes marked locomotor stimulation in monoamine-depleted mice. J Neural Transm 75:221–226, 1989

Carlsson A, Lindquist M: Effect of chlorpromazine and haloperidol on formation of 3-methoxytyramine and normetanephrine in mouse brain. Acta Pharmacol Toxicol 20:140–144, 1963

Carraway R, Leeman SE: The isolation of a new hypotensive peptide neurotensin, from bovine hypothalamus. J Biol Chem 248:6854–6861, 1973

Casacchia M, Casati C, Fazio C: P-chlorophenylalanine in schizophrenia. Biol Psychiatry 10:109–110, 1975

Ceulemans DLS, Gelders Y, Hoppenbrouwers ML, et al: Effect of serotonin antagonism in schizophrenia: a pilot study with setoperone. Psychopharmacology (Berl) 85:329–332, 1985

Chang WH, Chen TY, Lin SK, et al: Plasma catecholamine metabolites in schizophrenics: evidence for the two-subtype concept. Biol Psychiatry 27:510–518, 1990

Chouinard G, Jones B, Remington G, et al: A Canadian multicenter placebo-controlled study of fixed doses of risperidone and haloperidol in the treatment of chronic schizophrenic patients. J Clin Psychopharmacol 13:25–40, 1993

Cohen RM, Semple WE, Gross M, et al: The effect of neuroleptics on dysfunction in a prefrontal substrate of sustained attention in schizophrenia. Life Sci 43:1141–1150, 1988

Cohen SL, Knight M, Tamminga CA, et al: Cholecystokinin effects on conditioned avoidance behavior, stereotypy and catalepsy. Eur J Pharmacol 83:213–222, 1982

Connell PH: Amphetamine Psychosis. Maudsley Monograph No 5. London, Chapman & Hall, 1958

Crawley JCW, Crow TJ, Johnstone EC, et al: Dopamine D_2 receptors in schizophrenia studied in vivo. Lancet 1:224, 1986

Creese I, Burt DR, Snyder SH: Dopamine receptor binding predicts clinical and pharmacological potencies of antischizophrenic drugs. Science 192:481–483, 1976

Cross AJ, Crow TJ, Owen F: [^{3}H]flupenthixol binding in post-mortem brains of schizophrenics: evidence for a selective increase in dopamine D_2 receptors. Psychopharmacology (Berl) 74:122–124, 1981

Crow TJ, Johnstone EC, Longden AJ, et al: Dopaminergic mechanisms in schizophrenia: the antipsychotic effect and the disease process. Life Sci 23:563–567, 1978

Crow TJ, Baker HF, Cross AJ, et al: Monoamine mechanisms in chronic schizophrenia: postmortem neurochemical findings. Br J Psychiatry 134:249–256, 1979

Daniel DG, Berman KF, Weinberger DR: The effect of apomorphine on regional cerebral blood flow in schizophrenia. Journal of Neuropsychiatry 1:377–384, 1989

Daniel DG, Weinberger DR, Jones DW, et al: The effect of amphetamine on regional cerebral blood flow during cognitive activation in schizophrenia. J Neurosci 11:1907–1917, 1991

Davidson M, Davis KL: A comparison of plasma homovanillic acid concentrations in schizophrenics and normal controls. Arch Gen Psychiatry 45:561–563, 1988

Davidson M, Kahn RS, Knott P, et al: The effect of neuroleptic treatment on plasma homovanillic acid concentrations and schizophrenic symptoms. Arch Gen Psychiatry 48:910–913, 1991

Davies BM, Beech HR: The effect of 1-arylcyclohexylamine (Sernyl) on twelve normal volunteers. Journal of Mental Science 106:912–924, 1960

Davis KL, Kahn RS, Ko GN, et al: Dopamine in schizophrenia: a review and reconceptualization. Am J Psychiatry 148:1474–1486, 1991

Deakin JF, Slater P, Simpson M, et al: Frontal cortical and left temporal glutamatergic dysfunction in schizophrenia. J Neurochem 52:1781–1786, 1989

Dearry A, Gingrich JA, Falardeau P, et al: Molecular cloning and expression of the gene for a human D_1 dopamine receptor. Nature 347:72–76, 1990

DeLisi LE, Neckers LM, Weinberger DR, et al: Increased whole blood serotonin concentrations in chronic schizophrenia patients. Arch Gen Psychiatry 17:471–477, 1981

DeLisi LE, Freed WJ, Gillin JC, et al: P-chlorophenylalanine trial in schizophrenic patients. Biol Psychiatry 17:471–477, 1982

de Wied D: Psychopathology as a neuropeptide dysfunction, in Characteristics and Function of Opioids. Edited by van Ree JM, Terenius L. Amsterdam, Netherlands, Elsevier/North-Holland Biomedical Press, 1978, pp 113–122

Domino EF, Luby E: Abnormal mental states induced by phencyclidine as a model of schizophrenia, in PCP (Phencyclidine): Historical and Current Perspectives. Edited by Domino EF. Ann Arbor, MI, NPP Books, 1981

Farde L, Wiesel F-A, Hall H, et al: D$_2$ dopamine receptors in neuroleptic-naive schizophrenic patients: a positron emission tomography study with [^{11}C]raclopride. Arch Gen Psychiatry 47:213–219, 1990

Farley IJ, Price KS, McCullough E, et al: Norepinephrine in chronic schizophrenia: above-normal levels in limbic forebrain. Science 200:456–458, 1978

Farley I, Shannak K, Hornykiewicz D: Brain monoamine changes in chronic paranoid schizophrenia and their possible relation to increased dopamine receptor sensitivity, in Receptors for Neurotransmitters and Peptide Hormones. Edited by Pepeu G, Kuhar M, Enna S. New York, Raven, 1980, pp 427–433

Ferrier IN, Roberts GW, Crow TJ, et al: Reduced cholecystokinin and somatostatin-like immunoreactivity in limbic lobe is associated with negative symptoms in schizophrenia. Life Sci 33:475–482, 1983

Fields RB, van Kammen DP, Peters JL, et al: Clonidine improves memory function in schizophrenia independently from change in psychosis. Schizophr Res 1:417–423, 1988

Freedman DX, Belendiuk K, Belendiuk GW, et al: Blood tryptophan metabolism in chronic schizophrenics. Arch Gen Psychiatry 38:655–659, 1981

Freedman R, Kirch D, Bell J, et al: Clonidine treatment of schizophrenia: double blind comparison to placebo and neuroleptic drugs. Acta Psychiatr Scand 65:35–45, 1982

Fuxe K, Agnati LF, Celani MF: Evidence for interactions between striatal cholecystokinin and glutamate receptors: CCK-8 in vitro produces a marked downregulation of [^{3}H]glutamate binding sites in striatal membranes. Acta Physiol Scand 118:75–77, 1983

Fyrö B, Wode-Helgodt B, Borg S, et al: The effect of chlorpromazine on homovanillic acid levels in cerebrospinal fluid of schizophrenic patients. Psychopharmacology (Berl) 35:287–294, 1974

Gaddum JH, Hameed KA: Drugs which antagonize 5-hydroxytryptamine. Br J Pharmacol 9:240–248, 1954

Garbutt JC, van Kammen DP: The interaction between GABA and dopamine: implications for schizophrenia. Schizophr Bull 9:336–353, 1983

Garelis E, Gillin JC, Wyatt RJ, et al: Elevated blood serotonin concentration in unmedicated chronic schizophrenic patients: a preliminary study. Am J Psychiatry 132:184–186, 1975

Gattaz WF, Gattaz D, Beckmann H: Glutamate in schizophrenics and healthy controls. Archiv für Psychiatrie und Nervenkrankheiten (Berl) 231:221–225, 1982a

Gattaz WF, Waldmeier P, Beckmann H: CSF monoamine metabolism in schizophrenia patients. Acta Psychiatr Scand 66:350–360, 1982b

Gelders Y, Ceulemans DLS, Reyntjens A, et al: Ritanserin, a selective serotonin antagonist in chronic schizophrenia (abstract). Proceedings of the
Fourth World Congress of Biological Psychiatry, Philadelphia, PA, September 1985a, p 417

Gelders Y, Ceulemans DLS, Reyntjens A, et al: The influence of selective
serotonin antagonism on conventional neuroleptic therapy. Proceedings
of the Fourth World Congress of Biological Psychiatry, Philadelphia, PA,
September 1985b

Geola FL, Hershman JM, Warwick R, et al: Regional distribution of
cholecystokinin-like immunoreactivity in the human brain. J Clin En-
docrinol Metab 53:270–275, 1981

Gerlach J, Thorsen K, Fog R: Extrapyramidal reactions and amine metabolites in cerebrospinal fluid during haloperidol and clozapine treatment of
schizophrenic patients. Psychopharmacology (Berl) 40:341–350, 1975

Gerner RH, Yamada T: Altered neuropeptide concentrations in cerebrospinal
fluid of psychiatric patients. Brain Res 238:298–302, 1982

Gomes UCR, Shanley BC, Potgieter L, et al: Noradrenergic overactivity in
chronic schizophrenia: evidence based on cerebrospinal fluid noradrenaline and cyclic nucleotide concentrations. Br J Psychiatry 137:346–351,
1980

Griffiths EC, McDermott JR, Smith AI: A comparative study of neurotensin
inactivation by brain peptidases from different vertebrate species. Comp
Biochem Physiol C 77:363–366, 1984

Heritch AJ: Evidence for reduced and dysregulated turnover of dopamine in
schizophrenia. Schizophr Bull 16:605–615, 1990

Hess EJ, Bracha HS, Kleinman JE, et al: Dopamine receptor subtype imbal-
ance in schizophrenia. Life Sci 40:1487–1497, 1987

Hietala J, Syvalahti E, Vuorio K, et al: Striatal dopamine D_2 receptor density
in neuroleptic-naive schizophrenics studied with positron emission tomography, in Biological Psychiatry, Vol 2. Edited by Racagni G,
Brunello N, Fukuda T. Amsterdam, Netherlands, Excerpta Medica,
1991, pp 386–387

Hokfelt T, Rehfeld JF, Skirboll LR, et al: Evidence for coexistence of dopamine and CCK in mesolimbic neurons. Nature 285:476–478, 1980

Hsiao JK, Colison J, Bartko JJ, et al: Monoamine neurotransmitter interactions in drug-free and neuroleptic-treated schizophrenics. Arch Gen
Psychiatry 50:606–614, 1993

Iqbal N, Asnis GM, Wetzler S, et al: The role of serotonin in schizophrenia:
new findings. Schizophr Res 5:181–182, 1991

Issa F, Gerhardt GA, Bartko JJ, et al: Cerebrospinal fluid biogenic amine
analysis in schizophrenia, a multidimensional approach, I: comparisons
with nonpsychiatric control subjects and off versus on neuroleptic
matched pairs analyses. Psychiatry Res 52:237–249, 1994a

Issa F, Kirch DG, Gerhardt GA, et al: Cerebrospinal fluid biogenic amine analysis in schizophrenia, a multidimensional approach, II: correlations with psychopathology. Psychiatry Res 52:251–258, 1994b

Jackman H, Luchins D, Meltzer HY: Platelet serotonin levels in schizophrenia: relationship to race and psychopathology. Biol Psychiatry 18:887–902, 1983

Janowsky DS, El-Yousef K, Davis JM, et al: Provocation of schizophrenic symptoms by intravenous administration of methylphenidate. Arch Gen Psychiatry 28:185–191, 1973

Javitt DC: Negative schizophrenic symptomatology and the PCP (phencyclidine) model of schizophrenia. Hillside Journal of Clinical Psychiatry 9:12–35, 1987

Javitt DC, Zukin SR: Role of excitatory amino acids in neuropsychiatric illness. J Neuropsychiatry Clin Neurosci 2:44–52, 1990

Jenner P, Sheehy M, Marsden CD: Noradrenaline and 5-hydroxytryptamine modulation of brain dopamine function: implications for the treatment of Parkinson's disease. Br J Clin Pharmacol 15 (suppl 2):277S–289S, 1983

Jimerson DC, Post RM, Stoddard FJ, et al: Preliminary trial of the noradrenergic agonist clonidine in psychiatric patients. Biol Psychiatry 15:45–57, 1980

Joseph MH, Baker HF, Crow TJ, et al: Brain tryptophan metabolism in schizophrenia: a postmortem study of metabolites on the serotonin and kynurenine pathways in schizophrenic and control subjects. Psychopharmacology (Berl) 62:279–285, 1979

Joyce JM, Lexow N, Bird E, et al: Organization of dopamine D_1 and D_2 receptors in human striatum: receptor autoradiographic studies in Huntington's disease and schizophrenia. Synapse 2:546–557, 1988

Joyce JN, Shane A, Lexow N, et al: Serotonin uptake sites and serotonin$_2$ receptors are altered in the limbic system of schizophrenics. Neuropsychopharmacology 8:315–336, 1993

Kafka MS, van Kammen DP: Alpha-adrenergic receptor function in schizophrenia: receptor number, cyclic adenosine monophosphate production, adenylate cyclase activity, and effects of drugs. Arch Gen Psychiatry 40:264–270, 1983

Kahn RS, Davidson M: On the value of measuring dopamine, norepinephrine and their metabolites in schizophrenia. Neuropsychopharmacology 8:93–95, 1993

Kahn RS, Siever LJ, Gabriel S, et al: Serotonin function in schizophrenia: effects of meta-chlorophenylpiperazine in schizophrenic patients and healthy subjects. Psychiatry Res 43:1–12, 1992

Kemali D, Del Vecchio M, Maj M: Increased noradrenaline levels in CSF and plasma of schizophrenic patients. Biol Psychiatry 17:711–717, 1982

Kilts CD, Bissette G, Cain ST, et al: Neuropeptide-dopamine interactions: focus on neurotensin, in Dopamine Systems and Their Regulation. Edited by Woodruff DN, Poats JA, Roberts PJ. London, Macmillan, 1986, pp 223–242

Kim JS, Kornhuber HH, Schmid-Burgk W, et al: Low cerebrospinal fluid glutamate in schizophrenic patients and a new hypothesis on schizophrenia. Neurosci Lett 20:379–382, 1980

King R, Faull KF, Stahl SM, et al: Serotonin and schizophrenia: correlations between serotonergic activity and schizophrenic motor behavior. Psychiatry Res 14:235–240, 1985

Kirkpatrick B, Buchanan RW, Waltrip RW, et al: Diazepam treatment of early symptoms of schizophrenic relapse. J Nerv Ment Dis 177:52–53, 1989

Kissling W, Moller HJ, Burk F, et al: Multicenter double-blind comparison between des-enkephalin-γ-endorphin (DEgE: Org 5878) and haloperidol concerning the efficacy and safety in the treatment of schizophrenia. Paper presented at the 14th Congress of Collegium Internationale Neuro-Psychopharmacologium, Florence, Italy, 1984

Kleinman JE, Govoni S, Memo M, et al: Cholecystokinin and calmodulin in schizophrenic brains. Paper presented at the 37th annual meeting of the Society of Biological Psychiatry, Toronto, Canada, May 12–16, 1982

Ko GN, et al: Lower α_2 agonist binding in schizophrenic brains. Abstracts of Panels and Posters, American College of Neuropsychopharmacology, December 1985, p 150

Konig P, Benzer MK, Fritzsche H: SPECT technique for visualization of cerebral dopamine D_2 receptors. Am J Psychiatry 148:1607–1608, 1991

Kornhuber J, Mack-Burkhardt F, Riederer P, et al: [3H]MK-801 binding sites in postmortem brain regions of schizophrenic patients. J Neural Transm 77:231–236, 1989a

Kornhuber J, Riederer P, Reynolds GP, et al: [^{3}H]spiperone binding sites in post-mortem brains from schizophrenic patients: relationship to neuroleptic drug treatment, abnormal movements, and positive symptoms. J Neural Transm 75:1–10, 1989b

Korpi ER, Kleinman JE, Goodman SI, et al: Serotonin and 5-hydroxyindoleacetic acid in the brains of suicide victims: comparison in chronic schizophrenic patients with suicide as cause of death. Arch Gen Psychiatry 43:594–600, 1986

Kovacs GL, Szabo G, Penke B, et al: Effects of cholecystokinin octapeptide on striatal dopamine metabolism and on apomorphine-induced stereotyped cage-climbing in mice. Eur J Pharmacol 69:313–319, 1981

Kraepelin E: Dementia Praecox and Paraphrenia. Huntington, NY, Robert E. Krieger, 1919

Lake CR, Sternberg DE, van Kammen DP, et al: Schizophrenia: elevated cerebrospinal fluid norepinephrine. Science 207:331–333, 1980

Laruelle M, Abi-Dargham A, Casanova MF, et al: Selective abnormalities of prefrontal serotonergic receptors in schizophrenia: a postmortem study. Arch Gen Psychiatry 50:810–818, 1993

Lindström LH: Low HVA and normal 5-HIAA CSF levels in drug-free schizophrenic patients compared to healthy volunteers: correlations to symptomatology and family history. Psychiatry Res 14:265–273, 1985

Lindström LH, Widerlöv E, Bissette G, et al: Reduced CSF neurotensin concentration in drug-free schizophrenic patients. Schizophr Res 1:55–59, 1988

Linnoila M: Reliability of norepinephrine and major monoamine metabolite measurements in CSF in schizophrenic patients. Arch Gen Psychiatry 40:1290–1298, 1983

Losonczy MF, Song IS, Mohs RC, et al: Correlates of lateral ventricular size in chronic schizophrenia. Am J Psychiatry 143:1113–1118, 1986

Luby ED, Cohen BD, Rosenbaum F, et al: Study of a new schizophreno-mimetic drug, Sernyl. Archives for Neurology and Psychiatry 81:363–369, 1959

Mackay AVP, Iversen LL, Rossor M, et al: Increased brain dopamine and dopamine receptors in schizophrenia. Arch Gen Psychiatry 39:991–997, 1982

Manchanda R, Hirsch SR, Barnes TRE: Criteria for evaluating improvement in schizophrenia in psychopharmacological research (with special reference to gamma endorphin fragments). Br J Psychiatry 153:354–358, 1988

Martinot JL, Peron-Magnan P, Huret JD, et al: Striatal D_2 dopaminergic receptors assessed with positron emission tomography and [^{76}Br]bromospiperone in untreated schizophrenic patients. Am J Psychiatry 147:44–50, 1990

Martinot JL, Paillère-Martinot ML, Loch C, et al: The estimated density of D_2 striatal receptors in schizophrenia: a study with positron emission tomography and ^{76}Br-bromolisuride. Br J Psychiatry 158:346–350, 1991

Mashal RD, Owen F, Deakin JFW, et al: The effects of cholecystokinin on dopaminergic mechanisms in rat striatum. Brain Res 277:375–376, 1983

Meltzer HY, Aurora RC: Skeletal muscle MAO activity in the major psychosis: relationship with platelet and plasma MAO activities. Arch Gen Psychiatry 37:333–339, 1980

Meltzer HY, Stahl SM: The dopamine hypothesis of schizophrenia: a review. Schizophr Bull 2:19–76, 1976

Memo M, Kleinman JE, Hanbauer I: Coupling of dopamine D_1 recognition sites with adenylate cyclase in nuclei accumbens and caudatus of schizophrenics. Science 221:1304–1307, 1983

Mesulam M: Frontal cortex and behavior (editorial). Ann Neurol 19:320–325, 1986

Mita T, Hanada S, Nishino N, et al: Decreased serotonin S_2 and increased dopamine D_2 receptors in chronic schizophrenics. Biol Psychiatry 21:1407–1414, 1986

Moises HW, Gelernter J, Giuffra LA, et al: No linkage between D_2 dopamine receptor gene region and schizophrenia. Arch Gen Psychiatry 48:643–647, 1991

Moore CM, Redmond OM, Buckley P, et al: In vivo proton NMR spectroscopy (STEAM) in patients with schizophrenia (abstract). Proceedings of the Society of Magnetic Resonance Imaging in Medicine, Berlin, Germany, 1992, p 1933

Naber D, Albus M, Burke H, et al: Neuroleptic withdrawal in chronic schizophrenia: CT and endocrine variables relating to psychopathology. Psychiatry Res 16:207–219, 1985

Nair NPV, Lal S, Bloom DM: Cholecystokinin and schizophrenia. Prog Brain Res 65:237–258, 1986

Nasrallah HA: [1]H nuclear magnetic resonance spectroscopy of the hippocampus in schizophrenia. Paper presented at the 145th annual meeting of the American Psychiatric Association, Washington, DC, May 1992

Nemeroff CB, Youngblood W, Manberg PJ, et al: Regional brain concentrations of neuropeptides in Huntington's chorea and schizophrenia. Science 221:972–975, 1983

Ninan PT, van Kammen DP, Scheinin M, et al: CSF 5-hydroxyindoleacetic acid levels in suicidal schizophrenic patients. Am J Psychiatry 141:566–569, 1984

Niznik HB, Van Tol HH: Dopamine receptor genes: new tools for molecular psychiatry. J Psychiatry Neurosci 17:158–180, 1992

Nyback H, Berggren BM, Hindmarsh T, et al: Cerebroventricular size and cerebrospinal fluid monoamine metabolites in schizophrenic patients and healthy volunteers. Psychiatry Res 9:301–308, 1983

Overall JE, Gorham DR: The Brief Psychiatric Rating Scale. Psychol Rep 10:799–812, 1962

Owen F, Cross AJ, Crow TJ, et al: Increased dopamine-receptor sensitivity in schizophrenia. Lancet 2:223–226, 1978

Panza G, Monzani E, Sacerdote P, et al: B-endorphin, vasoactive intestinal peptide and cholecystokinin in peripheral blood mononuclear cells from healthy subjects and from drug-free and haloperidol-treated schizophrenic patients. Acta Psychiatr Scand 85:207–210, 1992

Perry RH, Dockray GJ, Dimaline R, et al: Neuropeptides in Alzheimer's disease, depression and schizophrenia. J Neurol Sci 51:465–472, 1981

Perry TL: Normal cerebrospinal fluid and brain glutamate levels in schizophrenia do not support the hypothesis of glutamatergic neuronal dysfunction. Neurosci Lett 28:81–85, 1982

Pickar D, Labarca R, Doran AR, et al: Longitudinal measurement of plasma homovanillic acid levels in schizophrenic patients. Arch Gen Psychiatry 43:669–676, 1986

Pickar D, Breier A, Hsiao JK, et al: Cerebrospinal fluid and plasma monoamine metabolites and their relation to psychosis: implications for regional brain dysfunction in schizophrenia. Arch Gen Psychiatry 47:641–648, 1990

Post RM: CSF norepinephrine and dopamine-β-hydroxylase in affective illness and schizophrenia, in Recent Advances in Neuropsychopharmacology. Edited by Angrist BM, Burrows GD, Lader M, et al. New York, Pergamon, 1981, pp 283–288

Post RM, Fink E, Carpenter WT, et al: Cerebrospinal fluid amine metabolites in acute schizophrenia. Arch Gen Psychiatry 32:1063–1069, 1975

Potkin SG, Weinberger DR, Linnoila M, et al: Low CSF 5-HIAA in schizophrenic patients with enlarged cerebral ventricles. Am J Psychiatry 140:21–25, 1983

Quirion R: Autoradiographic distribution of [^{3}H]neurotensin receptors in rat brain: visualization by tritium-sensitive film. Peptides 4:609–615, 1983

Quirion R, Everist HD, Pert A: Nigrostriatal dopamine terminals bear neurotensin receptors but the mesolimbic do not. Society for Neuroscience Abstracts, 1982

Radhakishun FS, Westerink BHC, van Ree JM: Dopamine release in the nucleus accumbens of freely moving rats determined by on-line dialysis: effects of apomorphine and the neuroleptic-like peptide desenkephalin-γ-endorphin. Neurosci Lett 89:328–334, 1988

Reynolds GP, Rossor MN, Iversen LL: Preliminary studies of human cortical 5-HT$_2$ receptors and their involvement in schizophrenia and neuroleptic drug action. J Neural Transm 18 (suppl):273–277, 1983

Reynolds GP, Czudek C, Andrews HB: Deficit and hemispheric asymmetry of GABA uptake sites in the hippocampus in schizophrenia. Biol Psychiatry 27:1038–1044, 1990

Rimon R, Roos BE, Rakkolainen V, et al: The content of 5-HIAA and HVA in the CSF of patients with acute schizophrenia. J Psychosom Res 15:375–378, 1971

Roberts E: An hypothesis suggesting that there is a defect in the GABA system in schizophrenia, in Neuroscience Research Program Bulletin, Vol 10. Cambridge, MA, MIT Press, 1972, pp 468–482

Ronken E, Tonnaer JADM, de Boer T, et al: Autoradiographic evidence for binding sites for des-enkephalin-gamma-endorphin in rat forebrain. Eur J Pharmacol 162:189–191, 1989

Rosse RB, Theut SK, Banay-Schwartz M, et al: Glycine adjuvant therapy to conventional neuroleptic treatment in schizophrenia: an open-label, pilot study. Clin Neuropharmacol 12:416–424, 1989

Roth RH, Tam S-Y, Ida Y, et al: Stress and the mesocorticolimbic dopamine systems, in The Mesocorticolimbic Dopamine System. Edited by Kalivas PW, Nemeroff CB. New York, New York Academy of Sciences, 1988, pp 138–147

Scatton B, Worms P, Lloyd KG, et al: Cortical modulation of striatal function. Brain Res 232:331–343, 1982

Schneider LH, Alpert JE, Iversen SD: CCK-8 modulation of mesolimbic dopamine: antagonism of amphetamine stimulated behaviours. Peptides 4:749–753, 1983

Sedvall G, Fyrö B, Nyback H, et al: Mass fragmentometric determination of homovanillic acid in lumbar cerebrospinal fluid of schizophrenic patients during treatment with antipsychotic drugs. J Psychiatr Res 11:75–80, 1974

Seeman P: Elevated D_2 in schizophrenia: role of endogenous dopamine and cerebellum. Commentary on "The current status of PET scanning with respect to schizophrenia." Neuropsychopharmacology 7:55–57, 1992a

Seeman P: Dopamine receptor sequences: therapeutic levels of neuroleptics occupy D_2 receptors, clozapine occupies D_4. Neuropsychopharmacology 7:261–284, 1992b

Seeman P, Niznik HB: Dopamine receptors and transporters in Parkinson's disease and schizophrenia. FASEB J 4:2737–2744, 1990

Seeman P, Ulpian C, Bergeron C, et al: Bimodal distribution of dopamine receptor densities in brains of schizophrenics. Science 225:728–731, 1984

Seeman P, Bzowej NH, Guan HC, et al: Human brain D_1 and D_2 dopamine receptors in schizophrenia, Alzheimer's, Parkinson's, and Huntington's diseases. Neuropsychopharmacology 1:5–15, 1987

Seibyl JP, Krystal JN, Price LH, et al: Neuroendocrine and behavioral responses to MCPP in unmedicated schizophrenics and healthy subjects. Paper presented at the annual meeting of the American College of Neuropsychopharmacology, Maui, HI, December 1989

Sharma R, Javaid JI, Janicak P, et al: Plasma and CSF HVA before and after pharmacological treatment. Psychiatry Res 28:97–104, 1989

Sherman AD, Davidson AT, Baruah S: Evidence of glutamatergic deficiency in schizophrenia. Neurosci Lett 121:77–80, 1991

Shore D, Korpi ER, Bigelow LB, et al: Fenfluramine and chronic schizophrenia. Biol Psychiatry 20:329–352, 1985

Simpson GM, Kunz-Bartholini E, Watts TPS: A preliminary evaluation of the sedative effects of Catapres, a new antihypertensive agent, in chronic schizophrenic patients. J Clin Pharmacol 7:221, 1967

Stahl SM, Uhr SB, Berger PA: Pilot study on the effects of fenfluramine on negative symptoms in twelve schizophrenic inpatients. Biol Psychiatry 20:1098–1102, 1985

Stanley JA: In vivo proton magnetic resonance spectroscopy in never-treated schizophrenics. Paper presented at the 145th annual meeting of the American Psychiatric Association, Washington, DC, May 1992

Stein L, Wise CD: Possible etiology of schizophrenia: progressive damage to the noradrenergic reward system by 5-hydroxydopamine. Science 171:1032–1036, 1971

Sternberg DE, Charney DS, Heninger GR, et al: Impaired presynaptic regulation in schizophrenia: effects of clonidine in schizophrenic patients and normal controls. Arch Gen Psychiatry 39:285–289, 1982

Tassin JP, Kitabgi P, Tramu G, et al: Rat mesocortical dopaminergic neurons are mixed neurotensin/dopamine neurons: immunohistochemical and biochemical evidence. Ann N Y Acad Sci 537:531–533, 1988

Tatetsu S: Schizophrenia and methamphetamine psychosis: histopathological comparison, in World Issues in the Problems of Schizophrenia Psychoses. Edited by Fukuda T, Mitsuda H. New York, Igaku-Shoin, 1976, pp 109–114

Todrick A, Tait MB, Marshall EF: Blood platelet 5-HT levels in psychiatric patients. Journal of Mental Science 106:884–890, 1960

Toru M, Watanabe S, Shibuya H, et al: Neurotransmitters, receptors and neuropeptides in post-mortem brains of chronic schizophrenic patients. Acta Psychiatr Scand 78:121–137, 1988

Uhl GR, Snyder SH: Regional and subcellular distributions of brain neurotensin. Life Sci 19:1827–1832, 1977

Vanderhaeghen JJ, Lotstra F, Vierendeels G, et al: Cholecystokinins in the central nervous system and neurohypophysis. Peptides 2:81–88, 1981

van Kammen DP, Gelernter J: Biochemical instability in schizophrenia, II: the serotonin and gamma-aminobutyric acid system, in Psychopharmacology: The Third Generation of Progress. Edited by Meltzer HY. New York, Raven, 1987, pp 753–758

van Kammen DP, Sternberg DE, Hare TA, et al: CSF levels of gamma-aminobutyric acid in schizophrenia. Arch Gen Psychiatry 39:91–97, 1982

van Kammen DP, Mann LS, Sternberg DE, et al: Dopamine-β-hydroxylase activity and homovanillic acid in spinal fluid of schizophrenics with brain atrophy. Science 220:974–977, 1983

van Kammen DP, Rosen J, Peters J, et al: Are there state-dependent markers in schizophrenia? Psychopharmacol Bull 21:497–502, 1985

van Kammen DP, Yao JK, Goetz K, et al: Polyunsaturated fatty acids, prostaglandins, and schizophrenia. Ann N Y Acad Sci 559:411–423, 1989a

van Kammen DP, Peters JL, van Kammen WB, et al: Clonidine treatment of schizophrenia: can we predict treatment response? Psychiatry Res 27:297–311, 1989b

van Kammen DP, Peters J, Yao J, et al: Norepinephrine and relapse in chronic schizophrenia: negative symptoms revisited. Arch Gen Psychiatry 47:161–168, 1990

van Praag HM: CSF 5-HIAA and suicide in non-depressed schizophrenics. Lancet 2:977–978, 1983

van Ree JM, Caffe AR, Wolterink G: Non-opiate β-endorphin fragments and dopamine, III: γ-type endorphins and various neuroleptics counteract the hyperactivity elicited by intra-accumbens injection of apomorphine. Neuropharmacology 21:1111–1117, 1982a

van Ree JM, Innemee H, Louwerens JW, et al: Non-opiate β-endorphin fragments and dopamine, I: the neuroleptic-like γ-endorphin fragments interfere with behavioral effects elicited by low doses of apomorphine. Neuropharmacology 21:1095–1101, 1982b

van Ree JM, Wolterink G, Fekete M, et al: Non-opiate β-endorphin fragments and dopamine, IV: γ-endorphins may control dopaminergic systems in the nucleus accumbens. Neuropharmacology 21:1119–1127, 1982c

van Ree JM, Gaffori O, de Wied D: In rats, the behavioural profile of CCK-8 related peptides resembles that of antipsychotic agents. Eur J Pharmacol 93:63–78, 1983

van Ree JM, Verhoeven WMA, Claas FHJ, et al: Antipsychotic action of γ-type endorphins: animal and human studies. Prog Brain Res 65:221–235, 1986

Verbanck PMP, Lotstra F, Gilles C, et al: Reduced cholecystokinin immunoreactivity in the cerebrospinal fluid of patients with psychiatric disorders. Life Sci 34:67–72, 1984

Wang RY, White FJ: Cholecystokinin octapeptide excitation and dopamine inhibition of nucleus accumbens neurons in the rat (abstract). Proceedings of the Fifth International Catecholamine Symposium, 1983, pp 314–315

Waziri R: Glycine therapy of schizophrenia (letter). Biol Psychiatry 23:210–211, 1988

Waziri R, Baruah S, Hegwood TS, et al: Abnormal serine hydroxymethyl transferase activity in the temporal lobes of schizophrenics. Neurosci Lett 120:237–240, 1990

Weinberger DR: Implications of normal brain development for the pathogenesis of schizophrenia. Arch Gen Psychiatry 44:660–669, 1987

Weinberger DR, Berman KF, Illowsky BP: Physiological dysfunction of dorsolateral prefrontal cortex in schizophrenia, III: a new cohort and evidence for a monoaminergic mechanism. Arch Gen Psychiatry 45:609–615, 1988

Whitaker PM, Crow TJ, Ferrier IN: Tritiated LSD binding in frontal cortex in schizophrenia. Arch Gen Psychiatry 38:278–280, 1981

Widerlöv E: A critical appraisal of CSF monoamine metabolite studies in schizophrenia. Ann N Y Acad Sci 537:309–323, 1988

Widerlöv E, Lindstrom LH, Bissette G, et al: Subnormal CSF levels of neurotensin in a subgroup of schizophrenic patients: normalization after neuroleptic treatment. Am J Psychiatry 139:1122–1126, 1982

Widerlöv E, Kalivas PW, Lewis MH, et al: Influence of cholecystokinin on central monoaminergic pathways. Regul Pept 6:99–109, 1983

Winblad B, Bucht G, Gottfries CG, et al: Monoamines and monoamine metabolites in brains from demented schizophrenics. Acta Psychiatr Scand 60:17–28, 1979

Wolkowitz OM, Pickar D: Benzodiazepines in the treatment of schizophrenia: a review and reappraisal. Am J Psychiatry 148:714–726, 1991

Wolkowitz OM, Breier A, Doran A, et al: Alprazolam augmentation of antipsychotic effects of fluphenazine in schizophrenic patients: preliminary results. Arch Gen Psychiatry 45:664–671, 1988

Wong DF, Wagner HN Jr, Tune LE, et al: Positron emission tomography reveals elevated D_2 dopamine receptors in drug-naive schizophrenics. Science 234:1558–1563, 1986

Woolley DW: Evidence for the participation of serotonin in mental processes. Ann N Y Acad Sci 66:649, 1957

Woolley DW, Shaw E: Some antimetabolites of serotonin and their possible application to the treatment of hypertension. Journal of the American Chemical Society 74:2948–2949, 1952

Wyatt RJ: The dopamine hypothesis: Variations on a theme (II). Psychopharmacol Bull 22:923–927, 1986

Wyatt RJ, Vaughan T, Galater M, et al: Behavioral changes of chronic schizophrenic patients given L-5-hydroxytryptophan. Science 177:1124–1126, 1972

Wyatt RJ, Murphy DL, Belmaker R, et al: Reduced monoamine oxidase activity in platelets: a possible genetic marker for vulnerability to schizophrenia. Science 173:916–918, 1973

Wyatt RJ, Schwartz MA, Erdelyi E, et al: Dopamine β-hydroxylase activity in brains of chronic schizophrenic patients. Science 187:368–370, 1975

Zukin SR, Nussenzveig IZ, Javitt DC, et al: NMDA receptor stimulation in schizophrenia: candidate mechanisms and effect of oral glycine. Paper presented at the annual meeting of the American College of Neuropsychopharmacology, San Juan, Puerto Rico, December 1992

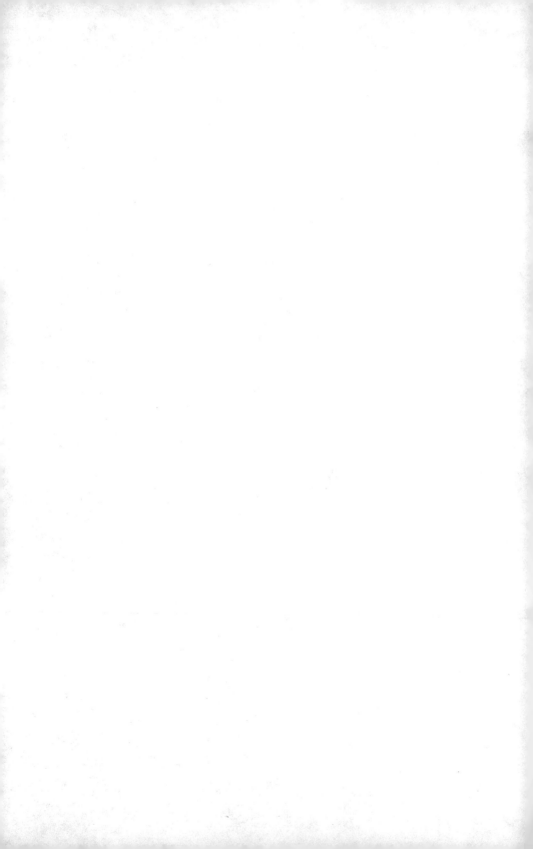

CHAPTER 2

Postmortem Brain Abnormalities in Schizophrenia

Bernhard Bogerts, M.D.,
and Peter Falkai, M.D.

Despite the development of modern brain-imaging methods such as computed tomography (CT) and magnetic resonance imaging (MRI), neuropathological studies will remain an indispensable tool in the search for biological correlates of schizophrenia. The limited resolution and contrast of modern brain-imaging methods make it difficult to locate and precisely delineate the smaller cell groups in the brain stem, limbic system, and hypothalamus that are important in current theories of the so-called endogenous psychoses. Moreover, to understand the nature of ventricular enlargement and tissue volume reduction, as demonstrated by many CT and MRI studies (see Chapter 10), studies of fine brain tissue structures at the histological and cellular levels are necessary.

This work was supported by Deutsche Forschungsgemeinschaft (Bo 799/1–3) and the Alfried-Krupp-von Bohlen und Halbach Stiftung.

Postmortem studies of brains from patients with dementia praecox were part of the first biological approaches to the disease. In 1897, Alzheimer described neuronal changes in the cortex that were clearly different from those he observed in senile dementias. In 1915, cortical atrophy in the association areas was reported by Southard. Buscaino (1924) described histopathological changes in the basal ganglia that he thought were responsible for catatonia-like and stereotyped behavior. The Vogts and their co-workers (Bäumer 1954; Fünfgeld 1925; Treff and Hempel 1958; Vogt and Vogt 1952) reported cell gaps and "dwarf cells" in the cortex and thalamus of schizophrenic patients.

These early findings in the cortex, basal ganglia, and thalamus later were heavily criticized by the influential neuropathologists Dunlap (1924) and Peters (1967), who regarded the reported structural changes in brains of schizophrenic individuals as postmortem artifacts or normal variants. After the first International Congress of Neuropathology in 1952, most neuropathologists and psychiatrists assumed that anatomical correlates could not be convincingly demonstrated in brains of schizophrenic individuals.

The failure of early neuropathological schizophrenia research to convincingly demonstrate neuropathological changes in schizophrenic patients becomes understandable given the following considerations:

1. According to Kraepelin's (1899) concept, dementia praecox was defined as a disease entity; hence, a specific brain pathology characteristic for all schizophrenic patients was expected, but not found.

2. In nearly all of the studies that were reported during the first half of the 20th century, structural brain abnormalities in schizophrenic patients were detected by qualitative tissue assessment; that is, researchers did not apply morphometric-statistical methods. Given the considerable variability of normal brain structure and the substantial overlap in neuroanatomy of schizophrenic patients and nonpsychiatric control subjects, as has been shown by recent brain-imaging and postmortem studies, the subtle abnormalities of macroscopic and microscopic brain anatomy today presumed to underlie schizophrenia are detectable only by applying optimal quantitative-morphometric and statistical procedures. Because these techniques were not available during the first half of the century, it is not surprising that only impressive morphological changes, as seen in Alzheimer's, Pick's, and Parkinson's diseases, were previously discovered.

3. Confounding variables have not always been taken into account. Such variables involve brain changes secondary to complicating neurological or vascular diseases, pre-agonal conditions (e.g., protracted coma), chronic diseases of peripheral organs, and time to fixation, as well as postmortem shrinkage and swelling of brain tissue (Casanova and Kleinman 1990; Peters 1967).
4. Because little was known about the neuroanatomy and physiology of the limbic system during the first half of the 20th century, the temporolimbic and related paralimbic structures that are now thought to play a crucial role in at least some schizophrenic symptoms were completely over-looked in the search for anatomical changes in schizophrenia.

Recent Neuropathological Findings in Schizophrenia

In this chapter, we summarize the more important neuropathological findings that, in our view, have contributed to a better understanding of the nature of schizophrenia. The reader is referred to two recent comprehensive reviews on the neuropathology of schizophrenia (Bogerts 1993; Bogerts and Lieberman 1993).

At present, interest in the neuropathology of schizophrenia is focused on three major types of findings:

- The increasing evidence of subtle structural changes in the limbic systems of schizophrenic patients
- The evidence for anatomical changes in structures outside the limbic system (e.g., in the cortex, brain stem, thalamus), although such anatomical changes have been less often investigated than have changes in limbic structures
- The theory that brain changes seen in postmortem brains as well as in CT and MRI scans reflect a disorder of early brain development

Structural Changes in the Limbic Systems of Schizophrenic Patients

Key structures of the limbic system are those situated in the medial temporal lobe—the hippocampus, parahippocampal gyrus, and amygdala. This brain region is closely interconnected with the septum-hypothalamus complex, prefrontal and orbital cortex, cingulate gyrus, nucleus accumbens, temporal pole, and polymodal sensory association cortex. Limbic functions are comprised of the coordination of cognitive and emotional activities, higher cortical integration and association of different sensory modalities, representation and analysis of environmental contexts, sensory gating, and the neuronal generation and control of basic drives and emotions (Gray 1982; Gray et al. 1991; McLean 1952; Mesulam 1986; Millner 1992; Schmajuk 1987). Increasing knowledge of limbic system physiology has yielded more plausible theories linking a broad spectrum of schizophrenic symptoms to dysfunctions of limbic and related structures (Bogerts 1985, 1991).

There are now more than 20 publications on structural changes in the limbic systems of schizophrenic patients. The findings in limbic brain regions include the following:

1. Reduced volumes or cross-sectional areas of the hippocampus, amygdala, and parahippocampal gyrus (Altshuler et al. 1990; Bogerts 1984; Bogerts et al. 1985, 1990b; Brown et al. 1986; Colter et al. 1987; Falkai and Bogerts 1986; Falkai et al. 1988a; Jeste and Lohr 1989)
2. Left temporal horn enlargement, which is consistent with tissue loss in the surrounding limbic structures (Bogerts et al. 1985; Brown et al. 1986; Crow et al. 1989; Heckers et al. 1990b)
3. Reduced cell numbers or cell sizes in the hippocampus or parahippocampal gyrus or entorhinal cortex (Benes et al. 1991b; Casanova et al. 1991; Falkai and Bogerts 1986; Falkai et al. 1988a; Jakob and Beckmann 1986; Jeste and Lohr 1989)
4. White-matter reductions in parahippocampal gyrus or hippocampus (Colter et al. 1987; Heckers et al. 1991b)
5. Disturbed architecture and abnormal cell arrangements in the hippocampus, entorhinal, cingulate, and orbital cortex (Arnold et al. 1991; Benes and Bird 1987; Conrad et al. 1991; Falkai and Bogerts 1989; Falkai et al. 1988b; Jakob and Beckmann 1986; Kovelman and Scheibel 1984; Senitz and Winkelmann 1991)
6. Increased vertical axon numbers and deficits in small interneurons in the cingulate gyrus (Benes et al. 1987, 1991a)
7. Increased incidence of a cavum septi pellucidi (Degreef et al. 1992)

Although the type and extent of the reported limbic system pathology in schizophrenia varies, and although there seems not to be a homogeneous pattern of limbic pathology in schizophrenia, the vast majority of researchers agree that there are subtle changes in limbic brain regions in a significant percentage of schizophrenic patients.

The limbic and paralimbic brain regions (i.e., hippocampus, amygdala, parahippocampal gyrus, entorhinal cortex, cingulate gyrus, orbital cortex, temporal pole) are to be regarded as highly organized supramodal association and integration areas (Gray 1982; Mesulam 1986; Millner 1992; Schmajuk 1987; van Hoesen 1982). Therefore, structural and functional deficits in these brain regions could be associated with the failure of many schizophrenic patients in the higher integrative and associative brain functions, leading to these patients' having distorted interpretations of external reality.

Postmortem Findings Outside Limbic Structures

Brain weight, cortex, and ventricles.   Brown et al. (1986), Bruton et al. (1990), and Pakkenberg (1987) reported a subtle but significant decrease (5%–8%) in schizophrenic patients' brain weights, and Bruton et al. (1990) reported a decrease in these patients' brain lengths. Heckers et al. (1991a), however, found nearly identical brain weights and hemispheric volumes in schizophrenic patients and nonpsychiatric control subjects.

Very few histopathological studies of the cortex have been performed in the new era of neuropathological schizophrenia research. Lower neuronal densities and deficits in small interneurons in the prefrontal cortex and anterior cingulate gyrus (Benes et al. 1986, 1991a) and reductions of cortical volume (12%) and central gray matter (6%; Pakkenberg 1987) have been described.

Pathology of the frontal cortex could well explain some psychopathological aspects of schizophrenia, such as negative symptoms and cognitive deficits. Frontal lobe syndromes caused by brain tumors, injuries, lobotomy, or Pick's disease are characterized by apathy, loss of drive, inappropriate affect, social withdrawal or disinhibition, poor judgment, and psychomotor retardation (Fuster 1989). Many of these symptoms are commonly seen in patients with negative schizophrenia.

It is, however, difficult to demonstrate ventricular enlargement—as revealed by CT and MRI studies—with postmortem methods because artificial brain shrinkage and widening of internal and external cerebrospinal fluid spaces occur during fixation and embedding of the brain. Moreover, ventricles are frequently compressed during the mechanical handling of the brain during autopsy.

Brain stem, basal ganglia, and thalamus.   With regard to the theoretical importance of the cerebral neurotransmitters—especially dopamine—in schizophrenia, it is surprising that only a few direct neurohistological studies of these cell groups in schizophrenic patients have been performed (Bogerts et al. 1983; Karson et al. 1991; Lohr and Jeste 1988). Because these brain stem neurotransmitter studies were based on small sample sizes and, therefore, have to be regarded as preliminary, they are not commented on here in more detail.

The basal ganglia, especially the striatum and pallidum, are regarded to be parts of the extrapyramidal and limbic system (Mesulam 1986) and are involved in the neuronal modulation of movement coordination. It is, therefore, conceivable that dysfunction of these brain parts plays a role in the pathogenesis of catatonic symptoms. Data from qualitative (Hopf 1954; Stevens 1982) and quantitative (Bogerts et al. 1986; Stevens 1986) postmortem studies support the notion that pallidum dysfunction might occur in catatonic schizophrenic patients.

Some neuropathological studies of the thalamus have been published. Treff and Hempel (1958) described a significant reduction of neurons in the mediodorsal nucleus of the thalamus of catatonic and paranoid patients. Similar results were later published by Pakkenberg (1990). Lesch and Bogerts (1984) reported a reduction of thalamic periventricular gray matter surrounding the third ventricle. In the most recent study of our new Düsseldorf brain collection, we (Bogerts et al., in press) found a significant (about 15%) volume reduction of the right and left thalamus in addition to smaller temporolimbic structures in a sample of 28 schizophrenic patients compared with 27 well-matched nonpsychiatric control subjects. Clinical symptoms associated with dysfunctions of the thalamus resemble the negative symptoms of schizophrenia (Lesch and Bogerts 1984). Thus, thalamic dysfunction might contribute to the pathophysiology of the disease.

Evidence for an Early Disorder of Brain Development

The majority of the investigators reporting structural changes in brains of schizophrenic patients seem to agree that the revealed subtle abnormalities were a result of a prenatal or perinatal disturbance of brain development. We found 23 studies in which the findings were consistent with a disorder of brain development (summarized in Table 2–1). Authors of 5 studies favored an inflammatory or degenerative brain disease (see Table 2–2), and authors of 13 studies did not give any comments on the etiology of the disease (Table 2–3).

The following neuropathological changes support the notion that, in at least a substantial proportion of the patients, the subtle structural changes described above result from an early disorder of brain development.

Absence of gliosis in limbic structures.   The absence of gliosis in a structurally changed brain region is compatible with a fixed, very early prenatal or genetic pathology. An earlier gliotic response to a perinatal lesion may disappear many years after the initial lesion (Friede 1989).

Although gliosis has been described qualitatively in periventricular and temporolimbic structures (Bruton et al. 1990; Nieto and Escobar 1972; Stevens 1982) as well as in the brain stem (Fisman 1975), the majority of the quantitative-statistical glial cell studies have indicated that the anatomical abnormalities described in the mesiotemporal structures, cingulate gyrus, and thalamus are not associated with gliosis and, therefore, might reflect a disorder of brain development (Benes et al. 1986, 1991a; Casanova 1991; Crow et al. 1989; Falkai and Bogerts 1986; Falkai et al. 1988a; Pakkenberg 1990; Roberts et al. 1987). There might, however, be a subgroup of patients with a reactive gliosis around the third ventricle, possibly caused by a later-acquired subtle brain lesion (Bogerts et al. 1990c).

Cytoarchitectural alterations in the hippocampus, cingulate gyrus, and entorhinal cortex.   Abnormal architectonic arrangements of

Table 2–1.   Studies in which structural brain abnormalities in schizophrenia were found consistent with a disorder of brain development

McLardy (1974)	Reduced thickness of the granule cell layer in the hippocampal formation
Kovelman and Scheibel (1984)	Disorientation of hippocampal pyramidal cells
Bogerts (1984); Bogerts et al. (1985)	Reduced volumes of hippocampus, parahippocampal gyrus, and amygdala
Benes et al. (1986, 1987)	Reduced neuronal density and cytoarchitectural disturbances in the prefrontal cortex, anterior cingulate, and primary motor cortex
Brown et al. (1986)	Reduction of brain weight and left parahippocampal cortex; temporal horn enlargement
Falkai and Bogerts (1986)	Reduction of hippocampal pyramidal cells without gliosis
Jakob and Beckmann (1986)	Abnormal sulcogyral pattern; cytoarchitectonic abnormalities in the rostral entorhinal cortex and ventral insular region
Altshuler et al. (1987)	Correlation between hippocampal pyramidal cell disarray and severity of clinical symptoms
Roberts et al. (1987)	No change in astrocyte densities in the temporal lobe
Falkai et al. (1988a)	Lower volume and cell densities in the entorhinal cortex without gliosis
Falkai et al. (1988b)	Increased prevalence of heterotopic cell clusters in the left entorhinal cortex
Crow et al. (1989)	Selective left temporal horn enlargement
Falkai and Bogerts (1989)	Abnormal location of entorhinal pre–alpha cell clusters
Altshuler et al. (1990)	Reduced cross-sectional area of right parahippocampal gyrus but not hippocampus; shape abnormalities in medial temporal structures
Bogerts et al. (1990b)	Reduced hippocampal volume
Pakkenberg (1990)	Reduction of total neuron and glial cell numbers in the mediodorsal thalamic nucleus and nucleus accumbens
Arnold et al. (1991)	Aberrant invaginations, disruption of cortical layers, and heterotopic displacement of neurons in superficial layers of the parahippocampal gyrus
Benes et al. (1991a)	Reduced pyramidal cell density in hippocampal CA1 segment; overall reduction of pyramidal cell size
Benes et al. (1991b)	Reduction of interneurons in layer II of the cingulate and the prefrontal cortex
Conrad et al. (1991)	Disarray of pyramidal cells in right hippocampus
Karson et al. (1991)	Increase of cholinergic neurons in the nucleus pedunculopontinus; decrease of catecholaminergic neurons in the locus coeruleus

Table 2–1.   Studies in which structural brain abnormalities in schizophrenia were found consistent with a disorder of brain development *(continued)*

Degreef et al. (1992)	Increased prevalence of a cavum septi pellucidi
Falkai et al. (1992a)	Reduction of left Sylvian fissure length; loss of physiological left-right Sylvian fissure asymmetry

single nerve cells, cell clusters, or cortical layers are a strong indicator of disturbed prenatal brain development (Evrard et al. 1989). Cytoarchitectural anomalies in brains of schizophrenic patients were described in the dentate gyrus (McLardy 1974) and the cornu ammonis (CA) segments (Conrad et al. 1991; Kovelman and Scheibel 1984; Senitz and Winkelmann 1991) of the hippocampal formation; in the frontal cortex and cingulate gyrus (Benes and Bird 1987; Benes et al. 1986); and in the entorhinal cortex (Arnold et al. 1991; Falkai and Bogerts 1989; Falkai et al. 1988b; Jakob and Beckmann 1986).

Increased incidence of a cavum septi pellucidi.   An obvious sign of abnormal brain development in schizophrenia is an increased prevalence of the cavum septi pellucidi in postmortem brains and CT and MRI studies of schizophrenic patients (Degreef et al. 1992; Lewis and Mezey 1985). In fetuses, the two layers of the septum pellucidum are separated by a cavity of varying size that begins to shrink before birth

Table 2–2.   Studies in which structural brain abnormalities in schizophrenia were found consistent with an inflammatory or progressive brain disease

Nieto and Escobar (1972)	Gliosis in periventricular and limbic structures
Fisman (1975)	Glial knots and perivascular infiltrations in the brain stem
Stevens (1982)	Gliosis in hypothalamus, midbrain, basal nucleus, medial thalamus, amygdala, and hippocampus
Nasrallah et al. (1983)	Gliosis in the corpus callosum of late-onset schizophrenic patients
Bruton et al. (1990)	Reduction of brain weight and length; increase of ventricular size; periventricular fibrous gliosis in some schizophrenic patients

Table 2–3.   Studies of structural brain abnormalities in schizophrenia in which no comments on the etiology of the disease were given

Dom et al. (1981)	Reduced microneuron density in the pulvinar of catatonic patients
Bogerts et al. (1983)	Reduced volume of the lateral substantia nigra, smaller neurons in dopaminergic A10 area
Lesch and Bogerts (1984)	Reduction of thickness of diencephalic periventricular gray matter
Colter et al. (1987)	Reduced parahippocampal white matter
Pakkenberg (1987)	Volume reduction of both hemispheres, cortex, and subcortical white matter
Lohr and Jeste (1988)	Reduced neuropil in the locus coeruleus
Christison et al. (1989)	No disarray of hippocampal pyramidal cells
Jeste and Lohr (1989)	Reduced hippocampal volume and pyramidal cell numbers
Heckers et al. (1990a)	Unchanged volume of parahippocampal gyrus
Heckers et al. (1990b)	Unchanged volume of hippocampus, amygdala, and ventricular system; increase of left ventricular volume in paranoid schizophrenia
Casanova et al. (1991)	Bilateral reduction of cells in the entorhinal cortex
Heckers et al. (1991a)	Bilateral volume increase of the corpus striatum; right-sided increase of pallidal volume; no differences in white matter and cortical volumes
Heckers et al. (1991b)	Reduction of hippocampal white matter; no differences in total cell numbers, cell density, and total volume of hippocampus

and disappears long before adulthood. The cavum persists in only a small percentage of adults. Degreef et al. (1992) reported a more than twofold increased prevalence of a cavum septi pellucidi in postmortem brains and a tenfold increase in MRI scans of schizophrenic patients.

Absence of normal structural cerebral asymmetry.   The normal structural asymmetry of the brain includes a larger left planum temporale, a longer left Sylvian fissure, and larger right frontal and temporal lobes (Galaburda et al. 1987). These asymmetries are already present at birth, having been genetically preprogrammed and having developed in the second and third trimester of pregnancy (Wada and Davies 1977).

Most of the above-mentioned postmortem studies (Tables 2–1 through 2–3) did not focus on left-right differences. Some investigators, however, have reported selective left temporal horn enlargement (Brown et al. 1986; Crow et al. 1989) or a tendency toward left but not right ventricular enlargement (Heckers et al. 1990b).

Crow (1990) postulated that schizophrenia was caused by a developmental anomaly of cerebral asymmetry, and suggested that temporal lobe asymmetries provide an important key to the etiology of the illness. This view has gained further support from recent reports of an absence of the normal Sylvian fissure asymmetry (Crow et al. 1992; Falkai et al. 1992) and of mesiotemporal (Bogerts et al. 1990a) and frontal lobe asymmetry (Bilder et al. 1994) in schizophrenic patients.

Concluding Remarks

One important difference between the schizophrenic disorders and the well-known neurodegenerative disorders is that in most schizophrenic patients, the structural changes in the brain are not progressive and were acquired very early in life (Bogerts 1989, 1993; Crow 1990; Jones and Murray 1991; Weinberger 1987). The magnitude of the pathology in schizophrenia is far less than that seen in Alzheimer's, Pick's, Parkinson's, or Huntington's disease. Limbic tissue volumes and cell numbers and sizes in schizophrenic patients differ only by some 10%–30% from those in normal/healthy control subjects, whereas *every* patient with one of the above-mentioned degenerative brain diseases has an obvious brain pathology. Furthermore, there is a considerable overlap between schizophrenic patients and control subjects, with only about one-fourth of the patients having values outside the range of those of the control subjects.

There are several theories that offer an explanation for the long latency between the early disturbance of brain development and the onset of the typical clinical symptoms in schizophrenic patients (Benes 1989; Bogerts 1989; Murray et al. 1991; Stevens 1992; Weinberger 1987). Common to all of these theories is that the investigators regard the structural abnormalities in brains of schizophrenic patients as vulnerability markers that predispose the brain to decompensate under the influence of additional factors—factors related to stress and to a vulnerable age period between puberty and old age.

Because no therapeutic method yet exists for reversing the structural deficits seen in many schizophrenic patients, treatment strategies should aim at reducing, by pharmacological and psychotherapeutic means, the effects of environmental stressors that decompensate brains vulnerable to schizophrenia because of a subtle abnormality of early brain development.

References

Altshuler LL, Conrad A, Kovelman JA, et al: Hippocampal pyramidal cell orientation in schizophrenia. Arch Gen Psychiatry 44:1094–1098, 1987

Altshuler LL, Casanova MF, Goldberg TE, et al: The hippocampus and parahippocampus in schizophrenic, suicide, and control brains. Arch Gen Psychiatry 47:1029–1034, 1990

Alzheimer A: Beitrage zur pathologischen Anatomie der Hirnrinde und zur anatomischen Grundlage der Psychosen. Monatsschrift für Psychiatrie und Neurologie 2:82–120, 1897

Arnold SE, Hyman BT, Van Hösen GW, et al: Some cytoarchitectural abnormalities of the entorhinal cortex in schizophrenia. Arch Gen Psychiatry 48:625–632, 1991

Bäumer H: Veranderungen des Thalamus bei Schizophrenie. J Hirnforsch 1:157–172, 1954

Benes FM: Myelination of cortical-hippocampal relays during late adolescence. Schizophr Bull 15:585–593, 1989

Benes FM, Bird ED: An analysis of the arrangement of neurons in the cingulate cortex of schizophrenic patients. Arch Gen Psychiatry 44:608–616, 1987

Benes FM, Davidson B, Bird ED: Quantitative cytoarchitectural studies of the cerebral cortex of schizophrenics. Arch Gen Psychiatry 43:31–35, 1986

Benes FM, Majocha R, Bird ED, et al: Increased vertical axon numbers in cingulate cortex of schizophrenics. Arch Gen Psychiatry 44:1017–1021, 1987

Benes FM, McSparren J, Bird ED, et al: Deficits in small interneurons in prefrontal and cingulate cortices of schizophrenic and schizoaffective patients. Arch Gen Psychiatry 48:996–1001, 1991a

Benes FM, Sorensen I, Bird ED: Reduced neuronal size in posterior hippocampus of schizophrenic patients. Schizophr Bull 17:597–608, 1991b

Bilder RM, Wu H, Bogerts B, et al: Absence of regional hemispheric volume asymmetries in first-episode schizophrenia. Am J Psychiatry 151:1437–1447, 1994

Bogerts B: Zur Neuropathologie der Schizophrenien. Fortschr Neurol Psychiatr 52:428–437, 1984

Bogerts B: Schizophrenien als Erkrankungen des limbischen Systems, in Basisstadien endogener Psychosen und das Borderline-Problem. Edited by Huber G. Stuttgart, Germany, Schattauer, 1985, pp 163–179

Bogerts B: Limbic and paralimbic pathology in schizophrenia: interaction with age and stress related factors, in Schizophrenia: Scientific Progress. Edited by Schulz SC, Tamminga CA. Oxford, UK, Oxford University Press, 1989, pp 216–227

Bogerts B: The neuropathology of schizophrenia: pathophysiological and neurodevelopmental implications, in Fetal Neural Development and Adult Schizophrenia. Edited by Mednick SA, Cannon TD, Barr CE. Cambridge, UK, Cambridge University Press, 1991, pp 153–173

Bogerts B: Recent advances in the neuropathology of schizophrenia. Schizophr Bull 19:431–435, 1993

Bogerts B, Lieberman J: Neuropathology in the study of psychiatric disease, in International Review of Psychiatry, Vol 1. Edited by Costa e Silva ACJ, Nadelson CC. Washington, DC, American Psychiatric Press, 1993, pp 515–555

Bogerts B, Häntsch H, Herzer M: A morphometric study of the dopamine-containing cell groups in the mesencephalon of normals, Parkinson patients and schizophrenics. Biol Psychiatry 18:951–971, 1983

Bogerts B, Meertz E, Schönfeldt-Bausch R: Basal ganglia and limbic system pathology in schizophrenia. Arch Gen Psychiatry 42:784–791, 1985

Bogerts B, Falkai P, Tutsch J: Cell numbers in the pallidum and hippocampus of schizophrenics, in Biological Psychiatry. Edited by Shagass C, Josiassen RC, Bridger WH, et al. Amsterdam, Netherlands, Elsevier, 1986, pp 1178–1180

Bogerts B, Ashtari M, Degreef G, et al: Reduced temporal limbic structure volumes on magnetic resonance images in first episode schizophrenia. Psychiatry Res: Neuroimaging 35:1–13, 1990a

Bogerts B, Falkai P, Haupts M, et al: Post-mortem volume measurements of limbic system and basal ganglia structures in chronic schizophrenics. Schizophr Res 3:295–301, 1990b

Bogerts B, David S, Falkai P, et al: Quantitative evaluation of astrocyte densities in schizophrenia. Paper presented at the 17th Congress of the Collegium Internationale Neuro-Psychopharmacologicum, Kyoto, Japan, September 1990c

Bogerts B, Falkai P, Greve B, et al: Reduced volumes of hippocampus and thalamus in schizophrenia: a morphometric study from the new Düsseldorf collection. Schizophr Res (in press)

Brown R, Colter N, Corsellis JAN, et al: Postmortem evidence of structural brain changes in schizophrenia: differences in brain weight, temporal horn area and parahippocampal gyrus compared with affective disorder. Arch Gen Psychiatry 43:36–42, 1986

Bruton CJ, Crow TJ, Frith CD, et al: Schizophrenia and the brain: a prospective clinico-neuropathological study. Psychol Med 20:285–304, 1990

Buscaino VM: Neue Tatsachen über die pathologische Histologie und die Pathogenese der Dementia praecox, der Amentia und der extrapyramidalen Bewegungsstörungen. Schweiz Arch Neurol Psychiatr 14:210–215, 1924

Casanova MF: Astrocytosis and schizophrenia. Schizophr Res 5:186–187, 1991

Casanova MF, Kleinman JE: The neuropathology of schizophrenia: a critical assessment of research methodologies. Biol Psychiatry 27:353–362, 1990

Casanova MF, Saunders R, Altshuler LL, et al: Entorhinal cortex pathology in schizophrenia and affective disorders, in Biological Psychiatry. Edited by Racagni G, Brunello N, Fukada T. Amsterdam, Netherlands, Elsevier, 1991, pp 504–506

Christison GW, Casanova MF, Weinberger DR, et al: A quantitative investigation of hippocampal pyramidal cell size, shape and variability of orientation in schizophrenia. Arch Gen Psychiatry 46:1027–1031, 1989

Colter N, Battal S, Crow TJ, et al: White matter reduction in the parahippocampal gyrus of patients with schizophrenia (letter). Arch Gen Psychiatry 44:1023, 1987

Conrad AJ, Abebe T, Austin R, et al: Hippocampal cell disarray in schizophrenia. Arch Gen Psychiatry 48:413–417, 1991

Crow TJ: Temporal lobe asymmetries as the key to the etiology of schizophrenia. Schizophr Bull 16:434–443, 1990

Crow TJ, Ball J, Bloom SR, et al: Schizophrenia as an anomaly of development of cerebral asymmetry. Arch Gen Psychiatry 46:1145–1150, 1989

Crow TJ, Brown R, Bruton CJ, et al: Loss of Sylvian fissure asymmetry in schizophrenia: findings in the Runwell 2 series of brains. Schizophr Res 6:152–153, 1992

Degreef G, Bogerts B, Falkai P, et al: Increased prevalence of the cavum septum pellucidum in MRI scans and postmortem brains of schizophrenic patients. Psychiatry Res 45:1–13, 1992

Dom R, de Saedeler J, Bogerts B, et al: Quantitative cytometric analysis of basal ganglia in catatonic schizophrenics, in Biological Psychiatry. Edited by Perris C, Struwe G, Jansson B. Amsterdam, Netherlands, Elsevier, 1981, pp 723–726

Dunlap CB: Dementia precox: some preliminary observations on brains from carefully selected cases, and a consideration of certain sources of error. Am J Psychiatry 80:403–421, 1924

Evrard P, Kadhim HJ, deSaint-Georges P, et al: Abnormal development and destructive processes of human brain during the second half of gestation, in Developmental Neurobiology. Edited by Evrard P, Minkowski A. New York, Raven, 1989, pp 21–41

Falkai P, Bogerts B: Cell loss in the hippocampus of schizophrenics. Eur Arch Psychiatry Neursci 236:154–161, 1986

Falkai P, Bogerts B: Morphometric evidence for developmental disturbances in brains of some schizophrenics. Schizophr Res 2:99, 1989

Falkai P, Bogerts B, Rozumek M: Cell loss and volume reduction in the entorhinal cortex of schizophrenics. Biol Psychiatry 24:515–521, 1988a

Falkai P, Bogerts B, Roberts GW, et al: Measurement of the alpha-cell migration in the entorhinal region: a marker for developmental disturbances in schizophrenia? Schizophr Res 1:157–158, 1988b

Falkai P, Bogerts B, Greve B, et al: Loss of Sylvian fissure asymmetry in schizophrenia: a quantitative postmortem study. Schizophr Res 7:23–32, 1992

Fisman M: The brain stem in psychosis. Br J Psychiatry 126:414–422, 1975

Friede RL: Developmental Neuropathology. Berlin, Springer, 1989

Fünfgeld E: Pathologisch-anatomische Untersuchungen bei Dementia praecox mit besonderer Berücksichtigung des Thalamus opticus. Zeitschrift für die gesamte Neurologie und Psychiatrie 95:411–463, 1925

Fuster JM: The Prefrontal Cortex. New York, Raven, 1989

Galaburda AM, Corsiglia J, Rosen GD, et al: Planum temporale asymmetry, reappraisal since Geschwind and Levitzky. Neuropsychologia 6:853–868, 1987

Gray JA: The Neuropsychology of Anxiety: An Enquiry Into the Function of the Septo-Hippocampal System. Oxford, UK, Oxford University Press, 1982

Gray JA, Feldon J, Rawlins JNP, et al: The neuropsychology of schizophrenia. Behav Brain Res 14:1–84, 1991

Heckers S, Heinsen H, Heinsen Y, et al: Morphometry of the parahippocampal gyrus in schizophrenics and controls: some anatomical considerations. J Neural Transm 80:151–155, 1990a

Heckers St, Heinsen H, Heinsen YC, et al: Limbic structures and lateral ventricle in schizophrenia. Arch Gen Psychiatry 47:1016–1022, 1990b

Heckers S, Heinsen H, Heinsen Y, et al: Cortex, white matter, and basal ganglia in schizophrenia: a volumetric postmortem study. Biol Psychiatry 29:556–566, 1991a

Heckers S, Heinsen H, Geiger B, et al: Hippocampal neuron number in schizophrenia. Arch Gen Psychiatry 48:1002–1008, 1991b

Hopf A: Orientierende Untersuchung zur Frage pathoanatomischer Veränderungen im Pallidum und Striatum bei Schizophrenie. J Hirnforsch 1:97–145, 1954

Jakob J, Beckmann H: Prenatal developmental disturbances in the limbic allocortex in schizophrenics. J Neural Transm 65:303–326, 1986

Jeste DV, Lohr JB: Hippocampal pathologic findings in schizophrenia: a morphometric study. Arch Gen Psychiatry 46:1019–1024, 1989

Jones P, Murray RM: The genetics of schizophrenia is the genetics of neurodevelopment. Br J Psychiatry 158:615–623, 1991

Karson CN, Garcia-Rill E, Biedermann JA, et al: The brain stem reticular formation in schizophrenia. Psychiatry Res: Neuroimaging 40:31–48, 1991

Kovelman JA, Scheibel AB: A neurohistological correlate of schizophrenia. Biol Psychiatry 19:1601–1621, 1984

Kraepelin E: Psychiatrie: Ein Lehrbuch für Studierende und Ärzte, 6th Edition. Leipzig, Germany, Barth, 1899

Lesch A, Bogerts B: The diencephalon in schizophrenia: evidence for reduced thickness of the periventricular grey matter. Eur Arch Psychiatry Neurosci 234:212–219, 1984

Lewis SW, Mezey GC: Clinical correlates of septum pellucidum cavities: an unusual association with psychosis. Psychol Med 15:43–54, 1985

Lohr JB, Jeste DV: Locus coeruleus morphometry in aging and schizophrenia. Acta Psychiatr Scand 77:689–697, 1988

McLardy T: Hippocampal zinc and structural deficit in brains from chronic alcoholics and some schizophrenics. Journal of Orthomolecular Psychiatry 4:32–36, 1974

McLean PD: Some psychiatric implications of physiological studies on frontotemporal portion of limbic system (visceral brain). Electroencephalogr Clin Neurophysiol 4:407–418, 1952

Mesulam MM: Patterns in behavioral neuroanatomy: association areas, the limbic system, and hemispheric specialization, in Principles of Behavioral Neurology. Edited by Mesulam MM. Philadelphia, PA, Davis, 1986, pp 1–70

Millner R: Cortico-Hippocampal Interplay and the Representation of Contexts in the Brain. Berlin, Springer, 1992

Murray RM, Jones P, O'Callaghan E: Fetal brain development and later schizophrenia, in Ciba Foundation Symposium 156: The Childhood Environment and Adult Disease. Chichester, UK, Wiley, 1991, pp 155–170

Nasrallah HA, McCalley-Whitters M, Rauscher FP, et al: A histological study of the corpus callosum in chronic schizophrenia. Psychiatry Res 8:151–160, 1983

Nieto D, Escobar A: Major psychoses, in Pathology of the Nervous System. Edited by Minkler J. New York, McGraw-Hill, 1972, pp 2654–2665

Pakkenberg B: Post-mortem study of chronic schizophrenic brains. Br J Psychiatry 151:744–752, 1987

Pakkenberg B: Pronounced reduction of total neuron number in mediodorsal thalamic nucleus and nucleus accumbens in schizophrenics. Arch Gen Psychiatry 47:1023–1028, 1990

Peters G: Neuropathologie und Psychiatrie, in Psychiatrie der Gegenwart, Bd 1/1A. Edited by Gruhle HW, Jung R, Mayer-Gross W, et al. Berlin, Springer, 1967, pp 286–298

Roberts GW, Colter N, Lofthouse R, et al: Is there gliosis in schizophrenia? investigations of the temporal lobe. Biol Psychiatry 22:1459–1468, 1987

Schmajuk NA: Animal models for schizophrenia: the hippocampally lesioned animal. Schizophr Bull 13:317–327, 1987

Senitz D, Winkelmann E: Neuronale Strukturanormalität im orbito-frontalen Cortex bei Schizophrenen. J Hirnforsch 32:149–158, 1991

Southard EEL: On the topographic distribution of cortex lesions and anomalies in dementia praecox with some account of their functional significance. American Journal of Insanity 71:603–671, 1915

Stevens JR: Neuropathology of schizophrenia. Arch Gen Psychiatry 39:1131–1139, 1982

Stevens JR: Clinicopathological correlations in schizophrenia. Arch Gen Psychiatry 43:715–716, 1986

Stevens JR: Abnormal reinnervation as a basis for schizophrenia: a hypothesis. Arch Gen Psychiatry 49:238–243, 1992

Treff WM, Hempel KJ: Die Zelldichte bei Schizophrenen und klinisch Gesunden. J Hirnforsch 4:314–369, 1958

van Hoesen GW: The parahippocampal gyrus: new observations regarding its cortical connections in the monkey. Trends Neurosci 5:345–350, 1982

Vogt C, Vogt O: Résultats de l'étude anatomique de la schizophrénie et d'autres psychoses dites fonctionelles faites à l'Institut du cerveau de Neustadt, Schwarzwald, in Proceedings of the First International Congress of Neuropathology, Vol 1. Turin, Italy, Rosenberg & Sellier, 1952, pp 515–532

Wada JA, Davies AE: Fundamental nature of human infant's brain asymmetry. Can J Neurol Sci 4:203–207, 1977

Weinberger DR: Implications of normal brain development for the pathogenesis of schizophrenia. Arch Gen Psychiatry 44:660–669, 1987

CHAPTER 3

The New Genetics of Schizophrenia

Michel Maziade, M.D., F.R.C.P.C., and
Vincent Raymond, M.D., Ph.D.

Although numerous questions remain regarding the genetic contribution in schizophrenia, recent findings indicate that genetic factors are involved in the etiology of schizophrenia, and that the syndrome is best understood as comprising several etiologically distinct subgroups (Gottesman 1991; Torrey 1992). These subgroups range from one in which genetics exclusively contribute to the etiology of the disease, to one in which there is no genetic contribution to the disease, to a probable subgroup in which an interaction of genetic and environmental factors contributes to the illness.

Major areas that require further study include the nature of the genetic components in schizophrenia, the distinction between the genetic form of the disease and its nongenetic counterparts, and the development of innovative methods to deal with the complexity of these genetic influences. Although the genetic component is frequently argued to be the single most clearly evident causative factor for schizophrenia, some investigators have expressed the view that the genetic contribution to the illness may be overestimated (Torrey 1992). The validity of either view can be proven primarily in future well-designed and systematic epidemiological studies that use novel molecular genetic techniques. The controversy surrounding the importance of genetic factors in schizophrenia has generated new strategies to uncover susceptibility genes.

Rather than give a comprehensive review of the genetics of schizophrenia, in this chapter we offer a selective overview of recent progress and understanding in this area.

Evidence of a Genetic Component for Schizophrenia

Although the mode of inheritance for schizophrenia is still unknown (McGue and Gottesman 1989), based on their recent review of 26 family studies, Kendler (1988a) and then Kendler and Diehl (1993) found that first-degree relatives are at greater risk for schizophrenia than individuals in the general population. The relatives of schizophrenic patients are 5 to 15 times more likely to develop the illness (Baron et al. 1985; Frangos et al. 1985; Kendler 1988b; Kendler et al. 1985; Tsuang et al. 1980). In addition, there appears to be a certain specificity as to which illness is being transmitted among relatives. Indeed, the risk of developing schizophrenia is greater for relatives of schizophrenic probands than it is for relatives of probands with a bipolar disorder. Moreover, studies of very large multi-generational families that are densely affected with schizophrenia in geographically or demographically isolated populations (e.g., Egeland and Hostetter 1983; Kennedy et al. 1988) and in various Western industrial nations (Sherrington et al. 1988) have presented congruent evidence that schizophrenia runs in families under the influence of a genetic predisposition. An example of such densely affected multi-generational families, which are currently being investigated by our group (Maziade et al., in press) in Eastern Quebec and Northern New Brunswick, is provided in Figure 3–1.

In addition to family and adoption studies, a review of twin studies also demonstrates that genetic factors play an important role in the etiology of schizophrenia. Twin studies reveal that the concordance

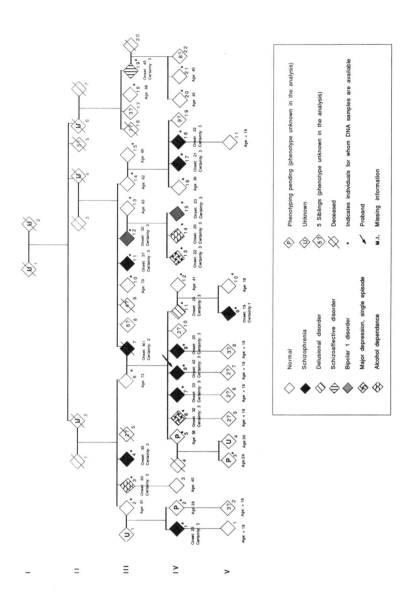

Figure 3–1. F 255 schizophrenia pedigree. To preserve confidentiality and anonymity for the family members, sex was disguised, birth order was changed, and five unaffected members were added. Level of diagnostic certainty: 3 = definitive; 2 = probable; 1 = possible.

rate for schizophrenia is higher in monozygotic (average 48%) than in dizygotic (average 17%) twins (see reviews by Fischer 1973; Gottesman and Shields 1972; Kendler 1988a, 1988b; Kendler and Robinette 1983; Tienari 1975). The study of discordant identical twins who were reared apart, and of a set of quadruplets concordant for variations of schizophrenia, also supports a genetic predisposition (Gottesman 1991). The study of a small but unique cohort of Danish schizophrenic twins and their offspring, conducted by Gottesman and Bertelsen (1989), provided compelling evidence for a genetic component in schizophrenia. These authors observed that the offspring of the phenotypically normal monozygotic co-twins of schizophrenic patients had the same risk of developing schizophrenia as children of schizophrenic patients (17%) (see Table 3–1). This finding indicates that the genotype for schizophrenia can remain dormant and be transmitted and expressed in future generations.

Several genetic models have been proposed for schizophrenia. The single-major-locus model with nonfamilial environmental factors is likely for only a minor proportion of etiologic subgroups of schizophrenia (Gottesman 1991). There is general agreement (Rutter 1986; Weeks et al. 1990; Weiner 1985) that the most likely causative model for a major proportion of schizophrenia subgroups resides in a multifactorial threshold model (Gottesman and Shields 1967; Reich et al. 1975). In this model, one or more genes may confer a predisposition to the disease, with this genetic susceptibility being influenced by either physical or sociofamilial factors. Some authors consider these gene-environment interactions as influential (Lander 1988), whereas others regard them as playing a minor role (Kendler 1988a). Such environmental factors (e.g., stressful life events) could either facilitate the expression of the illness or exert a protective influence.

With regard to recent linkage studies, a genetic defect on chromosome 5 was first suggested by the co-occurrence of schizophrenia and dysmorphic features in a patient and his maternal uncle, who both had unbalanced translocations of chromosome 5 region q11–q13 to chromosome 1, creating a trisomy for region 5q11–q13 (Bassett et al. 1988). Although the mother carried a balanced translocation of chromosome 5 to chromosome 1, she was phenotypically normal. These observations led to several investigations that found evidence of link-

Table 3–1.   Schizophrenia and schizophrenia-like psychosis in offspring of schizophrenic twins

		Offspring	
		Schizophrenia and	
		schizophrenia-like	Morbid
Index parents	Number	psychosis	risk (%)
Monozygotic sample			
Schizophrenic twins (*n* = 11)	47	6	16.8
"Normal" co-twins (*n* = 6)	24	4	17.4
Dizygotic sample			
Schizophrenic twins (*n* = 10)	27	4	17.4
"Normal" co-twins (*n* = 20)	52	1	2.1

Source. Gottesman and Bertelsen (1989).

age between genetic markers on chromosome 5 and schizophrenia in different populations. Sherrington et al. (1988) first reported linkage in five Icelandic and two English schizophrenia families, with markers on 5q11–q13. When the diagnosis was restricted to schizophrenia, the lod score[1] reached 3.22. However, when diagnoses were extended to include the whole schizophrenia spectrum as well as other psychiatric disorders, the revised lod score was 6.49. These results were then believed to provide evidence for linkage between schizophrenia and this chromosomal region.

It is unfortunate that subsequent attempts have failed to confirm a linkage to 5q markers. Using a large Northern Swedish kindred affected with schizophrenia, Kennedy et al. (1988) were able to exclude the 5q11–q13 region. Several other groups (St. Clair et al. [1989] with Scottish pedigrees; McGuffin et al. [1990] with British families; and Aschauer et al. [1990], Crowe et al. [1991], and Detera-Wadleigh et al. [1989] with several American families) did not find evidence of linkage between schizophrenia and markers on chromosome 5q. This

---

[1]The lod score is the base 10 logarithm of the odds favoring linkage. Most researchers tend to consider a lod score of 3 or more as indicating a significant linkage with the disease.

failure to replicate promising preliminary findings has generated a beneficial reappraisal of the methodology used in psychiatric genetics.

There are several potential sources for the inconsistencies among linkage reports: 1) sample heterogeneity and complex mode of inheritance (with the concomitant possibility of falsely negative reports), 2) random procedural errors, and 3) nonrandom or systematic procedural errors. In order to replicate reported linkages and to search the human genome for disease loci, several researchers have proposed to undertake a fresh start using current technology on well-chosen samples of affected pedigrees (Gershon 1990; Gershon et al. 1990; Suarez et al. 1990).

The Degree of Etiologic Independence Between Schizophrenia and Bipolar Disorder

This question is important to the genetics of both schizophrenia and bipolar disorder, especially because of the inclusion, in prior linkage studies, of individuals with a schizoaffective diagnosis at the first diagnostic hierarchical level. The reliability of schizoaffective diagnoses was lower in the Amish study (Hostetter et al. 1983) and in the study by Maziade et al. (1992). As previously mentioned, there is a greater familial aggregation of affective disorders (as well as the spectrum of affective disorders) in the families of affective probands (Egeland and Hostetter 1983; Goldin and Gershon 1988; Rice et al. 1987; Weissman et al. 1984) and a similar greater familial aggregation of schizophrenia in the families of schizophrenic probands (Kendler 1988a), suggesting a separate etiology for each disorder. However, relatives of affective probands are, to a certain extent, more at risk of developing schizophrenia (Kendler et al. 1986) than population figures would predict. The rate of affective disorders in relatives of schizophrenic probands is also slightly increased (Baron et al. 1985; Frangos et al. 1985; Kendler et al. 1985, 1993).

At best, the transmission of genetic susceptibility to schizophrenia or bipolar disorder is a complex phenomenon that requires careful scrutiny as to the validity and stability of psychiatric diagnoses over many years (Lander 1988). The possibility that some etiologic (and genetic) overlap exists for a proportion of bipolar disorder and schizophrenic patients cannot be ruled out at present. The unreliability of schizoaffective diagnoses observed in genetic linkage studies (Maziade et al. 1992) and the controversy surrounding the existence of schizoaffective disorder as a distinct etiologic syndrome suggest that schizoaffective patients should be excluded from the first hierarchical diagnostic level in genetic linkage analyses of affected pedigrees.

Improving Methods for Identifying Schizophrenia Genes

A critical review of epidemiological and genetic studies of schizophrenia offers two main conclusions. First, as discussed above, a genetic component in schizophrenia is unequivocal despite ongoing debate (Gottesman 1991; Torrey 1992). Second, there is a general consensus (Baron et al. 1990a; Maziade et al. 1992; Owen 1992; Weeks et al. 1990) that the failure thus far to find or replicate consistent linkages is attributable to major methodological issues that have not received adequate attention. To correct this situation, future studies should include

- More stringent reliability criteria and characterization of schizophrenia phenotypes, given the sensitivity of linkage analysis to diagnostic misclassification (Baron et al. 1990a, 1990b; Egeland et al. 1990; Martinez et al. 1989; Maziade et al. 1992)
- Detailed clinical and epidemiological longitudinal data in addition to using official classification systems (e.g., DSM-III-R and DSM-IV [American Psychiatric Association 1987, 1994], Research Diagnostic Criteria [Spitzer et al. 1975], International Classification of Diseases, 10th Edition [World Health Organization 1992]) as well as continuous measures at the symptom level (Pauls 1993)
- Novel statistical methods that take into account inherent phenotypic variance and etiologic heterogeneity
- The development of strategies for detecting phenocopies
- Analyses at the symptom level in addition to the syndromal level (Baron et al. 1990a; Costello 1992)

- Avoidance of undetected bilineal transmission (Owen 1992) or recognition of bilineality (Gottesman 1991; Simpson et al. 1992)
- Blindness of investigators at the genotyping and phenotyping levels

A review of 38 linkage studies (Maziade et al. 1992) indicated that only a minority reported reliability for the diagnostic assessment procedure. From this review, Maziade et al. derived 13 methodological elements on which they based a comprehensive, consensus, best-estimate diagnostic procedure. Using this procedure, the assessment of 59 members of the pedigree sample showed that blindness to probands' and relatives' diagnostic condition has a statistically significant effect on reliability. Maziade et al.'s results indicated that investing in such a strict diagnostic procedure, with repeated reliability checks at different levels, and providing raw clinical information to a blind panel of research psychiatrists are warranted in order to ensure a satisfactory reliability in genetic studies.

Although strong evidence supports the recognition of schizophrenia and bipolar disorder as two distinct illnesses, a genetic overlap or a common etiologic zone for these two disorders is also possible. The latter possibility may have negatively influenced prior linkage studies, given that many of them included patients with schizoaffective disorder.

Using large extended pedigrees and using a greater number of smaller multiplex families are strategies that each present specific advantages and should be used together. The former is more powerful for detecting linkage (Baron et al. 1990a; Suarez et al. 1990). A disadvantage to using large extended pedigrees is that they are less generalizable.

A crucial issue resides in designing studies that aim to distinguish genetic types on clinical grounds (e.g., phenomenology, illness course, age at onset, treatment response), biological grounds (e.g., biochemical factors, neurophysiological factors), or both. By comparing one familial form of the disorder with other familial or nonfamilial forms on specific clinical parameters (DeLisi 1992), etiologic heterogeneity could be clarified (Baron et al. 1990a). Much work needs to be done in that respect. A recent review (Roy and Crowe 1994) of more than 50 studies on the distinction between sporadic (nonfamilial) and familial schizophrenia was inconclusive, mainly because of the invalidity of the sporadic-familial categorization, a problem attributable to methodological difficulties.

Future studies should use strategic combinations of association analyses[2] and linkage analysis (Owen and Mullan 1990; Pauls 1993). Recent work has, for example, successfully employed, sequentially, association and linkage analyses to demonstrate tight linkage to the apolipoprotein AI-CIII-AIV gene cluster on chromosome 11q23–q24 in a subset of families with familial combined hyperlipidemia (Wojciechowski et al. 1991).

Rather than concentrating genetic research efforts on schizophrenia or bipolar disorder exclusively, there is a definite advantage to studying pedigrees with either illness, as such an approach allows for the possibility of a best-estimate diagnostic procedure to be performed blind to the probands' and relatives' diagnoses.

The search for the co-occurrence of cytogenetic anomalies and schizophrenia transmitted within the same family can help identify vulnerability genes (Bassett 1992), particularly when the search is integrated in a regional systematic screening of densely affected pedigrees. The leads arising from cytogenetic anomalies are invaluable but require careful scrutiny if there are a small number of clearly affected subjects within the pedigree, or if there is a lack of specificity of the disorders associated with the karyotypic anomaly (Maziade et al. 1993). An example of this was reported by St. Clair and colleagues (1990), who found an association, within a family, of a balanced autosomal translocation t(1,11) with several mental disorders.

To summarize, the usual methods for identifying the genes for susceptibility to schizophrenia and bipolar disorder require reappraisal in the following four areas:

1. More attention needs to be given to phenotype definition and reliability.
2. Multiple and varied sampling strategies should be used in conjunction with appropriate epidemiological methods.

---

[2]Association analyses aim to test for an overrepresentation of a specific genetic marker in a group of schizophrenic patients compared with a nonpsychiatric control group.

3. There is a need to integrate reliable continuous measures at the symptom level and at the syndromal level.
4. In addition to using valid and reliable categorical and continuous measures of clinical phenotypes, there is a need to integrate measurements of environmental factors believed to be involved in the causative mechanisms of schizophrenia.

Novel Approaches to Finding Susceptibility Genes to Schizophrenia

In combination with appropriate epidemiological and statistical analytical procedures, the discovery of polymorphic DNA markers makes it now possible to initiate a systematic search, using linkage analysis, for mutations causing schizophrenia. Although schizophrenia does not show Mendelian inheritance, pioneering work on other complex non-Mendelian disorders (e.g., type I [insulin-dependent] diabetes in the mouse [Todd et al. 1991]; type II [non–insulin-dependent] diabetes of the young in humans); hypertension in the rat [Jacob et al. 1991]) has demonstrated the feasibility of successfully applying gene mapping techniques to complex non-Mendelian pathologies.

In fact, genetic mapping provides a powerful strategy for the study of inherited diseases in humans, as genes can be localized by linkage analysis and then cloned based on their chromosomal position. The well-proven restriction fragment length polymorphism linkage analysis technique, first described by Botstein et al. (1980), has helped to localize the chromosomal regions of genes for several hereditary diseases with no previously known biochemical or etiologic information. This technology first provided an invaluable tool for localizing chromosomal loci for simple Mendelian diseases such as Huntington's disease (Gusella et al. 1983), cystic fibrosis (Tsui et al. 1985; White et al. 1985), von Recklinghausen's disease (Barker et al. 1987; Seizneinger et al. 1987), and fragile X syndrome. The assignment of these loci were major breakthroughs, leading to the genes associated with each specific disease.

To find evidence of linkage between genetic markers and susceptibility genes to schizophrenia, two strategies can be exploited: 1) the candidate gene–region approach, and 2) the systematic screening of the entire human genome to search for linked markers. The first strategy was exemplified in the studies of 30 international families for linkage of 5q (Aschauer et al. 1990; Crowe et al. 1991; Detera-Wadleigh et al. 1989; Kennedy et al. 1988; McGuffin et al. 1990; Sherrington et al. 1988; St. Clair et al. 1989). Other families have also been tested for linkage with several candidate genes.

The dopamine hypothesis of schizophrenia (Seeman 1987; see also Chapter 1) and the increased dopamine D_2 receptor densities in untreated schizophrenic patients (Seeman et al. 1984) support the dopamine D_2 receptor gene as a good candidate gene for the illness. Following this line of discovery, Moises et al. (1991) assessed linkage between markers located in the D_2 dopamine receptor locus (DRD_2) and schizophrenia. Using multipoint linkage analysis, they found no linkage between the DRD_2 region and schizophrenia (Moises et al. 1991). A total of five genes for dopamine receptors have now been cloned. Using these five loci as candidate genes, Coon et al. (1993) tested nine multigenerational families for linkage. Results were consistently negative, indicating that a defect at any of the actual receptor sites was unlikely to be a major contribution to schizophrenia in the nine families studied (Coon et al. 1993). Although mutations at the dopamine receptor loci may not be involved in the genesis of schizophrenia, other neurotransmitter systems may influence dopaminergic transmission. The serotoninergic, gamma-aminobutyric acid (GABA)-ergic, and acetylcholinergic systems thus become candidate loci to be tested.

Two recent major advances in molecular biology have made possible the rapid development of highly informative markers for genetic mapping and linkage analysis of complex diseases. With the use of these new markers, the systematic screening of the entire human genome now becomes feasible in a time frame of several months to 1–2 years.

First, in 1985 it was discovered that short segments of DNA could be amplified in vitro from a template using DNA polymerase and temperature cycling, by polymerase chain reaction (PCR) (Mullis 1990). PCR has revolutionized the molecular analysis of genetic disorders because it allows for the detection and analysis of specific gene sequences without requiring the application of cloning or blotting procedures.

Second, in 1989 several laboratories used PCR to demonstrate a high level of polymorphism or allelic variation in small regions of repetitive DNA known as *microsatellites* (Litt and Luty 1989; Weber and May 1989). Microsatellites consist of 10–50 copies of motifs from 1–6 base pairs that can occur in perfect tandem repetition. Microsatellites have been shown to be abundant in the human genome and are very informative, with multiple alleles per locus. With such markers, the parents are most often heterozygous at the locus; furthermore, the segregation of the alleles can be observed unambiguously in the progeny (Hyer et al. 1991). The availability of a more detailed human genome map at a 4- to 6-centimorgan (cM) resolution (meaning that one marker is available every 5 million nucleotides on average) can now be exploited (Weissenbach et al. 1992). The search for a genetic marker in multiplex pedigrees affected by schizophrenia will help to distinguish different subgroups etiologically, clarify nosology, and eventually discover interactions with environmental factors.

Effects of Schizophrenia and Antipsychotic Drugs on Gene Expression

It is now well recognized that a variety of neurochemical systems can induce the expression not only of genes involved in neuronal plasticity but also of a series of genes encoding longer-lasting neuropeptides like somatostatin, corticotropin-releasing hormone, thyrotropin-releasing hormone, and enkephalin. Among these genes, c-fos proto-oncogene is probably one of the best understood and can thus be used as a paradigm. The term *fos* was first used to describe the oncogene encoded by the Finkel-Biskis-Jenkins murine osteosarcoma virus. The normal cellular sequences from which the viral oncogene was derived are referred to as the *fos proto-oncogene* or *c-fos,* and its expression is highly regulated at many cellular levels.

Another gene known to be altered during neurotransmission is the *jun proto-oncogene.* It is believed that c-fos and c-jun may be involved in processes mediating long-term alterations important for behavior. In fact, Graybiel et al. (1990) showed that amphetamine and cocaine induce drug-specific activation of the c-fos gene in striosome-matrix compartments and limbic subdivisions of the striatum. These authors proposed that the differential activation of c-fos by psychostimulants may be an early step in a drug-specific molecular cascade contributing to acute and long-lasting psychostimulant-induced behavioral changes.

In order to decipher the mechanisms by which antipsychotic drug actions are translated into therapeutic effects, several groups have oriented their research to receptor-mediated regulation of gene expression. Some have investigated the specificity of c-fos induction as well as that of another gene named Zif268 after acute administration of several antipsychotic drugs in the rat (Nguyen et al. 1992). Nguyen and colleagues demonstrated that antipsychotic drugs with potent dopaminergic D_2 receptor antagonist properties, such as haloperidol, induced both c-fos and Zif268 mRNA in the caudate putamen; however, the atypical antipsychotic drug clozapine induced Zif268 but not c-fos in that region. In contrast, both drugs induced c-fos protein in the nucleus accumbens (Nguyen et al. 1992). Furthermore, Robertson and Fibiger (1992) reported patterns of clozapine- and haloperidol-induced c-fos immunoreactivity in the caudate putamen and nucleus accumbens that were similar to those described above. Because c-fos is induced by both dopamine agonists and dopamine antagonists, a major challenge is to understand how specificity is achieved. Further research on neural gene expression will likely provide important insights into the therapeutic mechanisms of action of these drugs.

Conclusion

Indisputably, the combination of new epidemiological methods with innovative molecular biology techniques generates hope for major discoveries in the genetics of major psychoses, with potential medical and socioeconomic repercussions for diagnostic tests and curative treatments.

References

American Psychiatric Association: Diagnostic and Statistical Manual of Mental Disorders, 3rd Edition, Revised. Washington, DC, American Psychiatric Association, 1987

Aschauer HN, Aschauer-Treiber G, Isenberg KE, et al: No evidence for linkage between chromosome 5 markers and schizophrenia. Hum Hered 40:109–115, 1990

Barker D, Wright E, Nguyen K, et al: Gene for von Recklinghausen neurofibromatosis is in the pericentrometric region of chromosome 17. Science 236:1100–1102, 1987

Baron M, Gruen R, Rainer JD, et al: A family study of schizophrenic and normal control probands: implications for the spectrum concept of schizophrenia. Am J Psychiatry 142:447–454, 1985

Baron M, Endicott J, Ott J: Genetic linkage in mental illness: limitations and prospects. Br J Psychiatry 157:645–655, 1990a

Baron M, Hamburger R, Sandkuyl LA, et al: The impact of phenotypic variation on genetic analysis: application to X-linkage in manic-depressive illness. Acta Psychiatr Scand 82:196–203, 1990b

Bassett AS: Chromosomal aberrations and schizophrenia: autosomes. Br J Psychiatry 161:123–134, 1992

Bassett AS, McGillivray BC, Jones BD, et al: Partial trisomy chromosome 5 cosegregating with schizophrenia. Lancet 1:799–801, 1988

Botstein D, White RL, Skolnick M, et al: Construction of a genetic linkage map in man using restriction fragment length polymorphisms. Am J Hum Genet 32:314–331, 1980

Coon H, Byerley W, Holik J, et al: Linkage analysis of schizophrenia with five dopamine receptor genes in nine pedigrees. Am J Hum Genet 52:327–334, 1993

Costello CG: Research on symptoms versus research on syndromes: arguments in favour of allocating more research time to the study of symptoms. Br J Psychiatry 160:304–308, 1992

Crowe RR, Black DW, Wesner R, et al: Lack of linkage to chromosome 5q11–q13 markers in six schizophrenia pedigrees. Arch Gen Psychiatry 48:357–361, 1991

DeLisi LE: The significance of age of onset for schizophrenia. Schizophr Bull 18:209–215, 1992

Detera-Wadleigh SD, Goldin LR, Sherrington R, et al: Exclusion of linkage to 5q11–q13 in families with schizophrenia and other psychiatric disorders. Nature 340:391–393, 1989

Egeland JA, Hostetter AM: Amish study, I: affective disorders among the Amish, 1976–1980. Am J Psychiatry 140:56–61, 1983

Egeland JA, Sussex JN, Endicott J, et al: The impact of diagnoses on genetic linkage study for bipolar affective disorders among the Amish. Psychiatric Genetics 1:5–18, 1990

Fischer M: Genetic and environmental factors in schizophrenia. Acta Psychiatr Scand Suppl 38:238, 1973

Frangos E, Athanassenas G, Tsitourides S, et al: Prevalence of DSM-III schizophrenia among the first-degree relatives of schizophrenic probands. Acta Psychiatr Scand 72:382–386, 1985

Gershon ES: Genetic linkage and complex diseases: a comment. Genet Epidemiol 7:21–23, 1990

Gershon ES, Martinez M, Goldin LR, et al: Genetic mapping of common diseases: the challenges of manic-depressive illness and schizophrenia. Trends Genet 6:282–287, 1990

Goldin LR, Gershon ES: The genetic epidemiology of major depressive illness, in American Psychiatric Press Review of Psychiatry, Vol 7. Edited by Frances AJ, Hales RE. Washington, DC, American Psychiatric Press, 1988, pp 149–168

Gottesman II: Schizophrenia Genesis: The Origins of Madness. New York, WH Freeman, 1991

Gottesman II, Bertelsen A: Confirming unexpressed genotypes for schizophrenia: risks in the offspring of Fischer's Danish identical and fraternal discordant twins. Arch Gen Psychiatry 46:867–872, 1989

Gottesman II, Shields J: A polygenic theory of schizophrenia. Proc Natl Acad Sci U S A 58:199–205, 1967

Gottesman II, Shields J: Schizophrenia and Genetics: A Twin Study Vantage Point. New York, Academic Press, 1972

Graybiel AM, Moratalla R, Robertson HA: Amphetamine and cocaine induce drug-specific activation of the c-fos gene in striosome-matrix compartments and limbic subdivisions of the striatum. Proc Natl Acad Sci U S A 87:6912–6916, 1990

Gusella JF, Wexler NS, Conneally PM, et al: A polymorphic DNA marker genetically linked to Huntington's disease. Nature 306:234–238, 1983

Hostetter AM, Egeland JA, Endicott J: Amish study, II: consensus diagnoses and reliability results. Am J Psychiatry 140:62–66, 1983

Hyer RN, Julier C, Buckley JD, et al: High-resolution linkage mapping for susceptibility genes in human polygenic disease: insulin-dependent diabetes mellitus and chromosome 11q. Am J Hum Genet 48:243–257, 1991

Jacob HJ, Lindpaintner K, Lincoln SE: Genetic mapping of a gene causing hypertension in the stroke-prone spontaneously hypertensive rat. Cell 67:213–224, 1991

Kendler KS: The genetics of schizophrenia and related disorders: a review, in Relatives at Risk for Mental Disorder. Edited by Dunner DL, Gershon ES, Barrett JE. New York, Raven, 1988a, pp 247–266

Kendler KS: The genetics of schizophrenia: an overview, in Handbook of Schizophrenia, Vol 3: Nosology, Epidemiology and Genetics of Schizophrenia. Edited by Tsuang MMT, Simpson JC. Amsterdam, Netherlands, Elsevier, 1988b, pp 437–462

Kendler KS, Diehl SR: The genetics of schizophrenia: a current genetic-epidemiologic perspective. Schizophr Bull 19:261–285, 1993

Kendler KS, Robinette CD: Schizophrenia in the National Academy of Sciences National Research Council twin registry: a 16-year update. Am J Psychiatry 140:1551–1563, 1983

Kendler KS, Gruenberg AM, Tsuang MT: Psychiatric illness in first-degree relatives of schizophrenic and surgical control patients. Arch Gen Psychiatry 42:770–779, 1985

Kendler KS, Gruenberg AM, Tsuang MT: DSM-III family study of the nonschizophrenic psychotic disorders. Am J Psychiatry 143:1098–1105, 1986

Kendler KS, McGuire M, Gruenberg AM, et al: The Roscommon family study, I: methods, diagnosis of probands, and risk of schizophrenia in relatives. Arch Gen Psychiatry 50:527–540, 1993

Kennedy JL, Giuffra LA, Moises HW, et al: Evidence against linkage of schizophrenia to markers on chromosome 5 in a northern Swedish pedigree. Nature 336:167–170, 1988

Lander ES: Splitting schizophrenia. Nature 336:105–106, 1988

Litt M, Luty JA: A hypervariable microsatellite revealed by in vitro amplification of a dinucleotide repeat within the cardiac muscle actin gene. Am J Hum Genet 44:397–401, 1989

Martinez M, Khlat M, Leboyer M, et al: Performance of linkage analysis under misclassification error when the genetic model is unknown. Genet Epidemiol 6:253–258, 1989

Maziade M, Roy MA, Fournier JP, et al: Reliability of best-estimate diagnosis in genetic linkage studies of major psychoses: results from the Quebec pedigree studies. Am J Psychiatry 149:1674–1686, 1992

Maziade M, De Braekeleer M, Genest P, et al: A balanced 2:18 translocation and familial schizophrenia: falling short of an association. Arch Gen Psychiatry 50:73–75, 1993

Maziade M, Raymond V, Cliche D, et al: Linkage results on 11q21–q22 in Eastern Quebec pedigrees densely affected by schizophrenia. Am J Med Genet (in press)

McGue M, Gottesman II: A single dominant gene still cannot account for the transmission of schizophrenia. Arch Gen Psychiatry 46:478–479, 1989

McGuffin P, Sargeant M, Hetti G: Exclusion of a schizophrenia susceptibility gene from the chromosome 5q11–q13 region: new data and a reanalysis of previous reports. Am J Hum Genet 47:524–535, 1990

Moises HW, Gelernter J, Giuffra LA: No linkage between D₂ dopamine receptor gene region and schizophrenia. Arch Gen Psychiatry 48:643–647, 1991

Mullis KB: The unusual origin of the polymerase chain reaction. Sci Am 262:36–43, 1990

Nguyen TV, Kosofsky BE, Birnbaum R, et al: Differential expression of c-fos and Zif268 in rat striatum after haloperidol, clozapine, and amphetamine. Proc Natl Acad Sci U S A 89:4270–4274, 1992

Owen MJ: Will schizophrenia become a graveyard for molecular geneticists? Psychol Med 22:289–293, 1992

Owen MJ, Mullan MJ: Molecular genetic studies of manic-depression and schizophrenia. Trends Neurosci 13:29–31, 1990

Pauls DL: Behavioral disorders: lessons in linkage. Nature Genetics 3:4–5, 1993

Pulver AE, Bale SJ: Availability of schizophrenic patients and their families for genetic linkage studies: findings from the Maryland epidemiology sample. Genet Epidemiol 6:671–680, 1989

Reich T, Cloninger CR, Guze SB: The multifactorial model of disease transmission, I: description of the model and its use in psychiatry. Br J Psychiatry 127:1–10, 1975

Rice J, Reich T, Andreasen NC, et al: The familial transmission of bipolar illness. Arch Gen Psychiatry 44:441–447, 1987

Robertson GR, Fibiger HC: Neuroleptics increase c-fos expression in the forebrain: contrasting effects of haloperidol and clozapine. Neuroscience 46:315–328, 1992

Roy MA, Crowe RR: Validity of the familial and sporadic subtypes of schizophrenia. Am J Psychiatry 151:805–814, 1994

Rutter M: Child psychiatry: the interface between clinical and developmental research. Psychol Med 16:151–169, 1986

Seeman P: Dopamine receptors and the dopamine hypothesis of schizophrenia. Synapse 1:133–152, 1987

Seeman P, Ulpian C, Bergeron C, et al: Bimodal distribution of dopamine receptor densities in brains of schizophrenics. Science 225:728–730, 1984

Seizneinger BR, Rouleau GA, Ozelius LJ, et al: Genetic linkage of von Recklinghausen neurofibromatosis to the nerve growth factor receptor gene. Cell 49:589–594, 1987

Sherrington R, Brynjolfsson J, Petursson H, et al: Localization of a susceptibility locus for schizophrenia on chromosome 5. Nature 336:164–167, 1988

Simpson SG, Folstein SE, Meyers DA, et al: Assessment of lineality in bipolar I linkage studies. Am J Psychiatry 149:1660–1665, 1992

Spitzer RL, Endicott J, Robins E: Research Diagnostic Criteria (RDC) for a Selected Group of Functional Disorders. New York, Biometrics Research, New York State Psychiatric Institute, 1975

St. Clair D, Blackwood D, Muir W: No linkage of chromosome 5q11–q13 markers to schizophrenia in Scottish families. Nature 339:305–309, 1989

St. Clair D, Blackwood D, Muir W, et al: Association within a family of a balanced autosomal translocation with major mental illness. Lancet 336:13–16, 1990

Suarez BK, Reich T, Rice JP, et al: Genetic linkage and complex diseases: a comment. Genet Epidemiol 7:37–40, 1990

Tienari P: Schizophrenia in Finnish male twins, in Studies of Schizophrenia. Edited by Lader MH. Ashford, Kent, UK, Headley Brothers, 1975, pp 29–35

Todd JA, Aitman TJ, Cornall RJ, et al: Genetic analysis of autoimmune type I diabetes mellitus in mice. Nature 351:542–547, 1991

Torrey EF: Are we overestimating the genetic contribution to schizophrenia? Schizophr Bull 18:159–170, 1992

Tsuang MT, Winokur G, Crowe RR: Morbidity risks of schizophrenia and affective disorders among first degree relatives of patients with schizophrenia, mania, depression and surgical conditions. Br J Psychiatry 137:497–504, 1980

Tsui L, Buchwald M, Barker D: Cystic fibrosis locus defined by a genetically linked polymorphic DNA marker. Science 230:1054–1057, 1985

Weber J, May P: Abundant class of human DNA polymorphisms which can be typed using the polymerase chain reaction. Am J Hum Genet 44:388–396, 1989

Weeks DE, Brzustowicz L, Squires-Wheeler E, et al: Report of a workshop on genetic linkage studies in schizophrenia. Schizophr Bull 16:673–685, 1990

Weiner H: Schizophrenia: etiology, in Comprehensive Textbook of Psychiatry, 4th Edition. Edited by Kaplan HI, Sadock BJ. Baltimore, MD, Williams & Wilkins, 1985

Weissenbach J, Gyapay G, Dib C, et al: A second-generation linkage map of the human genome. Nature 359:795–801, 1992

Weissman MM, Gershon ES, Kidd KK, et al: Psychiatric disorders in the relatives of probands with affective disorders. Arch Gen Psychiatry 41:13–21, 1984

White RL, Woodward S, Leppert M, et al: A closely linked genetic marker for cystic fibrosis. Nature 318:382–384, 1985

Wojciechowski AP, Farrall M, Cullen P, et al: Familial combined hyperlipidemia linked to the apolipoprotein AI-CIII-AIV gene cluster on chromosome 11q23–q24. Nature 349:161–164, 1991
World Health Organization: International Classification of Diseases, 10th
Edition. Geneva, Switzerland, World Health Organization, 1992

SECTION II

Clinical and Diagnostic Issues in Schizophrenia

CHAPTER 4

The Diagnosis of Schizophrenia

Michael Flaum, M.D.

In approaching the topic of the diagnosis and classification of schizophrenia, it is helpful to begin with a recognition of three inexorable facts (N. C. Andreasen, personal communication, December 1988): First, schizophrenia is probably not a single disorder. Second, whatever it is, we don't know what it is. Third, diagnostic criteria are therefore arbitrary and are likely to change over time as we begin to understand more about the disorder's mechanisms.

In medicine, physicians recognize specific symptoms (i.e., nonspecific markers of disease [e.g., a cough]), syndromes (i.e., groups of symptoms that tend to co-occur [e.g., a cough, a fever, and chills]), and diseases (i.e., syndromes in which the pathophysiological mechanisms are understood, such as pneumococcal pneumonia). In psychiatry, it is critical to remember that most of the psychiatric diagnostic categories are still at the syndromal level rather than the disease level. Ultimately, it is hoped that psychiatric diagnostic nosology will pro-

This research was supported in part by National Institute of Mental Health Grants MHCRC43271 and MH47200.

ceed from a syndromal to a disease level through the process of validating existing categories. Until that time, the field is left with "tentative agreements to agree" as to where the boundaries between categories of mental disorders can be drawn.

My goal in this chapter is to provide an overview of the current nosology of schizophrenia. I begin by tracing the roots of the nosology for schizophrenia; I then discuss the advantages and disadvantages of existing operationalized diagnostic criteria systems in diagnosing schizophrenia, and finally conclude with a discussion of the DSM-IV (American Psychiatric Association 1994) criteria for schizophrenia, focusing on how and why they differ from previous classifications.

Historical Background of Nosology of Schizophrenia

Influential Figures in Defining Schizophrenia

The contemporary construct of schizophrenia derived from a blend of multiple influences. Numerous individuals have contributed to this blend, but perhaps none were as influential as Kraepelin, Bleuler, and Schneider.

Emil Kraepelin (1856–1926) approached the definition and classification of psychiatric disorders from a neurobiological perspective similar to that used by many contemporary neuropsychiatrists. He followed a large cohort of severely mentally ill patients over a period of several decades and maintained extensive notes regarding their symptoms and course of illness. Kraepelin's ultimate goal was to relate the observed clinical phenomena to their underlying neurobiological mechanisms and thereby identify valid disease entities. He assembled a widely respected group of neuroscientists, including Alzheimer, Broadman, and Nissel, who employed newly developed techniques (e.g., various staining procedures) to study the brain. Although his group did not realize its goals, through his study of phenomenology, Kraepelin was able to provide a nosological framework for psychotic disorders that has stood the test of time. Perhaps his greatest contribution to psychiatric nosology was his emphasis on the importance of the longitudinal course rather than the cross-sectional symptomatology in classification (Kraepelin et al. 1919). He recognized that although patients may present with a wide variety of features in the context of psychosis (e.g., catatonia, hebephrenia, paranoia—all of which had been previously described as separate syndromes), some of them followed a markedly episodic course with good interepisodic functioning, whereas others followed a primarily chronic and deteriorating course. Noting that patients whose courses were more episodic tended to have more prominent mood symptoms during their periods of acute exacerbation, he dichotomized psychotic patients into those with "manic-depressive insanity" versus those with "dementia praecox" (later renamed *schizophrenia* by Bleuler). This dichotomy between schizophrenia and mood-related psychotic disorders has been maintained in almost every nosological system that has evolved subsequently.

Eugen Bleuler (1857–1939) approached the study of psychotic disorders from a more psychological model. Unlike Kraepelin, who emphasized the importance of longitudinal course, Bleuler described a set of symptoms that he believed to be characteristic or "fundamental" to the disorder he renamed schizophrenia—symptoms that could be observed in one form or another at any point during the course of the illness (Bleuler 1911/1950). These symptoms, commonly referred to as *the four A's,* include affective flattening, associative loosening, ambivalence, and autism. Bleuler described *affective flattening* as a marked diminution in emotional expressiveness; *associative loosening* as disorganization in thought processes; *ambivalence* as the inability to initiate and follow through on even simple tasks; and *autism* as a profound degree of social and interpersonal unrelatedness. Thus, in defining schizophrenia, Bleuler focused on what today are considered negative symptoms rather than on positive symptoms, such as hallucinations and delusions. Indeed, Bleuler markedly broadened Kraepelin's concept of dementia praecox by including relatively mild and nonpsychotic forms (e.g., simple schizophrenia without symptoms such as hallucinations or delusions) and by stressing cross-sectional rather than longitudinal features. Bleuler was extremely influential, especially in the United States, during the middle decades of this century.

Kurt Schneider (1887–1967), on the other hand, was highly influential in Europe and Britain at around the same time. Like Bleuler, he stressed the importance of certain characteristic symptoms that could be observed cross-sectionally and deemphasized the importance of course (Schneider 1959). However, the specific symptoms that Schneider described as fundamental were quite different from those described by Bleuler. They included positive symptoms (e.g., hearing multiple voices commenting on or conversing about one's behavior; experiencing one's thoughts as being broadcast and heard by others; experiencing the feeling of being controlled by external forces) along with a series of other delusions and hallucinations that had as a common theme an impaired ability to differentiate internal versus external experiences or self versus other. These symptoms, which Schneider referred to as *first-rank symptoms* of schizophrenia (also commonly referred to as *Schneiderian symptoms*), were conceptualized as characteristic, if not pathognomonic, of the disorder. Although several subsequent studies have shown this not to be the case, these symptoms remain prominently featured in many classification systems for schizophrenia (Andreasen and Akiskal 1983; Carpenter et al. 1973b; Flaum et al. 1991; Silverstein and Harrow 1981).

The Impact of Construct Diversity on Diagnostic Reliability

As shown above, by the middle part of the 20th century, schizophrenia had been defined in many different ways, yielding quite a divergence of constructs. It is not surprising, therefore, that a series of studies done in the 1950s, 1960s, and 1970s revealed that diagnosticians often disagreed when diagnosing schizophrenia (Beck et al. 1962; Kreitman et al. 1961); that is, diagnostic reliability was extremely low. An important example of such a study was the United States–United Kingdom study (Cooper et al. 1972), in which the relative rates of schizophrenia and mood disorders were examined in hospitals in New York and London. Schizophrenia was found to be much more common than mood disorders in New York, whereas in London, schizophrenia was diagnosed about as frequently as mood disorders. If such geographic variation indeed proved to be the case, it would have important implications regarding the etiology of the disease (e.g., genetic factors, culture-bound factors). However, when research psychiatrists applied standardized operational criteria to all cases (United States–United Kingdom Cross-National Project 1974), the relative rates of schizophrenia and affective disorder were almost identical across the two sites.

Results from other studies (for a review, see Andreasen and Flaum 1991) have indicated that the prevalence of schizophrenia is relatively constant throughout the world, although the construct (and therefore the diagnosis) differs markedly across geographic boundaries (Carpenter et al. 1973a). Still other studies have demonstrated that the schizophrenia construct also has changed over time (Kuriansky et al. 1974). For example, in one New York hospital, the rates of schizophrenia over a 10-year period in the 1950s almost doubled from the rates found in the same hospital the previous decade. Such a dramatic change in prevalence over time, if true, would suggest an etiology such as viral syndromes (e.g., post–influenza epidemic). However, once again, when research psychiatrists applied operationalized diagnostic criteria to the medical records, no difference in incidence was observed (Kuriansky et al. 1974). Instead, they found that it was the construct of schizophrenia that had broadened over time, rather than any real change in the prevalence of the syndrome.

The Introduction of Operationalized Diagnostic Criteria

By the 1970s, studies like those mentioned above had underscored the need for a common language in psychiatry. The goal of optimizing diagnostic reliability was important not only for facilitating research but also for clinical and administrative purposes. One method of improving diagnostic reliability that had been used by the research community for some time involved the application of operationalized diagnostic criteria systems, based on the theory that diagnoses generated through the application of specific algorithms of signs and symptoms are more likely to be consistent across individuals and over time than those assigned on the basis of a theoretical construct or personal belief. It was in this context that the 1970s saw a proliferation of criteria-based diagnostic systems. Examples include the Feighner criteria (also known as the St. Louis or Washington University criteria;

Feighner et al. 1972), the New Haven Schizophrenia Index (Astrachan et al. 1972), the Flexible System (Carpenter et al. 1973a), the Research Diagnostic Criteria (Spitzer et al. 1975), the CATEGO System (Wing et al. 1974), and the Taylor and Abrams criteria (Taylor and Abrams 1978). Although the use of each of these sets of operationalized diagnostic criteria did increase the likelihood that two diagnosticians applying them would arrive at the same diagnosis, they each defined very different groups of patients as schizophrenic (Stephens et al. 1982). For example, when the New Haven Schizophrenia Index was applied to a sample of 283 hospitalized patients, 88% were classified as schizophrenic, whereas only 38% were so classified by the Feighner criteria. Thus, although the use of operationalized diagnostic systems improved reliability among those who used each particular system, it did not lead to a greater consensus as to where the boundaries between mental disorders should be drawn.

DSM-III and DSM-III-R

The Impact of DSM-III

The introduction of DSM-III (American Psychiatric Association 1980) changed this situation dramatically. For the first time, clinicians and researchers throughout the United States and, indeed, throughout much of the world began applying the same set of operationalized diagnostic criteria in defining psychiatric disorders. This practice served not only to facilitate clinical and research communication through enhanced reliability but also to promote an emphasis on empirical data, bringing psychiatry back into the mainstream of other medical disciplines.

The DSM-III criteria for schizophrenia did not represent a choice among existing constructs so much as a blend of various historical influences. For example, Kraepelin's contribution was reflected in the requirement for some evidence of chronicity (i.e., criterion C, which required a duration of at least 6 months of continuous illness to make the diagnosis of schizophrenia). Bleuler's influence was noted in the inclusion of loosening of associations and affective disturbances among the characteristic symptoms (criterion A6). Schneider's influence was evidenced in the inclusion of several of his "first-rank" symptoms among those listed in criteria A (e.g., A1, A4). This combined approach to setting criteria partly reflected the fact that the DSM-III system was generated by a consensus among experts rather than by a single person, as well as the explicit intention that the new system was to be an atheoretical system with the goal of reliably defining syndromal categories rather than describing validated disease processes. The process of validating these tentatively defined syndromes would be the ongoing task of the field.

The Disadvantages of DSM-III

The degree to which DSM-III was incorporated into research and clinical use reflects the important gap that it filled. However, even though that impact cannot be underestimated, there were some disadvantages to this phenomenon. The main problem with the wide acceptance of DSM-III was that it tended to lure both clinicians and researchers into a mistaken sense of comfort that they knew more than they did. Simply having all of the categories neatly and precisely laid out in a manual that was ubiquitously employed made it easy for users to forget that these were indeed "tentative agreements to agree." This was especially true for people just learning about psychiatric disorders, or those only peripherally involved in mental health, who often mistook the diagnostic manual for a textbook of psychiatry. Such misconceptions led to the impression, often false, that the signs and symptoms included in diagnostic algorithms were descriptive as well as defining features of the disorders. In fact, signs and symptoms included in diagnostic algorithms were often chosen based on a variety of psychometric properties, such as reliability or specificity, rather than because they were perceived as fundamental or particularly descriptive of the disorder. Therefore, although DSM-III provided psychiatry with a common language, it also set the stage for an environment that was ripe for reification and pseudoprecision, and introduced important changes in the concept of what was fundamental or core to schizophrenia.

DSM-III-R

The introduction of DSM-III-R (American Psychiatric Association 1987) further muddied the waters. Although the rationale for its introduction was to fine-tune the diagnostic system set forth in DSM-III, it was ultimately received by much of the psychiatric community as a full-blown revision, making the field extremely wary of subsequent revisions (e.g., DSM-IV).

For the diagnoses of schizophrenia and related psychotic disorders, two major changes were introduced in DSM-III-R (Kendler et al. 1989). First, the construct of the paranoid subtype of schizophrenia was changed so that it no longer reflected the content of the delusions or hallucinations (i.e., delusions and hallucinations of a paranoid nature), but rather reflected a subtype of schizophrenia in which there was relative preservation of affective and cognitive functioning. Paranoid schizophrenia came to be defined as a subtype that was characterized by prominent delusions, hallucinations, or both, that usually involved a single, coherent theme (although not necessarily one of paranoid content), without prominent disturbances in affect or prominently disorganized speech or behavior.

The second important change in DSM-III-R was that operationalized criteria for schizoaffective disorder were introduced. In DSM-III, this category was included in the manual without diagnostic criteria and was meant to be used only in those instances in which "the clinician is unable to make differential diagnosis with any degree of certainty between affective disorder and either schizophreniform disorder or schizophrenia" (American Psychiatric Association 1980, p. 202). However, in order to facilitate research on this confusing category, specific criteria for schizoaffective disorder were introduced in DSM-III-R. These criteria required concurrent psychotic symptoms and a full mood syndrome (either mania or depression) along with a period of psychotic symptoms without prominent mood symptoms during the same episode. Further, it was specified that mood symptoms had to be present for a substantial portion of the total duration of illness. The introduction of this category served the function of facilitating research, although it continued to be a confusing and difficult diagnosis to apply clinically.

DSM-IV

The Controversy Surrounding the Timing of DSM-IV

As DSM-III-R was introduced in 1987, many in both the clinical and the research mental health communities protested that any further revisions in the DSM system should be delayed for a substantial period of time so that an adequate database could be gathered using any one system (Zimmerman 1988). Two major arguments were advanced for an earlier introduction of DSM-IV (Frances et al. 1989). The first was that DSM-III had been finalized in the late 1970s and was based on a relatively limited amount of empirical evidence. The field had grown substantially over the ensuing 15 years, and it was felt that the information acquired during this period should be incorporated into the nosological system. Proponents of DSM-IV suggested that approximately 15 years was an appropriate amount of time in which to introduce major revisions, and that DSM-III-R was never intended to be a substitute for a new round of major revisions.

The second major motivation for introducing DSM-IV by the mid-1990s had to do with concordance with the international system. The 10th Edition of the International Classification of Diseases (ICD-10; World Health Organization 1992), the other system widely used throughout the world, included a section on the classification of mental disorders (see ICD-10, Chapter V, "Mental and Behavior Disorders (Including Disorder of Psychological Development): Diagnostic Criteria for Research"). The introduction of DSM-II in 1968 had coincided with the eighth revision of the ICD system, and the introduction of DSM-III, with the ninth revision. It had long been the intention of the American Psychiatric Association (APA) to continue to revise DSM in parallel with ICD so as to optimize concordance between the systems. ICD-10 was introduced in 1992, and the APA's plan was to introduce the next major DSM revision at the same time.

This controversy over the timing of DSM-IV was debated in the literature, as well as through a referendum subject to the approval of all APA members. Ultimately, the decision was made to proceed with the revision as scheduled.

The DSM-IV Process: Three Stages of Empirical Evidence Gathering

The APA task force to study diagnosis and nomenclature impaneled 13 work groups composed of nationally recognized experts in each category of disorders covered in the manual. The work group for psychotic disorders was chaired by Nancy Andreasen, and included John Kane, Samuel Keith, Kenneth Kendler, and Tom McGlashan. A large number of advisors were also designated to each work group.

The first task of each of the work groups was to identify those aspects of the DSM-III-R criteria that might be subject to change. Reasons for considering a change included any evidence that the current criteria 1) were not performing optimally in either clinical or research settings, 2) did not optimally reflect the current state of knowledge, or 3) differed markedly from the proposed ICD-10 criteria. The work group on psychotic disorders also paid particular attention to issues of user friendliness and the educational value of the criteria (i.e., that the diagnostic criteria be adequately descriptive, conceptually clear, and easy to remember and apply). The APA task force made it clear that a high threshold for changes would be required (Frances et al. 1989); a substantial amount of empirical evidence would be expected prior to introducing any change in criteria that might substantially affect case classification.

Three stages of empirical review were followed by each work group. The first involved review of the existing literature. For example, among the issues identified by the DSM-IV work group for psychotic disorders was the question of whether the minimum threshold for the overall duration of symptoms should be shortened in order to be more consistent with the ICD-10 criteria, which require a total duration of 1 month of illness. A literature review was conducted on the predictive validity of the 6-month duration criteria and, based on this review alone, the work group reached consensus that the 6-month–duration criteria should be maintained in DSM-IV (Keith and Matthews 1991). However, there were several issues raised for which the existing literature was inadequate in providing guidance. For example, questions were raised as to which symptoms should be included in criteria A (active symptoms list) and the effects on case classification of adding or deleting any of the symptoms delineated in DSM-III-R. These types of specific questions were addressed by the next two phases of empirical data analysis, which included 1) a reanalysis of existing data sets that had been gathered for other reasons, and 2) prospectively conducted field trials.

A large number of existing phenomenological databases were identified with which the effects of proposed revisions in criteria could be efficiently explored. Specifically, the impact of adding, deleting, or changing the criteria A symptoms on case classification could be approximated by applying diagnostic algorithms to such existing phenomenological databases. These analyses demonstrated, for example, that the addition of "disorganized behavior" to the list of active symptoms would not substantially broaden case classification for schizophrenia, although it would serve to make the criteria more descriptive of the disorder (Andreasen and Flaum 1991). These types of analyses allowed the work group to generate three sets of option criteria for DSM-IV, whose performance characteristics could then be empirically examined and compared with those of DSM-III, DSM-III-R, and ICD-10 criteria in focused field trials (Flaum and Andreasen 1991; Kendler 1990).

For the psychotic disorders field trial, a total of 450 patients were evaluated across nine sites (seven within and two outside of the United States). In order to maintain the focus on the population of interest, the primary inclusion criterion for the field trial was the presence of at least one prominent positive or negative symptom at the time of the evaluation. Almost all patients were interviewed by two raters, half in a conjoint interview and the other half by independent raters on consecutive days, in order to gather both interrater and test-retest reliability data. Raters used a semistructured interview instrument created specifically for this project, which elicited each of the signs and symptoms necessary to make a diagnosis according to each of the criteria sets being evaluated.

Primary Issues Evaluated

In addition to general performance characteristics (e.g., overall diagnostic reliability, rates of case classification, user friendliness), a number of specific issues were evaluated in the data reanalyses and field trials. Three issues that were deemed of primary importance to examine in these later stages of data analysis were

1. Which symptoms should be included among the characteristic list and, specifically, to what extent should negative symptoms be emphasized?
2. Should the required duration of active symptoms (i.e., criteria A symptoms) be increased from 1 week to 1 month?
3. Could the criteria for schizophrenia be simplified in order to be made more conceptually clear and easier to use and remember without sacrificing reliability or changing case classification rates?

The process of resolving each of these issues and the resulting decisions are described below.

Characteristic symptoms of schizophrenia.   Criteria A in both DSM-III and DSM-III-R described "active" or "characteristic" symptoms. In DSM-III-R, these included delusions; prominent hallucinations; loosening of associations, or incoherence; catatonic behavior; and flat or inappropriate affect. Two or more of these symptoms were required to be present in order to satisfy these criteria. Further, if the delusions were bizarre, or the hallucinations consisted of voices commenting on or conversing about the subject's behavior, only one such symptom was required. Thus, there was an increased weighting on Schneiderian first-rank symptoms.

Were these the characteristic symptoms of schizophrenia? The answer to this question depends on what is meant by "characteristic." Does it mean "common"? "Specific"? Does it mean "core" or "fundamental" to the disorder in some way? In the process of the data reanalysis, the work group looked at some of these questions. For example, in Figure 4–1 the relative frequency of each of these symptoms among three large independent samples of patients evaluated at the University of Iowa between 1985 and 1990, all of whom met either DSM-III or DSM-III-R criteria for schizophrenia, is shown. Admittedly, the strategy for selecting the patient group was somewhat circular in that the patients had to have some of these symptoms of the disorder in order to meet the diagnosis; nevertheless, this study did reveal some interesting aspects in terms of the descriptive value of the current criteria. The work group found that delusions were quite common, prominent hallucinations occurred in approximately half of the patients, and flat and inappropriate affect were fairly common, but that incoherence, marked formal thought disorder, and catatonic behavior were rare. When the rates of the A2 and A3 criteria (i.e., the Schneiderian first-rank symptoms) were examined, it was clear that these symptoms occurred in only about 20%–30% of patients across all three samples (see Figure 4–2). When negative symptoms were examined (see Figure 4–3), it was found that they were essentially ubiquitous. Thus, although nonspecific, negative symptoms were extremely common among people who met diagnostic criteria for schizophrenia, negative symptoms did not feature prominently within the diagnostic algorithm. Specifically, flat affect was the only negative symptom included in DSM-III and III-R.

In light of the historical importance of negative symptoms, the

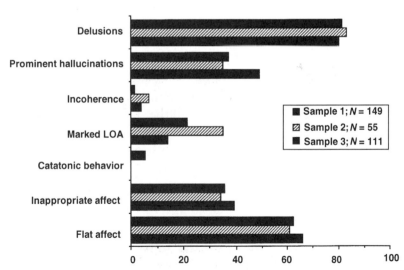

Figure 4–1. Frequency of DSM-III-R criterion A-1 symptoms among three independent samples of schizophrenic patients diagnosed according to DSM-III-R. Symptoms were rated on the Scale for the Assessment of Positive Symptoms (Andreasen 1984) and the Scale for the Assessment of Negative Symptoms (Andreasen 1983). LOA = loosening of associations.

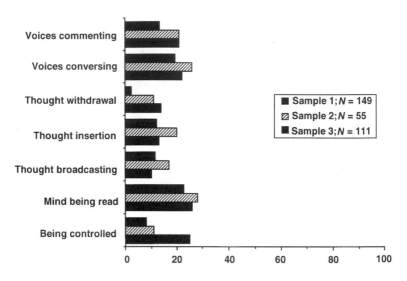

Figure 4–2. Frequency of DSM-III-R criteria A-2 and A-3 symptoms among three independent samples of schizophrenic patients diagnosed according to DSM-III-R. Symptoms were rated on the Scale for the Assessment of Positive Symptoms (Andreasen 1984) and the Scale for the Assessment of Negative Symptoms (Andreasen 1983).

increased attention being paid to them in research over the past decade, and the work group's intent to make the criteria optimally descriptive and educationally useful, the group was inclined to increase the emphasis on negative symptoms in the DSM-IV criteria. The group's concerns with taking this action had to do with reliability; positive symptoms tend to be more discontinuous with normality, whereas negative symptoms tend to be more on a continuum. Therefore, it would seem that it would be easier to dichotomize positive symptoms as present or absent than it would be to do the same for negative symptoms.

In order to further investigate the impact of including more negative symptoms in the criteria, the work group examined the reliability of both positive and negative symptoms in the field trials (Flaum et al., in press). It found that, indeed, hallucinations and delusions were rated with the highest degree of reliability (i.e., intraclass r's > 0.7), with the reliability of negative symptoms being somewhat lower (intraclass r's on the order of 0.5–0.6). However, the reliability rating for negative symptoms was in the same range as the work group observed for other positive symptoms, such as disorganized behavior or inappropriate affect. The issue that the work group had to determine was whether the addition of negative symptoms to the active symptom list would decrease the overall reliability in making the diagnosis of schizophrenia.

The three new sets of option criteria for DSM-IV that were tested in the field trial emphasized negative symptoms to varying degrees, including one in which they were emphasized quite heavily. It was found that the reliability did not differ significantly among any of the three option criteria sets, and indeed was in the acceptable range across all six criteria sets tested ($\kappa > 0.7$ for interrater and > 0.6 for test-retest). Similarly, case classification rates were minimally different across the criteria sets. Thus, the work group concluded that the active symptom list could be made more descriptive and educationally meaningful without compromising reliability or case classification. For all of these reasons, the decision was made to include a greater emphasis on negative symptoms in criteria A for the diagnosis of schizophrenia in DSM-IV (see Table 4–1).

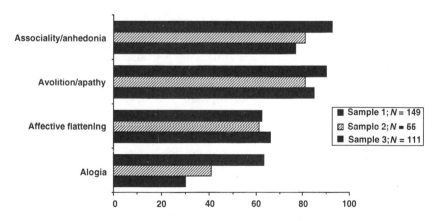

Figure 4–3. Frequency of negative symptoms among three independent samples of schizophrenic patients diagnosed according to DSM-III-R. Symptoms were rated on the Scale for the Assessment of Negative Symptoms (Andreasen 1983).

Table 4–1.   DSM-IV diagnostic criteria for schizophrenia

A. *Characteristic symptoms:* Two (or more) of the following, each present for a significant portion of time during **a 1-month period** (or less if successfully treated):
    (1) delusions
    (2) hallucinations
    (3) **disorganized speech** (e.g., frequent derailment, incoherence)
    (4) **grossly disorganized** or catatonic behavior
    (5) **negative symptoms (i.e., affective flattening, alogia, or avolition)**
[Note: Only one A symptom is required if delusions are bizarre or hallucinations consist of a voice keeping up a running commentary on the person's behavior or thoughts, or two or more voices conversing with each other.]
B. *Social/occupational dysfunction:* For a significant portion of the time since the onset of the disturbance, one or more major areas of functioning such as work, interpersonal relations or self-care is markedly below the level achieved prior to the onset (or when the onset is in childhood or adolescence, failure to achieve expected level of interpersonal, academic, or occupational achievement.
C. *Duration:* Continuous signs of the disturbance persist for at least 6 months. This 6-month period must include at least 1 month of symptoms that meet criteria A (i.e., active phase symptoms), and may include periods of prodromal or residual symptoms. During these prodromal or residual periods, the signs of the disturbance may be manifested by only negative symptoms or two or more symptoms listed in criteria A present in an attenuated form (e.g., odd beliefs, unusual perceptual experiences).
D. *Schizoaffective and mood disorder exclusion:* Schizoaffective disorder and mood disorder with psychotic features have been ruled out because either 1) no major depressive or manic episodes have occurred concurrently with the active phase symptoms, or 2) if mood episodes have occurred during active phase symptoms, their total duration has been brief relative to the duration of the active and residual periods.
E. *Substance/general medical condition exclusion:* The disturbance is not attributable to the direct effects of a substance (e.g., drugs of abuse, medication) or a general medical condition.
F. *Relationship to a pervasive developmental disorder:* If there is a history of autistic disorder or another pervasive developmental disorder, the additional diagnosis of schizophrenia is made only if prominent delusions or hallucinations are also present for at least a month (or less, if successfully treated).

Classification of longitudinal course (can be applied only after at least 1 year has elapsed since the initial onset of active-phase symptoms):

Episodic with interepisode residual symptoms (episodes are defined by the reemergence of prominent psychotic symptoms); *also specify if:* with prominent negative symptoms

Episodic with no interepisode residual symptoms

Continuous (prominent psychotic symptoms are present throughout the period of observation); *also specify if:* with prominent negative symptoms

Single episode in partial remission; *also specify if:* with prominent negative symptoms

Single episode in full remission

Other or unspecified pattern

Note. Words in boldface type reflect differences from DSM-III-R.
Source. American Psychiatric Association 1994, pp. 285–286.

One-week versus 1-month duration of active symptoms. In the DSM-III-R criteria, active symptoms were required for at least 1 week (or less, if successfully treated). The work group considered expanding the duration threshold for active symptoms to 1 month for two reasons. First, doing so would make the DSM system more compatible with the ICD-10 criterion, which requires 1 month of active symptoms. Second, doing so would address concerns about false-positive diagnoses of schizophrenia. This was especially the case in light of the number of commonly used substances of abuse that can result in psychotic symptoms (e.g., cocaine, amphetamines). The concern from a clinical perspective was that a patient could present emergently with psychotic symptoms secondary to drug abuse—symptoms that would be difficult to distinguish from those of early-onset schizophrenia. If these symptoms were to persist, and if this individual's history of illicit drug use was not definitively established, the presumptive diagnosis of schizophreniform disorder might be made. Then, most likely, the patient would be started on antipsychotic medications, which in turn could cause the appearance of negative-like symptoms, providing further presumptive evidence for the schizophrenia diagnosis. Indeed, once a diagnosis of schizophrenia or even schizophreniform disorder appears in a medical record, it may have long-standing implications for medical and psychosocial management. Given the impact of this diagnosis, the work group felt that false positives should be avoided if possible.

The field trial allowed the work group to ask the question, What would be the effect on case classification if the only difference between the DSM-IV and the DSM-III-R criteria for schizophrenia was the one change in the duration criterion of active symptoms from 1 week to 1 month? The group found that a small, but substantial, number of cases would be affected by this one change. Specifically, about 8% of people who currently meet DSM-III-R criteria for schizophrenia would end up being diagnosed as having an otherwise unspecified psychosis if this change were made. Not surprisingly, it is the first-episode cases that make up the bulk of that 8%; indeed, up to 20%–25% of the first-episode cases in the field trial study would have had to be differentially classified if this change were made.

The next question had to do with whether changing the criterion on duration of active symptoms was a valid change: Do patients who are differentially classified differ in any way from those who are unaffected by such a change? In order to examine this, the work group compared those who would be reclassified with those who would not on a large number of phenomenological course variables, such as age at onset, duration of hospitalizations, overt severity of illness, functional status, and occupational status. It was interesting to note that the two groups differed only on variables relating to alcohol and substance use. Those excluded by the longer duration threshold for active symptoms were more likely to have a history of both alcohol and substance abuse than those unaffected by this change. This lent support to the idea that such a change would decrease the number of false-positive diagnoses of schizophrenia secondary to substance-induced psychoses. Ultimately, the work group recommended that the longer duration criterion be incorporated into the DSM-IV criteria. Therefore, a total of 1 month of active symptoms is now required in order to make the diagnosis of schizophrenia. The parenthetical remark "unless successfully treated" (meaning that if it is the clinician's judgment that in the absence of effective treatment, psychotic symptoms would have persisted for a month or more, the diagnosis can be made in light of a shorter duration) remains in DSM-IV.

Simplifying the complexity of the schizophrenia diagnosis.   The diagnostic criteria for schizophrenia in DSM-III-R were criticized for being overly complicated and difficult to remember. For example, the active symptom lists include A1, A2, and A3 criteria: either two symptoms of A1 or one symptom of A2 or A3 was required. Making matters worse was the fact that there was redundancy among these criteria: the A2 criterion listed specific types of delusions and the A3 criterion listed specific types of hallucinations, yet both delusions and hallucinations appeared in the A1 criterion. In light of these problems, the work group raised the question as to whether the criteria could be simplified without substantially sacrificing reliability or changing case classification.

    To look at this, an approach similar to that used for the duration question was implemented. The work group determined the number of cases that would be affected if the only change made was eliminating the A2 and A3 criteria (i.e., eliminating increased diagnostic weighting on specific types of delusions and hallucinations). Once again, the group found a small, but substantial, minority of cases that would be affected by such a change—approximately 9%.

The next question was whether this was a valid change: Did the individuals affected differ in any meaningful way from those unaffected? Unlike the results found for the duration criterion, the work group found absolutely no difference between those who would be excluded by such a change and those unaffected, suggesting that although appealing for the sake of user friendliness and simplicity, such a change would not be valid. Therefore, the consensus was to maintain the increased weighting on the first-rank Schneiderian symptoms. However, a simple formatting change was introduced to render the criteria less complicated while maintaining the same basic algorithm: rather than having separate A2 and A3 criteria, DSM-IV includes a parenthetical remark at the end of the simplified Criteria A that states, "If delusions are bizarre or hallucinations consist of multiple voices conversing or commenting upon the person's behavior, then only one criteria A symptom is required."

The result of this rather minor change is that when readers look at criteria A for schizophrenia as they appear in DSM-IV, there is an implied, inherent conceptual structure that was lacking in previous versions. Each of the major symptoms represents a function that is evaluated separately during a typical mental status examination: perception (hallucinations), inferential thinking (delusions), speech and thought (disorganized speech), behavioral organization (disorganized or catatonic behavior), and negative symptoms.

Other Requirements for the Diagnosis of Schizophrenia in DSM-IV

In addition to characteristic symptoms persisting for at least 1 month (in the absence of effective treatment), the diagnosis of schizophrenia is made if

- There is clear evidence of impairment in social and occupational functioning (criterion B)

- There is some evidence of a continued disturbance for at least 6 months (criterion C)
- The disorder is not better accounted for by a mood disorder (criterion D), substance use or a general medical condition (criterion E), or an autistic disorder (criterion F)

Criteria B and C.   The requirement for social and occupational dysfunction and an overall duration criterion of 6 months reflect the Kraepelinian emphasis on chronicity and ongoing impairment in functioning as defining features of schizophrenia. ICD-10 does not embrace these concepts; indeed, according to that system, the diagnosis of schizophrenia can be made in the presence of 1 month of active symptoms that are not attributable to a mood or organic disorder. In the DSM system, there must be a clear degree of dysfunction in social, occupational, or educational functioning that represents a change from a preestablished baseline. In the case of childhood or adolescent onset, a change from preestablished baseline is not required, but it must be clear that the patient is not achieving at the social, occupational, or educational level that would be expected for someone of his or her age and cultural group.

The overall duration criterion requires that there be some evidence of ongoing illness for at least 6 months. This must include at least 1 month of active symptoms (unless successfully treated, as noted above) and may also include a period of prodromal or residual symptoms. Prodromal and residual symptoms may include attenuated forms of the active symptoms delineated in criteria A and may be limited to negative symptoms. The overall duration criterion in DSM-IV is unchanged in intent from that of DSM-III-R, but once again is simpler and easier to use in that it no longer includes a subcriterion for determining the presence of a prodromal or residual phase. Reliability of determining the presence or duration of prodromal symptoms was found to be only fair, and the overall diagnostic reliability was not lowered by simplifying the criterion as it appears in DSM-IV.

Criteria D–F.   The criterion requiring a differential with mood and schizoaffective disorder in DSM-IV is essentially unchanged from that in DSM-III-R. As noted above, this diagnosis can be difficult to apply practically. One reason for this difficulty is that many—if not the majority of—patients with schizophrenia experience prominent mood symptoms (usually depressive) at some point during the course of the disorder. The critical element in the differential is the temporal relationship between mood and psychotic symptomatology. If characteristic symptoms of schizophrenia (i.e., criteria A symptoms) appear only in the context of a full mood episode (either depression or mania), the diagnosis is that of mood disorder with psychotic features. If mood symptoms are brief relative to the schizophrenic symptoms, the diagnosis is that of schizophrenia. In such a case, the clinician may further specify a "depressive disorder not otherwise specified," if clinically relevant. The diagnosis of schizoaffective disorder is reserved for those cases in which the relative duration of mood and schizophrenic symptomatology is approximately equivalent throughout the course of any episode of the disorder.

Another reason for the difficulties in applying these criteria is that it is often unclear what an "episode" means in a disorder that may be quite chronic. An attempt was made to clarify this concept in DSM-IV by stipulating that the diagnosis of schizoaffective disorder applies to an episode rather than a lifetime course, recognizing that in some cases these will be the same (i.e., in individuals who never achieve complete remission).

The word "organic" has been stricken from the DSM-IV language because it was perceived to perpetuate a mind-body dichotomy inconsistent with the thrust of contemporary thinking in psychiatry. It is now commonly recognized that disorders such as schizophrenia most likely have an organic basis, even though the specifics have not yet been elucidated. In place of "organic," the term "secondary" is used in DSM-IV. If there is evidence that a schizophrenic-like disorder was initiated and maintained by a known endogenous or exogenous factor, it is now termed a "psychotic disorder secondary to [that factor]" in the case of a general medical condition (e.g., "psychotic disorder secondary to hyperthyroidism"). If the presumed etiologic factor involves substance use, the DSM-IV language is "[the specific substance]–induced psychotic disorder."

Finally, according to the DSM-IV system, schizophrenia is not diagnosed in the context of autistic disorder unless hallucinations or delusions are prominent. This exclusion criterion becomes particularly important in the evaluation of children in light of the expanded criteria A because children with pervasive developmental disorders will not uncommonly manifest disorganized behavior and negative symptoms such as social withdrawal.

Subtypes and Course Modifiers in DSM-IV

The traditional subtypes of paranoid, catatonic, disorganized, undifferentiated, and residual schizophrenia have been maintained in DSM-IV with minimal changes from DSM-III-R. A review of the literature showed that the paranoid versus nonparanoid distinction was the most valid, but that the evidence for the validity of the remaining subtypes was less compelling. A variety of other options were explored, including the incorporation of a tridimensional model of subtypes consisting of psychotic (hallucinations and delusions), disorganized (disorganized speech and behavior), and deficit (primary negative) symptoms as the defining features over the longitudinal course of the disorder. The performance characteristics of this newly proposed subtyping scheme proved to be problematic (e.g., low reliability, substantial overlap, discordance with ICD-10) and, therefore, the traditional system was retained in DSM-IV. The tridimensional model was placed in the appendix, indicating the need for further research.

Course modifiers were amended in order to be more clinically useful and more consistent with ICD-10. Rather than classifying course in terms of chronicity and acuity (e.g., chronic with acute exacerbation) as had been the case in DSM-III and DSM-III-R, the pattern of symptoms over time may now be specified in the fifth digit.

Other Related Diagnoses in DSM-IV

Schizophrenia is differentiated from schizophreniform disorder and brief psychotic disorder primarily on the basis of overall duration. If criteria A symptoms persist for less than 1 month, in the absence of any of the exclusionary criteria, with a full return to premorbid level of functioning, the diagnosis is *brief psychotic disorder*. This category replaces what had been referred to as brief reactive psychosis in DSM-

III and DSM-III-R. If the symptoms appear to be clearly related to a stressful event, the specifier "reactive type" is added. If the disorder persists for more than 1 month, but less than 6 months, the diagnosis is *schizophreniform disorder*. In many cases, both of these diagnostic categories will serve as transitional diagnoses for new-onset cases of schizophrenia.

Delusional disorder is defined by the presence of nonbizarre delusions that persist for at least 1 month and that are not accompanied by other characteristic signs or symptoms of schizophrenia. Nonbizarre delusions are those that are plausible within an individual's subculture, such as the belief that one's spouse is being unfaithful or that one is being followed by the CIA. Although such beliefs may result in a substantial degree of social or occupational dysfunction, that dysfunction must be clearly attributable to the impact of the delusion for this diagnosis to be made (i.e., criterion B for schizophrenia should not be fulfilled independently of the delusion). As in the case of schizophrenia, it must be clear that the delusion is not secondary to a mood disorder, substance use, or a general medical condition in order for the diagnosis of delusional disorder to be made.

Finally, a residual category of *psychotic disorder not otherwise specified* is retained in the DSM-IV for those cases in which the clinician recognizes the prominence of psychotic features but is unable to further specify diagnosis because of a lack of or contradictory information, atypicality of presentation, or other factors that would make a more specific diagnosis premature.

Concluding Remarks

In this chapter I have attempted to present a balanced view of the value and limitations of the current diagnostic criteria for schizophrenia in the context of a historical perspective. It is suggested that the more systematically psychiatrists can apply diagnoses, both in clinical and in research settings, the better it will be for patient care and for the advancing of psychiatry's understanding of the mechanisms underlying these disorders.

For those disorders in medicine for which the mechanism has been elucidated (e.g., pneumococcal pneumonia), making an accurate diagnosis indeed represents the most important part of what the care provider does for the patient. Once having done so, appropriate treatment can be prescribed and followed. In psychiatry, making the diagnosis is just the beginning. Diagnostic determinations group individuals into categories that are still relatively broad and that are almost certainly heterogeneous with respect to underlying etiology and mechanisms. The researcher must consider this heterogeneity in designing and interpreting studies and must avoid the tendency to restrict the designs to comparisons of schizophrenic patients as a group with some control or comparison group on the variable of interest. Similarly, the clinician must be mindful of this heterogeneity in that the disease is likely to reflect heterogeneity in treatment response and course. The process of making an accurate diagnosis is, therefore, a critical beginning, but by no means an end, in the practice of psychiatry.

References

American Psychiatric Association: Diagnostic and Statistical Manual of Mental Disorders, 2nd Edition. Washington, DC, American Psychiatric Association, 1968

American Psychiatric Association: Diagnostic and Statistical Manual of Mental Disorders, 3rd Edition. Washington, DC, American Psychiatric Association, 1980

American Psychiatric Association: Diagnostic and Statistical Manual of Mental Disorders, 3rd Edition, Revised. Washington, DC, American Psychiatric Association, 1987

American Psychiatric Association: Diagnostic and Statistical Manual of Mental Disorders, 4th Edition. Washington, DC, American Psychiatric Association, 1994

Andreasen NC: The Scale for the Assessment of Negative Symptoms (SANS). Iowa City, IA, University of Iowa, 1983

Andreasen NC: The Scale for the Assessment of Positive Symptoms (SAPS). Iowa City, IA, University of Iowa, 1984

Andreasen NC, Akiskal HS: The specificity of Bleulerian and Schneiderian symptoms: a critical reevaluation. Psychiatr Clin North Am 6:41–54, 1983

Andreasen NC, Flaum M: Schizophrenia: the characteristic symptoms. Schizophr Bull 17:27–49, 1991

Astrachan BM, Harrow M, Adler D, et al: The checklist for the diagnosis of schizophrenia. Br J Psychiatry 121:529–539, 1972

Beck AT, Ward CH, Mendelson M: Reliability of psychiatric diagnosis, II: a study of consistency of clinical judgments and ratings. Am J Psychiatry 119:351–357, 1962

Bleuler E: Dementia Praecox or The Group of Schizophrenias (1911). Translated by Zinkin J. New York, International Universities Press, 1950

Carpenter WT, Strauss JS, Bartko JJ: Flexible system for the diagnosis of schizophrenia: report from the World Health Organization International Pilot Study of Schizophrenia. Science 182:1275–1278, 1973a

Carpenter WT Jr, Strauss JS, Muleh S: Are there pathognomonic symptoms in schizophrenia? an empirical investigation of Schneider's first-rank symptoms. Arch Gen Psychiatry 28:847–852, 1973b

Cooper JE, Kendell RE, Gurland BJ, et al: Psychiatric Diagnosis in New York and London (Maudsley Monograph No 20). London, Oxford University Press, 1972

Feighner JP, Robins E, Guze SB, et al: Diagnostic criteria for use in psychiatric research. Arch Gen Psychiatry 26:57–63, 1972

Flaum M, Andreasen NC: Diagnostic criteria for schizophrenia and related disorders: options for DSM-IV. Schizophr Bull 17:133–142, 1991

Flaum M, Arndt S, Fleming F, et al: The reliability and frequency of "first-rank" symptoms in schizophrenia: implications for DSM-IV (abstract). International Congress on Schizophrenia Research, Tucson, Arizona, April 1991

Flaum M, Amador XA, Bracha HS, et al: The field trials for schizophrenia and other psychotic disorders in DSM-IV. Am J Psychiatry (in press)

Frances AJ, Widiger TA, Pincus HA: The development of DSM-IV. Arch Gen Psychiatry 46:373–375, 1989

Keith SJ, Matthews SM: The diagnosis of schizophrenia: a review of onset and duration issues. Schizophr Bull 17:51–67, 1991

Kendler KS: Toward a scientific psychiatric nosology: strengths and limitations. Arch Gen Psychiatry 47:969–973, 1990

Kendler KS, Spitzer RL, Williams JBL: Psychotic disorders in DSM-III-R. Am J Psychiatry 146:953–962, 1989

Kraepelin E, Barclay RM, Robertson GM: Dementia Praecox and Paraphrenia. Edinburgh, Scotland, E & S Livingstone, 1919

Kreitman N, Sainsbury P, Morrissey J, et al: The reliability of psychiatric assessment: an analysis. Journal of Mental Science 107:887–908, 1961

Kuriansky JB, Deming WE, Gurland BJ: On trends in the diagnosis of schizophrenia. Am J Psychiatry 131:402–408, 1974

Professional staff of the United States–United Kingdom Cross-National Project: The diagnosis and psychopathology of schizophrenia in New York and London. Schizophr Bull 11:80–102, 1974

Schneider K: Clinical Psychopathology. Translated by Hamilton MW. New York, Grune & Stratton, 1959

Silverstein ML, Harrow M: Schneiderian first-rank symptoms in schizophrenia. Arch Gen Psychiatry 38:288–293, 1981

Spitzer RL, Endicott J, Robins E: Research Diagnostic Criteria. New York, New York State Psychiatric Institute, Biometrics Research Division, 1975

Stephens JH, Astrup C, Carpenter WT, et al: A comparison of nine systems to diagnosis of schizophrenia. Psychiatry Res 6:127–143, 1982

Taylor M, Abrams R: The prevalence of schizophrenia: a reassessment using modern diagnostic criteria. Am J Psychiatry 135:945–948, 1978

Wing JK, Cooper JE, Sartorius N: The Description and Classification of Psychiatric Symptoms: An Instruction Manual for the PSE and CATEGO System. Cambridge, UK, Cambridge University Press, 1974

World Health Organization: International Classification of Diseases, 10th Edition. Geneva, Switzerland, World Health Organization, 1992

Zimmerman M: Why are we rushing to publish DSM-IV? Arch Gen Psychiatry 45:1135–1138, 1988

CHAPTER 5

Conceptual Models of the Relationship Between Positive and Negative Symptoms

Rajiv Tandon, M.D.; Michael D. Jibson, M.D., Ph.D.;
Stephan F. Taylor, M.D.; and John R. DeQuardo, M.D.

H omogeneity in psychiatric disorders is rare; variations in phenomenology, course, treatment response, and underlying disease mechanisms create a complex picture of mental disorders.

Schizophrenia is one of the most variable of psychiatric disorders; in fact, variability is considered by some experts to be an intrinsic feature of schizophrenic illness (Van der Velde 1976; Wyatt et al. 1988). Ever since Kraepelin (1919/1971) and Bleuler (1911/1950) consolidated the concepts of dementia praecox and schizophrenia almost a century ago, several approaches have been devised to understand and explain the enormous heterogeneity of schizophrenic illness. Clinicians and investigators have struggled to identify the syndrome's core in terms of its symptomatology, genetic liability, association with various neurobiological abnormalities, treatment response, longitudinal course, and outcome. Explanations of schizophrenic symptoms have usually been founded on one of two broad strategies: descriptive categorization or neurobiological categorization. However, another explanation for the syndrome, in which schizophrenic symptoms have been dichotomized as either positive or negative, is unique in that it attempts to incorporate both psychopathological and neurobiological dimensions of the illness.

Positive symptoms in schizophrenia refer to the presence of behaviors and functions that otherwise would not normally be present (e.g., delusions, hallucinations). *Negative symptoms* refer to the absence or diminution of behaviors and functions that are usually present (i.e., apathy, amotivation, anhedonia, avolition, blunted affect, emotional withdrawal, and impoverished speech and thinking). Early theoreticians, including Kraepelin and Bleuler, considered negative symptoms to represent the fundamental or core psychopathology of the illness. Over the years, however, the importance of negative symptoms has been progressively downplayed. Instead, increasing emphasis has been placed on positive symptoms, as epitomized by the publication and almost universal acceptance of Schneider's (1959) checklist of "first rank" schizophrenic symptoms, which consisted exclusively of positive symptoms. Factors contributing to this trend of favoring positive symptoms included 1) the difficulty in reliably defining and documenting negative symptoms; 2) the more florid expression of positive symptoms; and 3) the revolution in the treatment of schizophrenia brought about by the introduction of antipsychotic medications, which produce their most dramatic improvement in positive symptoms.

Despite their widespread acceptance, however, positive symptoms were unable to provide an adequate characterization of schizophrenia. In fact, they were found to correlate poorly with chronicity and deterioration, features that were considered central to traditional definitions of schizophrenia. Furthermore, the almost universal presence and relative persistence of negative symptoms, combined with the fact that negative symptoms represent the most debilitating and refractory aspect of schizophrenic psychopathology, made them difficult to ignore. Strauss et al. (1974) reintroduced the positive–negative symptom distinction to the study of schizophrenia in the early 1970s;

further impetus for recent empirical work was provided by Crow (1980) and Andreasen (1982), both of whom explored the utility of schizophrenic subtypes based on the positive–negative symptom distinction.

In contrast to positive symptoms, negative symptoms have generally been found to be

- More chronic and persistent
- Less responsive to neuroleptic treatment
- Associated with abnormal premorbid adjustment and poor social functioning
- Accompanied by a greater likelihood of cognitive impairment and computed tomographic evidence of cerebral atrophy
- Associated with poor outcome

Although dopaminergic hyperactivity (the dominant neurobiological hypothesis of schizophrenic pathophysiology) was found to provide a reasonable explanation for positive symptoms, this mechanism provided an inadequate explanation for negative symptoms. Attempts to understand these different profiles led to the suggestion that positive symptoms were related to dopaminergic hyperactivity and negative symptoms were linked to structural brain abnormalities (Crow 1980).

The positive–negative syndrome dichotomy has been increasingly prioritized as an organizing principle in schizophrenia over the past decade, as attested to by the profusion of studies in this area. Although exciting and long overdue, this inundation of the field by multiple competing concepts and definitions has led to much confusion. Consequently, a clarification of these concepts with particular reference to their implied pathophysiologies and implications for treatment may be useful.

Our purpose in this chapter is not to provide a comprehensive review of all pathophysiological mechanisms implicated in the production of positive and negative symptoms in schizophrenia; Chapters 1, 2, and 10 provide a more thorough overview from neurochemical and neuromorphological perspectives. Instead, in this chapter we review the major conceptual frameworks that have been proposed for understanding the relationship between positive and negative symptoms in schizophrenia in terms of their underlying theoretical assumptions, pathophysiological mechanisms proposed, and treatment implications. Finally, an overall model for the evaluation of negative symptoms is presented and its treatment implications discussed.

Models for Conceptualizing the Relationship Between Positive and Negative Syndromes

Negative Versus Positive Versus Mixed Schizophrenia

This model, developed by Andreasen (1982), was based on the assumption that positive and negative symptoms are dichotomous, and that their presence defines two distinct types of schizophrenic patients—*positive patients* and *negative patients*—with unique pathophysiology. Differentiation between these subtypes could be made cross-sectionally; furthermore, it was assumed that these subtypes were longitudinally stable (i.e., a positive patient would always remain a positive patient and, conversely, a negative patient would remain a negative patient). The *mixed type* was presumed to constitute a small percentage of schizophrenic patients with both positive and negative symptoms. Although the underlying pathophysiological basis of the positive and negative schizophrenic subtypes was never explicitly stated, it was implied in this model that dopaminergic hyperactivity characterized the positive subtype, and structural brain abnormalities characterized the negative subtype. From a treatment standpoint, positive patients were considered to be responsive to neuroleptics and, therefore, a neuroleptic treatment regimen was the treatment of choice; negative patients were considered to be refractory to neuroleptics and, as a result, no specific treatment regimen was recommended for this group.

In actual fact, the mixed type was found to constitute a majority of schizophrenic patients (Andreasen et al. 1990); furthermore, the positive–negative–mixed subtyping was not found to be longitudinally stable (see Chapter 6). Consequently, strict positive–negative subtyping of schizophrenic illness as originally proposed by this model is not presently considered viable or valid.

Type I Versus Type II Schizophrenia

Crow (1980) used the distinction between positive and negative symptoms to postulate two types of schizophrenia: *type I,* characterized by positive symptoms, absence of intellectual impairment, normal brain structure, and good response to neuroleptics; and *type II,* characterized by prominent negative symptoms, intellectual deterioration, enlarged cerebral ventricles, and poor response to neuroleptics. Crow originally conceived the type I and type II forms to be different stages of schizophrenic illness, with type II reflecting a more chronic, deteriorated stage; patients could progress from type I to type II, but not the other way around (Crow 1983). Pathophysiological and treatment implications of the type I–type II dichotomy were part of their very definition.

Subsequently, Crow (1985) suggested that the positive and negative symptoms reflected two syndromes that were relatively independent processes and that could coexist in the same patient but follow different time courses. He also suggested that they were different manifestations of the activity of the same pathogen. Crow hypothesized that dopaminergic hyperactivity was the underlying basis of the type I (positive) syndrome, which consequently responded well to neuroleptic treatment, and that cerebral atrophy and other structural brain abnormalities were the underlying pathophysiology of the type II (negative) syndrome.

The syndromatic view of positive and negative symptoms (i.e., that positive and negative symptoms reflect distinct dimensions of schizophrenic illness that are not mutually exclusive) is now generally well accepted and has been further developed in the following models.

Deficit Versus Nondeficit Schizophrenia

Carpenter et al. (1985) highlighted the fact that negative symptoms did not compose a homogeneous entity, and further emphasized the need to distinguish between primary and secondary negative symptoms. *Primary negative symptoms* refer to negative symptoms that are intrinsic to schizophrenic illness, whereas *secondary negative symptoms* refer to negative symptoms occurring in association with (and presumably caused by) positive symptoms, depression, extrapyramidal side effects, environmental deprivation, and so on. Carpenter et al. suggested that secondary negative symptoms were usually responsive to treatment of the underlying cause (e.g., positive symptoms, depression). They further suggested a number of possible pathophysiological mechanisms for primary negative symptoms, including brain amine deficiency and frontal lobe dysfunction. They indicated that the precise mechanism underlying primary negative symptoms was not known and that there was no available intervention with established efficacy in treating primary symptoms.

Carpenter et al. (1988) subsequently refined this concept and suggested a subclassification between deficit and nondeficit schizophrenia. They reiterated the distinction between primary and secondary negative symptoms, and further differentiated primary negative symptoms into *nonenduring or (psychotic) phasic primary negative symptoms* and *enduring or deficit primary negative symptoms.* They suggested that the presence of deficit symptoms defined a subgroup of schizophrenic patients, and indicated that some specific pathophysiological process, whose nature was unknown, caused the deficit symptoms and was present only in this subgroup of schizophrenic patients. It was further suggested that there was no effective treatment for deficit symptoms.

In a further refinement of the concept, Carpenter and Buchanan (1989) hypothesized that deficit processes were one of five distinct domains of psychopathology in schizophrenia; each domain presumably had a unique underlying pathophysiology and thus merited independent investigation and could be used to subgroup cohorts of schizophrenic patients. The other four domains were delusions and hallucinations, cognitive impairment, dissociative affective processes, and neurological processes.

This model is perhaps the most widely used framework for understanding negative symptoms at the present time, as it incorporates several useful refinements of the original positive–negative symptom dichotomy. A careful examination of these refinements and the theoretical, pathophysiological, and treatment implications of this model may be useful.

First, this model differentiates between primary and secondary negative symptoms. The fact that many different factors in schizophrenia can contribute to the phenotypic expression of negative symptoms, which are indistinguishable except when one considers the overall clinical picture (Carpenter 1991; Sommers 1985; Tandon and Greden 1990), is an important point to note. Whether one can reliably differentiate between primary and secondary negative symptoms, however, is questionable. Furthermore, even though depression, extrapyramidal syndromes, positive symptoms, the deficit process, and so on can all separately cause phenotypic negative symptoms, it is possible that all these etiologic agents act via a common mechanism (Berman and Weinberger 1990; Bermanzohn and Siris 1992; Tandon and Greden 1989, 1991). Although the distinction between primary and secondary negative symptoms is logical and makes good common sense, operationalizing this distinction is problematic.

A second important refinement of this model is that it incorporates a longitudinal perspective. Deficit symptoms are delineated not merely by the absence of other etiologic factors (i.e., those that cause secondary negative symptoms) but also by the need for a minimum 1-year duration. The distinction between nonenduring, transient (psychotic-phasic) and enduring, deficit primary negative symptoms is important; it implies that there may be two separate pathophysiological processes (both unique to schizophrenia and part of the core illness) that contribute to the production of negative symptoms at different stages of the schizophrenic illness. The distinction between nonenduring and enduring primary negative symptoms appears to be valid, in that these types of primary negative symptoms have distinct clinical and neurobiological correlates (Tandon et al. 1990).

It is not clear, however, whether enduring negative symptoms constitute a homogeneous entity. It is well known that a significant proportion of schizophrenic patients exhibit poor premorbid functioning (mainly because of negative symptoms); it is also known that schizophrenic illness is characterized by a progressive deterioration, mainly through a worsening of negative symptoms (McGlashan and Fenton 1993), particularly in the first 5 years or so of the illness

(M. Bleuler 1978; Ciompi 1983). It is possible (but certainly not established) that the same mechanism contributes to the production of both premorbid and deteriorative components of enduring negative symptoms. In fact, the data suggest that premorbid and deteriorative enduring negative symptoms may reflect different pathophysiological mechanisms (Bilder et al. 1985; DeQuardo et al. 1994).

Finally, it is not clear whether deficit symptoms (even if one accepts that they can be reliably defined) delineate a distinct subgroup of schizophrenic patients who are different in important ways (e,g., in terms of genetics, neurobiology) from other schizophrenic patients. Although the distinction between deficit and nondeficit subtypes has been heuristically useful in the study of the etiology, pathophysiology, course, and treatment of schizophrenia, that distinction is far less useful in the description of individual patients. Indeed, the ubiquity of deficit symptoms among schizophrenic patients strongly argues in favor of a dimensional view, in which the degree of deficit, rather than the presence or absence of deficit, is described. This question is unresolved and clearly needs further study.

Other Models for Categorizing Schizophrenic Illness Based on Positive and Negative Symptoms

Other models of categorizing schizophrenic illness either are not as well developed as the models discussed above or are only indirectly based on positive–negative symptoms; consequently, they are only briefly mentioned here.

Keefe et al. (1988) proposed a distinction between Kraepelinian and non-Kraepelinian schizophrenia, based on the outcome of the illness (i.e., the presence or absence of deterioration and severe debilitation). Keefe and colleagues associated Kraepelinian schizophrenia with more severe negative symptoms, greater familial loading of schizophrenia spectrum disorders, structural brain abnormalities, and poor response to treatment. There is some overlap between the positive–negative and the Kraepelinian–non-Kraepelinian dichotomy in that there are some common correlates of negative and Kraepelinian schizophrenia. More extensive studies indicate, however, that this overlap is superficial and that Kraepelinian patients have severe, relatively treatment-refractory positive and negative symptoms (Keefe et al. 1991; Tapp et al. 1992).

Schizophrenic patients have been classified on the basis of neuroleptic treatment response into treatment-responsive and treatment-refractory subgroups. Although there is some obvious overlap here with the positive–negative classification, the two classification schemes do not directly match one another.

Kay (1990) and co-workers have repeatedly emphasized the distinction between negative symptoms in acute phases and negative symptoms in chronic phases of schizophrenic illness; this distinction is essentially analogous to the nonenduring–enduring primary negative symptom distinction referred to above.

Liddle (1987) suggested that the positive symptom syndrome has two separate components comprising three syndromes: 1) reality distortion (delusions–hallucinations), 2) disorganization (thought disorder–conceptual disorganization), and 3) negative symptoms. Factor analytical studies have provided limited support to this three-syndrome model (Arndt et al. 1991; Bilder et al. 1985). Liddle and co-workers provided preliminary data suggesting distinct neurobiological underpinnings (on the basis of positron-emission tomography studies) for these three syndromes. Although this model is promising, studies of its utility and validity are presently in their initial stages.

Making Sense of It All: How to Conceptualize Negative Symptoms

The negative symptom construct and the positive–negative syndrome distinction provide a useful organizing framework for understanding the heterogeneity of schizophrenic illness. However, the multiplicity of related but different conceptualizations of this construct (summarized above) leads to confusion. How does one piece together a simple, meaningful framework that incorporates current knowledge and has clear pathophysiological and treatment implications? In attempting to provide such a framework, we offer the following summary of current facts about negative symptoms:

1. Negative symptoms constitute an integral component of schizophrenic psychopathology. They may also occur in other psychiatric disorders or conditions, meaning that negative symptoms are not specific to schizophrenia.

2. There is convincing evidence that a negative syndrome exists. Although specific definitions may vary, there is a core negative syndrome profile consisting of affective blunting, emotional withdrawal, alogia, anhedonia, avolition, apathy, and amotivation.

3. Substantial data support the distinction between positive and negative syndromes. The two syndromes appear to have distinct clinical and neurobiological correlates, separate temporal sequences in the context of schizophrenic illness (elaborated in Chapter 6), and different prognostic implications and course.

4. The positive and negative syndromes are not, however, mutually exclusive and often coexist in the same patient. In a given schizophrenic patient, relative proportions and actual magnitude of positive and negative syndromes vary throughout the course of the illness. Consequently, cross-sectional classification of schizophrenic patients on the basis of the presence or absence of negative symptoms is meaningless. Such subtyping has not been found to be longitudinally stable (a point discussed at length in Chapter 6).

   Positive and negative syndromes may best be viewed as separate dimensions of schizophrenic illness, present to some degree in all patients, but with relatively independent clinical presentations, courses, and pathophysiology. The diagnosis of schizophrenia, in contrast to the diagnosis of other disorders, requires pathology along both dimensions. The positive and negative dimensions vary throughout the course of the illness, giving rise to the variety of clinical presentations seen cross-sectionally among schizophrenic patients and seen longitudinally in the same patient over the course of the illness.

5. Negative symptoms are not a unitary construct. They can be presented as a consequence of a variety of conditions that occur during the course of schizophrenic illness, including core schizophrenic pathology, depression, antipsychotic medication–induced extrapyramidal side effects, and so on (see Figure 5–1). As discussed previously, it is quite possible that a final common pathophysiological pathway may mediate negative symptoms attributable to multiple etiologic agents. Distinguishing among these etiologic factors is not easy, but an awareness of the contributing factors can provide a useful treatment framework.

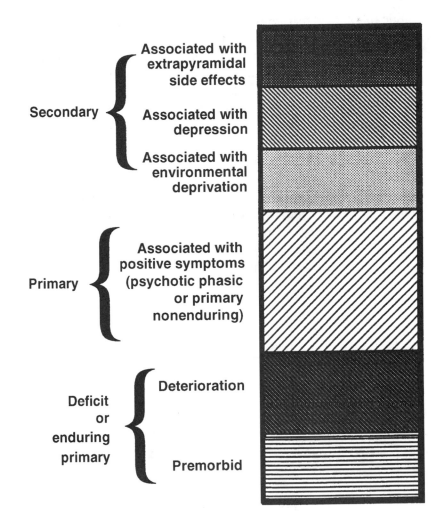

Figure 5–1. Components of negative symptoms in schizophrenia.

6. Effective treatment of secondary negative symptoms involves effective treatment of the suspected etiologic factor. For example, if a full-blown depressive syndrome is believed to underlie apparent negative symptoms in a particular schizophrenic patient, effective antidepressant treatment would be the treatment of choice.

7. From a longitudinal perspective, there appear to be three components of primary negative symptoms (see also Figure 5–2): 1) a premorbid component (i.e., negative symptoms that are present prior to the first psy-

chotic episode and that are associated with poor premorbid functioning); 2) a psychotic-phasic or nonenduring component (i.e., negative symptoms that occur only in association with positive symptoms and that are restricted to the period around a psychotic exacerbation of schizophrenic illness); and 3) a postpsychotic deterioration component (i.e., persistent negative symptoms that occur after a psychotic episode and that reflect deterioration and decline from premorbid levels of functioning). The pathophysiological basis of these components may differ; similarly, there may be different treatment strategies that are appropriate for these distinct elements of primary negative symptoms.

Although the mechanisms underlying these three components of primary negative symptoms have not been precisely delineated, it appears reasonable that possibly irreversible structural brain abnormalities (as reflected, for example, in atrophy of certain brain structures or ventricular enlargement) contribute to the premorbid and deteriorative components

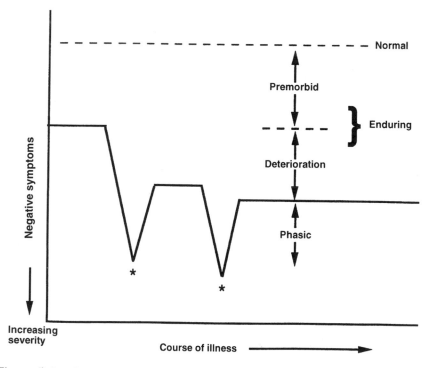

Figure 5–2. Components of primary negative symptoms in schizophrenia.
∗ = psychotic exacerbation.

and that reversible neurochemical changes (for example, cholinergic hyperactivity [Tandon and Greden 1989]) contribute to the psychotic-phasic component.

8. Negative symptoms are not completely refractory to neuroleptic treatment. In fact, there is strong evidence that negative symptoms do improve in the course of neuroleptic treatment (Meltzer 1990; Meltzer et al. 1986; Tandon and Greden 1989; Tandon et al. 1993a; van Kammen et al. 1987). Such improvement occurs in the acute phase of the illness and appears to covary with a concomitant improvement in positive symptoms (Meltzer 1990; Tandon and Greden 1989; van Kammen et al. 1987). This covariance suggests that improvement in these (psychotic-phasic, transient, nonenduring) primary negative symptoms is secondary to improvement in positive symptoms; alternatively, it suggests that related, but different, neurochemical mechanisms underlie positive symptoms and psychotic-phasic, nonenduring negative symptoms (e.g., concomitant dopaminergic and cholinergic hyperactivity underlie positive and negative symptoms, respectively, as proposed by Tandon and Greden [1989]).

9. Clozapine has been proposed to be uniquely effective in treating primary negative symptoms. Recent data suggest that the apparent greater efficacy of clozapine in treating negative symptoms may be attributable to its lower propensity to cause extrapyramidal side effects. This agent has also demonstrated greater clinical efficacy in treating positive symptoms in otherwise treatment-refractory patients. Recent data suggest that improvement in negative symptoms during clozapine therapy covaries with concomitant improvement in positive symptoms (Kane 1993; Tandon et al. 1993b). There is no evidence that clozapine benefits enduring or deficit negative symptoms; in fact, results of a recent study (Breier et al. 1992) suggested that clozapine may actually adversely affect deficit symptoms.

10. There appears to be no effective pharmacological treatment for premorbid primary negative symptoms. Cognitive retraining and other rehabilitative strategies for treating this component are being developed; currently, these strategies are investigational.

11. Although there is no effective pharmacological treatment for deteriorative negative symptoms, it may be possible to prevent or delay the development of such symptoms by rapid effective treatment of schizophrenia in the psychotic phase of the illness (this issue is discussed at length in Chapter 16).

Conclusion

The positive–negative syndrome distinction is an important organizing construct in understanding the heterogeneity of schizophrenia. There are multiple competing concepts (and terms) describing this syndrome that are not interchangeable. Negative symptoms themselves are heterogeneous, with multiple contributing factors. Although many pathophysiological mechanisms have been implicated in the expression of negative symptoms, none of these can be considered definitive. A longitudinal perspective and the framework of the overall clinical state are important in the assessment and effective management of negative symptoms.

References

Andreasen NC: Negative symptoms in schizophrenia: definition and reliability. Arch Gen Psychiatry 39:784–788, 1982

Andreasen NC, Flaum M, Swayze VW II, et al: Positive and negative symptoms in schizophrenia: a critical reappraisal. Arch Gen Psychiatry 47:615–621, 1990

Arndt S, Alliger RJ, Andreasen NC: The distinction of positive and negative symptoms: the failure of a two-dimensional model. Br J Psychiatry 158:317–322, 1991

Berman KF, Weinberger DR: Prefrontal dopamine and defect symptoms in schizophrenia, in Negative Schizophrenic Symptoms: Pathophysiology and Clinical Implications. Edited by Greden JF, Tandon R. Washington, DC, American Psychiatric Press, 1990, pp 81–95

Bermanzohn PC, Siris SC: Akinesia: a syndrome common to parkinsonism, retarded depression, and negative symptoms of schizophrenia. Compr Psychiatry 33:221–231, 1992

Bilder RM, Mukherjee S, Rieder RO, et al: Symptomatic and neuropsychological components of defect states. Schizophr Bull 11:409–419, 1985

Bleuler E: Dementia Praecox or The Group of Schizophrenias (1911). Translated by Zinkin J. New York, International Universities Press, 1950

Bleuler M: The Schizophrenic Disorders: Long-Term Patient and Family Studies. Translated by Clemens SM. New Haven, CT, Yale University Press, 1978

Breier A, Buchanan RW, Kirkpatrick B, et al: Clozapine in schizophrenic outpatients: efficacy, long-term outcome, and predictors. Scientific Abstracts of the annual meeting of the American College of Neuropsychopharmacology, San Juan, Puerto Rico, December 14–18, 1992

Carpenter WT Jr: Psychopathology and common sense: where we went wrong with negative symptoms. Biol Psychiatry 29:735–737, 1991

Carpenter WT Jr, Buchanan RW: Domains of psychopathology relevant to the study of etiology and treatment of schizophrenia, in Schizophrenia: Scientific Progress. Edited by Schulz SC, Tamminga CT. New York, Oxford University Press, 1989, pp 13–22

Carpenter WT Jr, Heinrichs DW, Alphs LD: Treatment of negative symptoms. Schizophr Bull 11:440–452, 1985

Carpenter WT Jr, Heinrichs DW, Wagman AMI: Deficit and nondeficit forms of schizophrenia: the concept. Am J Psychiatry 145:578–583, 1988

Ciompi L: Schizophrenic deterioration. Br J Psychiatry 143:79–80, 1983

Crow TJ: Molecular pathology of schizophrenia: more than one disease process. BMJ 280:66–68, 1980

Crow TJ: Schizophrenic deterioration. Br J Psychiatry 143:80–81, 1983

Crow TJ: The two-syndrome concept: origins and current status. Schizophr Bull 11:471–486, 1985

DeQuardo JR, Goldman R, Tandon R, et al: Ventricular enlargement, cognitive function, educational achievement, and premorbid function in schizophrenia. Biol Psychiatry 35:517–524, 1994

Kane JM: New developments in the pharmacologic treatment of schizophrenia. J Psychiatr Res 27:349–353, 1993

Kay SR: Longitudinal course of negative symptoms in schizophrenia, in Negative Schizophrenic Symptoms: Pathophysiology and Clinical Implications. Edited by Greden JF, Tandon R. Washington DC, American Psychiatric Press, 1990, pp 21–40

Keefe RSE, Mohs RC, Davidson M, et al: Kraepelinian schizophrenia: a subgroup of schizophrenia? Psychopharmacol Bull 24:56–61, 1988

Keefe RSE, Lobel DS, Mohs RC, et al: Diagnostic issues in chronic schizophrenia: Kraepelinian schizophrenia, undifferentiated schizophrenia, and state-independent negative symptoms. Schizophr Res 4:71–79, 1991

Kraepelin E: Dementia Praecox and Paraphrenia (1919). Translated by Barclay RM. New York, Krieger, 1971

Liddle PF: The symptoms of chronic schizophrenia: a re-examination of the positive-negative symptom dichotomy. Br J Psychiatry 151:145–151, 1987

McGlashan TH, Fenton WS: Subtype progression and pathophysiologic deterioration in early schizophrenia. Schizophr Bull 19:71–84, 1993

Meltzer HY: Pharmacological treatment of negative symptoms, in Negative Schizophrenic Symptoms: Pathophysiology and Clinical Implications. Edited by Greden JF, Tandon R. Washington DC, American Psychiatric Press, 1990, pp 215–231

Meltzer HY, Sommers AA, Luchins DJ: The effect of neuroleptics and other psychotropic drugs on negative symptoms in schizophrenia. J Clin Psychopharmacol 6:329–338, 1986

Schneider K: Clinical Psychopathology. Translated by Hamilton MW. New York, Grune & Stratton, 1959

Sommers AA: "Negative symptoms": conceptual and methodological problems. Schizophr Bull 11:364–379, 1985

Strauss JS, Carpenter WT Jr, Bartko JJ: The diagnosis and understanding of schizophrenia, III: speculations on the processes that underlie schizophrenic symptoms and signs. Schizophr Bull 11:61–75, 1974

Tandon R, Greden JF: Cholinergic hyperactivity and negative schizophrenic symptoms. Arch Gen Psychiatry 46:745–753, 1989

Tandon R, Greden JF: Conclusion: is integration possible? in Negative Schizophrenic Symptoms: Pathophysiology and Clinical Implications. Edited by Greden JF, Tandon R. Washington DC, American Psychiatric Press, 1990, pp 233–239

Tandon R, Greden JF: Negative symptoms of schizophrenia: need for conceptual clarity. Biol Psychiatry 30:321–325, 1991

Tandon R, DeQuardo JR, Goldman R: Psychotic phasic and deficit enduring subtypes of negative symptoms: biological markers and relationship to outcome (abstract). Biol Psychiatry 27:101A–102A, 1990

Tandon R, Ribeiro SCM, Goldman R, et al: Covariance of positive and negative symptoms during neuroleptic treatment in schizophrenia: a replication. Biol Psychiatry 34:495–497, 1993a

Tandon R, Goldman R, DeQuardo JR, et al: Positive and negative symptoms covary during clozapine treatment in schizophrenia. J Psychiatr Res 27:341–347, 1993b

Tapp A, Tandon R, Dudley E, et al: Clinical characteristics of Kraepelinian and nonKraepelinian schizophrenia: overlap with positive–negative dichotomy. Scientific Abstracts of Schizophrenia 1992, Vancouver, Canada, July 19–22, 1992

Van der Velde CD: Variability in schizophrenia, reflection of a regulatory disease. Arch Gen Psychiatry 33:489–496, 1976

van Kammen DP, Hommer DW, Malas KL: Effect of pimozide on positive and negative symptoms in schizophrenia: are negative symptoms state-dependent? Neuropsychobiology 18:113–117, 1987

Wyatt RJ, Alexander RC, Egan MF, et al: Schizophrenia, just the facts. Schizophr Res 1:3–18, 1988

CHAPTER 6

Epidemiology of Positive and Negative Symptoms in Schizophrenia

Heinz Häfner, M.D., Ph.D., Drs.h.c.,
and Kurt Maurer, Ph.D.

What Are Negative Symptoms?

The global notion of "positive versus negative symptoms" dates back to the British psychiatrist J. R. Reynolds (1858) and the neurologist J. H. Jackson (1889), who used the term later than Reynolds (see Berrios 1991). The distinction between positive and negative symptoms in schizophrenia was first proposed by Wing and Brown (1970). They distinguished between the florid or positive symptoms of a psychotic episode and the *clinical poverty syndrome* of chronic schizophrenia, characterized by emotional apathy, slowness of thought and movement, underactivity, lack of drive, poverty of speech, and social withdrawal. Referring to the work of Venables and colleagues (Venables 1957; Venables and Wing 1962), in which negative symptoms could be interpreted as a protective mechanism against hyperarousal, Wing (1978) assumed causal relationships between the two symptom dimensions. Together with Brown (Wing and Brown 1970), he also showed that an understimulating hospital environment was capable of exacerbating negative symptoms, whereas mild social stimulation could improve them, though not to any dramatic extent.

In 1974, Strauss et al. suggested that the two symptom dimensions represented independent processes with different underlying pathophysiologies in schizophrenia. Their hypothesis gave a strong impetus to the development of etiologic concepts about schizophrenia. The most outstanding examples of follow-up to Strauss et al.'s ideas were the dichotomous models proposed by Crow (1980b; type I and type II schizophrenia) and Andreasen and Olsen (1982; positive, negative, and mixed schizophrenia). But the situation in real life appeared to be more complex than represented in either of these two models (Andreasen et al. 1991).

Carpenter et al. (1991) went one step further by differentiating primary and secondary negative symptoms. The criteria for primary or deficit negative symptoms—1) that they be stable over time, 2) that they not be secondary to environmental factors, and 3) that they not respond to neuroleptic medication—were based on the assumption of different etiologies for which no external criteria were yet available apart from therapy response. According to these authors, secondary negative symptoms were not causally associated with the disease process. At the current state of knowledge, Carpenter et al.'s criteria merely serve as a basis for tentative hypotheses (e.g., which items or factors pertaining to the negative syndrome are stable over time, and which items or factors vary with neuroleptic treatment and environmental factors).

Definition and Measurement of the Negative Syndrome

The most widely used scales for measuring schizophrenic symptoms are Andreasen's Scale for the Assessment of Negative Symptoms (SANS; Andreasen 1983) and Scale for the Assessment of Positive Symptoms (SAPS; Andreasen 1984), Lewine et al.'s (1983) scale for the assessment of negative and positive symptoms, and Kay et al.'s Positive and Negative Syndrome Scale (PANSS; 1987). All of these scales are derived from generally accepted psychopathology rating scales or assessment interviews (for reviews, see Barnes 1989; Pogue-Geile and Zubin 1988).

The SANS describes five major negative symptoms—affective blunting, alogia, avolition-apathy, anhedonia, and attentional impairment—each comprising two to seven items and a global rating. The SANS has proven reliable in cross-sectional, longitudinal, and correlation studies, although the results of these studies have not yet allowed a post hoc validation of the underlying constructs (Andreasen et al. 1991). The heuristic nature of the "negative syndrome" construct does not rule out the possibility that, instead of being unitary, the syndrome might after all contain several components. Possible components of the negative syndrome might be 1) persistent symptoms correlating with premorbid social and cognitive deficiencies or corollaries of neuropsychologically measurable deficits attributable to brain lesions; 2) variable symptoms representing direct expressions of the psychotic process; 3) residual states of psychotic episodes (in Kraepelin's sense), accumulating to a deficit state over time; and 4) coping behavior employing negative symptoms, such as avoidance of social contact or social and emotional withdrawal as a protective mechanism against relapses (Carpenter et al. 1985; Strauss 1987).

Attempts at Validating the Positive-Negative Syndrome Constructs Based on External Criteria

The usual definition of negative symptoms as deficits of normal functioning—as opposed to positive symptoms as phenomena normally absent—is a commonsense statement. The positive-negative distinction, essentially heuristic in nature (Andreasen 1985; Sommers 1985), has acquired clinical relevance because of the association of negative symptoms with the so-called residual or deficit states or defects (Andreasen 1982; Huber et al. 1980; Lewine and Sommers 1985) and the association of positive symptoms with the psychotic phases of illness; however, considerable overlap occurs between these two types of symptoms. For these reasons, great interest has been taken in the validation of the constructs on external criteria and the discovery of the underlying pathophysiological mechanisms and, hence, Crow's hypotheses (1980a, 1980b, 1991).

Research on the association of negative symptoms to cognitive deficits measurable by neuropsychological tests has yielded mainly positive results: "in general, cognitive tasks that emphasize speed and effortful processing appear to be most closely associated with negative symptoms" (Pogue-Geile and Zubin 1988, p. 32). However, a precise characterization of the negative symptoms representing expressions of cognitive deficits is still lacking.

Another objectively assessable external criterion is structural brain abnormalities. In some studies focusing on the subtypes of schizophrenia, brain-imaging techniques, such as computed tomography (CT) and magnetic resonance imaging (MRI) scans, have shown structural brain anomalies to be frequent in patients with prominent negative symptoms (Andreasen and Olsen 1982; Andreasen et al. 1991; Bogerts et al. 1991; Gross et al. 1982; Johnstone et al. 1976; Weinberger 1987). However, the findings have been conclusive neither with respect to the presence of an association between brain abnormalities and negative symptoms nor with respect to the areas affected in the brain. Several studies have found no association, or even a significant negative correlation, between negative symptom measures and measures of ventricular enlargement (see Pogue-Geile and Zubin 1988).

Consequently, positive CT or MRI findings have so far failed to validate the negative syndrome as a whole.

At the neurobiological level, Crow (1980b) assumed that positive symptoms might be produced by a dopamine hypersensitivity or excessive dopamine turnover, whereas negative symptoms—as the expressions of structural brain abnormalities—should not be related to dopaminergic neurotransmission at all, and thus should be unresponsive to neuroleptic medication or dopamine agonists. However, high amphetamine dosages appear to be capable of producing both positive and negative symptoms, whereas low dosages bring about only partial improvement in negative symptoms (Angrist et al. 1980, 1982; Goldberg 1985). On the other hand, high-dosage neuroleptic medications can provoke negative symptoms, such as reduced facial expression and poverty of speech, which would clearly be medication induced.

Because of a lack of precise in vivo symptom measures and artifactual considerations, postmortem studies provide only partial insight into the number of D_2 receptors associated with negative or positive symptoms in schizophrenia (Crow 1991; Glowinski et al. 1988).

Specificity of Negative Symptoms to Schizophrenia

Several studies have reported that overall negative symptom ratings in depressed inpatients are as high as or even higher than those of hospitalized schizophrenic patients. This applies especially to the symptoms of affective blunting, reduced facial expression, and anhedonia (Andreasen 1979; Berenbaum et al. 1987; Boeringa and Castellani 1982; Chaturvedi et al. 1985; Kulhara and Chadda 1987; Sommers 1985). The frequency of negative symptoms in schizophrenia has also been compared with their frequency in Parkinson's disease (Alpert and Rush 1983) and in schizoid-schizotypal personality disorder (Sommers 1985; for further discussion, see Tsuang et al. 1991); with extrapyramidal symptom ratings as indicators of neuroleptic side effects; and with ratings in long-term inpatients to assess institutionalization effects (Sommers 1985).

The overall result of studies, then, has been that negative symptom measures do not constitute a distinguishing characteristic of schizophrenia. This statement probably masks differences in detail, because the above studies did not pay attention to different stages of illness. In fact, Pogue-Geile and Harrow (1984) demonstrated that schizophrenic patients do show significantly higher levels of negative symptoms 1 year after hospital discharge than do depressed patients. This could suggest that, no matter how nonspecific it may be, the negative syndrome in schizophrenia differs from that observed in affective disorder patients in terms of its course pattern and probably also its underlying pathophysiology.

Although not appearing to be specific to schizophrenia, negative symptoms might be direct expressions of the schizophrenic disease process. The specificity of negative symptoms might be determined by their course pattern, as is the case for the specificity of the periodic attacks of fever in vivax malaria.

Negative and Positive Symptom Traits in Adult Populations

The continuity models, which postulate psychosis as the extreme end of a scale measuring schizophrenia-like personality traits (Gottesman and Shields 1972; Häfner 1988; Kretschmer 1921; Kringlen 1987; Meehl 1962; Parnas 1986), and the vulnerability hypothesis (Zubin and Spring 1977) have spurred population studies aimed at identifying individuals vulnerable to psychotic breakdowns. Apart from Eysenck's psychoticism dimension (P-scale of the Eysenck Personality Questionnaire; Eysenck and Eysenck 1975), which is based on a global construct that was not designed specifically for schizophrenia, all the scales used for this purpose have been developed primarily on the basis of positive symptoms (Bentall and Slade 1985; Eckblad and Chapman 1983; Tsuang et al. 1991). Claridge and Broks' Schizotypal Personality Questionnaire (1984) was modeled on eight DSM-III (American Psychiatric Association 1980) criteria for schizotypal personality disorders, of which at least two—social isolation and inadequate rapport and constricted affect—can be subsumed under the negative spectrum of symptoms. Chapman and colleagues' Social and Physical Anhedonia Scale (1976) is the only instrument that assesses a selective component of negative symptoms exclusively.

The results obtained with these assessment instruments are more or less comparable in quantitative terms, although the scales include different items out of the total spectrum of the symptoms associated with schizophrenia and may be based on different concepts. The prevalence rates reported range from 3% to 8% for the categories identified in adult populations by using various case definitions and threshold values. In addition to two other independent factors, Bentall and co-workers (1989) identified an anhedonia factor, which has consistently been reported in several other studies (Claridge 1990; Foulds and Bedford 1975; Raine and Allbutt 1989). No findings have come to our notice that would confirm an elevated risk for schizophrenia in individuals with an elevated anhedonia value or in individuals with schizoid or schizotypal personality disorder in the general population.

Genetic Transmission of Negative and Positive Syndromes

Twin studies.   Only a few twin studies have investigated the concordance of negative subtypes or negative subthreshold pathology under different definitions (Dworkin and Lenzenweger 1984; McGuffin et al. 1987, 1991; Siever and Gunderson 1979; Torgersen 1985). Obstacles that cannot be overcome satisfactorily in such studies are the low lifetime stability of the negative and particularly the positive syndrome (McGuffin et al. 1991) and the rarity of purely negative cases. The results indicate only a weak tendency to homotypy (McGuffin et al. 1987).

More clear-cut is the difference between monozygotic and dizygotic twins in schizotypal personality disorder, as defined by both symptom dimensions (Siever and Gunderson 1979; Torgersen 1985). The most pronounced results have been reported by Dworkin and Lenzenweger (1984). Rating negative symptoms on the basis of the SANS in 302 case histories from five twin studies (Fischer 1973; Gottesman and Shields 1972; Kringlen 1967; Slater 1953; Tienari 1963), these researchers obtained the highest concordance rates in monozygotic twins when the number of negative symptoms was high, and the lowest rates with positive symptoms.

Family studies.   Epidemiological family studies that have included all first-degree relatives of representative samples of schizophrenic patients are rare. In his review of eight family studies, Kendler (1988) mentioned three such studies. Maier et al.'s (1993) methodologically well-designed family study is another such study. Because several family studies conducted with less-sophisticated methodologies have concurrently yielded similar results—namely, significantly elevated rates of schizotypal personality disorder, ranging from 4.2% to 14.6%, in the first-degree relatives of schizophrenic patients (Baron et al. 1985; Kendler et al. 1981, 1984, 1985; Tsuang et al. 1991), the association of this subthreshold disorder with the schizophrenic genotype can no longer be doubted. Kendler et al. (1983) assessed the criteria for schizotypal personality disorder separately and found that four negative symptoms (social isolation, constricted affect, suspiciousness, and odd speech) showed markedly higher familiality than was shown by the positive-symptom criteria. Tsuang et al. (1991), too, using more precise SANS- and SAPS-based definitions, found that in relatives of schizophrenic patients, the prevalence of negative symptoms was significantly higher than that of positive symptoms. In an attempt to test Crow's dichotomy hypothesis, Tsuang et al. (1991), using a simple model of quantitative difference between negative and positive symptoms on a continuum of genetic liability rather than a model of two independent factors, were able to achieve a considerably better fit with the family data (Tsuang et al. 1991).

High-risk and adoption studies.   The third approach to testing hypotheses are high-risk (Mednick and Schulsinger 1980; Mednick et al. 1978) and adoption studies (Gunderson et al. 1983; Kendler et al. 1981; Kety 1988). The largest sample with the longest follow-up is the group of adopted-away offspring of schizophrenic mothers included in the Danish adoption study (Kendler et al. 1981; Kety 1988). When the investigation started in 1962, the sample consisted of 207 individuals at a mean age of 15 years. Further diagnostic assessments followed 5, 10, and 25 years later, up to a mean age of 40 years (Parnas et al. 1991). The Present State Examination (PSE; Wing et al. 1974) was first administered at the 10-year follow-up. Gunderson et al. (1983) reanalyzed the data from the Danish adoption study in terms of symptoms, discriminating between the biological parents of schizophrenic patients and nonpsychiatric control subjects. In contrast to psychosis-like positive symptoms, social isolation, deficient interpersonal relations, and impoverished affective experience proved to have high discriminative power. In an independent analysis of the Danish data, Kendler et al. (1982) and later also Parnas (1986) found that passive behavior and social withdrawal in the first 2 years of life differentiated the biological relatives of schizophrenic and control adoptees.

The results of twin, family, high-risk, and adoption studies seem to suggest that pronounced negative, rather than purely or predominantly positive, symptoms seem to represent a genetically transmitted form of the disorder, or at least a weak indicator of the schizophrenic genotype, in individuals who are not mentally ill.

Prevalence of Negative Symptoms in Schizophrenia

Epidemiological investigations of negative symptoms in schizophrenia require the collection of objective, precise, and reliable data on the morbidity variables. In addition, sufficiently large, representative samples covering the total risk period and comprising all first-onset cases from a fairly stable and demographically well-studied population in a defined period of time should be used.

The question of whether all individuals with a diagnosis of schizophrenia develop negative symptoms has considerable theoretical implications. Implicit or explicit in all the dichotomous models mentioned is the assumption that a substantial proportion of schizophrenic patients develop no or only a few negative symptoms. In fact, all studies providing data relevant to this question show that either positive or negative symptoms or both can be found in subsamples of schizophrenic patients at any one time. Nevertheless, the question is not easy to answer epidemiologically, given that cross-sectional studies are of low informative value when applied to an irregularly recurring disease like schizophrenia in which the two symptom dimensions probably do not run parallel courses. Rather, assessment of the lifetime risk for the occurrence of negative symptoms would be needed, an undertaking that could be accomplished only by following representative samples of first-admission schizophrenic patients for as long a period of time as possible.

Negative Symptoms at First Admission (Cross-Sectional Studies)

First-admission studies in schizophrenia have the advantage of allowing the investigation of approximately identical phases of illness, as it is the first acute episode that usually leads to the first hospital admission. This was the case in 87% of our "age, beginning, and course" (ABC) schizophrenia sample of 276 first-admission and directly investigated cases from a total population of about 1.5 million (Häfner et al.

1993b). At index admission, the patients were interviewed with the PSE; subsequently, behavioral ratings on the basis of the Psychological Impairments Rating Schedule (PIRS; Biehl et al. 1989a, 1989b) and SANS assessments (Andreasen 1983) were performed.

Of the 20 negative SANS symptoms (the global rating of the five sections was not considered), a mean of 6.7 symptoms (median = 6.0) was present at first admission. One patient showed a maximum of 19 symptoms. Only 19 patients (7.0%) of the sample did not present any negative symptoms (exceeding a threshold > 1) at first admission. Seventy-four (27.4%) patients had 10 or more negative symptoms. From these results we concluded that negative symptoms constitute an almost obligatory component of the symptomatology in the first psychotic episode.

The mean number of negative symptoms was determined by the section means of 2.06 for affective blunting, 0.67 for alogia, 1.33 for avolition-apathy, 2.06 for anhedonia, and 0.68 for attentional impairment. However, before being interpreted, the section means were corrected for the different numbers of symptoms included in each SANS section. The corrected average percentages of symptoms observed were 29.3% for affective blunting, 16.8% for alogia, 44.3% for avolition-apathy, 51.3% for anhedonia, and 34.0% for attentional impairment. Hence, the negative symptoms most frequent at this stage of illness belonged to the domain of anhedonia and avolition-apathy.

Age-at-Onset Differences in Negative and Positive Symptoms

The influence of age at onset on measures of negative symptomatology has not yet been studied systematically, although it played a role in Crow's (1980b) and Murray and Lewis's (1987) dichotomy models, including the traditional assumption that late-onset schizophrenia is associated with more affective and fewer negative symptoms. Reviewing more than 30 European studies on late-onset schizophrenia (age at onset > 40 years), Harris and Jeste (1988) found negative symptoms to be more frequent.

To compare symptomatology between age groups, we divided our ABC sample of 276 first-admission schizophrenic patients into three subsamples fairly equal in size (12–24 years; 25–34 years, and 35–59 years). After the alpha error was addressed by applying a split-half technique, only small differences emerged in the prevalence of negative and positive symptoms between the age groups, with poor concentration showing a maximum in the intermediate-age subsample, reduced facial expression being found in the youngest-age subsample, and positive Schneiderian first-rank symptoms showing no difference by age at all. Most of the age differences observed concerned nonspecific secondary symptoms, with anxiety items being most frequent in the youngest group and items of depression being most frequent in the intermediate group. With positive symptoms—delusions in particular—a trend toward a more differentiated elaboration and externalization with age emerged. This trend was reflected in the maximum of systematized paranoid delusions in the oldest group.

Our results demonstrated that age at onset does not have any substantial effect on the negative symptomatology in the early phase of the disorder. Hence, the results did not support the dichotomous models in which age at onset is postulated as a discriminating criterion (i.e., Crow's type I versus type II schizophrenia and Murray and Lewis's neurodevelopmental versus affective disorder models).

Sex Differences in Negative and Positive Symptoms

Although the prevailing opinion holds that negative symptoms are more frequent in male schizophrenic patients and positive symptoms more common in female schizophrenic patients, Pogue-Geile and Zubin (1988) concluded that none of the few studies that allowed adequate comparisons showed a significant excess of negative symptoms in males. Lewine and Meltzer (1984) even observed significantly more negative symptoms in females. Summarizing the results of these studies is difficult, however, as different measures of negative symptoms and heterogeneous stages of illness were included.

We analyzed sex differences at first admission in data from our ABC sample (51.8% females, 48.2% males). After the application of the split-half technique to eliminate the alpha error, no differences emerged in the 10 most frequent symptoms, in any negative symptoms, or in any positive symptoms of first rank. The only significant

($P \leq .01$) difference was found with positive symptoms and concerned the content of delusions. Sexual delusions occurred rarely and delusions of pregnancy occurred never in males, whereas in females both types of delusions were significantly more frequent. The most pronounced sex difference emerged in social behavior. Eleven socially negative behavioral items (e.g., self-neglect, poor social adjustment, loss of interest in getting a job or in going back to work or study, social inattentiveness, social withdrawal) were significantly more frequent in males, whereas the PIRS item "social overcompliance" was significantly more frequent in females. The group of socially negative behavioral items is closely associated with the negative syndrome, and some of the items are in fact included in the assessment instruments, particularly the SANS. Because no sex differences in the total scores of the negative core symptoms (e.g., affective blunting, anhedonia, alogia) emerged at the time of first admission, we were fairly confident that the differences observed pertained to illness behavior. They probably arose from innate male and female behavioral differences reflected in other domains of life as well as in the different frequency of asocial behavior and crimes of violence.

Epidemiology of the Early Course of Negative and Positive Symptoms

The earliest symptomatology of schizophrenia is of great interest because it might provide more direct clues to the disease process and the underlying pathophysiology than are provided by symptomatology later in the course of the illness, as the later course is influenced by coping behavior, environmental factors, and biological factors to a greater extent than is the earlier course.

An exact determination of the onset of schizophrenia is difficult. Because of the extremely low incidence rates of about 10 per 100,000 and the high proportion of nonspecific early courses of about 70% of schizophrenic patients, a purely prospective design is impracticable (Häfner and Maurer 1993). Undisputed is the fact that the disease is present prior to the first hospital admission for schizophrenia and in some cases for several years prior to the first contact with mental health professionals.

In the first systematic study on this topic, Lindelius (1970) found a mean period of latency of 4.4 years between the first appearance of positive symptoms and first admission (for a review, see Angermeyer and Kühn 1988). The 23.2 months reported by Lewine (1980) and the 1 year observed by Loebel et al. (1992) were preceded by substantial prepsychotic periods. The length of the pretreatment period in the early course of schizophrenia is a powerful predictor of the course of the first psychotic episode (Loebel et al. 1992). The untreated period depends on the type, extent, and social conspicuousness of symptoms, the availability of mental health services, and the help-seeking behavior of the population.

Whereas Kraepelin (1909–1915) and Bleuler (1911) described nonspecific symptoms such as increased irritability, capriciousness, and mood disturbances in the beginning of schizophrenia, Janzarik (1968) and Huber et al. (1979) observed that affective blunting, avolition-apathy, and disturbances of concentration and thinking frequently preceded the psychotic episode.

To assess the beginning and early course of schizophrenia, we used the standardized Interview for the Retrospective Assessment of the Onset of Schizophrenia (IRAOS; Häfner et al. 1992a), which we developed on the basis of a selection of internationally accepted instruments (e.g., PSE, SANS). Three different sources of information—the patient, a close relative, and objective data such as case records—were used to determine the first occurrence and the accumulation of symptoms until first hospital admission. Using a broad definition of diagnosis, we found that negative symptoms appeared first in 70% of the cases, positive and negative symptoms appeared simultaneously (within a month) in 20% of the cases, and positive symptoms appeared first in 10% of the cases. In the early course of schizophrenia, two phases were identified: a prepsychotic one with predominantly negative and nonspecific symptoms and a mean duration of 3.1 years (median = 1.1 years) and a subsequent psychotic one with a mean duration of only 1.6 years (median = 0.1 years) until productive symptoms reached their maximum (Zedlick et al. 1993). The differences between the means and medians reflected strongly skewed distributions, in which phases of short duration predominated and very long ones were rare (maximum duration of nonspecific—including negative—symptomatology was 28.6 years; maximum duration of positive symptomatology was 23.7 years).

When the accumulation of the two symptom dimensions was depicted as cumulative scores of 13 negative and 17 positive symptoms from the IRAOS, the increase in the number of negative symptoms was at first slow; however, as the time of the first admission drew closer, it gained momentum and became exponential (see Figure 6–1). Positive symptoms followed with a marked delay, and their accumulation was almost parallel to that of negative symptoms in the period immediately preceding first admission. Comparisons of these cumulative patterns of increase across the age and sex groups did not reveal relevant differences (Häfner et al. 1992b).

Variability or Persistence of Negative Symptoms Over the Long-Term Course

If negative symptoms are viewed as resulting from structural brain abnormalities (as per Crow 1980a, 1980b), they should either persist or gradually increase with the duration of the disease. The few studies

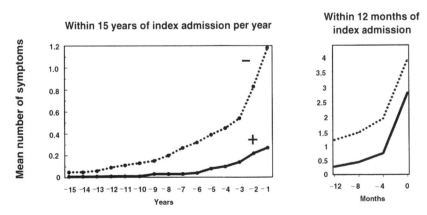

Figure 6–1. Cumulative values of persistent positive and negative symptoms up to first hospital admission for schizophrenia ($N = 236$).
Source. Häfner et al. 1993a.

assessing negative symptoms in schizophrenic patients receiving long-term hospital care (Knight et al. 1979; Roff and Knight 1978) have demonstrated higher values in later than in earlier stages of the disorder, thus supporting the residual-state or defect hypothesis. But these findings do not provide any evidence for case-related increases in negative symptoms.

Pogue-Geile and Harrow (1985) and Biehl et al. (1986) studied the persistence of positive and negative symptoms in the course of schizophrenia by following more or less representative samples prospectively for 2 and 5 years, respectively, and by including non-readmitted cases in their analyses. In both studies, the authors found that negative symptom ratings were reduced by about half at the first follow-up assessment, which occurred at 12 months (Pogue-Geile and Harrow study) and 6 months (Biehl et al. study) after first admission. Thereafter, the mean scores remained stable. On the basis of similar observations, Kay et al. (1986) hypothesized that negative symptoms assessed in the acute episode might be quite different from those assessed during other phases of the disorder.

In our ongoing study, we have assessed a subsample ($n = 133$) from our comprehensive ABC sample of first-admission schizophrenic patients three times: at 6 months, 1 year, and 2 years after index admission (see Figure 6–2). The results have confirmed Biehl et al.'s (1986) findings of initially high positive and negative symptom scores, their decrease by the 6-month assessment, and the subsequent stability of the mean scores throughout the 2-year follow-up period. In Table 6–1, the percentages of patients with symptoms from the five SANS sections at two consecutive cross-sectional assessments are given. Also illustrated is how the percentages varied as a result of changes in individual symptom prevalence (i.e., as a result of the disappearance or persistence of symptoms). After remission of the acute episode, negative symptoms were relatively frequent in the 2 years following first admission. At any follow-up assessment, affective blunting was present in about 40%–50% of the cases, avolition-apathy in 40%–60%, and anhedonia in 50%–60%, with alogia (10%–25%) and attentional impairment (20%–30%) being comparatively rare.

In contrast to the relatively constant proportions of patients with negative symptoms at any follow-up visit, a relatively large proportion

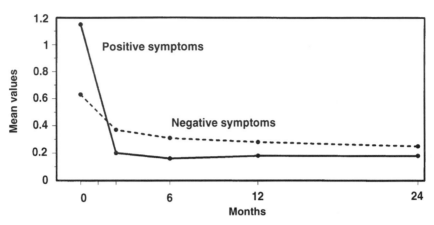

Figure 6–2. Mean values of factor analytic scores for positive and negative symptoms over 2 years. Data are from the course sample of the Mannheim Age, Beginning, and Course (ABC) Schizophrenia Study (n = 133).
Source. Häfner et al. 1993a.

of patients had fluctuating symptomatology. Half of the patients who had symptoms of blunted affect at 1-year follow-up did not show any such symptoms 1 year later. The same was true for alogia and avolition-apathy. Only anhedonia showed a markedly higher degree of persistence, but it was not possible to determine whether this symptom was attributable to secondary phenomena—for example, such as social impairment—or whether it represented a primary personality trait.

In contrast to this finding of high individual variability of negative symptoms, achieved on a sample assessed comprehensively at short intervals, Pfohl and Winokur (1982) and Johnstone et al. (1986), studying patients who had been continuously hospitalized for several years, found lower remission rates of 6% and 35%, respectively, for affective flattening and 29% and 19%, respectively, for poverty of speech in their study samples. It must be stressed that these findings were based on a selected sample of mainly chronic schizophrenic patients characterized by residual states, whereas a considerable proportion of our sample of first-hospitalization cases was bound to remit without developing any residual symptoms.

Despite the high proportion of transitions between the case subjects with and without negative symptoms, the five SANS section scores and the two factor-analytically derived subscores (Rey et al. 1992) were highly significantly associated with the scores at the next follow-up (Table 6–2). The correlation coefficients for t_0 and t_1 were significantly lower, whereas those for the 6-month and the 1-year follow-up were substantially higher (.57 and .68, respectively), except for alogia. What has been said about the section scores basically applies as well to the two factor-analytic scores of anhedonia and affective blunting (see Rey et al. 1992). From these results, we concluded that negative symptoms occurring in the psychotic episode are a poor predictor of later recurrence or persistence of negative symptomatol-

Table 6–1. Percentages of cases from follow-up subsample (n = 133) of the Mannheim Age, Beginning, and Course (ABC) Schizophrenia Study with negative symptoms (SANS global ratings) and changes therein at consecutive assessments

Global rating	Period of change	t	+[a]	−[b]	t + 1
Blunted affect	$t_{0/1}$	45.5	15.8	15.8	45.5
	$t_{1/2}$	47.8	10.0	10.0	47.8
	$t_{2/3}$	50.6	14.1	24.7	40.0
Alogia	$t_{0/1}$	26.7	5.0	18.8	12.9
	$t_{1/2}$	12.2	13.3	7.8	17.8
	$t_{2/3}$	18.8	4.7	12.9	10.6
Avolition	$t_{0/1}$	62.4	13.9	28.7	47.5
	$t_{1/2}$	48.9	11.1	10.0	50.0
	$t_{2/3}$	47.1	10.6	20.0	37.6
Anhedonia	$t_{0/1}$	61.4	11.9	22.8	50.5
	$t_{1/2}$	52.2	12.2	7.8	56.7
	$t_{2/3}$	57.6	8.2	15.3	50.6
Attention	$t_{0/1}$	31.6	9.2	15.3	25.5
	$t_{1/2}$	30.2	8.1	12.8	25.6
	$t_{2/3}$	26.3	6.3	13.8	18.8

Note. **Definition of timepoints:** t_0 = at index admission; t_1 = 6 months after index admission; t_2 = 1 year after index admission; t_3 = 2 years after index admission. **Periods of change:** $t_{0/1}$ = from t_0 to t_1 (t = t_0; t + 1 = t_1). $t_{1/2}$ = from t_1 to t_2 (t = t_1; t + 1 = t_2). $t_{2/3}$ = from t_2 to t_3 (t = t_2; t + 1 = t_3). SANS: Scale for the Assessment of Negative Symptoms (Andreasen 1983).
[a]Percentage of patients without negative symptoms at t and with negative symptoms at t + 1.
[b]Percentage of patients with negative symptoms at t and without negative symptoms at t + 1.
Source. For data: Häfner et al. 1993a.

Table 6–2.   Stability (Pearson correlations) of five (additive) SANS section scores and two factor-analytic scores

Symptom	$t_{0/1}$	$t_{1/2}$	$t_{2/3}$	$t_{0/2}$
Section scores				
Blunted affect	.38*	.57*	.42*	$.14^{ns}$
Alogia	.36*	.38*	.37*	.30*
Avolition	.35*	.66*	.53*	.33*
Anhedonia	.39*	.68*	.61*	.44*
Attention	.32*	.62*	.56*	.34*
Factor scores				
Anhedonia	.40*	.71*	.63*	.46*
Blunted affect	.35*	.58*	.42*	$.18^{ns}$

Note. **Definition of timepoints:** t_0 = at index admission; t_1 = 6 months after index admission; t_2 = 1 year after index admission; t_3 = 2 years after index admission. **Significance levels of Pearson correlations:** ns = not significant; * = $P \leq .01$. **Pearson correlations of negative symptoms:** at t_0 and t_1: $t_{0/1}$; at t_1 and t_2: $t_{1/2}$; at t_2 and t_3: $t_{2/3}$; at t_0 and t_2: $t_{0/2}$. SANS: Scale for the Assessment of Negative Symptoms (Andreasen 1983).
Source. For data: Häfner et al. 1993a.

ogy and, consequently, of an unfavorable long-term course, whereas the occurrence of negative symptoms in nonpsychotic phases is a powerful predictor of such subsequent events.

Independence of Positive and Negative Symptom Dimensions

In most cross-sectional studies conducted among schizophrenic patients, positive and negative symptoms have turned out to be statistically independent (Bilder et al. 1985). However, Pogue-Geile and Zubin's (1988) conclusion that this independence "suggests that the direct pathophysiologies of the two syndromes differ" (p. 16) is to be taken with caution. In an illness running an irregular course through episodes, intervals, and different degrees of residual states, the heterogeneity of the stages assessed can mask relationships between the two symptom dimensions that might otherwise be discernible as cross-sectional or longitudinal relationships if the stages of illness were homogeneous.

Independence is assumed in the dichotomous models proposed by Crow (1980a, 1980b) and Murray and Lewis (1987), whereas Andreasen and colleagues, who originally presumed a negative correlation between the two syndromes, now consider interdependence possible (Andreasen et al. 1991).

Another factor contributing to the heterogeneity of research results is that, as our findings presented in Table 6–3 show, a theory of either dependence or independence can be supported, depending on how the syndromes are operationalized. When cumulative scores of 13 negative and 17 positive PSE items were used, significantly positive, though low, correlations emerged throughout, except for the assessment at first admission; this finding was similar to that obtained on the early, preclinical course (Häfner and Maurer 1991). Additionally, we used the operationalization of Biehl et al. (1989b), who took from the Psychological Impairments Rating Schedule (PIRS) 30 positive and 20 negative items, thus forming two sum-scores—POSY (positive symptoms score) and NESY (negative symptoms score). for these operationalizations of functional impairments, the correlations dropped below the level of significance and were nearly zero at the 2-year follow-up. In the World Health Organization disability study (Maurer and Häfner 1991), both the PSE and the PIRS scores had yielded a similar result.

Table 6–3. Dependence or independence of positive and negative symptoms: comparison of factor-analytic PSE symptom scores and clinical (intuitive) PIRS impairment scores

	t_0	t_1	t_2	t_3
Reported PSE symptoms				
$r\pm$	$.15^{ns}$	$.27^*$	$.45^*$	$.46^*$
Observed PIRS impairments				
$r\pm$	$.10^{ns}$	$.18^{ns}$	$.14^{ns}$	$.01^{ns}$

Note. **Definition of timepoints:** t_0 = at index admission; t_1 = 6 months after index admission; t_2 = 1 year after index admission; t_3 = 2 years after index admission. **Other:** $r\pm$ = Pearson correlation of positive and negative symptoms: ns = not significant; $^*P \le .01$. PSE: Present State Examination (Wing et al. 1974); PIRS: Psychological Impairments Rating Schedule (Biehl et al. 1989a, 1989b).
Source. For data: Häfner et al. 1993a.

The Prognostic Value of Negative and Positive Symptoms

Negative symptoms—blunted affect in particular—have long been assumed to be a poor prognostic sign not only of later functioning, but also of the long-term course and outcome of schizophrenia, including positive symptomatology. The prognostic value of positive symptoms has always been regarded as low (Schubart et al. 1987).

We tested this assumption on data from our ABC cohort, trying to determine whether positive and negative symptoms at first admission correlate with positive and negative symptoms later in the course. As demonstrated in Table 6–4, no significant correlations emerged between negative symptoms at first admission and positive symptoms in the later course at any follow-up visit over a 2-year period. In contrast, early positive symptoms turned out to be positively and significantly correlated with later negative symptoms almost throughout follow-up, with the coefficients, ranging from .20 to .30, being rather low. This result contradicted the finding of the prospective Disability Study—

Table 6–4.   Pearson correlations between early positive symptoms and later negative symptoms and between early negative symptoms and later positive symptoms measured by PSE

Positive symptoms	Negative symptoms		
	t_1	t_2	t_3
t_0	.21*	.26**	.20^{ns}
t_1	–	.28**	.25*
t_2	–	–	.30**
Negative symptoms	Positive symptoms		
	t_1	t_2	t_3
t_0	.01^{ns}	.09^{ns}	.08^{ns}
t_1	–	.04^{ns}	.13^{ns}
t_2	–	–	.12^{ns}

Note. **Definition of timepoints:** t_0 = at index admission; t_1 = 6 months after index admission; t_2 = 1 year after index admission; t_3 = 2 years after index admission. **Significance levels of Pearson correlations:** ns = not significant; * = $P \le .05$; ** = $P \le .01$. PSE: Present State Examination (Wing et al. 1974).
Source. For data: Häfner et al. 1993a.

which included seven cross-sectional assessments in 5 years (see Maurer and Häfner 1991)—that negative symptoms predicted later positive symptoms. This discrepancy has yet to be explained.

Patterns of Course of Negative Symptoms

To obtain a more differentiated picture of the course of negative symptoms, we set up empirical course categories on the basis of the SANS global ratings. At each follow-up, the presence of negative symptoms exceeding a critical threshold value (rating > 1) was assessed. The categories used were

- Type 1—free of symptom (i.e., the symptom was not present at any follow-up)
- Type 2—nonrecurring (i.e., the symptom was observed once, but had disappeared by the 2-year follow-up)
- Type 3—recurring (i.e., the symptom was present at several follow-ups)
- Type 4—continuous (i.e., the symptom was present at all four follow-ups).

As shown in Table 6–5, the continuous pattern (Type 4) was the rarest. As in other analyses, too, the persistence indicator was at its highest in anhedonia, which in one-quarter of the cases showed the continuous pattern of course. Avolition-apathy displayed a continuous course in 15% of the cases only, and blunted affect, in 10%. These

Table 6–5. SANS course types over 2 years (percentages)

SANS global rating	Type 1	Type 2	Type 3	Type 4
Blunted affect	25.3	51.9	12.7	10.1
Alogia	53.2	40.5	3.8	2.5
Avolition	13.9	55.7	15.2	15.2
Anhedonia	19.0	40.5	13.9	26.6
Attention	50.0	38.9	4.2	6.9

Note. **Definition of course types (based on SANS global ratings):** Type 1 = free of symptoms; Type 2 = nonrecurring; Type 3 = recurring; Type 4 = continuous. SANS: Scale for the Assessment of Negative Symptoms (Andreasen 1983).
Source. For data: Häfner et al. 1993a.

results once again clearly contradicted the hypothesis postulating predominantly stable personality traits or largely stable brain lesions as causes underlying the negative symptomatology. However, it cannot be ruled out that negative symptomatology as a whole or components of it become increasingly stable over a lengthy illness course.

The above finding—achieved at the level of the global ratings of the five SANS sections—was confirmed at the item level. The proportion of continuous courses was still smaller here. Apart from the two anhedonia items (recreational interests and activities [16.5%] and relationships with friends and peers [15.2%]), all the other items yielded percentages below 10%. Five symptoms (poor eye contact, affective nonresponsivity, and the alogia symptoms except poverty of speech) did not show a continuous type of course in any of the cases included.

Conclusion

Schizophrenia as broadly defined starts with negative symptoms in 70% of cases and with positive symptoms in only 10% of cases. There is a significant positive correlation between the two symptom measures in the early preclinical course, although the coefficients are relatively low. After the first psychotic episode, negative symptoms remit by a mean of about 50%. In the post–first-episode course, too, variability exceeds persistence. The few epidemiological studies conducted have indicated slight increases in the means over the first 5 years after first admission. Whether that trend continues or changes its direction in the post–5-year course is not known.

Patients' age at onset and sex do not appear to have any major effect on the type and extent of negative symptoms at first admission, in contrast with findings on patients undergoing long-term institutional care. But social behavior, showing limited overlap with the common operationalizations of the negative syndrome, appears to differ considerably between the sexes in the preclinical course. The predominance of socially negative behavior in male schizophrenic patients and of social overcompliance in female schizophrenic patients probably reflects normal male and female behavioral stereotypes and not sex differences in the disease process.

As far as hypotheses about the positive and negative syndromes are concerned, research has failed to confirm the dichotomous models of schizophrenia (Andreasen and Olsen 1982; Crow 1980a, 1980b; Murray and Lewis 1987). The same is true for the postulations about two independent neurophysiological processes as the underlying causes of the positive and the negative syndromes (Carpenter et al. 1991; Strauss and Carpenter 1974).

A consistent finding of genetic-epidemiological studies is that in nonschizophrenic relatives or probands at risk, case definitions based on negative symptom measures yield better fits with heritability models than case definitions based on subliminal positive symptom measures. This finding and the major role negative symptoms play in the early course of schizophrenia suggest that, despite their unestablished specificity to schizophrenia, negative symptoms contain the core syndrome of the disease. Whether this statement also applies to positive symptoms more specific to schizophrenia has yet to be clarified.

References

Alpert M, Rush M: Comparison of affects in Parkinson's disease and schizophrenia. Psychopharmacol Bull 19:118–120, 1983

American Psychiatric Association: Diagnostic and Statistical Manual of Mental Disorders, 3rd Edition. Washington, DC, American Psychiatric Association, 1980

Andreasen NC: Affective flattening and criteria for schizophrenia. Am J Psychiatry 136:944–947, 1979

Andreasen NC: Negative symptoms in schizophrenia: definition and reliability. Arch Gen Psychiatry 39:784–788, 1982

Andreasen NC: The Scale for the Assessment of Negative Symptoms (SANS). Iowa City, IA, University of Iowa, 1983

Andreasen NC: The Scale for the Assessment of Positive Symptoms (SAPS). Iowa City, IA, University of Iowa, 1984

Andreasen NC: Positive versus negative schizophrenia: a critical evaluation. Schizophr Bull 11:380–389, 1985

Andreasen NC, Olsen S: Negative versus positive schizophrenia: definition and validation. Arch Gen Psychiatry 39:789–794, 1982

Andreasen NC, Flaum M, Arndt S, et al: Positive and negative symptoms: assessment and validity, in Negative Versus Positive Schizophrenia. Edited by Marneros A, Andreasen NC, Tsuang MT. Berlin, Springer, 1991, pp 28–51

Angermeyer MC, Kühn L: Gender differences in age at onset of schizophrenia: an overview. Eur Arch Psychiatry Clin Neurosci 237:351–364, 1988

Angrist BM, Rotrosen J, Gershon S: Differential effects of amphetamine and neuroleptics on negative versus positive symptoms in schizophrenia. Psychopharmacology 72:17–19, 1980

Angrist BM, Peselow E, Rubinstein M, et al: Partial improvement in negative schizophrenic symptoms after amphetamine. Psychopharmacology 78:128–130, 1982

Barnes TRE: Negative symptoms in schizophrenia. Br J Psychiatry 155 (suppl 7):8–135, 1989

Baron M, Gruen R, Rainer JD, et al: A family study of schizophrenic and normal control probands: implications for the spectrum concept of schizophrenia. Am J Psychiatry 145:447–455, 1985

Bentall PR, Slade PD: Reliability of a scale measuring disposition towards hallucinations: a brief report. Personality and Individual Differences 6:527–529, 1985

Bentall RP, Claridge GS, Slade PD: The multidimensional nature of schizotypal traits: a factor analytic study with normal subjects. Br J Clin Psychol 28:363–375, 1989

Berenbaum SA, Abrams R, Rosenberg S, et al: The nature of emotional blunting: a factor analytic study. Psychiatry Res 20:57–67, 1987

Berrios GE: Positive and negative signals: a conceptual history, in Negative Versus Positive Schizophrenia. Edited by Marneros A, Andreasen NC, Tsuang MT. Berlin, Springer, 1991, pp 8–27

Biehl H, Maurer K, Schubart C, et al: Prediction of outcome and utilization of medical services in a prospective study of first onset schizophrenics. Eur Arch Psychiatr Neurosci 236:139–147, 1986

Biehl H, Maurer K, Jablensky A, et al: The WHO psychological impairments rating schedule (WHO/PIRS), I: introducing a new instrument for rating observed behaviour and the rationale of the psychological impairment concept. Br J Psychiatry 155:68–70, 1989a

Biehl H, Maurer K, Jung E, et al: The WHO psychological impairments rating schedule (WHO/PIRS), II: impairments in schizophrenics in cross-sectional and longitudinal perspective—the Mannheim experience in two independent samples. Br J Psychiatry 155:71–77, 1989b

Bilder RM, Mukherjee S, Rieder RO, et al: Symptomatic and neuropsychological components of defect states. Schizophr Bull 11:409–417, 1985

Bleuler E: Dementia praecox oder Gruppe der Schizophrenien, in Handbuch der Psychiatrie. Edited by Aschaffenburg G. Leipzig, Germany, Deuticke, 1911, pp 1–420

Boeringa JA, Castellani S: Reliability and validity of emotional blunting as a criterion for diagnosis of schizophrenia. Am J Psychiatry 139:1131–1135, 1982

Bogerts B, Falkai P, Degreef G, et al: Neuropathological and brain imaging studies in positive and negative schizophrenia, in Negative Versus Positive Schizophrenia. Edited by Marneros A, Andreasen NC, Tsuang MT. Berlin, Springer, 1991, pp 292–316

Carpenter WT, Heinrichs DW, Alphs LD: Treatment of negative symptoms. Schizophr Bull 11:440–452, 1985

Carpenter WT, Buchanan RW, Kirkpatrick B, et al: Negative symptoms: a critique of current approaches, in Negative Versus Positive Schizophrenia. Edited by Marneros A, Andreasen NC, Tsuang MT. Berlin, Springer, 1991, pp 126–133

Chapman LJ, Chapman JP, Raulin ML: Scales for physical and social anhedonia. J Abnorm Psychol 85:374–382, 1976

Chaturvedi SK, Prasad Rao G, Mathai JP, et al: Negative symptoms in schizophrenia and depression. Indian Journal of Psychiatry 27:237–241, 1985

Claridge GS: Can a disease model of schizophrenia survive? in Reconstructing Schizophrenia. Edited by Bentall RP. London, Routledge, 1990, pp 157–183

Claridge GS, Broks P: Schizotypy and hemisphere function, 1: theoretical considerations and the measurement of schizotypy. Personality and Individual Differences 5:633–648, 1984

Crow T: Molecular pathology of schizophrenia: more than one disease process? BMJ 280:66–68, 1980a

Crow T: Positive and negative schizophrenic symptoms and the role of dopamine. Br J Psychiatry 137:383–386, 1980b

Crow T: The demise of the Kraepelinian binary concept and the aetiological unity of the psychoses, in Negative Versus Positive Schizophrenia. Edited by Marneros A, Andreasen NC, Tsuang MT. Berlin, Springer, 1991, pp 425–440

Dworkin RH, Lenzenweger MF: Symptoms and the genetics of schizophrenia: implications for diagnosis. Am J Psychiatry 141:1541–1546, 1984

Eckblad M, Chapman LJ: Magical ideation as an indicator of schizotypy. J Consult Clin Psychol 51:215–225, 1983

Eysenck HJ, Eysenck SBG: Manual of the Eysenck Personality Questionnaire. London, Hodder & Stoughton, 1975

Fischer M: Genetic and environmental factors in schizophrenia: a study of schizophrenic twins and their families. Acta Psychiatr Scand Suppl 238:1–158, 1973

Foulds GA, Bedford A: Hierarchy of classes of personal illness. Psychol Med 5:181–192, 1975

Glowinski J, Hervé D, Tassin JP: Heterologous regulation of receptors on target cells of dopamine neurons in the prefrontal cortex, nucleus accumbens and striatum. Ann N Y Acad Sci 137:112–123, 1988

Goldberg SC: Negative and deficit symptoms in schizophrenia do respond to neuroleptics. Schizophr Bull 11:453–456, 1985

Gottesman II, Shields J: Schizophrenia and Genetics: A Twin Study Vantage Point. New York, Academic Press, 1972

Gross G, Huber G, Schüttler R: Computerized tomography studies on schizophrenic diseases. Archiv für Psychiatrie und Nervenkrankheiten 231:519–526, 1982

Gunderson JG, Siever LJ, Spaulding E: The search for a schizotype: crossing the border again. Arch Gen Psychiatry 40:15–22, 1983

Häfner H: What is schizophrenia? Eur Arch Psychiatr Neurosci 238:63–72, 1988

Häfner H, Maurer K: Are there two types of schizophrenia? true onset and sequence of positive and negative syndromes prior to first admission, in Negative Versus Positive Schizophrenia. Edited by Marneros A, Andreasen NC, Tsuang MT. Berlin, Springer, 1991, pp 134–159

Häfner H, Maurer K: Methodenprobleme der Erforschung von Krankheitsbeginn und Frühverlauf am Beispiel der Schizophrenie. Fundamenta Psychiatrica 7:1–12, 1993

Häfner H, Riecher-Rössler A, Hambrecht M, et al: IRAOS: an instrument for the assessment of onset and early course of schizophrenia. Schizophr Res 6:209–223, 1992a

Häfner H, Riecher-Rössler A, Maurer K, et al: First onset and early symptomatology of schizophrenia. Eur Arch Psychiatry Neurosci 242:109–118, 1992b

Häfner H, Riecher-Rössler A, an der Heiden W, et al: Generating and testing a causal explanation of the gender difference in age at first onset of schizophrenia. Psychol Med 23:925–940, 1993a

Häfner H, Maurer K, Löffler W, et al: The influence of age and sex on the onset and early course of schizophrenia. Br J Psychiatry 162:80–86, 1993b

Harris MJ, Jeste DV: Late-onset schizophrenia: an overview. Schizophr Bull 14:39–55, 1988

Huber G, Gross G, Schüttler R: Schizophrenie. Eine Verlaufs- und sozialpsychiatrische Langzeitstudie. Berlin, Springer, 1979

Huber G, Gross G, Schüttler R, et al: Longitudinal studies of schizophrenic patients. Schizophr Bull 6:592–605, 1980

Jackson JH: On postepileptic states: a contribution to the comparative study of insanities. Journal of Mental Science 34:490–500, 1889

Janzarik W: Schizophrene Verläufe. Berlin, Springer, 1968

Johnstone EC, Crow TJ, Frith CD, et al: Cerebral ventricular size and cognitive impairment in chronic schizophrenia. Lancet 2:924–926, 1976

Johnstone EC, Owens DGC, Frith CD, et al: The relative stability of positive and negative features in chronic schizophrenia. Br J Psychiatry 150:60–64, 1986

Kay SR, Fiszbein A, Lindenmayer J-P, et al: Positive and negative syndromes in schizophrenia as a function of chronicity. Acta Psychiatr Scand 74:507–518, 1986

Kay SR, Fiszbein A, Opler LA: The positive and negative syndrome scale (PANSS) for schizophrenia. Schizophr Bull 13:261–276, 1987

Kendler KS: The genetics of schizophrenia: an overview, in Handbook of Schizophrenia, Vol 3: Nosology, Epidemiology and Genetics of Schizophrenia. Edited by Tsuang MT, Simpson JC. Amsterdam, Netherlands, Elsevier, 1988, pp 437–462

Kendler KS, Gruenberg AM, Strauss JS: An independent analysis of the Copenhagen sample of the Danish adoption study of schizophrenia, II: the relationship between schizotypal personality disorder and schizophrenia. Arch Gen Psychiatry 38:982–984, 1981

Kendler KS, Gruenberg AM, Strauss JS: An independent analysis of the Copenhagen sample of the Danish adoption study of schizophrenia, V: the relationship between childhood social withdrawal and adult schizophrenia. Arch Gen Psychiatry 39:1257–1261, 1982

Kendler KS, Gruenberg AM, Tsuang MT: The specificity of DSM-III schizotypal symptoms. Abstracts of the 135th Annual Meeting of the American Psychiatric Association, Washington, DC, May 1983

Kendler KS, Masterson CC, Ungaro R, et al: A family history study of schizophrenia-related personality disorders. Am J Psychiatry 141:424–427, 1984

Kendler KS, Masterson CC, Davis KL: Psychiatric illness in first-degree relatives of patients with paranoid psychosis, schizophrenia, and medical illness. Br J Psychiatry 147:524–531, 1985

Kety SS: Schizophrenic illness in the families of schizophrenic adoptees: findings from the Danish national sample. Schizophr Bull 14:217–222, 1988

Knight RA, Roff JD, Barnett J, et al: Concurrent and predictive validity of thought disorder and affectivity: a 22-year follow-up of acute schizophrenics. J Abnorm Psychol 88:1–12, 1979

Kraepelin E: Psychiatrie, Vols 1–4. Leipzig, Germany, Barth, 1909–1915

Kretschmer E: Körperbau und Charakter. Berlin, Springer, 1921

Kringlen E: Heredity and environment in the functional psychoses: an epidemiological twin study. London, Heinemann, 1967

Kringlen E: Contributions of genetic studies on schizophrenia, in Search for the Causes of Schizophrenia. Edited by Häfner H, Gattaz WF, Janzarik W. Berlin, Springer, 1987, pp 123–142

Kulhara P, Chadda R: A study of negative symptoms in schizophrenia and depression. Compr Psychiatry 28:229–235, 1987

Lewine RRJ: Sex differences in age of symptom onset and first hospitalization in schizophrenia. Am J Orthopsychiatry 50:316–322, 1980

Lewine RRJ, Meltzer HY: Negative symptoms and platelet monoamine oxidase activity in male schizophrenic patients. Psychiatry Res 12:99–109, 1984

Lewine RRJ, Sommers AA: Clinical definitions of negative symptoms as a reflection of theory and methodology, in Controversies in Schizophrenia: Changes and Constancies. Edited by Alpert M. New York, Guilford, 1985, pp 267–279

Lewine RRJ, Fogg L, Meltzer HY: Assessment of negative and positive symptoms in schizophrenia. Schizophr Bull 9:368–376, 1983

Lindelius R: A study of schizophrenia. Acta Psychiatr Scand Suppl 216:9–125, 1970

Loebel AD, Lieberman JA, Alvir JMJ, et al: Duration of psychosis and outcome in first-episode schizophrenia. Am J Psychiatry 149:1183–1188, 1992

Maier W, Lichtermann D, Minges J, et al: Continuity and discontinuity of affective disorders and schizophrenia: results of a controlled family study. Arch Gen Psychiatry 50:871–883, 1993

Maurer K, Häfner H: Dependence, independence or interdependence of positive and negative symptoms, in Negative Versus Positive Schizophrenia. Edited by Marneros A, Andreasen NC, Tsuang MT. Berlin, Springer, 1991, pp 160–182

McGuffin P, Farmer AE, Gottesman II: Is there really a split in schizophrenia? the genetic evidence. Br J Psychiatry 150:581–592, 1987

McGuffin P, Harvey I, Williams M: The negative/positive dichotomy: does it make sense from the perspective of the genetic researcher? in Negative Versus Positive Schizophrenia. Edited by Marneros A, Andreasen NC, Tsuang MT. Berlin, Springer, 1991, pp 250–264

Mednick SA, Schulsinger F: Longitudinal research in early detection and prevention of mental illness, in Psychiatrische Verlaufsforschung: Methoden und Ergebnisse. Edited by Schimmelpenning GW. Bern, Germany, Huber, 1980, pp 37–57

Mednick SA, Schulsinger F, Teasdale TW, et al: Schizophrenia in high-risk children: sex differences in predisposing factors, in Psychiatrische Verlaufsforschung: Methoden und Ergebnisse. Edited by Serban G. New York, Brunner/Mazel, 1978, pp 169–204

Meehl P: Schizotaxia, schizotypy, schizophrenia. Am Psychol 17:827–838, 1962

Murray RM, Lewis SW: Is schizophrenia a neurodevelopmental disorder? BMJ 295:681–682, 1987

Parnas J: Risk Factors in the Development of Schizophrenia: Contributions From a Study of Children of Schizophrenic Mothers. Copenhagen, Laegeforeningens Forlag, 1986

Parnas J, Jacobsen B, Schulsinger H: Lifetime DSM-III-R diagnostic outcome in children of schizophrenic mothers and its relationship to diagnostic methodology. Paper presented at the International Congress on Schizophrenia and Affective Psychoses, Nosology in Contemporary Psychiatry, Geneva, Switzerland, September 12–14, 1991

Pfohl B, Winokur G: The evolution of symptoms in institutionalized hebephrenic/catatonic schizophrenics. Br J Psychiatry 141:567–572, 1982

Pogue-Geile MF, Harrow M: Negative and positive symptoms in schizophrenia and depression: a follow-up. Schizophr Bull 10:371–387, 1984

Pogue-Geile MF, Harrow M: Negative symptoms in schizophrenia: their longitudinal and prognostic importance. Schizophr Bull 11:427–439, 1985

Pogue-Geile MF, Zubin J: Negative symptomatology and schizophrenia: a conceptual and empirical review. International Journal of Mental Health 16:3–45, 1988

Raine A, Allbutt J: Factors of schizoid personality. Br J Clin Psychol 28:31–40, 1989

Rey E-R, Birnbaum D, Koppe T, et al: Ein statistisches Modell zur Interaktion von Negativsymptomatik, Krankheitsbewältigung und sozialer Unterstützung sowie dessen prognostische Bedeutung für den Krankheitsverlauf, in Verlaufsprozesse schizophrener Erkrankungen. Edited by Brenner HD, Böker W. Bern, Germany, Verlag Hans Huber, 1992, pp 91–111

Reynolds JR: On the pathology of convulsions, with special reference to those of children. Liverpool Med Chir J 2:1–14, 1858

Roff JD, Knight R: Young adult schizophrenics: prediction of outcome and antecedent childhood factors. J Consult Clin Psychol 46:947–952, 1978

Schubart C, Krumm B, Biehl H, et al: Factors influencing the course and outcome of symptomatology and social adjustment in first-onset schizophrenics, in Search for the Causes of Schizophrenia. Edited by Häfner H, Gattaz WF, Janzarik W. Berlin, Springer, 1987, pp 98–106

Siever LJ, Gunderson JG: Genetic determinants of borderline conditions. Schizophr Bull 5:59–86, 1979

Slater E: Psychotic and Neurotic Illness in Twins. Medical Research Council Special Report Series No 278. London, Her Majesty's Stationery Office, 1953

Sommers AA: "Negative symptoms": conceptual and methodological problems. Schizophr Bull 11:364–379, 1985

Strauss JS: Processes of healing and chronicity in schizophrenia, in Search for the Causes of Schizophrenia. Edited by Häfner H, Gattaz WF, Janzarik W. Berlin, Springer, 1987, pp 75–87

Strauss JS, Carpenter WT Jr: Characteristic symptoms and outcome in schizophrenia. Arch Gen Psychiatry 30:429–434, 1974

Strauss JS, Carpenter WT Jr, Bartko JJ: The diagnosis and understanding of schizophrenia, III: speculations on the processes that underlie schizophrenic symptoms and signs. Schizophr Bull 11:61–76, 1974

Tienari P: Psychiatric illness in identical twins. Acta Psychiatr Scand Suppl 171:9–195, 1963

Torgersen S: Relationship of schizotypal personality disorder to schizophrenia: genetics. Schizophr Bull 11:554–563, 1985

Tsuang MT, Gilbertson MW, Faraone SV: Genetic transmission of negative and positive symptoms in the biological relatives of schizophrenics, in Negative Versus Positive Schizophrenia. Edited by Marneros A, Andreasen NC, Tsuang MT. Berlin, Springer, 1991, pp 265–291

Venables PH: A short scale for rating "activity withdrawal" in schizophrenia. Journal of Mental Science 103:197–199, 1957

Venables PH, Wing JK: Level of arousal and the subclassification of schizophrenia. Arch Gen Psychiatry 7:114–119, 1962

Weinberger DR: Implications of normal brain development for the pathogenesis of schizophrenia. Arch Gen Psychiatry 44:660–669, 1987

Wing JK: Clinical concepts of schizophrenia, in Schizophrenia: Towards a New Synthesis. Edited by Wing JK. New York, Grune & Stratton, 1978, pp 1–51

Wing JK, Brown GW: Institutionalism and Schizophrenia. London, Cambridge University Press, 1970

Wing JK, Cooper JE, Sartorius N: The Description and Classification of Psychiatric Symptoms: An Instruction Manual for the PSE and CATEGO System. Cambridge, UK, Cambridge University Press, 1974

Zedlick D, Maurer K, Löffler W, et al: Der Frühverlauf der Schizophrenie und seine Beziehung zu Alter, Geschlecht und Diagnose bei stationärer Erstaufnahme. Neuropsychiatrie 7:183–196, 1993

Zubin J, Spring B: Vulnerability—a new view of schizophrenia. J Abnorm Psychol 86:103–126, 1977

CHAPTER 7

Depression in Schizophrenia

Samuel G. Siris, M.D.

B ased on the diagnostic perspective developed over the past century, affective disorders traditionally have been considered distinct from schizophrenia. There is no doubt that, throughout the history of psychiatric nosology, the clarity generated by this separation has yielded crucial insights into the realms of psychopathology, pathophysiology, behavioral genetics, and many aspects of psychiatric prognosis and clinical care. Furthermore, the order that has been imposed on the entire field by the achievement of this separation of the two entities, originally described by Kraepelin (1919), has been central to many of the successes of 20th century psychiatry.

Nevertheless, over the years, careful clinical descriptions have continued to document the finding that, no matter how meticulously or by what criteria the diagnosis of schizophrenia was made, many individuals with this disorder manifest symptomatology highly reminiscent of clinical depression during the longitudinal course of their illnesses. Although this course-related depression in schizophrenia has been described by different names, the descriptor that has come into the most standard usage—and the one included in the International Classification of Diseases, 10th Edition (ICD-10; World Health Organization 1992)—is *postpsychotic depression*. In this chapter, therefore, I focus on the concept of course-related postpsychotic depression in schizophrenia, as distinct from depressive symptomatology that may occur during flagrant episodes of psychosis, the latter being a topic best considered in the context of schizoaffective disorder and its differential diagnosis.

Epidemiology of Secondary Depression in Schizophrenia

Numerous studies, employing a wide variety of diagnostic criteria, have investigated the incidence and prevalence of course-related depressions in schizophrenia (McGlashan and Carpenter 1976; Plasky 1991; Siris 1991). Although the rates of the occurrence of depression in schizophrenia have ranged from 7% to 70%—depending on the patient sample studied, the interval examined, and the exact definition of depression used—it is noteworthy that in all studies of the issue at least some proportion of patients are assessed as suffering from depressive symptomatology. The modal rate of occurrence of secondary depression in these investigations has been that 25% of schizophrenic patients are reported to manifest this condition to a significant extent. In contrast to the situation in acute psychosis, in which affective symptomatology is thought to represent a favorable sign, depressive symptomatology occurring in the longitudinal phase of schizophrenia is likely to be an indicator of a more negative outcome (Mandel et al. 1982).

Recognition of depression in schizophrenia is important not only because of the morbidity of the disorder and the fact that it may represent a treatable aspect of the patient's condition, but also because mortality may be associated with depression as well. Depressive symptomatology has been linked to suicidal ideation and behavior in schizophrenic patients (Barnes et al. 1989; Drake et al. 1985; Roy et al. 1983), and it has been estimated that approximately 10% of schizophrenic patients' lives terminate in suicide (Caldwell and Gottesman 1990; Miles 1977).

Differential Diagnosis of Secondary Depression in Schizophrenia

One of the issues most frequently raised in conjunction with depression occurring in the course of schizophrenia is whether it is a side effect of neuroleptic treatment. Several early reports suggested this; however, results of most recent studies seem to confirm that depression can occur independently from the effects of neuroleptics (Hirsch et al. 1989; Siris 1991).

These more recent studies have been of three types. One type of investigation involved the monitoring of depressive symptomatology in acutely psychotic schizophrenic patients as they began treatment with neuroleptic agents (Green et al. 1990; Hirsch et al. 1989); the result of these studies was the finding that depression actually decreases over time. A second type of study compared neuroleptic-treated schizophrenic patients with non–neuroleptic-treated control patients, with the result being that there was as much or more depressive symptomatology found among the patients who did not receive neuroleptics (Hirsch et al. 1989; Hogarty and Munetz 1984). A third type of investigation compared depressed versus nondepressed schizophrenic patients and found that the depressed group had not received more neuroleptic medication than the nondepressed group (Barnes et al. 1989; Siris et al. 1988a).

Nevertheless, apart from the findings noted above, there are two important side effects to treatment with neuroleptics—akinesia and akathisia—that can present clinical phenocopies to depression in schizophrenia and that therefore must be recognized in order to be properly treated.

Neuroleptic-Induced Akinesia

Akinesia is a term that has been used in two ways to describe extrapyramidally based neuroleptic side effects. One definition involves a reduction in accessory motor movements, and as such is a component of neuroleptic-induced parkinsonism (see Chapter 22). The other definition of akinesia involves a reduction in the ability to initiate or sustain motor behaviors (Rifkin et al. 1975; Van Putten and May 1978). Although this latter definition also has an extrapyramidal basis, it warrants separate consideration because it can occur in the absence of other extrapyramidal signs. When this happens, the patient appears to behave like "a bump on a log" or as if his or her "starter motor is broken." Such patients may, for example, respond fairly adequately when spoken to, but be unlikely to initiate conversation. Similarly, they may sit and watch television in an ordinary fashion, but then remain in their chairs when the show is over, continuing to watch whatever comes on next rather than moving on to some other activity or changing the channel to a more interesting program. In this state, patients may experience motor behavior as particularly effortful, although the interpretation given to this subjective experience by schizophrenic individuals may be variable, including laziness, sleepiness, or ineptitude.

Obviously, this akinetic nonspontaneity can easily be mistaken for depression, especially when the patient is questioned and reports boredom, lack of pleasure, or self-blame as a consequence. Indeed, a full symptomatic expression of depression can be manifest in the context of akinesia (Bermanzohn and Siris 1992; Martin et al. 1985; Siris 1987), and the difference may only be noted when the depressive symptomatology dramatically resolves following treatment considered to be specific for akinesia.

The most parsimonious way to treat neuroleptic-induced akinesia, of course, is by reduction of the dosage of neuroleptic medication. At times, however, this is either impractical or inadequate. Adjunctive antiparkinsonian medication is therefore often the treatment of choice for akinesia. Often, full doses of antiparkinsonian agents are required to treat akinesia, although when response occurs to those agents it is generally complete within a few days to a week. Indeed, because of the insidious nature of akinesia's development, the subtlety of its presentation, and the fact that it can so easily be mistaken for the negative symptoms of schizophrenia, an argument can be made that prophylactic antiparkinsonian treatment is warranted along with neuroleptic medication indefinitely, as long as the treating clinician remains alert to the possible side effects of antiparkinsonian medications themselves (Lavin and Rifkin 1991).

Neuroleptic-Induced Akathisia

The neuroleptic-induced extrapyramidal side effect of *akathisia* can also be mistaken for depression in schizophrenia. That is because the motor restlessness syndrome of akathisia (described in detail in Chapter 22) can be accompanied by intense states of dysphoria (Van Putten 1975). Anhedonia is often present, and the restlessness of akathisia can easily be mistaken for depressive agitation. Indeed, suicidal thoughts and behavior have been described as being associated with akathisia as well (Drake and Ehrlich 1985; Shear et al. 1983).

The treatment of akathisia involves lowering the level of neuroleptic medication either independently or in conjunction with adjunctive treatment with benzodiazepines, antiparkinsonian agents, or propranolol (Fleischhacker et al. 1990); this regimen is described in more detail in Chapter 22.

Situational Depression in Schizophrenia

The appearance of depressive symptoms in schizophrenia, of course, can also result from acute or chronic disappointment syndromes. Although acute disappointment reactions can look very similar to depression in cross-section, and especially so in patients with schizophrenia who may have relatively poor communication skills and be somewhat idiosyncratic in the way they express themselves, this state is notable for its transiency and the fact that it resolves relatively quickly and completely with the passage of time.

Chronic disappointment reactions, also conceptualized as the *demoralization syndrome* (Klein 1974), can be more difficult to differentiate from enduring depression in these individuals. Certainly schizophrenic patients may have much to be discouraged about in the way in which their lives are evolving. They may be in mourning for lost friends, lost successes, lost self-esteem, lost opportunities, or lost dreams. Battered by repeated failures, pessimism may have overtaken their fragile motivational fabric, leading to a demoralization syndrome that is similar to depression in many phenotypic respects, except that it generally lacks the vegetative symptoms that would be necessary for the diagnosis of a full depressive syndrome.

Negative Symptoms of Schizophrenia

Negative symptoms of schizophrenia can share many features with depression (Andreasen and Olsen 1982; Carpenter et al. 1985; Siris et al. 1988b). These features include anhedonia, anergia, lack of interest, and withdrawal. The cardinal feature of blunted affect, thought to be a core feature of the negative symptom syndrome, is not a typical feature of postpsychotic depression. Instead, patients with postpsychotic depression would be expected to manifest a "blue mood." Certainly, the differential diagnosis of negative symptoms and postpsychotic depression can be a difficult one in some cases of schizophrenia, and, indeed, depending on the definitions used, it may be appropriate to consider both syndromes to be present phenomenologically in a number of cases. (For further discussion of negative symptoms, the reader is referred to Chapters 5 and 6.)

Depressive Symptomatology During Psychotic Decompensation

Another time when a phenotypic expression of depression can occur in schizophrenia is during the evolution of an episode of psychosis (Docherty et al. 1978; Herz and Melville 1980). During the course of impending relapse, schizophrenic patients often become withdrawn and dysphoric. Furthermore, they may manifest sleep, appetite, and energy level changes that can be impossible to distinguish from those known to occur in depression. Cross-sectional diagnosis of this state in patients, therefore, can be quite difficult. With the passage of time, however, usually within the course of 1–2 weeks, the diagnosis becomes clear.

Obviously, the emergence of a new episode of psychosis is a crucial differential diagnosis to make from the phenotypically similar states of neuroleptic-induced akinesia, negative schizophrenic symptoms, or postpsychotic depression. This is so because an attempt to treat an emergent psychotic episode with a reduction of neuroleptic medication could exacerbate the patient's course. Similarly, many case reports of psychosis resulting from attempts to treat depression in schizophrenia with antidepressant medications could be the result of interventions at the time of this clinical state. As a result of this possibility, the recommended treatment for any state of newly emergent depressive symptomatology in schizophrenia is a period of intensified observation. Within 1–2 weeks, an incipient episode of psychosis will declare itself with the emergence of frank psychotic symptomatology. After that interval, appropriate treatment interventions can then be initiated as suits the situation.

Organically Based Causes of Depression

Underlying medical conditions can cause a depressive syndrome in schizophrenic patients in the same way that they can in non-schizophrenic individuals (Bartels and Drake 1988). Carcinomas, endocrinopathies, anemias, and neurological disorders are common medical conditions that can present as clinical depression, but there are others as well. The occurrence of depression in the course of schizophrenia, therefore, is cause for a thorough medical evaluation to identify a possible organic cause of the depressive symptomatology.

In addition, some commonly prescribed medications can lead to side effects that may present as phenocopies of depression. Beta-blockers and various other medications used in the treatment of hypertension are well known to cause depressive symptoms. Minor tranquilizers can lead to depressive states. On the other hand, the discontinuation of certain medications (e.g., stimulants, corticosteroids) can also lead to depression.

Substances of abuse can lead to states of depression on the basis of their acute use, chronic use, or discontinuation. Alcohol is the most commonly abused substance and is known to predispose the user to depressive states during or after intoxication or with chronic use. During the withdrawal phase from cocaine, a depression-like state emerges. Chronic use of cannabis can result in an anergic state similar in many respects to depression. Although a variety of illegal drugs can lead to depressive states during or after use, the completely legal drug caffeine can also be involved in dysphoric states—either the anxious-dysphoric state that may occur at times of peak use or the anergic-dysphoric state that can occur during periods of withdrawal. Nicotine withdrawal can also be associated with substantial dysphoria. Again, the crucial first step in making a differential diagnosis is to consider substance involvement in relationship to the presenting depression.

Treatment of the Postpsychotic Depression Syndrome

After all cases of depression associated with organic causes, neuroleptics, and purely situationally reactions have been dealt with, there still remains a substantial proportion of schizophrenic patients who present longitudinally with the symptomatology of secondary depression. A central question raised for clinicians in encountering these patients is whether the use of antidepressant medications is indicated in these cases.

As noted above, it is prudent first to monitor such patients for 1–2 weeks in order to ascertain that the seeming depression is not a stage in the process of psychotic decompensation. Also, if the depression represents a disappointment reaction to a specific situation, it will resolve by itself over this interval. This waiting period can be put to good use, however, by institution of a medical workup and substance abuse evaluation to determine if organic factors may be involved in the depressive state.

If the workup is negative for organic factors and a stable state of postpsychotic depression is found to exist, the next step of treatment is to attempt to rule out the akinesia syndrome. First, of course, it is important to ensure that the patient is being treated with the lowest effective dosage of neuroleptic medication. Then, if depression-like symptoms persist, full doses of antiparkinsonian agents may be required to rule out akinesia, especially in the absence of anticholinergic side effects, since marked interindividual variation can exist in the rate at which these medications are metabolized (Tune and Coyle 1980). If the condition is akinesia, it will generally respond to adequate antiparkinsonian intervention within a week.

If the patient's postpsychotic depression continues to persist after 1–2 weeks, it is appropriate to consider adjunctive antidepressant medication while maintaining the patient on his or her neuroleptic regimen. The use of various antidepressants has been described in the literature, with mixed results (Siris 1991). Among these studies, the most positive results were obtained with imipramine being added gradually (i.e., in increments of 50 mg/day each week) up to a final dosage of 200 mg or more and maintained for a full 6- to 9-week trial period (Siris et al. 1987). It is unclear, however, from the results of the Siris et al. (1987) study, whether imipramine specifically is truly superior to other adjunctive antidepressant medications for postpsychotic depression, because the methodology followed in the Siris et al. trial differed from that used in other trials in a number of additional respects, such as the precise definition of the depressive state, the nature of the neuroleptic employed, the stringency of the attempt to rule out the akinesia syndrome during the pretrial interval, and the fact that an antiparkinsonian agent was continued throughout the adjunctive antidepressant treatment phase.

Among those patients with postpsychotic depression who do respond to adjunctive antidepressant medications, it is likely that long-term maintenance treatment with the antidepressants is the indicated course. This recommendation must be taken with caution, however, because there has been only one prospective double-blind study of this issue (Siris et al. 1994), and the benefits of long-term maintenance antidepressant treatment must be weighed against any side effects that the medications may generate. In Siris et al.'s (1994) study, however, such side effects were not found to be a limiting factor.

Summary

Secondary depression occurring during the longitudinal course of schizophrenia has been noted to be present in approximately 25% of cases and to be associated with significant morbidity, functional impairment, and even mortality. The differential diagnosis of this condition includes a stage of decompensation into a new episode of psychosis, neuroleptic-induced akinesia and akathisia, acute disappointment reactions to specific situations, the demoralization syndrome, negative symptoms of schizophrenia, medical conditions, side effects of nonpsychiatric medications, and substance abuse states. Appropriate treatment occurs when the clinician considers each of these potential differential diagnoses and, after ruling out each of them in otherwise stable patients, only then proceeds to a trial of adjunctive antidepressant medication.

References

Andreasen NC, Olsen S: Negative symptoms in schizophrenia: definition and reliability. Arch Gen Psychiatry 39:789–794, 1982

Barnes TRE, Curson DA, Liddle PF, et al: The nature and prevalence of depression in chronic schizophrenic inpatients. Br J Psychiatry 154:486–491, 1989

Bartels SJ, Drake RE: Depressive symptoms in schizophrenia: comprehensive differential diagnosis. Compr Psychiatry 29:467–483, 1988

Bermanzohn PC, Siris SG: Akinesia: a syndrome common to parkinsonism, retarded depression, and negative symptoms. Compr Psychiatry 33:221–232, 1992

Caldwell CB, Gottesman II: Schizophrenics kill themselves too: a review of risk factors for suicide. Schizophr Bull 16:571–589, 1990

Carpenter WT Jr, Heinrichs DW, Alphs LD: Treatment of negative symptoms. Schizophr Bull 11:440–452, 1985

Docherty HP, van Kammen DP, Siris SG, et al: Stages of onset of schizophrenic psychosis. Am J Psychiatry 135:420–426, 1978

Drake RE, Ehrlich J: Suicide attempts associated with akathisia. Am J Psychiatry 142:499–501, 1985

Drake RE, Gates C, Whitaker A, et al: Suicide among schizophrenics: a review. Compr Psychiatry 26:90–100, 1985

Fleischhacker WW, Roth SD, Kane JM: The pharmacologic treatment of neuroleptic-induced akathisia. J Clin Psychopharmacol 10:12–21, 1990

Green MF, Nuechterlein KH, Ventura J, et al: The temporal relationship between depressive and psychotic symptoms in recent-onset schizophrenia. Am J Psychiatry 147:179–182, 1990

Herz M, Melville C: Relapse in schizophrenia. Am J Psychiatry 137:801–805, 1980

Hirsh SR, Jolley AG, Barnes TRE, et al: Dysphoric and depressive symptoms in chronic schizophrenia. Schizophr Res 2:259–264, 1989

Hogarty GE, Munetz MR: Pharmacogenic depression among outpatient schizophrenic patients: a failure to substantiate. J Clin Psychopharmacol 4:12–27, 1984

Klein DF: Endogenomorphic depression: a conceptual and terminological revision. Arch Gen Psychiatry 31:447–454, 1974

Lavin MR, Rifkin A: Prophylactic antiparkinson drug use, II: withdrawal after long-term maintenance therapy. J Clin Pharmacol 31:769–777, 1991

Mandel MR, Severe JB, Schooler NR, et al: Development and prediction of postpsychotic depression in neuroleptic-treated schizophrenics. Arch Gen Psychiatry 39:197–203, 1982

Martin RL, Cloninger RC, Guze SB, et al: Frequency and differential diagnosis of depressive syndromes in schizophrenia. J Clin Psychiatry 46 (suppl 11, sec 2):9–13, 1985

McGlashan TH, Carpenter WT Jr: Postpsychotic depression in schizophrenia. Arch Gen Psychiatry 33:231–239, 1976

Miles C: Conditions predisposing to suicide: a review. J Nerv Ment Dis 164:221–246, 1977

Plasky P: Antidepressant usage in schizophrenia. Schizophr Bull 17:649–656, 1991

Rifkin A, Quitkin F, Klein DF: Akinesia: a poorly recognized drug-induced extrapyramidal behavioral disorder. Arch Gen Psychiatry 32:672–674, 1975

Roy A, Thompson R, Kennedy S: Depression in chronic schizophrenia. Br J Psychiatry 142:465–470, 1983

Shear MK, Frances A, Weiden P: Suicide associated with akathisia and depot fluphenazine treatment. J Clin Psychopharmacol 3:235–236, 1983

Siris SG: Akinesia and post-psychotic depression: a difficult differential diagnosis. J Clin Psychiatry 48:240–243, 1987

Siris SG: Diagnosis of secondary depression in schizophrenia: implications for DSM-IV. Schizophr Bull 17:75–98, 1991

Siris SG, Morgan V, Fagerstrom R, et al: Adjunctive imipramine in the treatment of post-psychotic depression: a controlled trial. Arch Gen Psychiatry 44:533–539, 1987

Siris SG, Strahan A, Mandeli J, et al: Fluphenazine decanoate dose and severity of depression in patients with post-psychotic depression. Schizophr Res 1:31–35, 1988a

Siris SG, Adan F, Cohen M, et al: Post-psychotic depression and negative symptoms: an investigation of syndromal overlap. Am J Psychiatry 145:1532–1537, 1988b

Siris SG, Bermanzohn PC, Mason SE, et al: Maintenance imipramine therapy for secondary depression in schizophrenia. Arch Gen Psychiatry 51:109–115, 1994

Tune L, Coyle JT: Serum levels of anticholinergic drugs in the treatment of acute extrapyramidal side effects. Arch Gen Psychiatry 37:293–297, 1980

Van Putten T: The many faces of akathisia. Compr Psychiatry 16:43–47, 1975

Van Putten T, May PRA: "Akinetic depression" in schizophrenia. Arch Gen Psychiatry 35:1101–1107, 1978

World Health Organization: International Classification of Diseases, 10th Edition. Geneva, Switzerland, World Health Organization, 1992

CHAPTER 8

Diagnostic and Treatment Issues in Late-Onset Schizophrenia

Ira M. Lesser, M.D., and
J. Randolph Swartz, M.D.

The fact that a chapter on late-onset schizophrenia is included in this book is an answer to the question posed in an article written less than a decade ago, "Can Schizophrenia Begin After Age 44?" (Rabins et al. 1984). The debate about whether schizophrenic disorders can present late in life has a long history in European and British psychiatry, and a shorter history in American psychiatry (Bridge and Wyatt 1980a, 1980b; Gold 1984; Harris and Jeste 1988; Volavka 1985). In this chapter, we

- Review the history of diagnostic considerations regarding psychoses of late life
- Describe the many changes in nomenclature of late-onset schizophrenia seen over the last century
- Outline the epidemiology and clinical characteristics of late-onset schizophrenia and compare these with the early-onset disorder
- Describe findings from neuroimaging
- Review the scant literature on treatment of these patients

A Historical Perspective

Relying on vast clinical experience and astute powers of observation, Kraepelin (1919) organized the classification of psychoses to which psychiatry largely adheres today. His use of the term *dementia praecox* to denote an illness that begins early in life and leads to a chronic progressive course contrasted with his experience that the psychosis began after age 40 years in about 10% of patients. The majority of these later-onset cases had paranoid symptoms at their core. Kraepelin made the distinction between *paranoid schizophrenia,* which followed the deteriorating course of other schizophrenic illnesses; *paraphrenia,* which shared some symptoms with paranoid schizophrenia but showed less disorder of volition and emotion and did not have a deteriorating course; and *paranoia,* which presented without hallucinations.

Controversy about this distinction ensued, and follow-up studies of Kraepelin's patients (Mayer 1921; Roth 1955) noted that many patients with paraphrenia did, indeed, become chronically ill and were difficult to distinguish from patients labeled paranoid schizophrenic. Kay and Roth (Kay 1963; Kay and Roth 1961; Roth 1955) were proponents of the concept that older patients could present with a nonorganic psychosis of a predominantly paranoid type. They called these patients *late paraphrenics* and distinguished them from patients categorized as having affective psychosis, senile psychosis, arteriosclerotic psychosis, and acute confusion. In modern nomenclature, the late paraphrenic patients would probably be classified either as schizophrenic or as having a delusional disorder (Grahame 1984). Post (1966) argued for another classification system for patients presenting with paranoid symptoms after age 50. He divided these patients' presentations into paranoid hallucinosis, schizophreniform syndrome, and schizophrenic syndrome, with the latter classification being reserved for patients with Schneiderian first-rank symptoms. On follow-up, however, no clear differences emerged between these groups.

The debate about whether individuals could undergo the onset of a schizophrenic disorder later in life was reflected in DSM-III (American Psychiatric Association 1980), in which it was categorically stated that symptoms of schizophrenia must begin prior to age 45; a clinical picture identical to schizophrenia that began after age 45 was called *atypical psychosis*. However, with more recent interest in the study of disorders that occur in later life, that position was reversed in DSM-III-R (American Psychiatric Association 1987), into which a diagnosis of *schizophrenic disorder, late-onset type,* was incorporated. Some investigators, however, continue to hold out for the retention of the diagnosis of paraphrenia (Munro 1991).

In summary, that there exists a psychotic illness that begins after the age of 50, is typically paranoid in flavor, has no obvious organic etiology, and often leads to a state of chronicity is not in doubt. On the other hand, there is little agreement on what to call this disorder, with many clinicians unhappy with the current classification system.

Epidemiology of Late-Onset Schizophrenia

There are problems inherent to assessing the epidemiology of psychiatric disorders in elderly individuals: accurate delineation of when symptoms began; inaccuracy with recollection and often a lack of collateral information; and underreporting of symptoms by elderly individuals. Nevertheless, a variety of studies, including a recent review by Castle and Murray (1993), have attempted to assess the incidence of late-onset schizophrenia. In a review of 13 studies conducted between 1955 and 1984, Harris and Jeste (1988) reported that approximately 13% of all schizophrenic patients had the onset of symptoms in their fifth decade, 7% in their sixth decade, and 3% thereafter.

Post (1980) studied late-onset schizophrenia in hospitalized patients and found an annual incidence of 0.02% among patients over age 65. Christenson and Blazer (1984) evaluated *generalized persecutory ideation* with the paranoid scale of the Mini-Mult (Kincannon 1968), a shortened version of the Minnesota Multiphasic Personality Inventory (MMPI; Hathaway and McKinley 1943). They found that 40 (4%) of 997 people over age 65 studied had significant generalized persecutory ideation. According to the Epidemiologic Catchment Area (ECA) Study (Robins and Regier 1991), 5.2% of all schizophrenic patients had an onset between ages 40 and 45 (Keith et al. 1991);

no data were recorded regarding onset after 45 years of age because DSM-III did not allow for a diagnosis of schizophrenia to be made after age 45.

Data regarding how many of these cases currently are treated as outpatients or inpatients are not available. However, it is estimated that 12% of nursing home residents and 35% of public psychiatric hospital patients are elderly schizophrenic patients, although many developed the illness prior to age 45 (Gurland and Cross 1982).

Potential risk factors for developing late-onset schizophrenia seem to be impairment in sensory modalities and gender. In the Christenson and Blazer (1984) study, 78% of the patients with persecutory ideation had some degree of impaired vision, 58% had impaired hearing, and 52% exhibited some cognitive impairment. Preliminary data from the Suffolk County Mental Health Project (Bromet et al. 1992), in which first-admission psychosis is being evaluated, have indicated that there have been twice as many female as male patients admitted with psychosis who were over age 40. These sensory impairments and gender differences also were reported in the clinical studies cited below. The following case example illustrates some of the considerations related to clinical presentation of, differential diagnosis of, and treatment planning for patients with late-onset psychoses; these issues are discussed further in this chapter.

Case Example

A 58-year-old woman was admitted to the hospital after a 2-week period during which she lost her car, purse, and clothes, and found herself in a park in a confused state. She reported that for months she had been seeing images and hearing voices. The first image began one day when she turned off the television set but continued to see scenes of the movie she had been watching. This seeing images persisted with many objects that she would observe. She felt that these scenes were pictures from her previous life and believed that the images were reincarnated from previous generations, visible through hemoglobin in her eyes. At times she would hear voices, with up to five voices arguing back and forth.

This patient's speech was normal, with no looseness of associations, and her cognition was intact. She had no prior psychiatric history and was medically healthy and taking no medications. She had worked up until several months prior to evaluation as a data processor and prior to that as a laboratory technician. She had been divorced for about 8 years and had three children.

Laboratory examination revealed no abnormalities. Computed tomography (CT) and magnetic resonance imaging (MRI) scans of the brain were normal. An electroencephalogram was read as normal; however, a topographic brain mapping study revealed focal slowing in the left occipital area during both awake and drowsy states. A cerebral blood flow study showed focal hypoperfusion in the right parieto-occipital lobe with a smaller area of hypoperfusion in the same area on the left. Neuropsychological testing showed mild impairment of visual-constructional abilities.

Treatment with aspirin for the cerebral insufficiency resulted in improvement in the visual disturbances. However, despite treatment with neuroleptics, the auditory hallucinations and delusional material remained.

Clinical Picture

Differing nomenclature, difficulties in defining the exact age at onset, comorbidity with memory impairment and medical illnesses, and lack of follow-up studies make the careful study of late-onset schizophrenia difficult. (For a review of the methodological pitfalls and a summary of the current literature on clinical aspects, see the review by Harris and Jeste [1988].)

In DSM-III-R, no distinction is made (other than age at onset) between diagnostic criteria for early- and for late-onset schizophrenia. Authors of several studies (e.g., Jeste et al. 1988; Pearlson et al. 1989) have suggested that although there are clinical similarities between early- and late-onset schizophrenia, there also are different symptom pictures associated with the two. The most consistent differences appear to be a lack of formal thought disorder (e.g., looseness of associations, bizarre or non–goal-directed speech) and an absence of affective flattening in the late-onset as compared with the earlier-onset patients. The frequency of delusions and hallucinations seems to be similar between the groups, with the predominant delusion in the older patient being persecutory in nature. In contrast to patients diagnosed with delusional disorder, some of the late-onset schizophrenic patients display bizarre and elaborate delusional systems. In the Pearlson et al. (1989) study, auditory hallucinations were prominent, and visual hallucinations (61%) and tactile hallucinations (44%) were also frequent.

First-rank symptoms were found in about one-third of both late- and early-onset schizophrenic patients (Pearlson et al. 1989). As noted above, formal thought disorder has been found to be relatively rare (5%–15%) in the late-onset patients. In modern-day parlance, the frequency of positive symptoms seems to be similar in early- and late-onset patients, whereas negative symptoms are less frequent in the late-onset patients. Pearlson et al. (1989) also studied an older group of patients with early-onset schizophrenia; they reported that these patients appeared more like younger early-onset patients than like their age-matched, late-onset counterparts.

Some investigators have focused on sensory impairment as an associated or possible etiologic factor in the development of late-onset psychosis (Cooper and Curry 1976; Herbert and Jacobson 1967; Kay and Roth 1961; Naguib and Levy 1987; Post 1966; Prager and Jeste 1993). Significant hearing impairment is most common, occurring in up to 30% of patients; visual disturbances are the next most common impairment. The resulting isolation associated with such impairments may be related to the prominence of delusions regarding being spied upon, hearing things in adjoining rooms or dwellings, and visual misperceptions.

Investigators (Herbert and Jacobson 1967; Kay 1963; Pearlson et al. 1989) also have addressed the premorbid personality and function-ing of patients later diagnosed as having late-onset schizophrenia or paraphrenia. Although such assessment often is difficult, there is con-siderable agreement that many of these patients displayed paranoid or schizoid personality styles earlier in life, were married less frequently than nonpsychiatric control subjects or age-matched patients with affective illness, and had more childless marriages than age-matched controls. It is interesting that these same studies indicated that women are overrepresented in studies of late-onset schizophrenic patients, even after taking into account their greater longevity.

The course of late-onset schizophrenia resembles that of its earlier-onset counterpart in terms of a typical pattern of chronicity. However, there is not necessarily a deteriorating pattern. The longest follow-up studies (Herbert and Jacobson 1967; Kay and Roth 1961; Post

1966)—done at a time when the patients might not have received aggressive treatment, which could have biased the results—all reported a poor prognosis, although not a reduced life expectancy. Hymas et al. (1989) reported on a 3½-year follow-up of patients diagnosed as having late-onset paraphrenia. They found that improvement was seen in symptoms responsive to neuroleptics (e.g., delusions, hallucinations), although 45% still had paranoid symptoms and 29% had auditory hallucinations despite adequate treatment. Conversely, 35% had deterioration in memory function and 60% had some cognitive impairment. No patient required long-term hospitalization, and most were able to live somewhat independently.

The case example reported above is not atypical in terms of its clinical symptomatology. However, the picture could fit any number of diagnoses described above: paraphrenia, late paraphrenia, paranoid hallucinosis, or late-onset schizophrenia. Typically, the clinical phenomenology is organized to make a diagnosis based upon the system in fashion at the time.

The Role of Brain Pathology

Whenever one studies an illness demonstrating a change of behavior later in life, it is imperative to assess brain structure and function. This is particularly true in schizophrenia, because typically the illness begins much earlier in life. Indeed, throughout the literature on late-onset schizophrenia, references are made to potential organic etiologies. With the use of modern neuroimaging technology, substantial subgroups of patients with late-onset psychoses (over one-half in some studies) have been shown to have structural or functional brain abnormalities or both when compared with age-matched nonpsychiatric control subjects (Lesser et al. 1993).

Perhaps the most widely reported structural brain finding in late-onset schizophrenic patients has been increased ventricle-to-brain ratio (VBR) as seen on computed tomography (CT) or magnetic resonance imaging (MRI) scans (Krull et al. 1991; Naguib and Levy 1987; Pearlson et al. 1987; Rabins et al. 1987). It is interesting that this abnormality has also been widely found in younger and chronically ill schizophrenic patients (Andreasen et al. 1982; Johnstone et al. 1976; Weinberger et al. 1979). One study (Howard et al. 1992) reported that patients without Schneiderian first-rank symptoms had larger ventricles than both patients who had these symptoms and nonpsychiatric control subjects.

The consequences of enlarged ventricles in these older patients have not been established. In the follow-up study by Hymas et al. (1989), discussed above, ventricular enlargement had no bearing on the clinical course or outcome, nor did it predict cognitive deterioration.

In addition to these attempts to quantify ventricular and sulcal size, investigators have evaluated other structural changes in patients with late-onset psychosis, most notably changes in subcortical white matter and cortical gray matter. With few exceptions, there has been remarkable agreement that there are significantly greater numbers of late-onset psychotic patients showing large areas of white-matter hyperintensities compared with age-matched nonpsychiatric control subjects (Breitner et al. 1990; Flint et al. 1991; Lesser et al. 1991, 1992; Miller and Lesser 1988; Miller et al. 1991b). This has been true whether the diagnosis was schizophrenia, paranoia (delusional disorder), or a psychotic disorder not otherwise specified. However, these findings also have been reported in patients with late-onset depression in the absence of psychosis (Coffey et al. 1990), so there is no specificity in terms of diagnosis.

Another modality used to evaluate brain function has been studies of regional cerebral blood flow (rCBF). Our research group (Miller et al. 1992) found significant abnormalities in rCBF as seen with single photon emission computed tomography (SPECT) in late-onset psychotic patients when compared with nonpsychiatric control subjects. Of 20 such patients, only 5 had normal SPECT scans. In contrast, normal scans were seen in 26 out of 30 control subjects. The most common areas of hypoperfusion seen were in the frontal and temporal lobes (found in over 80% of patients), with the majority of patients showing multiple areas of hypoperfusion. A few patients also had hypoperfusion in the basal ganglia. In some patients, the areas of hypoperfusion correlated with large structural abnormalities visible on MRI, whereas in others the hypoperfusion had no structural correlate.

In this latter group of patients, the blood flow abnormalities may have reflected functional rather than gross structural changes. Although all brain areas were affected more in patients than in control subjects, anterior portions of the brain were affected to a greater degree. This study needs to be replicated, as it lacked quantification and the patients were not free of medication. Furthermore, the specificity of these findings remains to be determined, as there is emerging evidence (Lesser et al. 1994) that patients with depression also show abnormalities on SPECT, primarily in the frontal and temporal regions.

An important consideration in patients with late-onset schizophrenia is that significant numbers of these patients progress to states of dementia (Craig and Bregman 1988; Holden 1987; Lesser et al. 1989; Miller et al. 1991a, in press). Holden (1987) reported that 35% of 37 late-onset paraphrenic patients went on to develop dementia within 3 years of follow-up. It is unfortunate that no detailed neuropsychological evaluations were performed on these patients at baseline to determine whether some may have had cognitive deficits at the time of diagnosis. In a retrospective chart review, Craig and Bregman (1988) reported that, on follow-up, 10 of 15 state hospital inpatients who had a clinical diagnosis of late-onset schizophrenia or paranoid disorder and were also nonresponsive to treatment developed severe cognitive deterioration, with one patient eventually receiving a neuropathological diagnosis of Alzheimer's disease. In these studies, the patients were typically chronically ill and hospitalized. We (Lesser et al. 1989; Miller et al. 1991a, 1993) have shown that patients with a psychosis of short duration and displaying only mild cognitive impairment at baseline, but showing abnormal cerebral blood flow on SPECT, may go on to develop degenerative dementias, either of the Alzheimer or of the frontal lobe degeneration type. Thus, mounting evidence suggests that a subgroup of patients with late-onset psychosis are in the prodromal stages of a dementing illness, with the behavioral abnormality as the presenting symptom, prior to severe language or memory involvement.

Even if the hypothesis that brain abnormalities have an etiologic role in late-onset disease is accepted, another consideration to be taken into account is that other factors must interact with these brain changes to determine the form that the illness takes, or indeed whether there are any behavioral disturbances at all. Factors such as family history, premorbid functioning, cognitive deficits, medical illnesses, social supports, degree of sensory loss, and so on all could interact with similar disordered brain function to produce a different clinical picture. Unfortunately, there are no studies that collect data simultaneously from these varied perspectives.

Thorough evaluation of the case example reported above revealed that there was significant brain pathology (i.e., areas of hypoperfusion and slowing on electroencephalogram in the parieto-occipital region) indicative of cerebral ischemia. A less comprehensive workup would not have led to an accurate assessment of the pathological processes involved. This case highlights the interplay between cerebral pathology and psychosis, and shows that clinical symptomatology can have various etiologies that often are hard to delineate.

Treatment

Given that psychosis in elderly individuals, even more so than in younger patients, may have medical illnesses or medication side effects as etiologic factors, it is imperative that a thorough medical workup, including neuroimaging, be completed before treatment planning begins. The case reported above dramatically reinforces this idea and highlights that treatment must be focused on the etiology of particular symptoms. The treatment plan, once established, should almost always include both psychopharmacological and psychosocial modalities. We now highlight those areas of treatment that are particularly germane to older patients, rather than discuss these modalities in a comprehensive manner.

The primary pharmacological approach involves neuroleptic medication; several studies have documented their effectiveness in late-onset schizophrenia (Herbert and Jacobson 1967; Jeste et al. 1988; Post 1966; Rabins et al. 1984; Raskind et al. 1979). For example, Post (1966) showed that adequate dosages of trifluoperazine or thioridazine were more effective than either placebo or no treatment, with resulting decreases in psychotic symptoms and time spent in hospital, but little improvement in insight or social adjustment. Raskind et al.

(1979) showed intramuscular depot fluphenazine enanthate to be more effective than oral haloperidol in the outpatient care of elderly schizophrenic patients, mostly because of improved compliance. Rabins et al. (1984) found that a combination of neuroleptics and psychosocial therapies resulted in complete alleviation of symptoms or significant symptomatic improvement in 30 of 35 late-onset paraphrenic patients.

The issue of dosage has been addressed in several studies. Jeste et al. (1988) showed that the mean daily chlorpromazine equivalent dosage required for treatment response was much lower for patients with late-onset schizophrenia (192 mg/day) than for those with early-onset schizophrenia (841 mg/day). There is a suggestion that among schizophrenic patients over the age of 40, women require higher neuroleptic dosages than do men to achieve similar treatment responses (Seeman 1983).

A concern when treating elderly individuals is their sensitivity to many side effects of traditional neuroleptics, possibly because of the resultant higher blood levels of medication. Several studies have reported that elderly individuals develop higher plasma levels than do younger patients on comparable neuroleptic dosages (Jeste et al. 1981; Maartenson and Roos 1973; Yesavage et al. 1981), although not all researchers agree with this (Davis et al. 1982; Forsman and Ohman 1977). Some authors have suggested that age-related differences in side effect sensitivity occur at the pharmacodynamic (i.e., receptor) rather than the pharmacokinetic level (Raskind and Risse 1986). For example, it has been reported that central nervous system (CNS) cholinergic function decreases with age (Vernadakis 1985). Neuroleptics, particularly the low-potency ones, have considerable anticholinergic properties, which may result in elderly individuals having increased sensitivity to these effects and lead to cognitive impairments, perhaps even delirium (Vernadakis 1985). Similar mechanisms may be responsible for the increase in extrapyramidal side effects, as discussed below.

Elderly individuals also are very sensitive to other anticholinergic side effects, such as urinary retention, constipation, impaired visual accommodation, and dry mouth. Other concerns are orthostatic hypotension from α_1 receptor blockade and excess sedation from histamine$_1$ receptor blockade. Changes detectable on electrocardiograms can occur, such as tachycardia resulting from both anticholinergic effects and increased catecholamine levels. Other arrhythmias may occur because of altered potassium metabolism (Wragg and Jeste 1988). Elderly individuals also are sensitive to interdrug interactions, particularly cumulative sedative effects (Sargenti et al. 1988). These side effects and interactions put elderly patients at increased risk for falls and subsequent hip fractures.

Certain extrapyramidal symptoms, such as drug-induced parkinsonism (e.g., tremor, cogwheel rigidity, bradykinesia) and tardive dyskinesia, occur more frequently in older schizophrenic patients (Young and Meyers 1991). However, acute dystonic reactions, most common in young men, are rare in elderly individuals (Jeste et al. 1986). Most studies have found a higher incidence of drug-induced parkinsonism among psychotic patients over age 40 (Ayd 1976; Peabody et al. 1987; Salzman 1984), although one study reported the opposite (Moleman et al. 1986). This increased risk among elderly individuals may be attributable to age-related CNS changes—such as degeneration of the nigrostriatal pathway (Meyers and Kalayam 1989) or decreased dopamine receptors in the caudate nucleus (Thompson et al. 1983)—or may result from an underlying, unrecognized idiopathic parkinsonism exacerbated by neuroleptics (Levinson and Simpson 1987). Drug-induced parkinsonism in elderly individuals should be treated by lowering the neuroleptic dosage rather than by adding anticholinergic medications (Raskind and Risse 1986).

Although akathisia is common across all age groups, it is frequently underrecognized in elderly individuals (Wragg and Jeste 1988). Akathisia needs to be differentiated from worsening psychotic agitation; treatment for the former is decreased neuroleptic dosage whereas treatment for the latter is increased dosage. If misdiagnosed, elderly individuals may be subject to increasing dosages of neuroleptics, leading to a worsening of akathisia and other medication complications as discussed above.

Tardive dyskinesia (TD; see Chapter 25) is of particular concern when treating late-onset schizophrenia. There is an increased susceptibility to TD associated with aging that is not related to dosage or duration of treatment (Jeste and Wyatt 1987), with elderly women having a higher risk of developing severe TD than elderly men (Kane and Smith 1982). Elderly patients with TD are more likely to have oral-facial dyskinesias, whereas younger patients more often display limb dyskinesias (Jeste and Wyatt 1987). The differential diagnosis of TD in elderly individuals includes age-related spontaneous dyskinesias as well as oral dyskinesias secondary to loose-fitting dentures. Vigilance in preventing TD in elderly patients is important, because there is less chance for improvement following neuroleptic withdrawal in elderly compared with younger patients (Smith and Baldessarini 1980).

Despite the commonly held view that the neuroleptic malignant syndrome (NMS) occurs predominantly in younger patients, this potentially lethal condition is indeed a possible complication among older patients. Addonizio (1987) reported 18 cases of NMS occurring in patients over age 59, 14 of whom were being treated with dosages of neuroleptics that were relatively high for older patients. Of particular concern is the possibility that the early signs of NMS may go unrecognized in elderly individuals (Wragg and Jeste 1988). In addition, older patients often have preexisting renal, pulmonary, and cardiac disease, possibly placing them at increased risk for the more severe complications of NMS, such as renal failure attributable to myoglobinuria, pneumonia, pulmonary emboli, and cardiac failure.

Because of increased sensitivity to side effects of traditional neuroleptics, the emerging new generation of atypical neuroleptics may be of particular use in elderly individuals. These medications, including, among others, amperozide, clozapine, raclopride, remoxipride, risperidone, and savoxepine, are less likely to cause drug-induced parkinsonism or TD (Meltzer 1992). However, these compounds have not been evaluated for the treatment of late-onset schizophrenia in any known studies.

It is important to include psychosocial treatments as an integral part of the treatment plan. Psychosocial therapies, such as individual supportive therapy, group therapy for patients as well as for caregivers, and family therapy, help lower relapse rates and also improve patients' social adjustment outside the hospital. These treatments should focus on problem solving for the tasks of daily life and on socialization issues. Attempting to decrease the loneliness and isolation of these patients is important. In addition, behavioral therapies have proven effective in the elderly population, particularly in the treatment of agitation (Burgio and Burgio 1986; Hussian 1984; Wisocki 1984; Wragg and Jeste 1988); indeed, several studies have claimed that behavioral therapy aids in the reduction of psychotic symptoms in elderly individuals (Pinkston and Linsk 1984).

There are few controlled studies using both pharmacological and psychosocial therapies in treatment of patients with late-onset schizophrenia. As with younger patients, the florid psychotic symptoms are more easily controlled, whereas fixed delusions, paranoid thoughts, and social withdrawal are more problematic. An aggressive treatment plan should be made for late-onset schizophrenic patients that integrates psychosocial modalities with pharmacology (with the clinician being mindful of the problems with medications in elderly individuals) and that has as its goal the preservation of functioning and independence in these patients.

As interest in psychiatric disorders of elderly individuals expands, we are hopeful that data regarding more specific etiologies and, therefore, treatment strategies will be forthcoming.

References

Addonizio G: Neuroleptic malignant syndrome in elderly patients. J Am Geriatr Soc 35:1011–1012, 1987

American Psychiatric Association: Diagnostic and Statistical Manual of Mental Disorders, 3rd Edition. Washington, DC, American Psychiatric Association, 1980

American Psychiatric Association: Diagnostic and Statistical Manual of Mental Disorders, 3rd Edition, Revised. Washington, DC, American Psychiatric Association, 1987

Andreasen NC, Smith MR, Jacoby CG, et al: Ventricular enlargement in schizophrenia: definition and prevalence. Am J Psychiatry 139:292–296, 1982

Ayd FJ: A survey of drug-induced extrapyramidal reactions. JAMA 175:1045–1060, 1976

Breitner JCS, Husain MM, Figiel GS, et al: Cerebral white matter disease in late-onset paranoid psychosis. Biol Psychiatry 28:266–274, 1990

Bridge TP, Wyatt RJ: Paraphrenia: paranoid states of late life, I: European research. J Am Geriatr Soc 28:193–200, 1980a

Bridge TP, Wyatt RJ: Paraphrenia: paranoid states of late life, II: American research. J Am Geriatr Soc 28:201–205, 1980b

Bromet EJ, Schwartz JE, Fennig S, et al: The epidemiology of psychosis: the Suffolk County mental health project. Schizophr Bull 18:243–255, 1992

Burgio LD, Burgio KL: Behavioral gerontology: application of behavioral methods to the problems of older adults. J Appl Behav Anal 19:321–328, 1986

Castle DJ, Murray RM: The epidemiology of late-onset schizophrenia. Schizophr Bull 19:691–700, 1993

Christenson R, Blazer D: Epidemiology of persecutory ideation in an elderly population in the community. Am J Psychiatry 141:1088–1091, 1984

Coffey CE, Figiel GS, Djang WT, et al: Subcortical hyperintensity on magnetic resonance imaging: a comparison of normal and depressed elderly subjects. Am J Psychiatry 47:187–189, 1990

Cooper AF, Curry AR: The pathology of deafness in paranoid and affective psychoses of later life. J Psychosom Res 20:97–105, 1976

Craig TJ, Bregman Z: Late onset schizophrenia-like illness. J Am Geriatr Soc 36:104–107, 1988

Davis JM, Segal NL, Lesser JM: Use of antipsychotic drugs in the elderly, in Treatment of Psychopathology in the Aging. Edited by Eisdorfer C, Fann WE. New York, Springer-Verlag, 1982, pp 8–28

Flint AJ, Rifat SL, Eastwood MR: Late-onset paranoia: distinct from paraphrenia? International Journal of Geriatric Psychiatry 6:103–109, 1991

Forsman A, Ohman R: Applied pharmacokinetics of haloperidol in man. Current Therapeutic Research 21:396–411, 1977

Gold DD: Late age of onset schizophrenia: present but unaccounted for. Compr Psychiatry 25:225–237, 1984

Grahame PS: Schizophrenia in old age (late paraphrenia). Br J Psychiatry 145:493–495, 1984

Gurland BJ, Cross PS: Epidemiology of psychopathology in old age. Psychiatr Clin North Am 5:11–26, 1982

Harris MJ, Jeste DV: Late-onset schizophrenia: an overview. Schizophr Bull 14:39–55, 1988

Hathaway SR, McKinley JC: Minnesota Multiphasic Personality Inventory. Minneapolis, MN, University of Minnesota, 1943.

Herbert ME, Jacobson S: Late paraphrenia. Br J Psychiatry 113:461–469, 1967

Holden NL: Late paraphrenia or the paraphrenias? a descriptive study with a 10-year follow-up. Br J Psychiatry 150:635–639, 1987

Howard RJ, Forstl H, Almeida O, et al: Computer-assisted CT measurements in late paraphrenics with and without Schneiderian first-rank symptoms: a preliminary report. International Journal of Geriatric Psychiatry 7:35–38, 1992

Hussian RA: Behavioral geriatrics. Prog Behav Modif 16:159–183, 1984

Hymas N, Naguib M, Levy R: Late paraphrenia—a follow-up study. International Journal of Geriatric Psychiatry 4:23–29, 1989

Jeste DV, Wyatt RJ: Aging and tardive dyskinesia, in Schizophrenia and Aging. Edited by Miller NE, Cohen GD. New York, Guilford, 1987, pp 275–286

Jeste DV, Delisi LE, Zalcman S, et al: A biochemical study of tardive dyskinesia in young male patients. Psychiatry Res 4:327–331, 1981

Jeste DV, Wisniewski AA, Wyatt RJ: Neuroleptic-associated tardive syndromes. Psychiatr Clin North Am 9:183–192, 1986

Jeste DV, Harris MJ, Pearlson GD, et al: Late-onset schizophrenia: studying clinical validity. Psychiatr Clin North Am 11:1–13, 1988

Johnstone EC, Frith CD, Crow TJ, et al: Cerebral ventricular size and cognitive impairment in chronic schizophrenia. Lancet 2:924–926, 1976

Kane JM, Smith JM: Tardive dyskinesia: prevalence and risk factors, 1959 to 1979. Arch Gen Psychiatry 39:473–481, 1982

Kay DWK: Late paraphrenia and its bearing on the aetiology of schizophrenia. Acta Psychiatr Scand 39:159–169, 1963

Kay DWK, Roth M: Environmental and hereditary factors in the schizophrenias of old age ("late paraphrenia") and their bearing on the general causation in schizophrenia. Journal of Mental Science 107:649–686, 1961

Keith SA, Regier DA, Rae DS: Schizophrenic disorders, in Psychiatric Disorders in America—The Epidemiological Catchment Area Study. Edited by Robins LN, Regier DA. New York, Free Press, 1991, pp 33–52

Kincannon JC: Predictions of the standard MMPI scale scores from 71 items: the Mini-Mult. J Consult Clin Psychol 32:319–325, 1968

Kraepelin E: Dementia Praecox and Paraphrenia. Edinburgh, E & S Livingstone, 1919

Krull AJ, Press G, Dupont R, et al: Brain imaging in late-onset schizophrenia and related psychoses. International Journal of Geriatric Psychiatry 6:651–658, 1991

Lesser IM, Miller BL, Boone KB, et al: Psychosis as the first manifestation of degenerative dementia. Bulletin of Clinical Neuroscience 54:59–63, 1989

Lesser IM, Miller BL, Boone KB, et al: Brain injury and cognitive function in late-onset psychotic depression. J Neuropsychiatry Clin Neurosci 3:33–40, 1991

Lesser IM, Jeste DV, Boone KB, et al: Late-onset psychotic disorder, not otherwise specified: clinical and neuroimaging findings. Biol Psychiatry 31:419–423, 1992

Lesser IM, Miller BL, Swartz JR, et al: Brain imaging in late-life schizophrenia and related psychoses. Schizophr Bull 19:773–782, 1993

Lesser IM, Mena I, Boone KB, et al: Reduction of cerebral blood flow in older depressed patients. Arch Gen Psychiatry 51:677–686, 1994

Levinson DF, Simpson GM: Antipsychotic drug side effects, in Psychiatry Update: American Psychiatric Association Annual Review, Vol 6. Edited by Hales RE, Frances AJ. Washington, DC, American Psychiatric Press, 1987, pp 704–723

Maartenson E, Roos BE: Serum levels of thioridazine in psychiatric patients and healthy volunteers. Eur J Clin Pharmacol 6:181–186, 1973

Mayer W: Ueber paraphrena psychosen (On paraphrenic psychoses). Zeitschrift fur die Gesamte Neurologie und Psychiatrie 71:187–206, 1921

Meltzer HY (ed): Novel Antipsychotic Drugs. New York, Raven, 1992

Meyers B, Kalayam B: Update in geriatric psychopharmacology. Adv Psychosom Med 19:114–137, 1989

Miller BL, Lesser IM: Late-life psychosis and modern neuroimaging. Psychiatr Clin North Am 11:33–46, 1988

Miller BL, Cummings JL, Villanueva-Meyer J, et al: Frontal lobe degeneration: clinical, neuropsychological, MRI and SPECT characteristics. Neurology 41:1374–1382, 1991a

Miller BL, Lesser IM, Boone KB, et al: Brain lesions and cognitive function in late-life psychosis. Br J Psychiatry 158:76–82, 1991b

Miller BL, Lesser IM, Mena I, et al: Regional cerebral blood flow in late-life-onset psychosis. Neuropsychiatry, Neuropsychology, and Behavioral Neurology 5:132–137, 1992

Miller BL, Chang L, Mena I, et al: Progressive right frontotemporal degeneration: clinical, neuropsychological and SPECT characteristics. Dementia 4:204–213, 1993

Moleman P, Janzen G, von Bargen BA, et al: Relationship between age and incidence of parkinsonism in psychiatric patients treated with haloperidol. Am J Psychiatry 143:232–234, 1986

Munro A: A plea for paraphrenia. Can J Psychiatry 36:667–672, 1991

Naguib M, Levy R: Late paraphrenia: neuropsychological impairment and structural brain abnormalities on computed tomography. International Journal of Geriatric Psychiatry 2:83–90, 1987

Peabody CA, Warner D, Whiteford HA, et al: Neuroleptics and the elderly. J Am Geriatr Soc 35:233–238, 1987

Pearlson GD, Garbacz D, Tompkins RH, et al: Lateral cerebral ventricular size in late onset schizophrenia, in Schizophrenia and Aging. Edited by Miller NE, Cohen GD. New York, Guilford, 1987, pp 246–248

Pearlson GD, Kreger L, Rabins PV, et al: A chart review study of late-onset and early onset schizophrenia. Am J Psychiatry 146:1568–1574, 1989

Pinkston EM, Linsk NL: Behavioral family interventions with the impaired elderly. Gerontologist 24:576–583, 1984

Post F: Persistent Persecutory States of the Elderly. Oxford, Pergamon Press, 1966

Post F: Paranoid, schizophrenia-like, and schizophrenic states in the aged, in Handbook of Mental Health and Aging. Edited by Birren JE, Sloane RB. Englewood Cliffs, NJ, Prentice Hall, 1980, pp 591–615

Prager S, Jeste DV: Sensory impairment in late-life schizophrenia. Schizophr Bull 19:755–772, 1993

Rabins P, Pauker S, Thomas J: Can schizophrenia begin after age 44? Compr Psychiatry 25:290–293, 1984

Rabins P, Pearlson G, Jayaram G, et al: Increased ventricle-to-brain ratio in late-onset schizophrenia. Am J Psychiatry 144:1216–1218, 1987

Raskind MA, Risse SC: Antipsychotic drugs and the elderly. J Clin Psychiatry 47 (suppl 5):17–22, 1986.

Raskind M, Alvarez C, Herlin S: Fluphenazine enanthate in the outpatient treatment of late paraphrenia. J Am Geriatr Soc 27:459–463, 1979

Robins LN, Regier DA (eds): Psychiatric Disorders in America—The Epidemiological Catchment Area Study. New York, Free Press, 1991

Roth M: The natural history of mental disorder in old age. Journal of Mental Science 101:281–301, 1955

Salzman C: Clinical Geriatric Psychopharmacology. New York, McGraw-Hill, 1984

Sargenti CJ, Rizos AL, Jeste DV: Psychotropic drug interactions in the patient with late-onset psychosis and mood disorder: part I. Psychiatr Clin North Am 11:235–252, 1988

Seeman MV: Interaction of sex, age, and neuroleptic dose. Compr Psychiatry 24:125–128, 1983

Smith JM, Baldessarini RJ: Changes in prevalence, severity, and recovery in tardive dyskinesia with age. Arch Gen Psychiatry 37:1368–1373, 1980

Thompson TL, Moran MG, Nies AS: Psychotropic drug use in the elderly: part II. N Engl J Med 308:194–199, 1983

Vernadakis A: The aging brain. Clin Geriatr 1:61–94, 1985

Volavka J: Late-onset schizophrenia: a review. Compr Psychiatry 26:148–156, 1985

Weinberger DR, Torrey EF, Neophytides NN, et al: Lateral cerebral ventricular enlargement in chronic schizophrenia. Arch Gen Psychiatry 36:735–739, 1979

Wisocki PA: Behavioral approaches to gerontology. Prog Behav Modif 16:121–157, 1984

Wragg RE, Jeste DV: Neuroleptics and alternative treatments. Psychiatr Clin North Am 11:195–213, 1988

Yesavage JA, Holman CA, Cohn R: Correlation of thiothixene serum levels and age. Psychopharmacology 74:170–172, 1981

Young RC, Meyers BS: Psychopharmacology, in Comprehensive Review of Geriatric Psychiatry. Edited by Sadavoy J, Lazarus LW, Jarvik LF. Washington, DC, American Psychiatric Press, 1991, pp 435–467

CHAPTER 9

Neuropsychological Function in Schizophrenia

Anne L. Hoff, Ph.D.

C ognitive dysfunction in schizophrenia was noted as early as Kraepelin (1919), who commented on the "disorder of attention" in schizophrenia. K. Goldstein (1959) observed that schizophrenic patients had a loss of abstract attitude. Although it was commonly assumed that cognitive failures were functional deficits, deficits secondary to reductions in motivation, or the effects of long-term institutionalization, only recently have neurocognitive deficits in schizophrenia been considered to be a central feature of the illness and related to structural changes in the brain (reviewed by Seidman 1983) or abnormal brain metabolism (Paulman et al. 1990; Weinberger et al. 1986). The focus of this chapter is on the nature of cognitive deficits in schizophrenia; the timing of onset of cognitive failure and whether it is progressive; the relationship of demographic, symptomatic, and medication variables to cognitive dysfunction in schizophrenia; and the issue of whether neurocognitive

The author would like to acknowledge the assistance of Dr. Lynn E. DeLisi in the preparation of this chapter, and the support of the author's research by the National Alliance for Research on Schizophrenia and Depression.

dysfunction can be remediated by cognitive rehabilitation or medication approaches.

The Nature of Cognitive Dysfunction in Schizophrenia

Early neuropsychological studies of schizophrenia (see Heaton et al. 1978) focused largely on a level-of-function approach to differentiate schizophrenic patients from patients with brain damage on a host of neuropsychological measures. In general, acute schizophrenic patients or other psychotic patients had performances superior to those of patients with organic brain dysfunction, whereas chronic schizophrenic patients performed similarly to those with brain dysfunction. Heaton et al. (1978) asserted that these two groups could not be differentiated from one another at more than a chance level (54%). Some of these studies were limited by the unreliability of patient diagnosis. Patients with schizophrenia were also compared with patients whose organic brain dysfunction had multiple etiologies and courses of illness. Nonetheless, these studies were valuable in establishing that some schizophrenic patients had serious and disabling cognitive dysfunction.

The work of Flor-Henry et al. (1975) on temporal lobe epilepsy was seminal in the stimulation of neuropsychological research focusing on whether psychiatric illnesses had characteristic patterns of test results reflective either of a disturbance in functional lateralization or of damage to one cerebral hemisphere or the other (see also Flor-Henry and Yeudall 1979). In general, it was postulated that schizophrenia was a disturbance involving left hemisphere dysfunction, whereas bipolar affective disorder and other affective disorders were more related to right hemispheric impairment (Flor-Henry and Yeudall 1979). More recently, researchers (Kolb and Whishaw 1983; Taylor and Abrams 1984) have moved from inferences about the left or right side of the brain to hypotheses about cognitive dysfunction in schizophrenia related more to involvement of the anterior versus posterior regions of the brain, as well as to more medial and inferior structures such as the temporal cortex and hippocampal regions of the brain.

Because there have been a plethora of studies on many aspects of cognition in schizophrenia, it is probably most parsimonious to consider their categorization by functional domain. The following summary includes the areas of cognition that have received the most attention in the literature.

Language Function

There has been a long-standing controversy over whether schizophrenic language is like that of aphasia, in which brain pathology affecting language mechanisms is a key factor (Chaika 1974), or whether language dysfunction in schizophrenia is more of an epiphenomenon secondary to a central disturbance in thought or related to a general information-processing deficit (Asarnow and Watkins 1982). Some researchers (Andreasen and Grove 1979; Halpern and McCartin-Clark 1984) have found that schizophrenic individuals, unlike those with aphasia, have no difficulties with simple language measures of syntax, fluency, or naming. Faber and colleagues (Faber and Reichstein 1981; Faber et al. 1983) reported that patients with formal thought disorder, when compared with those without thought disorder, produce errors on measures of language not dissimilar to those produced by fluent aphasic individuals. Landre et al. (1992) confirmed these findings in a carefully defined subgroup of speech-disordered schizophrenic patients. In summary, schizophrenic and aphasic language can be phenomenologically similar, but a review of the literature indicates that only a subgroup of schizophrenic patients resemble aphasic individuals in both their reception and production of speech (Andreasen and Grove 1979; Landre et al. 1992).

Morice and colleagues (Morice and Ingram 1983; Morice and McNichol 1986) found that when free speech samples of schizophrenic patients were compared with those of nonpsychiatric control subjects, the patient group demonstrated a reduction in syntactic complexity, as manifested by simpler and shorter sentences, fewer dependent and embedded clauses, less depth of embedding, and greater verbal dysfluency. More recently, K. King et al. (1990) provided evidence for deterioration in the syntax of schizophrenic individuals over a 2- to 3-year period. In line with Landre et al.'s (1992) suggestion that language disorder in schizophrenia is part of a more generalized cognitive deficit, Frith and Allen (1988) argued that deficits in schizophrenic language were caused by errors in performance rather than by linguistic incompetence. Morice (1986) suggested that changes in the structural complexity in language were possibly related to prefrontal cortical dysfunction. Although it is unclear what the neuropathological substrate is for thought disorder or language dysfunction in schizophrenia, more recent brain morphology studies of the areas critical to language function (Crow et al. 1992; Hoff et al. 1992a; Rossi et al. 1992), such as the planum temporale in schizophrenia, may be useful in elucidating the nature of language dysfunction in schizophrenia.

Executive Function

The behavior of schizophrenic patients—in particular, those with negative symptoms—has been noted to bear a strong resemblance to the behavior of patients with disorders of the frontal cortex (Levin 1984); both syndromes are remarkable for apathy, lack of motivation, flat affect, disorders of attention, difficulties in the formulation of plans for goal-directed behavior, deficient concept formation, inability to maintain and change cognitive set, and perseverative tendencies. Probably the most influential study on frontal lobe function in schizophrenia was the Weinberger et al. (1986) study. In that study, schizophrenic patients were observed to exhibit a hypofrontality pattern on a positron-emission tomography (PET) scan during the Wisconsin Card Sorting Test (Heaton 1981), a test that measures abstract thinking and the ability to shift mental sets by asking subjects to match cards on the basis of color, shape, and number. The results were interpreted as evidence of impairment of the dorsolateral prefrontal cortex in schizophrenic individuals.

Goldberg and colleagues (1987) provided further evidence for the intransigence of the frontal lobe deficit by attempting to teach schizophrenic individuals how to perform the card sort testing by giving them explicit card-by-card instructions. When these instructions were withdrawn, the subjects immediately returned to their baseline performances. However, several other investigators have disputed the putative inability of schizophrenic individuals to perform the Wisconsin Card Sorting Test and have reported that instructional cues (Goldman et al. 1992), monetary reinforcement (Summerfelt et al. 1991), or combinations of monetary reinforcement and instructional cues (Bellack et al. 1990; Green et al. 1992) significantly improve patient performance. In the Bellack et al. (1990) study, these improvements were sustained the next day, when no additional cues were provided. Differences between these studies may be attributable to a more severely ill population in the Goldberg et al. (1987) study than in other studies and to differences in test administration between the various studies.

These studies question to some degree the ubiquity of the frontal lobe deficit in schizophrenic individuals. For example, in a group of stable outpatient schizophrenic individuals, only 35% scored in the impaired range on the Wisconsin Card Sorting Test (Braff et al. 1991), a performance similar to that of 29% of outpatient first-episode patients tested at 2-year follow-up in another study (Hoff et al. 1992b). In a group of 56 schizophreniform patients, frontal lobe functions were reported to be significantly impaired, but there was no evidence that they were relatively more impaired than functions of language, verbal memory, spatial memory, concentration, or motor performance (Hoff et al. 1992a). Saykin et al. (1991) also did not find evidence for selectivity of frontal lobe function in their group of unmedicated (and probably less severely ill) patients. Thus, it appears that frontal lobe function, as measured by the Wisconsin Card Sorting Test, is likely to be a more prominent feature among severely ill schizophrenic inpatients and perhaps one-third of stable outpatients. Indeed, there is evidence among paranoid schizophrenic individuals for an association of perseverative responding on the Wisconsin Card Sorting Test with negative symptoms, slowed reaction time, and more hospitalizations (Butler et al. 1992). Inpatient status and lower overall intellectual functioning has also been associated with impairment on the card sorting test (Heinrichs 1990); severity of positive symptoms was related to poorer card sorting test performance in another study (Morrison-Stewart et al. 1992).

The specificity of frontal lobe deficits to schizophrenia has also been questioned. Morice (1990) and Yurgelun-Todd and Levin (1988) have suggested that bipolar patients perform as poorly as schizophrenic patients on the card sorting test, which may indicate that prefrontal cortical dysfunction is more a correlate of general psychosis. Of course there are other purported cognitive measures of frontal lobe function, such as word or design fluency tests (Lezak 1983), the Categories Test and Trailmaking Test from the Halstead-Reitan Test Battery (Reitan and Wolfson 1985), the Stroop Test (Stroop 1935), tests of olfactory identification (Kopala and Clark 1990) and delayed recall (Freedman and Oscar-Berman 1986), and measures of temporal ordering and frequency estimation (Smith and Milner 1988). Given the relatively large size of the frontal cortex, it is not surprising that putative measures do not correlate significantly with one another (Goldberg et al. 1988; Seidman et al. 1992). Attempts to establish convergent and divergent validity for tests of executive function may contribute to the better understanding of frontal lobe dysfunction in schizophrenia (Sullivan et al. 1993).

Memory

Given that recent evidence has indicated that schizophrenic individuals have postmortem changes in the temporal and hippocampal areas of the brain indicative of neurodevelopmental pathology (Bogerts et al. 1985; Kovelman and Scheibel 1984), and that MRI studies have also documented reductions in size of the hippocampus, amygdala, and whole temporal lobes in schizophrenic patients (Dauphinais et al. 1990; DeLisi et al. 1991; Shenton et al. 1992; Suddath et al. 1989), it seems logical that schizophrenic patients would have memory difficulties. There have been numerous studies attempting to elucidate the nature of this dysfunction (reviewed in Koh 1978). Koh suggested that schizophrenic individuals have difficulty with recall but not with recognition, whereas Calev et al. (1983) suggested that schizophrenic patients' difficulties with memory were attributable to organizational deficits present at the time of encoding. Calev (1984) further indicated that chronically ill patients may have deficits in both recognition and recall. Some investigators (McKenna et al. 1990; Tamlyn et al. 1992) claim that the memory dysfunction in schizophrenia is not dissimilar to the classical amnestic syndrome of preserved immediate memory and deficient long-term memory. With regard to modality of information, it appears that schizophrenic patients are equally impaired on recall of both verbal and visual information (Calev et al. 1987; Gold et al. 1992a).

More recent studies have been aimed at demonstrating that automatic and unconscious (as opposed to effortful and conscious) processes, such as implicit learning (Schmand et al. 1992a), procedural learning (Schmand et al. 1992b), and semantic priming (Schwartz et al. 1992; Vinogradov et al. 1992), are essentially intact in schizophrenic patients, although Gold et al. (1992b) found deficits in both effortful and automatic memory processes. The latter authors concluded that both temporal and frontal lobe mechanisms are involved in memory dysfunction in schizophrenia. Indeed, there is a growing body of literature (Goldman-Rakic 1990; Park and Holzman 1992) that suggests that prefrontal cortical dysfunction contributes to deficits in *working memory*—conceptualized as an on-line, continually updated storage bank of information that guides the individual's responses in problem solving.

It is likely that, as is the case in much of the psychiatric literature, disparate findings regarding memory are related to differences in patient samples on such dimensions as illness severity. The challenge for those studying memory deficits in schizophrenia will be to examine large samples of schizophrenic patients that are heterogeneous in clinical presentation and illness severity on a broad range of memory tasks, thus tapping many levels of memory functioning.

Attention

Early work by Shakow (1962) using a simple reaction-time paradigm, and by Kornetsky and Mirsky (1966) using the Continuous Performance Test (CPT; Rosvold et al. 1956), highlighted the notion that schizophrenic patients have a central deficit in sustained attention. Since then, paradigms using backward masking, the span of apprehension test, and other information-processing tasks (for a review of the literature, see Nuechterlein and Dawson 1984) have demonstrated that schizophrenic individuals perform more poorly than control subjects on elementary information-processing tasks that are likely to involve the sensory register or short-term store (Atkinson and Shiffrin 1968). These deficits may be related to a reduction in processing capacity, abnormal allocation of attention, or poor regulation of arousal (Kahneman 1973). At any rate, such deficits in elementary information processing occur in remitted schizophrenic patients (Asarnow and MacCrimmon 1982), first-degree relatives of schizophrenic patients (Asarnow et al. 1977), and individuals with subclinical schizophrenic thinking (Asarnow et al. 1983). Saccuzzo and Braff (1986) found that informational processing deficits also occur in schizoaffective and bipolar patients, suggesting that processing deficits are more reflective of psychotic illness and may be a fundamental trait of schizophrenic spectrum disorders. Some investigators have found that patients with negative symptoms have relatively poorer information processing than positive-symptom patients (Green and Walker 1986; Weiner et al. 1990).

In summary, the elementary impairments that schizophrenic patients have on simple tasks of information processing speak to a more generalized trait disturbance, perhaps related to more inferior neural systems regulating arousal or to prefrontal regulatory influence. Given these more elementary impairments, it is not surprising that deficits in cognition have been found in almost every functional domain. Studies that use a number of methodologies, including attentional, higher order cognitive, brain morphology, electrophysiological, and metabolic measures, will be needed to clarify and integrate findings from the literature on attention, memory, language, and executive dysfunction in schizophrenia.

Onset and Course of Cognitive Dysfunction in Schizophrenia

There is evidence from studies of preschizophrenic children that cognitive and intellectual deficits are present in early childhood, existing well in advance of the onset of schizophrenic illness (Aylward et al.

1984; Erlenmeyer-Kimling et al. 1984). In addition, studies of military inductees (Mason 1956; Miner and Anderson 1958) have demonstrated that individuals who later developed schizophrenia could be differentiated from normal inductees on preinduction ability testing. Further, an additional decline of cognitive function associated with the onset of illness is evident when comparing military test scores in schizophrenic patients before and after illness onset (Schwartzman and Douglas 1962). As mentioned previously, first-episode schizophreniform patients demonstrated significant deficits on measures of language, executive function, memory, attention-concentration, and motor speed, indicating that substantial cognitive deficits are present at the onset of schizophrenic illness (Hoff et al. 1992a).

With regard to the course of cognitive function in schizophrenia, most of the current evidence indicates an absence of deterioration over the course of the illness, with the exception of small subgroups of patients (reviewed by Heaton and Drexler 1987). In fact, most of the evidence supports findings either of no change or of improvement in cognition over the course of illness. From a cross-sectional study, Hoff et al. (1992b) reported that first-episode schizophrenic patients were as cognitively impaired as patients with chronic schizophrenia. In some preliminary longitudinal findings, first episode schizophrenic patients demonstrated improvements on measures of executive function, concentration, and motor speed after 2 years of illness (Hoff et al. 1992a).

Preliminary evidence indicates that cognitive improvements may be related to symptom reduction. However, there is also some evidence that cognitive improvement can occur long after recovery from an acute psychotic episode, and that this improvement is unrelated to symptom reduction (Sweeney et al. 1991a). Cognitive improvement may be related to reductions in medication or a restabilization of brain physiology related to psychotropic treatment.

Goldstein and colleagues (G. Goldstein and Zubin 1990; G. Goldstein et al. 1991) also found little evidence for cognitive deterioration in schizophrenia. Only a schizophrenic group with documented neurological dysfunction (e.g., head trauma, epilepsy, vascular disorders) showed evidence of deterioration, suggesting a possible interactive effect of neurological factors, the schizophrenic illness, and the aging process in producing this deterioration.

Relationship of Demographic, Clinical, and Medication Factors to Cognitive Dysfunction in Schizophrenia

Effects of Gender

There have been very few neuropsychological studies on differences between male and female schizophrenic patients. Haas et al. (1991) found that male schizophrenic patients were more impaired than females on measures of verbal memory, whereas Perlick et al. (1992a) found that female schizophrenic patients were more impaired than males on measures of conceptualization and attention. Hoff et al. (1991) found that female chronic schizophrenic patients were more impaired on executive functioning than males, but that first-episode females and males were equal on summary measures of neuropsychological functioning. Walker and Lewine (1993) attributed these differences to sampling biases due to the higher threshold for involuntary treatment of females than males. According to this theory, involuntarily committed female schizophrenic patients would be more impaired than males, whereas in better-outcome outpatient settings, female patients should be less impaired than males. J. Goldstein (1993) agreed that differences in sample characteristics could account for these disparate findings, but argued that severity-of-illness factors rather than help-seeking behavior accounted for the results. Clearly, more work is needed in this area.

Effects of Positive Versus Negative Symptoms

Consistent with the concept of type II schizophrenia, which is characterized by negative symptoms, poor outcome, and possible structural damage to the brain (Crow 1980), there have been a number of investigators who have found that negative symptoms are associated with cognitive dysfunction (Andreasen and Olsen 1982; Johnstone et al. 1976; Owens and Johnstone 1980). It is interesting that Perlick et al. (1992b) reported that this relationship held true only in female schizophrenic patients and that it was especially true for performance on measures of conceptual-executive and verbal frontal functioning.

In a well-designed study, Green and Walker (1985) found positive symptoms to be inversely associated with verbal memory deficits and negative symptoms to be associated with visual-motor and visual-spatial impairments. These findings were supported to some degree by those of Bilder et al. (1985), who found that a factor reflecting positive formal thought disorder was inversely related to performance on summary scales of language and memory; by Silverstein et al. (1991), who found that left hemisphere dysfunction was associated with positive thought disorder and right hemisphere and bilateral dysfunction, with negative symptoms; and by Mayer et al. (1985), who found that right hemisphere dysfunction was related to negative symptoms and flat affect. Thus, it is likely that different symptom clusters are related to different neuroanatomic substrates. Consistent with the above findings have been the results of studies comparing schizophrenic subtypes on cognitive measures, with indications that paranoid schizophrenic individuals perform better than nonparanoid schizophrenic individuals on measures of neuropsychological function (G. Goldstein and Halperin 1977), although these differences between subgroups are to some degree attenuated after controlling for medication and severity of illness (Bornstein et al. 1990)

Effects of Medication

There have been five recent reviews of the literature on the effects of psychotropic medications on cognition (Cassens et al. 1990; Heaton and Crowley 1981; D. J. King 1990; Medalia et al. 1988; Spohn and Strauss 1989). In general, acute administration of neuroleptics can impair measures of sustained attention and motor speed in schizophrenic individuals and nonpsychiatric control subjects, whereas chronic administration of neuroleptics either results in no change or an improvement on measures of attention/information processing and abstract thinking for schizophrenic patients. There is some evidence that chronic administration of neuroleptics reduces motor speed and dexterity in schizophrenic patients. Frith (1984) has argued that memory impairment in schizophrenia may be a function of anticholinergic medications, such as benztropine (Cogentin), when used adjunctively to reduce extrapyramidal side effects. Supporting this notion, Perlick et al. (1986) found that free recall was inversely related to serum anticholinergic levels.

Because neuroleptics themselves have varying degrees of anticholinergic activity, recent findings of reduced visual memory in clozapine-treated patients by Goldberg et al. (1993) and Hoff et al. (1993) are interesting in light of clozapine's strong anticholinergic profile. Sweeney et al. (1991b) suggested that poorer neuropsychological functioning is associated with higher levels of neuroleptic and anticholinergic medication after controlling for symptom severity and intellectual functioning. Berger et al. (1989) also reported that haloperidol adversely effects the ability of patients with spasmodic torticollis to make conceptual shifts on the Wisconsin Card Sorting Test.

Cognitive Remediation: Is There Any Hope?

Despite the progress that has been made in the last 10 years in the remediation of cognitive deficits of brain-damaged individuals—specifically, head-injured patients (Meier et al. 1987; Sohlberg and Mateer 1989)—there has been little application of these principles to the rehabilitation of cognitive deficits in schizophrenic patients. This lack of effort is probably in part attributable to the belief widely held by many practitioners that cognitive deficits are functional or secondary to the principal symptoms of thought disorder, or are artifacts related to both positive and negative symptoms or medication. Yet there is recent evidence that cognitive deficits are potent predictors of clinical outcome and can differentiate long-term inpatient or outpatient status (Perlick et al. 1992c, 1992d). Breier et al. (1991) specifically found that tests of frontal functioning were related to measures of social outcome.

Because cognitive deficits are a residual part of psychiatric illness and often limit vocational and social choices (Goldberg et al. 1990, 1993), it appears prudent to test the efficacy of cognitive remediation in schizophrenic illness. A number of investigators have recently made cogent arguments to this effect (Green 1993; Spring and Ravdin 1992), and a number of groups are attempting programs to target and remediate specific deficits. For example, Zec et al. (1988) developed the Executive Board System to improve problem solving and executive functioning. Others (Hermanutz and Gestrich 1991) have targeted attentional processes and have found that schizophrenic individuals can be trained to be less distractible in reaction-time tests.

Hogarty and Flesher (1992) argued that cognitive remediation with schizophrenic patients might not be profitable because schizophrenic patients have long-standing, pervasive cognitive deficits as well as poor motivation. These variables are predictive of poor outcome in brain injury rehabilitation. Nevertheless, until this area receives further study, definitive conclusions cannot be drawn. Both Spaulding (1992) and Jaeger et al. (1992) have presented informative reviews of the methodological difficulties to be overcome in studying the efficacy of cognitive rehabilitation in schizophrenia.

Another approach to the amelioration of cognition may be pharmacological. Goldberg et al. (1991) found that performance on the Wisconsin Card Sorting Test could be improved by the adjunctive use of amphetamines with standard neuroleptic treatment. Although these investigators did not recommend the clinical use of amphetamines with schizophrenic patients, they did suggest that dopamine agonists may have a role in future treatment.

Soper et al. (1990) theorized that reducing serotonergic levels in schizophrenic individuals by the administration of fenfluramine may benefit cognition, based on reported behavioral improvement in autistic patients. However, neuropsychological functioning worsened as a result of the fenfluramine treatment, but an interesting dissociation of serotonin levels and cognitive function was noted as the drug treatment lowered serotonin levels.

Additional pharmacological agents that might be useful for enhancing cognitive function in schizophrenic patients include the cholinomimetics. These have recently been shown to have some efficacy in a subgroup of dementia patients (Summers et al. 1986; also see review by Davidson et al. 1991). Although the etiology of schizophrenia is not thought to be related to cholinergic deficiency, anticholinergic effects of psychotropic medications may have an etiologic role in cognitive deficiencies in schizophrenia (Frith 1984) and could potentially be reversed by this group of medications.

References

Andreasen NC, Grove W: The relationship between schizophrenic language, manic language, and aphasia, in Hemisphere Asymmetries of Function in Psychopathology. Edited by Gruzelier J, Flor-Henry P. Amsterdam, Netherlands, Elsevier, 1979, pp 373–390

Andreasen NC, Olsen S: Ventricular enlargement in schizophrenia: relationship to positive and negative symptoms. Am J Psychiatry 139:297–302, 1982

Asarnow RF, MacCrimmon D: Attention/information processing, neuropsychological functioning, and thought disorder during the acute and partial recovery phases of schizophrenia: a longitudinal study. Psychiatry Res 7:309–319, 1982

Asarnow RF, Watkins J: Schizophrenic thought disorder: linguistic incompetence or information-processing impairment? The Behavioral and Brain Sciences 5:589–590, 1982

Asarnow RF, Steff R, MacCrimmon D, et al: An attentional assessment of foster children at risk for schizophrenia. J Abnorm Psychol 86:267–275, 1977

Asarnow RF, Nuechterlein K, Marder S: Span of apprehension, neuropsychological functioning, and indices of psychosis-proneness. J Nerv Ment Dis 171:662–669, 1983

Atkinson R, Shiffrin R: A proposed system and its control processes, in Advances in the Psychology of Learning and Motivation. Edited by Spence K, Spence J. New York, Academic Press, 1968

Aylward E, Walker E, Bettes B: Intelligence in schizophrenia: meta-analysis of the research. Schizophr Bull 10:430–459, 1984

Bellack AS, Mueser KT, Morrison R, et al: Remediation of cognitive deficits in schizophrenia. Am J Psychiatry 147:1650–1655, 1990

Berger H, Van Hoof J, Van Spaendonck K, et al: Haloperidol and cognitive shifting. Neuropsychologia 27:629–639, 1989

Bilder RM, Mukherjee S, Rieder RO, et al: Symptomatic and neuropsychological components of defect states. Schizophr Bull 11:409–419, 1985

Bogerts B, Meertz E, Schönfeldt-Bausch R: Basal ganglia and limbic system pathology in schizophrenia. Arch Gen Psychiatry 42:784–791, 1985

Bornstein RA, Nasrallah RA, Olson SC, et al: Neuropsychological deficit in schizophrenic subtypes: paranoid, nonparanoid, and schizoaffective subgroups. Psychiatry Res 31:15–24, 1990

Braff D, Heaton R, Kuck J, et al: The generalized pattern of neuropsychological deficits in outpatients with chronic schizophrenia with heterogeneous Wisconsin Card Sorting Test results. Arch Gen Psychiatry 48:891–898, 1991

Breier A, Schreiber J, Dyer J, et al: National Institute of Mental Health longitudinal study of chronic schizophrenia: prognosis and predictors of outcome. Arch Gen Psychiatry 48:239–246, 1991

Butler R, Jenkins M, Sprock J, et al: Wisconsin Card Sort Test deficits in chronic paranoid schizophrenia: evidence for a relatively discrete subgroup? Schizophr Res 7:169–176, 1992

Calev A: Recall and recognition in mildly disturbed schizophrenics: the use of matched tasks. Psychol Med 14:425–429, 1984

Calev A, Venables P, Monk A: Evidence for distinct verbal memory pathologies in severely and mildly disturbed schizophrenics. Schizophr Bull 9:247–264, 1983

Calev A, Korin Y, Kugelmass S, et al: Performance of chronic schizophrenics on matched word and design recall tasks. Biol Psychiatry 22:699–709, 1987

Cassens G, Inglis AK, Appelbaum PS, et al: Neuroleptics: effects on neuropsychological function in chronic schizophrenic patients. Schizophr Bull 16:477–499, 1990

Chaika E: A linguist looks at "schizophrenic" language. Brain Lang 1:257–276, 1974

Crow T: Molecular pathology of schizophrenia: more than one disease process? BMJ 280:66–68, 1980

Crow T, Brown R, Burton C, et al: Loss of sylvian asymmetry in schizophrenia: findings in the Runwell series of brains. Schizophr Res 6:152–153, 1992

Dauphinais I, DeLisi L, Crow T, et al: Reduction in temporal lobe size in siblings with schizophrenia: a magnetic resonance imaging study. Psychiatry Res 35:137–147, 1990

Davidson M, Stern RG, Bierer LM, et al: Cholinergic strategies in the treatment of Alzheimer's disease. Acta Psychiatr Scand Suppl 366:47–51, 1991

DeLisi L, Hoff A, Schwartz J, et al: Brain morphology in first-episode psychotic patients: a quantitative magnetic resonance imaging study. Biol Psychiatry 29:159–175, 1991

Erlenmeyer-Kimling L, Kestenbaum C, Bird H, et al: Assessment of the New York high risk project in sample A who are now clinically deviant, in Children at Risk for Schizophrenia: A Longitudinal Perspective. Edited by Watt N, Anthony E, Wynne L, et al. New York, Cambridge University Press, 1984, pp 34–44

Faber R, Reichstein M: Language dysfunction in schizophrenia. Br J Psychiatry 139:519–522, 1981

Faber R, Abrams R, Taylor M, et al: A comparison of schizophrenic patients with formal thought disorder and neurologically impaired patients with aphasia. Am J Psychiatry 140:1348–1351, 1983

Flor-Henry P, Yeudall L: Neuropsychological investigation of schizophrenia and manic-depressive psychoses, in Hemisphere Asymmetries of Function in Psychopathology. Edited by Gruzelier J, Flor-Henry P. Amsterdam, Netherlands, Elsevier, 1979, pp 341–362

Flor-Henry P, Yeudall L, Stefanyk W, et al: The neuropsychological correlates of the functional psychoses. IRCS Medical Science 3:34, 1975

Freedman M, Oscar-Berman M: Bilateral frontal lobe disease and selective delayed-response in humans. Behav Neurosci 100:337–342, 1986

Frith C: Schizophrenia, memory, and anticholinergic drugs. J Abnorm Psychol 93:339–341, 1984

Frith C, Allen H: Language disorders in schizophrenia and their implications for neuropsychology, in Schizophrenia: The Major Issues. Edited by Bebbington P, McGuffin P. Oxford, Heinemann Medical Books, 1988, pp 172–186

Gold J, Randolph C, Carpenter C, et al: The performance of patients with schizophrenia on the Wechsler Memory Scale-Revised. The Clinical Neuropsychologist 6:367–373, 1992a

Gold J, Randolph C, Carpenter C, et al: Forms of memory failure in schizophrenia. J Abnorm Psychol 101:487–494, 1992b

Goldberg T, Weinberger D, Berman K, et al: Further evidence for dementia of the prefrontal type in schizophrenia. Arch Gen Psychiatry 44:1008–1014, 1987

Goldberg T, Kelsoe J, Weinberger D, et al: Performance of schizophrenic patients on putative neuropsychological tests of frontal function. Int J Neurosci 42:51–58, 1988

Goldberg T, Ragland JD, Torrey EF, et al: Neuropsychological assessment of monozygotic twins discordant for schizophrenia. Arch Gen Psychiatry 47:1066–1072, 1990

Goldberg T, Bigelow LB, Weinberger DR, et al: Cognitive and behavioral effects of the coadministration of dexamphetamine and haloperidol in schizophrenia. Am J Psychiatry 148:78–84, 1991

Goldberg T, Greenberg R, Griffin S, et al: The effect of clozapine on cognition and psychiatric symptoms in patients with schizophrenia. Br J Psychiatry 162:43–48, 1993

Goldman R, Axelrod B, Tompkins L: Effect of instructional cues on schizophrenic patients' performance on the Wisconsin Card Sorting Test. Am J Psychiatry 149:1718–1722, 1992

Goldman-Rakic PS: Prefrontal cortical dysfunction in schizophrenia: the relevance of working memory, in Psychopathology and the Brain. Edited by Carroll B, Barrett J. New York, Raven, 1990, pp 1–23

Goldstein G, Halperin KM: Neuropsychological differences among subtypes of schizophrenia. J Abnorm Psychol 86:34–40, 1977

Goldstein G, Zubin J: Neuropsychological differences between young and old schizophrenics with and without associated dysfunction. Schizophr Res 3:117–126, 1990

Goldstein G, Zubin J, Pogue-Geile MF: Hospitalization and the cognitive deficits of schizophrenia: the influences of age and education. J Nerv Ment Dis 179:202–206, 1991

Goldstein J: Sampling biases in studies of gender and schizophrenia: a reply. Schizophr Bull 19:9–14, 1993

Goldstein K: Functional disturbances in brain damage, in American Handbook of Psychiatry. Edited by Arieti S. New York, Basic Books, 1959, pp 770–794

Green M: Cognitive remediation in schizophrenia: is it time yet? Am J Psychiatry 150:178–187, 1993

Green M, Walker E: Neuropsychological performance and positive and negative symptoms in schizophrenia. J Abnorm Psychol 94:460–469, 1985

Green M, Walker E: Symptom correlates of vulnerability to backward masking. Am J Psychiatry 143:181–186, 1986

Green M, Satz P, Ganzell S, et al: Wisconsin Card Sorting Test performance in schizophrenia: remediation of a stubborn deficit. Am J Psychiatry 149:62–67, 1992

Haas GL, Sweeney JA, Hien DA, et al: Sex differences in the course of schizophrenia. The Clinical Neuropsychologist 5:281–282, 1991

Halpern H, McCartin-Clark M: Differential language characteristics in adult aphasic and schizophrenic subjects. J Commun Disord 17:289–307, 1984

Heaton R: Wisconsin Card Sorting Test Manual. Odessa, TX, Psychological Assessment Resources, 1981

Heaton R, Crowley T: Effects of psychiatric disorders and their somatic treatments on neuropsychological test results, in Handbook of Clinical Neuropsychology. Edited by Filskov S, Boll T. New York, Wiley-Interscience, 1981, pp 481–525

Heaton R, Drexler M: Clinical neuropsychological findings in schizophrenia and aging, in Schizophrenia and Aging. Edited by Miller N, Cohen G. New York, Guilford, 1987, pp 145–161

Heaton R, Baade L, Johnson K: Neuropsychological test results associated with psychiatric disorders in adults. Psychol Bull 85:141–162, 1978

Heinrichs R: Variables associated with Wisconsin Card Sorting performance in neuropsychiatric patients referred for assessment. Neuropsychiatry, Neuropsychology, and Behavioral Neurology 3:107–112, 1990

Hermanutz M, Gestrich J: Computer-assisted attention training in schizophrenics. Eur Arch Psychiatry Clin Neurosci 240:282–287, 1991

Hoff AL, Riordan H, DeLisi L: Influence of gender on neuropsychological testing and MRI measures of schizophrenic inpatients. The Clinical Neuropsychologist 5:281, 1991

Hoff AL, Riordan H, O'Donnell D, et al: Neuropsychological functioning of first-episode schizophreniform patients. Am J Psychiatry 149:898–903, 1992a

Hoff AL, Riordan H, O'Donnell D, et al: Anomalous lateral sulcus asymmetry and cognitive function in first-episode schizophrenia. Schizophr Bull 18:257–272, 1992b

Hoff AL, Wieneke M, DeVilliers D, et al: Effect of clozapine on cognitive function. Paper presented at the annual meeting of the American Psychiatric Association, San Francisco, CA, May 1993

Hogarty GE, Flesher S: Cognitive remediation in schizophrenia: Proceed . . . with caution! Schizophr Bull 18:51–57, 1992

Jaeger J, Berns S, Tigner A, et al: Remediation of neuropsychological deficits in psychiatric populations: rationale and methodological considerations. Psychopharmacol Bull 28:367–390, 1992

Johnstone EC, Crow TJ, Frith C, et al: Cerebral ventricular size and cognitive impairment in chronic schizophrenia. Lancet 2:924–926, 1976

Kahneman D: Attention and Effort. Englewood Cliffs, NJ, Prentice-Hall, 1973

King DJ: The effect of neuroleptics on cognitive and psychomotor function. Br J Psychiatry 157:799–811, 1990

King K, Fraser I, Thomas P, et al: Re-examination of the language of psychotic subjects. Br J Psychiatry 156:211–215, 1990

Koh S: Remembering of verbal materials by schizophrenic adults, in Language and Cognition in Schizophrenia. Edited by Schwartz S. Hillsdale, NJ, Erlbaum, 1978, pp 59–99

Kolb B, Whishaw I: Performance of schizophrenic patients on tests sensitive to left or right frontal, temporal, or parietal function in neurological patients. J Nerv Ment Dis 171:435–443, 1983

Kopala LC, Clark C: Implications of olfactory agnosia for understanding sex differences in schizophrenia. Schizophr Bull 16:255–261, 1990

Kornetsky C, Mirsky A: On certain psychopharmacological and physiological differences between schizophrenics and normal persons. Psychopharmacology (Berl) 8:309–318, 1966

Kovelman J, Scheibel A: A neurohistological correlate of schizophrenia. Biol Psychiatry 19:1601–1621, 1984

Kraepelin E: Dementia Praecox and Paraphrenia. Edinburgh, Scotland, E & S Livingstone, 1919

Landre N, Taylor M, Kearns K: Language functioning in schizophrenic and aphasic patients. Neuropsychiatry, Neuropsychology, and Behavioral Neurology 5:7–14, 1992

Levin S: Frontal lobe dysfunctions in schizophrenia, II: impairments of psychological and brain functions. J Psychiatr Res 18:57–72, 1984

Lezak M: Neuropsychological Assessment. New York, Oxford University Press, 1983

Mason C: Pre-illness intelligence of mental hospital patients. Journal of Consulting Psychology 20:297–300, 1956

Mayer M, Alpert M, Stastny P, et al: Multiple contributions to clinical presentation of flat affect in schizophrenia. Schizophr Bull 11:420–426, 1985

McKenna P, Tamlyn D, Lund C, et al: Amnesic syndrome in schizophrenia. Psychol Med 20:967–972, 1990

Medalia A, Gold J, Merriam A: The effects of neuroleptics on neuropsychological test results of schizophrenics. Archives of Clinical Neuropsychology 3:249–271, 1988

Meier M, Benton A, Diller L: Neuropsychological Rehabilitation. New York, Churchill Livingstone, 1987

Miner J, Anderson J: Intelligence and emotional disturbance: evidence from Army and Veterans Administration records. J Abnorm Soc Psychol 56:75–81, 1958

Morice R: Beyond language—speculations on the prefrontal cortex and schizophrenia. Aust N Z J Psychiatry 20:7–10, 1986

Morice R: Cognitive inflexibility and pre-frontal dysfunction in schizophrenia and mania. Br J Psychiatry 157:50–54, 1990

Morice R, Ingram J: Language complexity and age of onset of schizophrenia. Psychiatry Res 9:233–242, 1983

Morice R, McNichol D: Language changes in schizophrenia: a limited replication. Schizophr Bull 12:239–251, 1986

Morrison-Stewart S, Williamson P, Corning W, et al: Frontal and non-frontal lobe neuropsychological test performance and clinical symptomatology in schizophrenia. Psychol Med 22:353–359, 1992

Nuechterlein K, Dawson M: Information processing and attentional functioning in the developmental course of schizophrenic disorders. Schizophr Bull 10:160–203, 1984

Owens D, Johnstone E: The disabilities of chronic schizophrenia—their nature and factors contributing to their development. Br J Psychiatry 136:384–395, 1980

Park S, Holzman PS: Schizophrenics show spatial working memory deficits. Arch Gen Psychiatry 49:975–982, 1992

Paulman R, Devoud M, Gregory R, et al: Hypofrontality and cognitive impairment in schizophrenia: dynamic single-photon tomography and neuropsychological assessment of schizophrenic brain function. Biol Psychiatry 27:377–399, 1990

Perlick D, Stastny P, Katz I, et al: Memory deficits and anticholinergic levels in schizophrenia. Am J Psychiatry 143:230–232, 1986

Perlick D, Mattis S, Stastny P, et al: Gender differences in cognition in schizophrenia. Schizophr Res 8:69–73, 1992a

Perlick D, Mattis S, Stastny P, et al: Negative symptoms are related to both frontal and nonfrontal neuropsychological measures in chronic schizophrenia. Arch Gen Psychiatry 49:245–246, 1992b

Perlick D, Stastny P, Mattis S, et al: Contribution of family, cognitive and clinical dimensions to long-term outcome in schizophrenia. Schizophr Res 6:257–265, 1992c

Perlick D, Mattis S, Stastny P, et al: Neuropsychological discriminators of long-term inpatient or outpatient status in chronic schizophrenia. J Neuropsychiatry Clin Neurosci 4:428–434, 1992d

Reitan R, Wolfson D: The Halstead-Reitan Neuropsychological Test Battery. Tucson, Neuropsychology Press, 1985

Rossi A, Stratta T, Mattei P, et al: Planum temporale in schizophrenia: a magnetic resonance imaging study. Schizophr Res 7:19–22, 1992

Rosvold HE, Mirsky AF, Sarason I, et al: A continuous performance test of brain damage. J Consult Clin Psychol 20:343, 1956

Saccuzzo DP, Braff DL: Information-processing abnormalities: trait- and state-dependent components. Schizophr Bull 12:447–459, 1986

Saykin AJ, Gur RC, Gur RE, et al: Neuropsychological function in schizophrenia: selective impairment in memory and learning. Arch Gen Psychiatry 48:618–624, 1991

Schmand B, Kop WJ, Kuipers T, et al: Implicit learning in psychotic patients. Schizophr Res 7:55–64, 1992a

Schmand B, Brand N, Kuipers T: Procedural learning of cognitive and motor skills in psychotic patients. Schizophr Res 8:157–170, 1992b

Schwartz BL, Rosse RB, Deutsch SI: Toward a neuropsychology of memory in schizophrenia. Psychopharmacol Bull 28:341–351, 1992

Schwartzman A, Douglas V: Intellectual loss in schizophrenia, part 1. Can J Psychol 16:161–168, 1962

Seidman L: Schizophrenia and brain dysfunction: an integration of recent neurodiagnostic findings. Psychol Bull 94:195–238, 1983

Seidman L, Talbot N, Kalinowski A, et al: Neuropsychological probes of fronto-limbic system dysfunction in schizophrenia: olfactory identification and Wisconsin Card Sorting performance. Schizophr Res 6:55–65, 1992

Shakow D: Segmental set: a theory of the formal psychological deficit in schizophrenia. Arch Gen Psychiatry 6:1–17, 1962

Shenton ME, Kikinis R, Jolesz FA, et al: Abnormalities of the left temporal lobe and thought disorder in schizophrenia. N Engl J Med 327:604–612, 1992

Silverstein ML, Marengo JT, Fogg L: Two types of thought disorder and lateralized neuropsychological dysfunction. Schizophr Bull 17:679–687, 1991

Smith M, Milner B: Estimation of frequency of occurrence of abstract designs after frontal or temporal lobectomy. Neuropsychologia 26:297–306, 1988

Sohlberg M, Mateer C: Introduction to Cognitive Rehabilitation. New York, Guilford, 1989

Soper HV, Elliot RO, Rejzer AA, et al: Effects of fenfluramine on neuropsychological and communicative functioning in treatment-refractory schizophrenic patients. J Clin Psychopharmacol 10:168–175, 1990

Spaulding W: Design prerequisites for research on cognitive therapy for schizophrenia. Schizophr Bull 18:39–50, 1992

Spohn H, Strauss M: Relation of neuroleptic medication to cognitive functions in schizophrenia. J Abnorm Psychol 98:367–380, 1989

Spring BJ, Ravdin L: Cognitive remediation in schizophrenia: should we attempt it? Schizophr Bull 18:15–20, 1992

Stroop J: Studies of interference in serial verbal reactions. J Exp Psychol 18:643–662, 1935

Suddath RL, Casanova MF, Goldberg TE, et al: Temporal lobe pathology in schizophrenia: a quantitative magnetic resonance imaging study. Am J Psychiatry 146:464–472, 1989

Sullivan E, Mathalon D, Zipursky R, et al: Factors of the Wisconsin Card Sorting Test as measures of frontal lobe function in schizophrenia and chronic alcoholism. Psychiatry Res 46:175–199, 1993

Summerfelt A, Alphs L, Funderburk F, et al: Impaired Wisconsin Card Sort performance in schizophrenia may reflect motivational deficits (letter). Arch Gen Psychiatry 48:282–283, 1991

Summers WK, Majovski LV, Marsh GM, et al: Oral tetrahydroaminoacridine in long-term treatment of senile dementia, Alzheimer type. N Engl J Med 315:1241–1245, 1986

Sweeney JA, Haas GL, Keilp JG, et al: Evaluation of the stability of neuropsychological functioning after acute episodes of schizophrenia: a one-year follow-up study. Psychiatry Res 38:63–76, 1991a

Sweeney JA, Keilp JG, Haas G, et al: Relationships between medication treatments and neuropsychological test performance in schizophrenia. Psychiatry Res 37:297–308, 1991b

Tamlyn D, McKenna PJ, Mortimer AM, et al: Memory impairment in schizophrenia: its extent, affiliations and neuropsychological character. Psychol Med 22:101–115, 1992

Taylor M, Abrams R: Cognitive impairment in schizophrenia. Am J Psychiatry 141:196–201, 1984

Vinogradov S, Ober BA, Shenaut GK: Semantic priming of word pronunciation and lexical decision in schizophrenia. Schizophr Res 8:171–181, 1992

Walker EF, Lewine RR: Sampling biases in studies of gender and schizophrenia. Schizophr Bull 19:1–7, 1993

Weinberger D, Berman K, Zec R: Physiologic dysfunction of dorsolateral prefrontal cortex in schizophrenia, I: regional cerebral blood flow evidence. Arch Gen Psychiatry 43:114–125, 1986

Weiner RU, Opler LA, Kay SR, et al: Visual information processing in positive, mixed, and negative schizophrenic syndromes. J Nerv Ment Dis 178:616–626, 1990

Yurgelun-Todd D, Levin S: Wisconsin Card Sort in schizophrenia and manic depressive illness. J Clin Exp Neuropsychol 10:71, 1988

Zec R, Gambach J, Myers D: Improved adaptive functioning in schizophrenic patients using the "Executive Board System." J Clin Exp Neuropsychol 10:20, 1988

Relationship of Structural Brain Changes to Antipsychotic Drug Response in Schizophrenia

Henry A. Nasrallah, M.D.

F ollowing the psychopharmacological revolution of the 1950s and 1960s that transformed the practice of psychiatry, the seedlings of another revolution were poised for sprouting during the 1970s. The first use of computed tomography (CT) to study the structure of the brain in schizophrenia (Johnstone et al. 1976) and the study of cerebral blood flow in relation to brain function in psychosis (Ingvar and Franzen 1974) served as the harbingers of the brain-imaging revolution in the 1980s. Many new findings and insights relating to brain structure and function in schizophrenia were generated with the applications of additional brain-imaging techniques, including magnetic resonance imaging (MRI), positron-emission tomography (PET), single photon emission computed tomography (SPECT), and magnetic resonance spectroscopy (MRS) (Abou-Saleh 1990).

Much has been learned about the clinical and biological correlates of structural brain abnormalities in schizophrenia. This is mainly because one of the earliest objectives of CT researchers was to examine the relationship between neuroanatomy and the clinical features of (including pharmacological response in) schizophrenia (Crow et al. 1982; Nasrallah et al. 1982; Weinberger et al. 1980). The type I and type II concepts of schizophrenia proposed by Crow (1980) were inspired by the early findings of what seemed to be atrophy in the brains of some schizophrenic patients but not others. Crow postulated that schizophrenic patients with cerebral structural pathology also had more negative symptoms, poor response to neuroleptic pharmacotherapy, and a deteriorating course. On the other hand, schizophrenic patients with no structural cerebral pathology were postulated to have more positive symptoms, good response to antipsychotic drugs, and better outcome. Although Crow's model could not explain all the complexities of the schizophrenic syndrome, it brought a welcome focus on the possible association between structural brain lesions and clinical response to antipsychotic medications in schizophrenia. Such an association can be of significant value to clinicians, both in the management of patients with schizophrenia and in considering alternatives for treatment.

In this chapter, I present an overview of the literature in which researchers have attempted to find a relationship between structural brain pathology and clinical response to standard or atypical neuroleptics in schizophrenia. I also address some related issues, such as the following:

- The possible relationships between what are now regarded as neurodevelopmental brain abnormalities in schizophrenia (Nasrallah 1993) and neurotransmitter systems, such as dopamine and serotonin
- Whether structural brain changes seen in some schizophrenic patients might possibly develop as a result of delayed or absent antipsychotic drug treatment, which would imply that untreated psychosis has neurotoxic effects
- Whether the link between structural brain changes and neuroleptic response is a spurious one
- How the clinical psychiatrist should use brain-imaging findings for the practical management of schizophrenic patients

Structural Brain Pathology in Schizophrenia

Several cortical and subcortical morphological abnormalities have been reported in schizophrenia (see summary in Table 10–1). The literature has focused mainly on cerebral ventricular dilatation and sulcal-fissure widening (Shelton and Weinberger 1986). For that reason, studies of neuroleptic response have focused almost entirely on these two morphological abnormalities, one being cortical (sulcal widening) and the other subcortical (ventricular enlargement). The literature reviewed below is therefore limited to those two types of lesions, since little if any work has been done on other structural abnormalities. At the time of the writing of this chapter, much attention was being focused on

Table 10–1.   Structural brain abnormalities reported in schizophrenia on computed tomography and magnetic resonance imaging scans

Cortical
  Widened fissures and sulci
  Decreased cranial volume
  Decreased gray matter volume
  Decreased brain volume
  Decreased frontal volume
  Decreased temporal volume
  Abnormal cerebral asymmetries
  Decreased tissue "density"

Limbic
  Decreased hippocampus volume
  Decreased parahippocampus volume
  Abnormal entorhinal cortex gyri and sulci

Subcortical
  Enlarged lateral ventricular volume
  Increased temporal horn of the lateral ventricles
  Enlarged third ventricular volume
  Increased frequency of cavum septum pellucidum
  Increased caudate nucleus volume
  Increased ventricular nucleus volume
  Decreased thalamic volume
  Increased corpus callosum thickness
  Increased callosal length

Cerebellar
  Vermal atrophy-hypoplasia
  Enlarged fourth ventricle

medial (limbic) temporal lobe structures (i.e., hippocampus, amygdala, parahippocampus, and entorhinal cortex), which tend to be "hypoplastic" in schizophrenia (see Chapter 2). It is possible that future studies of structural pathology and drug response in schizophrenia may focus on this region (Bogerts et al. 1993).

Studies of Structural Brain Pathology and Neuroleptic Drug Response in Schizophrenia

I present my review of studies on the relationship between structural brain abnormalities in schizophrenia and clinical response to neuroleptics in two main sections: cerebral ventricular enlargement and sulcal-fissure widening. Under each section, I present the literature in three subsections: studies showing a positive association, studies showing a negative association, and studies suggesting no relationship.

Cerebral Ventricular Enlargement

Essentially all of these studies focused on the lateral cerebral ventricles rather than the third ventricles.

Studies suggesting that large ventricular size (usually expressed as ventricle-to-brain ratio [VBR]) is associated with poor response to neuroleptics:

1. Weinberger et al. (1980) retrospectively examined 20 schizophrenic patients who had received at least 8 weeks of neuroleptic treatment following washout from their antipsychotic medication. The group with normal VBR was significantly less symptomatic after treatment (a 27.5-point drop in Brief Psychiatric Rating Scale [BPRS; Overall and Gorham 1962] score versus a 0.3-point drop for the large-VBR group [$P < .003$]).
2. Nasrallah et al. (1980) reexamined the VBR of seven patients who had failed to respond to the addition of the dopamine synthesis inhibitor α-methyl-p-tyrosine (AMPT) to their neuroleptic regimen. Six of the seven patients had ventricular enlargement. CT scans on those who responded to AMPT were not available for comparison.

3. Jeste et al. (1982) conducted a reexamination of those who responded and those who did not respond to neuroleptics in Weinberger et al.'s (1980) study. They found that 1 out of 8 patients who did respond had enlarged VBR versus 8 out of 12 patients who did not respond ($P < .03$).

4. Luchins et al. (1983) conducted a retrospective study of 35 schizophrenic patients treated with neuroleptics for at least 5 weeks. Ten patients had VBR greater than 1 standard deviation (SD) above that of the control subjects. The patients with smaller ventricles showed improvement ($P = .04$) on post hoc analysis of the Schedule for Affective Disorders and Schizophrenia–Change Version (SADS-C; Endicott and Spitzer 1978) for items relating to delusions of reference, persecution, psychomotor retardation, and catatonic and bizarre behavior.

5. Schulz et al. (1983) conducted a prospective study of 12 adolescents with schizophrenia, 8 of whom were drug naive. Testing on the BPRS was done at baseline and weekly for 2–6 weeks. Seven patients had abnormal VBR (greater than 2 SDs above the control mean) and 5 had normal VBR. The BPRS drop for the normal-VBR group was from 50.4 to 33.2 points, whereas the score for the abnormal-VBR group actually increased slightly but not significantly (from 40.0 to 40.9).

6. Luchins et al. (1984) reexamined the data from their 1983 study (described above) and obtained similar results.

7. Williams et al. (1985) rated the response in 40 patients on depot neuroleptics as good ($n = 11$), partial ($n = 12$), and poor ($n = 17$). The VBR was larger in those who responded poorly or only partially compared with those who responded well. The largest VBR was in the group of those who partially responded to treatment.

8. Pandurangi et al. (1989) conducted a prospective treatment study (2–7 weeks, mean of 3.7 weeks) with 19 schizophrenic patients. BPRS ratings were done at baseline and weekly. An amphetamine challenge test conducted with all patients revealed that those who worsened after amphetamine had smaller VBR and tended to show better response to neuroleptics ($P < .07$).

Studies suggesting that large ventricular size is associated with good response to neuroleptics:

1. Smith et al. (1983) treated 30 schizophrenic patients with either 20 mg of haloperidol or 100 mg of thioridazine for 3 weeks. Response was defined as a minimum of 50% decrease in the New Haven Schizophrenia

Index (Garver et al. 1977). There was a consistent, albeit nonsignificant, trend for patients with VBR above 5.7 to show greater response than patients with VBR less than 5.7.

2. Boronow et al. (1985) administered a double-blind, placebo-controlled drug treatment protocol in 30 patients with schizophrenia. All patients received more than 400 mg of chlorpromazine equivalents daily. Ratings were done on the BPRS. The only significant finding was that patients with large lateral ventricles showed more improvement in the withdrawal-retardation factor of the BPRS.

3. Smith et al. (1985) reexamined the data from their 1983 study (described above) and reported that ventricular enlargement tended to be positively correlated with clinical improvement in BPRS psychosis factor scores and negatively correlated with improvement in BPRS anergia scores.

Studies that found no relationship between ventricular enlargement and neuroleptic response:

1. Nasrallah et al. (1983b) classified the neuroleptic response of 55 schizophrenic patients as good, partial, or poor using the patients' medical records but without knowing the patient's VBR. Nineteen of the patients had a VBR greater than 2 SDs above the control mean. No significant differences were found in the proportion of those who responded well in the large- or normal-VBR groups.

2. Naber et al. (1985) assessed 36 patients during neuroleptic therapy and after 12 days of neuroleptic withdrawal, using the BPRS. The dosage and duration of neuroleptic therapy did not correlate with ventricular size or with any other CT variable.

3. Losonczy et al. (1986a), in a 6-week trial using a fixed-dosage schedule of haloperidol, found that none of the BPRS item scores or the total BPRS or Clinical Global Impression (CGI; Guy 1976) scores were related to VBR.

4. Pandurangi et al. (1986) rated response to treatment as none, mild, moderate, or high using the BPRS, and found no differences in drug response between schizophrenic patients with a large VBR ($n = 7$) and those with a normal VBR ($n = 13$). In this study, large VBR was defined as greater than 1 SD above the control mean.

5. Keefe et al. (1987) defined response to haloperidol as at least a 20% decrease in BPRS scores and a 2-point decrease in CGI score in 21 patients. They found no significant difference in treatment response be-

tween "Kraepelinian" schizophrenic patients (i.e., patients with large ventricles) and "non-Kraepelinian" schizophrenic patients.

6. Nimgaonkar et al. (1988) gave a minimum of 600 mg of chlorpromazine equivalents to 36 schizophrenic patients and measured serum dopamine-blocking activity with radioimmunoassay. Response was defined as having 80% improvement on the Montgomery Schizophrenia Scale (MSS; Montgomery et al. 1983), and nonresponse was defined as having less than 20% improvement. No difference was observed in mean VBR between those who did respond (n = 18; mean VBR = 10.2) and those who did not (n = 18; mean VBR = 9.7). In addition, there was no significant correlation between VBR and log-transformed change in MSS score.

7. Kaiya et al. (1989) divided 80 schizophrenic patients into those who responded excellently (n = 23), those who responded well (n = 51), and those who did not respond (n = 6). No difference in VBR was found among the groups.

8. Friedman et al. (1991) gave a trial of clozapine to treatment-resistant patients and classified them into those who did not respond, those who responded moderately well, and those who responded well based on the percentage of change in BPRS scores. They found no relationship between VBR and response to medication.

Sulcal-Fissure Widening[1]

Researchers in most of these studies assessed cortical atrophy using visual inspection ratings, but a few measured the actual width of the sulci and fissures.

Studies suggesting that sulcal-fissure widening is associated with poor response to neuroleptics:

1. Smith et al. (1983) rated clinical response in 30 schizophrenic patients treated with 20 mg of haloperidol or 100 mg of thioridazine daily for 3 weeks. Response was defined as a minimum of a 50% decrease in the New Haven Schizophrenia Index. Both the patients with severe cortical atrophy and those without any cortical atrophy had a poor clinical

---

[1] Also referred to as *cortical atrophy* by most of the studies.

response, but the best response was in the patients with mild cortical atrophy; that is, a curvilinear relationship was observed.

2. Vita et al. (1988) measured clinical response to neuroleptics using BPRS ratings after 4 weeks and 6 months of treatment. Both the atrophy ($n = 12$) and the no-atrophy ($n = 9$) groups improved after 4 weeks. However, after 6 months of neuroleptic treatment, the no-atrophy group continued to improve significantly more than at the 4-week level, whereas the atrophy group showed no additional improvement after the first 4 weeks.

3. Kaiya et al. (1989) retrospectively classified 80 patients as having an excellent response to neuroleptic treatment if positive symptoms disappeared after 3 months of antipsychotic drug treatment, as having a good response if partial improvement occurred, and as having failed treatment if no response occurred. Excellent drug response was associated with less cortical atrophy in the frontal lobe.

4. Friedman et al. (1991) examined response to clozapine in 34 treatment-resistant schizophrenic patients. Prefrontal sulcal prominence was rated from 0 to 3. The authors found a linear trend of declining prefrontal sulcal prominence across those who did not respond, those who responded moderately well, and those who responded well ($P = .004$). Multiple regression analysis showed that prefrontal sulcal prominence could predict BPRS score at the end of 6 weeks.

Studies suggesting that sulcal-fissure widening is associated with good response to neuroleptics:

1. Smith et al. (1983), as mentioned above, reported that patients with mild cortical atrophy had the best response to neuroleptics, whereas those without any cortical atrophy had a poorer response similar to that of patients with severe cortical atrophy.

Studies suggesting a lack of association between sulcal-fissure widening and clinical response to neuroleptics:

1. Nasrallah et al. (1983a) rated the response of 55 schizophrenic patients to neuroleptics (good response = all symptoms remitted; partial response = many symptoms remitted; poor response = most symptoms unchanged) over several episodes by reviewing their medical records. Patients were divided into those with ($n = 22$) and without ($n = 33$) sulcal

widening as shown on CT scans. Similar proportions of those with and those without sulcal widening (16% and 20%, respectively) had full response. No association was found between sulcal widening and response to neuroleptics.

2. Pandurangi et al. (1986) found no association between response to neuroleptic treatment and sulcal measures in 23 patients with schizophrenia.

3. Smith et al. (1987) found no difference in mean sulcal width between schizophrenic patients who responded well ($n = 20$) and those who responded poorly ($n = 19$) to neuroleptics when treated at a constant dosage of haloperidol 20 mg/day for 3 weeks.

4. Nimgaonkar et al. (1988) reported finding no significant correlation between the total score of sulcal widening and the log-transformed change in MSS score (T = .11) in 36 patients.

5. Using a stereological method, MacDonald et al. (1989) measured the sulcal-to-brain volume ratio in 27 patients who received a drug trial of pimozide versus flupenthixol. Response was measured on the Krawiecka scale (Krawiecka et al. 1977). No difference in response to neuroleptic medications was found between the large and the small sulcal-to-brain-volume ratios.

Structural Brain Abnormalities and Neurotransmitter Pathology in Schizophrenia

If structural brain abnormalities are associated with clinical response to antipsychotic drugs, then it can be inferred that structural abnormalities are associated with dysfunction in the neurotransmitter systems (i.e., dopamine and serotonin) that are the putative targets of antipsychotic drug actions. Antipsychotic medications are believed to exert at least part of their therapeutic effects by decreasing the activity of dopamine, possibly by blocking one or more of the five dopamine receptors that have been distinguished so far (especially the D_2 receptor for typical antipsychotics and the D_4 receptor for the atypical antipsychotics).

What is the evidence for this hypothesis? Direct data are not available, but there are some indirect data that might be relevant to this issue:

1. There appears to be a significant negative correlation between cerebrospinal fluid (CSF) homovanillic acid (HVA; a major metabolite of dopamine) and ventricular enlargement (Losonczy et al. 1986b), as well as a decrease in dopamine-β-hydroxylase and HVA in the CSF of schizophrenic patients with sulcal widening (van Kammen et al. 1983). Such findings imply that schizophrenic patients with structural brain abnormalities may have "*hypo*dopaminergia," but there is no direct evidence yet that schizophrenic patients without structural brain abnormalities have "*hyper*dopaminergia."

2. It has been proposed that schizophrenic patients with frontal lobe atrophy may have decreased cortical dopamine activity but increased (up-regulated) subcortical mesolimbic dopamine activity (Weinberger 1987). This might also explain the coexistence of positive symptoms (mesolimbic hyperdopaminergia) and negative symptoms (frontal cortical hypodopaminergia) in schizophrenia.

3. Several studies have found an association between obstetric complications (e.g., brain hypoxia) and structural brain abnormalities (Murray et al. 1988). It is therefore important to know what the effects of hypoxia on the developing brain are with regard to dopamine function. Researchers in several animal studies (Lun et al. 1986; Silverstein and Johnston 1984) have shown that perinatal hypoxia is associated with dopamine release.

4. One of the yet unanswered questions is how neurodevelopmental morphological changes in the limbic system (i.e., hippocampus, amygdala, parahippocampus, entorhinal cortex, anterior cingulate) in schizophrenia produce a neurochemical pathology in the mesolimbic dopamine system that in turn produces psychotic symptoms that require dopamine antagonists for therapy. One possible mechanism is that increased dopamine activity in the mesolimbic region of schizophrenia may be a compensatory mechanism (increased innervation) resulting from the loss of certain projections because of neurodevelopmental failures (Arnold et al. 1991).

Relationship of Delayed Antipsychotic Treatment to Structural Brain Abnormalities

An important body of literature is emerging, describing both retrospective and prospective studies, that indicates that a delay in the treatment of psychosis at its onset may result in resistance to treatment and poor outcome even after antipsychotics are eventually given (Wyatt 1991; see also Chapter 16). Recently, studies of first-episode schizophrenia patients have shown that those with the worst response to neuroleptic therapy were those with the longest duration of psychosis prior to receiving treatment (Loebel et al. 1992). There is also speculation as to whether active psychosis and hyperdopaminergia may be neurotoxic because of free-radical formation (Lohr 1991), which may also produce "progressive" ventricular enlargement early in the course of schizophrenia (Nasrallah 1991; Stevens 1991). As more investigators clarify the above issue, they might shed light on the relationship of structural brain abnormalities and clinical response to antipsychotic pharmacotherapy.

How the Clinical Psychiatrist Should Use Brain-Imaging Findings in Schizophrenia

Despite the lack of consistency in the literature regarding the relationship between structural brain abnormalities and therapeutic response to antipsychotic drugs in schizophrenia, there are several reasons why an MRI brain scan is useful in schizophrenia:

1. Every patient with a first lifetime psychotic episode deserves a full organic workup, including an MRI scan. Frontal tumors, metachromatic leukodystrophy, partial agenesis of the corpus callosum, and a variety of other organic lesions are not infrequently found and may change the diagnosis or contribute to alternative management.
2. The clinical psychiatrist has no means to quantify ventricular volume or sulcal widths. Most cortical and subcortical abnormalities in schizophrenia are detected only by statistical analysis of blind measurement. Most of the scans of schizophrenic patients are read as normal by neuroradiologists, except for the extreme cases of ventricular dilatation or cortical atrophy. Therefore, the clinical psychiatrist should give all patients with schizophrenia a course of antipsychotic therapy regardless of whether MRI findings do or do not point to an organic psychosis.
3. The initial MRI will serve as a valuable baseline for subsequent scans in case a major change in the patient's neurological or mental status occurs (e.g., polydipsia, tardive dyskinesia, hard neurological signs).

Conclusions

Despite evidence from some studies that schizophrenic patients with structural brain abnormalities are less likely to respond optimally to antipsychotic pharmacotherapy, this evidence is not incontrovertible, as many studies are not well designed or controlled, and there are several studies that show either no relationship between abnormalities and antipsychotics or a negative relationship. It is possible that as this research area matures, some guidelines may be developed. Until then, all patients should receive treatment with the understanding that some of those with large cerebral ventricles or sulcal widening may have a poorer response and may be at higher risk for extrapyramidal side effects, including tardive dyskinesia.

References

Abou-Saleh MT (ed): Brain imaging in psychiatry. Br J Psychiatry (suppl 9):1–101, 1990

Arnold SE, Hyman BT, Van Hösen GW, et al: Some cytoarchitectural abnormalities of the entorhinal cortex in schizophrenia. Arch Gen Psychiatry 48:625–632, 1991

Bogerts B, Lieberman JA, Ashtari M, et al: Hippocampus-amygdala volumes and psychopathology in chronic schizophrenia. Biol Psychiatry 33:236–246, 1993

Boronow J, Pickar D, Ninan PT, et al: Atrophy limited to the third ventricle in chronic schizophrenic patients. Arch Gen Psychiatry 42:266–271, 1985

Crow T: Molecular pathology of schizophrenia: more than one disease process? BMJ 280:66–68, 1980

Crow TJ, Cross AJ, Johnstone EC, et al: Two syndromes in schizophrenia and their pathogenesis, in Schizophrenia as a Brain Disease. Edited by Henn FA, Nasrallah HA. New York, Oxford University Press, 1982, pp 196–234

Endicott J, Spitzer RL: A diagnostic interview: the Schedule for Affective Disorders and Schizophrenia (SADS). Arch Gen Psychiatry 35:837–843, 1978

Friedman L, Knutson L, Shurell M, et al: Prefrontal sulcal prominence is inversely related to response to clozapine in schizophrenia. Biol Psychiatry 29:865–877, 1991

Garver DL, Dekirmenjian H, Davis JM, et al: Neuroleptic drug levels and therapeutic response: preliminary observations with red blood cell–bound butaperazine. Am J Psychiatry 134:304–307, 1977

Guy W (ed): ECDEU Assessment Manual for Psychopharmacology, Revised (DHEW Publ No ADM 76-388). Rockville, MD, U.S. Department of Health, Education and Welfare, 1976

Ingvar DH, Franzen G: Abnormalities of cerebral blood flow distribution in patients with chronic schizophrenia. Acta Psychiatr Scand 50:425–462, 1974

Jeste DV, Kleinman JE, Potkin SG, et al: Ex uno multi: subtyping the schizophrenic syndrome. Biol Psychiatry 17:199–222, 1982

Johnstone EC, Crow TJ, Frith CD, et al: Cerebral ventricular size and cognitive impairment in chronic schizophrenia. Lancet 2:924–926, 1976

Kaiya H, Uematsu M, Ofuji M, et al: Computerized tomography in schizophrenia: familial versus non-familial forms of illness. Br J Psychiatry 155:444–450, 1989

Keefe RSE, Mohs RC, Losonczy MF, et al: Characteristics of very poor outcome schizophrenia. Am J Psychiatry 144:889–895, 1987

Krawiecka M, Goldberg D, Vaughan M: A standardized psychiatric assessment scale for rating chronic psychotic patients. Acta Psychiatr Scand 55:299–308, 1977

Loebel AD, Lieberman JA, Alvir JMJ, et al: Duration of psychosis and outcome in first-episode schizophrenia. Am J Psychiatry 149:1183–1188, 1992

Lohr JB: Oxygen radicals and neuropsychiatric illness. Arch Gen Psychiatry 48:1097–1106, 1991

Losonczy MF, Song IS, Mohs RC, et al: Correlates of lateral ventricular size in chronic schizophrenia, I: behavioral and treatment response measures. Am J Psychiatry 143:976–981, 1986a

Losonczy MF, Song IS, Mohs RC, et al: Correlates of lateral ventricular size in chronic schizophrenia, II: biological measures. Am J Psychiatry 143:1113–1118, 1986b

Luchins DJ, Lewine RJ, Meltzer HY: Lateral ventricular size in the psychoses: relation to psychopathology and therapeutic and adverse response to medications. Psychopharmacol Bull 19:518–522, 1983

Luchins DJ, Lewine RRJ, Meltzer HY: Lateral ventricular size, psychopathology, and medication response in the psychoses. Biol Psychiatry 19:29–44, 1984

Lun A, Gross J, Beyer M, et al: The vulnerable period of perinatal hypoxia with regards to dopamine release and behavior in adult rats. Biomed Biochim Acta 45:619–627, 1986

MacDonald HL, Best JJK, Scottish Schizophrenia Research Group: The Scottish First Episode Schizophrenia Study, VI: computerized tomography brain scans in patients and controls. Br J Psychiatry 154:492–498, 1989

Montgomery SA, Taylor P, Montgomery D: Development of a schizophrenia scale sensitive to change. Neuropharmacology 17:1061–1063, 1983

Murray RM, Reveley AM, Lewis SW: Family history, obstetric complications and cerebral abnormality in schizophrenia, in Handbook of Schizophrenia, Vol 3: Nosology, Epidemiology and Genetics of Schizophrenia. Series edited by Nasrallah HA; volume edited by Tsuang MT, Simpson JC. Amsterdam, Netherlands, Elsevier, 1988, pp 563–578

Naber D, Albus M, Burke H, et al: Neuroleptic withdrawal in chronic schizophrenia: CT and endocrine variables relating to psychopathology. Psychiatry Res 16:207–219, 1985

Nasrallah HA: Progressive and static ventriculomegaly in schizophrenia: clinical and methodological variables. Schizophr Res 5:191–192, 1991

Nasrallah HA: Neurodevelopmental pathogenesis of schizophrenia. Psychiatr Clin North Am 16:269–280, 1993

Nasrallah HA, Kleinman JE, Weinberger DR, et al: Cerebral ventricular enlargement and dopamine synthesis inhibition in chronic schizophrenia (letter). Arch Gen Psychiatry 37:1427, 1980

Nasrallah HA, Jacoby CG, McCalley-Whitters M, et al: Cerebral ventricular enlargement in subtypes of chronic schizophrenia. Arch Gen Psychiatr 39:774–777, 1982

Nasrallah HA, Kuperman S, Jacoby CG, et al: Clinical correlates of sulcal widening in chronic schizophrenia. Psychiatry Res 10:237–242, 1983a

Nasrallah HA, Kuperman S, Hamra BJ, et al: Clinical differences between schizophrenic patients with and without large cerebral ventricles. J Clin Psychiatry 44:407–409, 1983b

Nimgaonkar VL, Wessely S, Tune LE, et al: Response to drugs in schizophrenia: the influence of family history, obstetric complications and ventricular enlargement. Psychol Med 18:583–592, 1988

Overall JE, Gorham DR: The Brief Psychiatric Rating Scale. Psychol Rep 10:799–812, 1962

Pandurangi AK, Dewan MJ, Boucher M, et al: A comprehensive study for chronic schizophrenic patients, II: biological, neuropsychological, and clinical correlates of CT abnormality. Acta Psychiatr Scand 73:161–171, 1986

Pandurangi AK, Goldberg SC, Brink DD, et al: Amphetamine challenge test, response to treatment, and lateral ventricle size in schizophrenia. Biol Psychiatry 25:207–214, 1989

Schulz SC, Sinicrope P, Kishore P, et al: Treatment response and ventricular brain enlargement in young schizophrenic patients. Psychopharmacol Bull 19:510–512, 1983

Shelton RC, Weinberger DR: X-ray computerized tomography in schizophrenia: a review and synthesis, in Handbook of Schizophrenia, Vol 1: The Neurology of Schizophrenia. Series edited by Nasrallah HA; volume edited by Nasrallah HA, Weinberger DR. Amsterdam, Netherlands, Elsevier, 1986, pp 207–250

Silverstein F, Johnston MV: Effects of hypoxia-ischemia on monoamine metabolism in the immature brain. Ann Neurol 15:342–347, 1984

Smith RC, Largen J, Calderon M, et al: CT scans and neuropsychological tests as predictors of clinical response in schizophrenics. Psychopharmacol Bull 19:505–509, 1983

Smith RC, Baumgartner R, Ravichandran GK, et al: Lateral ventricular enlargement and clinical response in schizophrenia. Psychiatry Res 14:241–253, 1985

Smith RC, Baumgartner R, Ravichandran GK, et al: Cortical atrophy and white matter density in the brain of schizophrenics and clinical response to neuroleptics. Acta Psychiatr Scand 75:11–19, 1987

Stevens JR: Schizophrenia: static or progressive pathophysiology. Schizophr Res 5:184–186, 1991

van Kammen DP, Mann LS, Sternberg DE, et al: Dopamine-β-hydroxylase activity and homovanillic acid in spinal fluid of schizophrenics with brain atrophy. Science 220:974–976, 1983

Vita A, Sacchetti E, Calzeroni A, et al: Cortical atrophy in schizophrenia: prevalence and associated features. Schizophr Res 1:329–337, 1988

Weinberger DR: Implications of normal brain development for the pathogenesis of schizophrenia. Arch Gen Psychiatry 44:660–669, 1987

Weinberger DR, Bigelow LB, Kleinman JE, et al: Cerebral ventricular enlargement in chronic schizophrenia: an association with poor response to treatment. Arch Gen Psychiatry 27:11–13, 1980

Williams AO, Reveley MA, Kolakowska T, et al: Schizophrenia with good and poor outcome, II: cerebral ventricular size and its clinical significance. Br J Psychiatry 146:239–246, 1985

Wyatt RJ: Neuroleptics and the natural course of schizophrenia. Schizophr Bull 17:325–351, 1991

CHAPTER 11

Gender Differences in Schizophrenia

Luc Nicole, M.D., F.R.C.P.C., and
Christian L. Shriqui, M.D., M.Sc, F.R.C.P.C.

D espite a predominance of male subjects in schizophrenia research studies (Wahl and Hunter 1992), there
have been numerous reports of gender differences in
the disorder. Sampling biases in studies of gender factors in schizophrenia are receiving increased attention (Hambrecht et al. 1992;
Walker and Lewine 1993). Gender and schizophrenia—once a neglected area of schizophrenia research—has recently become the focus
of several studies, review articles, and special journal themes (e.g.,
Volume 16, Number 2 (1990) of *Schizophrenia Bulletin* was entirely
devoted to the theme of gender and schizophrenia). However, much
of the information contained in these writings is dispersed throughout
the literature; in this chapter, we summarize the currently available
data on gender differences in schizophrenia.

This work was supported by a Scholarship Award from the Fonds de la Recherche en
Santé du Québec (FRSQ) to C. Shriqui. The authors thank Serge Champetier for
assistance in the manuscript preparation.

Incidence

Until recently, the incidence of schizophrenia was thought to be equal in both sexes (Wing 1987). Studies such as the World Health Organization study (Jablensky et al. 1992) and the National Institute of Mental Health Epidemiologic Catchment Area Study (Robins et al. 1984) did not report gender differences in the incidence rates of schizophrenia. Nevertheless, other studies have reported higher incidence rates in males, with a male-to-female incidence ratio ranging from 1.5:1 (NiNullain et al. 1987) to 2.5:1 (Nicole et al. 1992). After using various diagnostic criteria to reexamine the schizophrenic patients in these researchers' study samples, Iacono and Beiser (1992) still found a greater incidence of schizophrenia in males. Although the ratios given by NiNullain et al. and Nicole et al. appear to be genuine and not the result of study artifacts, there is an ongoing debate regarding the "true" incidence rate of schizophrenia in both sexes (Hambrecht et al. 1992).

Age at Onset

The age at onset for schizophrenia is generally reported to be earlier in males than in females (Häfner et al. 1989; Lewine 1988; Nicole 1992; Seeman 1982). However, we are aware of two studies in which this finding was not replicated (Leboyer et al. 1992; Thara and Rajkumar 1992).

Approximately two-thirds of males who develop schizophrenia, versus only one-third of females, are diagnosed prior to 25 years of age (Häfner et al. 1991a; Lewis 1992). Age at index hospitalization is often observed to be 4–5 years earlier for schizophrenic men (Angermeyer and Kühn 1988) than for women. However, this finding appears unrelated to gender differences in social tolerance or marital status (Häfner et al. 1989; Lewine 1988; Loranger 1984).

Despite cultural and demographic differences in schizophrenic patient samples and heterogeneity in the diagnostic criteria applied to schizophrenia, an earlier age at onset of illness in men than in women is the most frequently reported finding (Goldstein et al. 1989; Guereje 1991; Jablensky et al. 1992).

Familial Risk

A higher risk for schizophrenia is generally reported among first-degree relatives of female schizophrenic probands. However, heterogeneity in diagnostic groups and lack of both gender-matched samples and standardized diagnostic methods have limited the reliability of these findings. Bellodi et al. (1986) reported a risk of schizophrenia-spectrum disorders of 5.1% in the relatives of male schizophrenic probands as compared with 9.5% in the relatives of female schizophrenic probands. Similarly, in a study of 381 DSM-III (American Psychiatric Association 1980) schizophrenic probands (275 males and 106 females), Wolyniec et al. (1992) reported that the first-degree relatives of female schizophrenic probands have a higher risk of schizophrenia and nonaffective psychosis (5.0%) than the first-degree relatives of male schizophrenic probands (2.7%). Authors of other studies have reported similar findings (Goldstein et al. 1990; Lloyd et al. 1985; Nasrallah and Wilcox 1989).

Premorbid Characteristics

Premorbid social functioning is poorer in schizophrenic men than in women (Addington and Addington 1993; Klorman et al. 1977; Lewine 1981; McGlashan and Bardenstein 1990; Zigler and Levine 1973). Moreover, from their controlled study, Foerster et al. (1991) reported that both poor premorbid social functioning and schizoid and schizotypal personality traits are more frequent in men with schizophrenia than in either men or women with an affective disorder. Poorer premorbid intellectual functioning in male schizophrenic patients is also a reported but inconsistent finding (Aylward et al. 1984; McGlashan and Bardenstein 1990).

Symptomatology

Negative symptoms are reported to be more common in schizophrenic men (Addington and Addington 1993; Bardenstein and McGlashan 1990; Goldstein and Link 1988; Lewine 1985; McGlashan and Bardenstein 1990; Nasrallah and Wilcox 1989; Ring et al. 1991), whereas affective symptoms are more frequent in schizophrenic women (Bardenstein and McGlashan 1990).

Antisocial behavior is more frequent in schizophrenic men, whereas autodestructive behavior is more common in schizophrenic women (Bardenstein and McGlashan 1990; McGlashan and Bardenstein 1990).

Olfactory Function

Olfactory acuity or odor detection threshold has been reported as either increased or normal in schizophrenic patients (Bradley 1984; Isseroff et al. 1987). Since 1988, several studies have reported significant olfactory identification deficits occurring primarily in male schizophrenic patients (Hurwitz et al. 1988; Kopala et al. 1989, 1992; Seidman et al. 1992; Serby et al. 1990). Because human olfactory perception is closely linked to the functioning of the orbitofrontal lobes, investigation of olfactory function in schizophrenia has been suggested as a potential neuropsychological "probe" for the illness (Seidman et al. 1992). Clinical correlates of orbitofrontal dysfunction in schizophrenia have been associated with behavioral disinhibition, loosened social controls and judgment, sensitivity to interference, excitation, emotional lability, and impulse control disorders (Seidman et al. 1992).

Using the University of Pennsylvania Smell Identification Test (UPSIT; Doty et al. 1984), Hurwitz et al. (1988) reported significant olfactory deficits in a group of 18 schizophrenic patients. This result was independent of a medication effect, because neuroleptic-treated nonschizophrenic psychiatric patients performed similarly to subjects in a control group of healthy nonpsychiatric volunteers. In a subsequent study, Kopala et al. (1989) reported an olfactory deficit in 11 out of 26 male schizophrenic patients (42%) versus 1 out of 14 female schizophrenic patients. In this study, 100% of the 20 female control subjects and 96% (22 out of 23) of the male control subjects had normal olfactory function. The scores of a subsample of the male and female schizophrenic subjects tested for olfactory acuity were not significantly different from those of the control subjects.

The disassociation of olfactory acuity from olfactory identification suggests a central rather than peripheral origin for the olfactory agnosia. Using the UPSIT, Serby et al. (1990) reported the presence of an odor identification deficit in a group of 14 schizophrenic and 9 depressed men who had been off psychotropic medication for at least 10 days. In this study, the normal performance of both groups of patients in a forced-choice, yes-or-no odor discrimination paradigm raised the possibility that the poor test results on the UPSIT were the result of cognitive-attentional deficits.

Seidman et al. (1992) also examined olfactory identification using the UPSIT and the Wisconsin Card Sorting Test (Heaton 1985) in a group of 16 (15 male, 1 female) chronic schizophrenic patients and 17 (16 male, 1 female) age-matched nonpsychiatric control subjects. The authors found that, with the exception of the single schizophrenic woman, the olfactory identification deficits were confined to 69% of the schizophrenic men. In comparison with the performance of the control subjects, the schizophrenic patients' performance on the UPSIT and the Wisconsin Card Sorting Test (used to evaluate dorsolateral frontal lobe functioning) was significantly impaired. However, there was no correlation between UPSIT scores and Wisconsin Card Sorting Test performance in the schizophrenic group. Seidman and colleagues concluded that although olfactory identification deficits are prevalent in male schizophrenic patients, they appear to be independent of the cognitive-attentional deficits frequently associated with schizophrenia.

In a recent controlled study, Kopala et al. (1992) examined olfactory identification deficits in 40 (30 male, 10 female) neuroleptic-naive patients with schizophrenia and 58 (28 male, 30 female) age-matched nonpsychiatric control subjects. They reported no differences in olfactory acuity, but did find an olfactory agnosia present in

31% of the male schizophrenic sample. This finding would suggest that olfactory identification deficits in schizophrenia are independent of a neuroleptic medication effect.

Warner et al. (1990) reported no differences in olfactory identification ability in a total sample of 26 male subjects comprising 8 normal control subjects and 12 schizophrenic and 6 depressed patients taken off psychotropic medication for at least 2 weeks.

It has been suggested that the physiological action of sex hormones—particularly estradiol—on brain development plays a role in the gender differences in olfactory acuity observed in schizophrenic patients (Kopala and Clark 1990).

Neurodevelopmental Factors and Brain Structure

In a retrospective study, Nasrallah and Wilcox (1989) reported a greater frequency of early childhood brain injury in male than in female schizophrenic patients, whereas there was a greater frequency of family history of psychotic illness in female than in male schizophrenic patients. These results were consistent with the authors' hypothesis that neurological factors play a greater role in the development of schizophrenia in males.

Rossi et al. (1990) reported increased neurological soft signs in schizophrenic patients and their first-degree relatives. However, DeCataldo et al. (1992) found no gender difference in the total score of neurological soft signs in a sample of 43 males and 21 females with schizophrenia.

Structural brain differences between males and females with schizophrenia have been identified with computed tomography and magnetic resonance imaging scans. The findings have included gender differences in brain and cranium size and in corpus callosum thickness, as well as in lateral and third ventricle measurements (Andreasen et al. 1986; Nasrallah et al. 1986, 1990). However, these differences have not been consistently replicated (DeLisi et al. 1989), and opposite findings have also been reported (Nasrallah et al. 1990).

Variations in Medication Dosages and Treatment Response

Results from a majority of studies have indicated that schizophrenic women require lower dosages of neuroleptics than do schizophrenic men during the acute and maintenance phases of the illness (Chouinard et al. 1986; Kolakowska et al. 1985; Marriott and Hiep 1978; Seeman 1983a; Seeman and Lang 1990; Young and Meltzer 1980).

Maintenance neuroleptic dosages. In 1974, Hogarty et al. conducted a 2-year, placebo-controlled study examining the effects of maintenance neuroleptic treatment and sociotherapy in 374 schizophrenic patients; during that trial, 63% of male patients—as compared with 37% of female patients—relapsed while on chlorpromazine. The mean dosage levels of chlorpromazine were equivalent in both sexes during the first year of follow-up, but the male patients received higher dosages than the female patients during the second year. However, no differences in relapse rates between sexes could be observed in the placebo-treated group, a finding that indirectly supports the possibility of gender-related biological differences in neuroleptic response.

Type of neuroleptic used. In schizophrenic male and female patients, treatment response can vary according to the type of neuroleptic used. In a 4-week, double-blind, controlled trial comparing injectable fluspirilene with oral chlorpromazine, Chouinard et al. (1986) observed that male schizophrenic patients required a significantly higher mean dosage of fluspirilene than did female schizophrenic patients, whereas, for a similar therapeutic effect, no significant gender differences were observed for the chlorpromazine-treated group. The dosage difference in the fluspirilene-treated group could not be explained by sex differences in initial severity of illness, number of hospitalizations, weight, or side effects. In an earlier controlled trial using another diphenylbutylpiperidine, pimozide, in acute schizophrenic patients, Chouinard and Annable (1982) reported that female patients had a more favorable treatment response than male patients at similar mean dosages.

In an uncontrolled clinical trial, Lal and Nair (1992) evaluated the efficacy of methotrimeprazine used alone or in combination with other neuroleptics in 23 chronic treatment-refractory schizophrenic patients. Although scores on the Brief Psychiatric Rating Scale (Overall and Gorham 1962) prior to levomepromazine treatment were not obtained, 14 out of the 15 men and 2 out of the 8 women who entered in the study had improved at follow-up. However, this predominance of responsive male patients in treatment-refractory schizophrenia has not been replicated in clinical trials with clozapine (Meltzer 1992).

Age differences.   Marriott and Hiep (1978) examined patterns of drug monitoring at a depot phenothiazine clinic, finding that neuroleptic requirements between sexes vary according to age. In this study, men aged 20–40 years received significantly higher dosages of fluphenazine decanoate than women; a reduction in neuroleptic dosage was observed in older men between the ages of 51 and 70 years.

Treatment practices.   Apart from illness-related factors, the use of higher dosages of neuroleptics in young adult men with schizophrenia is influenced by treatment practices. Clinicians often consider age-related changes in drug metabolism, which explains the use of lower dosages of neuroleptics in elderly patients. Likewise, men are more likely to manifest aggressive behavior than women in the acute phase of schizophrenia; therefore, schizophrenic men may be perceived as being more dangerous than schizophrenic women, which may account for the use of higher dosages of neuroleptics in men (Addonizio and Susman 1991; Seeman 1983a, 1983b).

Kolakowska et al. (1985) examined neuroleptic responsiveness in 62 schizophrenic and 15 schizoaffective disorder patients and found that it was predominantly the female patients who responded well.

Psychopathology following withdrawal of medication.   Gender differences in psychopathology following neuroleptic withdrawal were reported in a study of 161 schizophrenic patients (105 males, 56 females) who were taken off their neuroleptic medication for 3 months (Abenson 1969). In the male patients, the greatest increase in psychopathology occurred with regard to paranoid ideation, thought disorder, and inappropriate behavior. In the women, the greatest increase in psychopathology was in social withdrawal. Although speculative, this result implies that a gradual reduction of neuroleptic dosage would be associated with a lesser risk of relapse of positive symptoms in schizophrenic women than in schizophrenic men.

Social and cultural factors.   Social and cultural influences may contribute to differences in treatment response patterns of schizophrenic men and women. Gender differences in neuroleptic drug compliance, propensity to experience side effects, maintenance of a stable therapeutic alliance, and acceptance of long-term neuroleptic drug therapy are understudied determinants of treatment response in schizophrenia.

Biological factors.   A neuroleptic-like effect of estrogen in the central nervous system might explain the use of lower antipsychotic dosages in schizophrenic women (Seeman 1982, 1983a; Seeman and Lang 1990). The dopamine antagonist activity of estrogen has been demonstrated in several animal studies (DiPaolo et al. 1981; Gordon et al. 1980; Raymond et al. 1978), and the decrease of estrogen levels in postmenopausal females has been associated with an increase in neuroleptic dosage requirements (Seeman 1983a).

Other biological factors that may influence dosage requirements of neuroleptics include sex differences in gastric emptying time, distribution of body fat, and cerebral blood flow (Seeman and Lang 1990). Sex differences in neuroleptic serum levels of schizophrenic patients have been related to the greater distribution volume and higher metabolic activity commonly found in men (Gaebel et al. 1992).

Neuroleptic Side Effects

Sex differences in acute and long-term extrapyramidal symptoms have often been reported. Female schizophrenic patients have a higher risk of developing drug-induced parkinsonism, akathisia, and tardive dyskinesia than male schizophrenic patients (American Psychiatric Association 1992; Ayd 1961; Casey 1991; Chouinard et al. 1980; Kane and

Smith 1982; Smith and Dunn 1979; Yassa and Jeste 1992), whereas male schizophrenic patients have an increased risk of acute and tardive forms of dystonia and of neuroleptic malignant syndrome (Addonizio and Susman 1991; Ayd 1961; Casey 1991; Gardos et al. 1987; Swett 1975).

Acute extrapyramidal symptoms are a major determinant of neuroleptic noncompliance (Casey 1991), and their recognition and management is of critical importance.

Sex differences in nonneurological side effects of neuroleptics are additional factors that can interfere with medication compliance. Women experience difficulty with weight gain and amenorrhea, whereas men have erection and ejaculation problems and decreased libido (Seeman 1983b). These side effects, particularly in males, must be inquired about directly or risk going unrecognized.

Suicide

Suicide is the leading cause of premature death among schizophrenic patients, with an estimated 10%–13% of these patients at risk for suicide (Caldwell and Gottesman 1990). In agreement with previous findings, Black and Fisher (1992) conducted a mortality study in 356 DSM-III-R (American Psychiatric Association 1987) schizophrenic patients followed over a 12-year period and found suicide to be the most common cause of death.

In the United States, the estimated male-to-female suicide ratio in the general population is about 3:1, whereas in the schizophrenic population it is closer to 2:1 (Caldwell and Gottesman 1990). Schizophrenic women have either an equal or a greater relative risk of suicide or suicide attempts than schizophrenic men, with results from several studies indicating a higher standardized mortality ratio in schizophrenic women than in men (Allebeck and Wistedt 1986; Black and Fisher 1992; Bleuler 1978; Caldwell and Gottesman 1990).

Nonetheless, although the mortality rates of schizophrenic women are high, in the majority of cases their deaths are from natural causes. Furthermore, most studies report a greater number of suicides in schizophrenic men than in women (Black and Fisher 1992; Breier and

Astrachan 1984; Nyman and Jonsson 1986; Roy 1986; Tsuang 1978). It is possible that schizophrenia decreases inhibitions to suicide in women (Caldwell and Gottesman 1990; Seeman 1986). In addition, female schizophrenic patients experience more affective symptoms than their male counterparts (Bardenstein and McGlashan 1990). Schizophrenic males who commit suicide share similar traits with males in the general population who kill themselves, including increased impulsivity and aggressiveness and low frustration tolerance (Seeman 1986). In addition, schizophrenic men use more lethal methods of suicide than schizophrenic women (Breier and Astrachan 1984).

Prognosis and Outcome

Although a more favorable outcome for schizophrenic women is reported in short-term follow-up studies (Angermeyer et al. 1989; Goldstein 1988; Goldstein and Link 1988; Hogarty et al. 1974; Kolakowska et al. 1985; Lewine 1981; Thara and Rajkumar 1992), this difference is less apparent in long-term follow-up studies (Bleuler 1974; Childers and Harding 1990; Ciompi 1980; Harding 1988; Huber et al. 1980).

In 1983, Salokangas reported his findings in a total sample of 175 schizophrenic patients followed for approximately 8 years after their first hospitalization. This study indicated that male patients had more frequent and prolonged hospitalization periods than female patients but used outpatient services less. In addition, social and work adjustment and psychosexual functioning were poorer in males than in females. Angermeyer and Kühn (1988) reported significantly fewer readmissions in schizophrenic women than in schizophrenic men in approximately half of the 12 studies they reviewed. About one-third of the approximately 30 studies in which the length of readmissions in schizophrenia was examined reported shorter hospital stays for female than for male patients, with the remaining two-thirds of the studies showing no significant differences between sexes. Similar results have been reported from subsequent studies examining the frequency and length of hospitalizations in schizophrenic men and women (Angermeyer et al. 1989; Goldstein 1988; Shepherd et al. 1989).

Other dimensions of good outcome in schizophrenia—such as marriage, work record, sociability, and a remitting course of illness— are generally superior in schizophrenic women (Seeman 1982).

Conclusion

Authors of several epidemiological studies have indicated a higher incidence rate of schizophrenia in males than in females, although some studies that controlled for errors in patient selection and other sources of artifacts reported an equal risk in both sexes (e.g., Hambrecht et al. 1992). Results of family studies have indicated that first-degree relatives of female schizophrenic probands are at increased risk to develop the illness.

In general, schizophrenic men have more frequent relapses, an earlier age at onset, and a more severe course of illness. Schizophrenic men also exhibit decreased levels of premorbid social adjustment, respond less favorably to neuroleptic medication, and tend to have an overall poorer prognosis than women.

Gender differences in schizophrenia have generated various speculations with regard to the etiology of the illness. Different social roles for men and women and a "protective" effect of estradiol in females have been suggested (Häfner et al. 1991b). However, a neurodevelopmental hypothesis suggests that men may be more vulnerable to developing schizophrenia because they have a slower pace of cerebral development, have increased lateralization of cerebral function, and are more prone to early brain injury and obstetric complications (Castle and Murray 1991; Nasrallah and Wilcox 1989).

Both biological (e.g., different distribution volumes in men and women, hormonal effects) and social (e.g., schizophrenic men possibly being perceived as potentially more aggressive or prone to behavioral disturbance) factors may influence neuroleptic dosage requirements in male and female schizophrenic patients. However, a neuroleptic dosage reduction, whenever possible, will often result in decreased neuroleptic side effects, better medication compliance, and improved quality of life to the patient.

Thus far, clinicians' knowledge of gender differences in schizophrenia has had a limited impact in the therapeutic management of schizophrenic men and women. Although practitioners need to consider gender-specific treatments and rehabilitation needs, Lewis (1992) reminds us that "gender, as with class and ethnicity, is an area with potential for creating generalization and myth" (p. 449).

References

Abenson MH: Drug withdrawal in male and female chronic schizophrenics. Br J Psychiatry 115:961–962, 1969

Addington J, Addington D: Premorbid functioning, cognitive functioning, symptoms and outcome in schizophrenia. J Psychiatry Neurosci 18:18–23, 1993

Addonizio G, Susman VL: Neuroleptic Malignant Syndrome: A Clinical Approach. St. Louis, MO, Mosby-Year Book, 1991

Allebeck P, Wistedt B: Mortality in schizophrenia: a ten-year follow-up based on the Stockholm County Inpatient Register. Arch Gen Psychiatry 43:650–653, 1986

American Psychiatric Association: Diagnostic and Statistical Manual of Mental Disorders, 3rd Edition. Washington, DC, American Psychiatric Association, 1980

American Psychiatric Association: Diagnostic and Statistical Manual of Mental Disorders, 3rd Edition, Revised. Washington, DC, American Psychiatric Association, 1987

American Psychiatric Association: Tardive Dyskinesia: A Task Force Report of the American Psychiatric Association. Edited by Kane JM, Jeste DV, Barnes TRE, et al. Washington, DC, American Psychiatric Association, 1992

Andreasen NC, Nasrallah HA, Dunn V, et al: Structural abnormalities in the frontal system in schizophrenia: a magnetic resonance imaging study. Arch Gen Psychiatry 43:136–144, 1986

Angermeyer MC, Kühn L: Gender differences in age at onset of schizophrenia: an overview. Eur Arch Psychiatry Clin Neurosci 237:351–364, 1988

Angermeyer MC, Goldstein JM, Kühn L: Gender differences in schizophrenia: rehospitalization and community survival. Psychol Med 19:365–382, 1989

Ayd FJ: A survey of drug-induced extrapyramidal reactions. JAMA 175:1054–1060, 1961

Aylward E, Walker E, Bettes B: Intelligence in schizophrenia: meta-analysis of the research. Schizophr Bull 10:430–459, 1984

Bardenstein KK, McGlashan TH: Gender differences in affective, schizoaffective and schizophrenic disorders: a review. Schizophr Res 3:159–172, 1990

Bellodi L, Bussoleni C, Scorza-Smeraldi R, et al: Family study of schizophrenia: exploratory analysis for relevant factors. Schizophr Bull 12:120–128, 1986

Black DW, Fisher R: Mortality in DSM-III-R schizophrenia. Schizophr Res 7:109–116, 1992

Bleuler M: The long-term course of the schizophrenic psychoses. Psychol Med 4:244–254, 1974

Bleuler M: The Schizophrenic Disorders: Long-Term Patient and Family Studies. Translated by Clemens SM. New Haven, CT, Yale University Press, 1978

Bradley EA: Olfactory acuity to a pheromonal substance and psychotic illness. Biol Psychiatry 19:899–905, 1984

Breier A, Astrachan B: Characterization of schizophrenic patients who commit suicide. Am J Psychiatry 141:206–209, 1984

Caldwell CB, Gottesman II: Schizophrenics kill themselves too: a review of risk factors for suicide. Schizophr Bull 16:571–589, 1990

Casey DE: Neuroleptic drug-induced extrapyramidal syndromes and tardive dyskinesia. Schizophr Res 4:109–120, 1991

Castle DJ, Murray RM: The neurodevelopmental basis of sex differences in schizophrenia. Psychol Med 21:565–575, 1991

Childers SE, Harding CM: Gender, premorbid social functioning, and long-term outcome in DSM-III schizophrenia. Schizophr Bull 16:309–318, 1990

Chouinard G, Annable L: Pimozide in the treatment of newly admitted schizophrenic patients. Psychopharmacol Bull 76:13–19, 1982

Chouinard G, Jones BD, Annable L, et al: Sex differences and tardive dyskinesia. Am J Psychiatry 137:507, 1980

Chouinard G, Annable L, Steinberg S: A controlled clinical trial of fluspirilene, a long-acting injectable neuroleptic, in schizophrenic patients with acute exacerbation. J Clin Psychopharmacol 6:21–26, 1986

Ciompi L: The natural history of schizophrenia in the long term. Br J Psychiatry 136:413–420, 1980

De Cataldo S, Rossi A, Di Michele V, et al: Soft neurological dysfunction and gender in schizophrenia. Br J Psychiatry 160:423–424, 1992

DeLisi LE, Dauphinais D, Hauser P: Gender differences in the brain: are they relevant to the pathogenesis of schizophrenia? Compr Psychiatry 30:197–208, 1989

DiPaolo T, Poyet P, Labrie F: Effect of chronic oestradiol and haloperidol treatment on striatal dopamine receptors. Eur J Pharmacol 73:105–106, 1981

Doty RL, Shaman P, Dann M: Development of the University of Pennsylvania Smell Identification Test: a standardized microencapsulated test of olfactory function. Physiol Behav 32:489, 1984

Foerster A, Lewis S, Owen M, et al: Premorbid adjustment and personality in psychosis: effects of sex and diagnosis. Br J Psychiatry 158:171–176, 1991

Gaebel W, Muller-Oerlinghausen B, Schley J: Early serum levels of neuroleptics do not predict therapeutic response in schizophrenia. Prog Neuropsychopharmacol Biol Psychiatry 16:891–900, 1992

Gardos G, Cole JO, Salomon M, et al: Clinical forms of severe tardive dyskinesia. Am J Psychiatry 144:895–902, 1987

Goldstein JM: Gender differences in the course of schizophrenia. Am J Psychiatry 145:684–689, 1988

Goldstein JM, Link BG: Gender and the expression of schizophrenia. J Psychiatry Res 22:141–155, 1988

Goldstein JM, Tsuang MT, Faraone SV: Gender and schizophrenia: implications for understanding the heterogeneity of illness. Psychiatry Res 28:243–253, 1989

Goldstein JM, Faraone SV, Chen WJ, et al: Sex differences in the familial transmission of schizophrenia. Br J Psychiatry 156:819–826, 1990

Gordon JH, Borison RL, Diamond BI: Modulation of dopamine receptor sensitivity by estrogen. Biol Psychiatry 15:389–396, 1980

Guereje O: Gender and schizophrenia: age at onset and sociodemographic attributes. Acta Psychiatr Scand 83:402–405, 1991.

Häfner H, Riecher A, Maurer K, et al: How does gender influence age at first hospitalization for schizophrenia? a translational case register study. Psychol Med 19:903–918, 1989

Häfner H, Behrens S, De Vry J, et al: Schizophrenia: gender and age: why is the onset of schizophrenia later in women? Biol Psychiatry 1:431–433, 1991a

Häfner H, Behrens S, De Vry J, et al: An animal model for the effects of estradiol on dopamine-mediated behavior: implications for sex differences in schizophrenia. Psychiatry Res 38:125–134, 1991b

Hambrecht M, Maurer K, Häfner H: Evidence for a gender bias in epidemiological studies of schizophrenia. Schizophr Res 8:223–231, 1992

Harding CM: Course types in schizophrenia: an analysis of European and American studies. Schizophr Bull 14:633–643, 1988

Heaton R: Wisconsin Card Sorting Test. Odessa, TX, Psychological Assessment Resources, 1985

Hogarty GE, Goldberg SC, Schooler NR, et al: Drug and sociotherapy in the aftercare of schizophrenic patients. Arch Gen Psychiatry 31:603–608, 1974

Huber G, Goss G, Schuttler R, et al: Longitudinal studies of schizophrenic patients. Schizophr Bull 6:592–605, 1980

Hurwitz T, Kopala LC, Clark C, et al: Olfactory deficits in schizophrenia. Biol Psychiatry 23:123–128, 1988

Iacono WG, Beiser M: Are males more likely than females to develop schizophrenia? Am J Psychiatry 149:1070–1074, 1992

Isseroff RD, Stoler M, Ophir D, et al: Olfactory sensitivity to androsterone in schizophrenic patients. Biol Psychiatry 22:922–925, 1987

Jablensky A, Sartorius N, Ernberg G, et al: Schizophrenia: manifestations, incidence and course in different cultures—a World Health Organization 10-country study. Psychol Med Monogr Suppl 20:1–97, 1992

Kane JM, Smith JM: Tardive dyskinesia: prevalence and risk factors, 1959 to 1979. Arch Gen Psychiatry 39:473–481, 1982

Klorman R, Strauss JS, Kokes RF: Premorbid adjustment in schizophrenia, III: the relationship of demographic and diagnostic factors to measures of premorbid adjustment in schizophrenia. Schizophr Bull 3:214–225, 1977

Kolakowska T, Williams AO, Ardern M, et al: Schizophrenia with good and poor outcome, I: early clinical features, response to neuroleptics and signs of organic dysfunction. Br J Psychiatry 146:229–239, 1985

Kopala LC, Clark C: Implications of olfactory agnosia for understanding sex differences in schizophrenia. Schizophr Bull 16:255–261, 1990

Kopala LC, Clark C, Hurwitz T: Sex differences in olfactory function in schizophrenia. Am J Psychiatry 146:1320–1322, 1989

Kopala LC, Clark C, Hurwitz T: Olfactory deficits in neuroleptic naive patients with schizophrenia. Schizophr Res 8:245–250, 1992

Lal S, Nair NPV: Is levomepromazine a useful drug in treatment-resistant schizophrenia? Acta Psychiatr Scand 85:243–245, 1992

Leboyer M, Filteau MJ, Jay M, et al: No gender effect on age at onset in familial schizophrenia? Am J Psychiatry 149:1409, 1992

Lewine RJ: Sex differences in schizophrenia: timing or subtypes? Psychol Bull 90:432–444, 1981

Lewine RJ: Schizophrenia: an amotivational syndrome in men. Can J Psychiatry 30:316–318, 1985

Lewine RJ: Gender and schizophrenia, in Handbook of Schizophrenia, Vol 3. Edited by Nasrallah HA. Amsterdam, Netherlands, Elsevier, 1988, pp 379–397

Lewis S: Sex and schizophrenia: vive la différence. Br J Psychiatry 161:445–450, 1992

Lloyd DW, Simpson JC, Tsuang MT: A family study of sex differences in the diagnosis of atypical schizophrenia. Am J Psychiatry 142:1366–1368, 1985

Loranger AW: Sex differences in age at onset of schizophrenia. Arch Gen Psychiatry 41:157–161, 1984

Marriott P, Hiep A: Drug monitoring at an Australian depot phenothiazine clinic. J Clin Psychiatry 39:206–207, 211–212, 1978

McGlashan TH, Bardenstein KK: Gender differences in affective, schizoaffective, and schizophrenic disorders. Schizophr Bull 16:319–329, 1990

Meltzer HY: Clozapine: pattern of efficacy in treatment-resistant schizophrenia, in Novel Antipsychotic Drugs. Edited by Meltzer HY. New York, Raven, 1992, pp 33–46

Nasrallah HA, Wilcox JA: Gender differences in the etiology and symptoms of schizophrenia. Genetic versus brain injury factors. Annals of Clinical Psychiatry 1:51–53, 1989

Nasrallah HA, Andreasen NC, Coffman JA, et al: A controlled magnetic resonance imaging study of the corpus callosum thickness in schizophrenia. Biol Psychiatry 21:274–282, 1986

Nasrallah HA, Schwarzkopf SB, Olson SC, et al: Gender differences in schizophrenia on MRI scans. Schizophr Bull 16:205–210, 1990

Nicole L: Schizophrénie: différences selon le sexe. Can J Psychiatry 37:116–120, 1992

Nicole L, Lesage A, Lalonde P: Lower incidence and increased male:female ratio in schizophrenia. Br J Psychiatry 161:556–557, 1992

NiNullain M, O'Hare A, Walsh D: Incidence of schizophrenia in Ireland. Psychol Med 17:943–948, 1987

Nyman A, Jonsson H: Patterns of self-destructive behavior in schizophrenia. Acta Psychiatr Scand 73:252–262, 1986

Overall JE, Gorham DR: The Brief Psychiatric Rating Scale. Psychol Rep 10:799–812, 1962

Raymond V, Beaulieu M, Labrie F, et al: Potent antidopaminergic activity of oestradiol at the pituitary level on prolactin release. Science 200:1173–1175, 1978

Ring N, Tantam D, Montague L, et al: Gender differences in the incidence of definite schizophrenia and atypical psychosis—focus on negative symptoms of schizophrenia. Acta Psychiatr Scand 84:489–496, 1991

Robins LN, Helzer JE, Weissman MM, et al: Lifetime prevalence of specific psychiatric disorders in three sites. Arch Gen Psychiatry 41:949–958, 1984

Rossi A, De Cataldo V, Di Michele V, et al: Neurological soft signs in schizophrenia. Br J Psychiatry 157:735–739, 1990

Roy A: Depression, attempted suicide, and suicide in patients with chronic schizophrenia. Psychiatr Clin North Am 9:193–206, 1986

Salokangas RKR: Prognostic implications of the sex of schizophrenic patients. Br J Psychiatry 142:145–151, 1983

Seeman MV: Gender differences in schizophrenia. Can J Psychiatry 27:107–112, 1982

Seeman MV: Interaction of sex, age, and neuroleptic dose. Compr Psychiatry 24:125–128, 1983a

Seeman MV: Schizophrenic men and women require different treatment programs. Journal of Psychiatric Treatment and Evaluation 5:143–148, 1983b

Seeman MV: Current outcome in schizophrenia: women versus men. Acta Psychiatr Scand 73:609–617, 1986

Seeman MV, Lang M: The role of estrogens in schizophrenia gender differences. Schizophr Bull 16:185–194, 1990

Seidman LJ, Talbot NL, Kalinowski AG, et al: Neuropsychological probes of fronto-limbic system dysfunction in schizophrenia: olfactory identification and Wisconsin card sorting performance. Schizophr Res 6:55–65, 1992

Serby M, Larson P, Kalkstein D: Olfactory sense in psychoses. Biol Psychiatry 28:830, 1990

Shepherd M, Watt D, Falloon I, et al: The natural history of schizophrenia: a five-year follow-up study of outcome and prediction in a representative sample of schizophrenics. Psychol Med Monogr Suppl 15:1–46, 1989

Smith JM, Dunn DD: Sex differences in the prevalence of tardive dyskinesia. Am J Psychiatry 136:1080–1082, 1979

Swett C: Drug-induced dystonia. Am J Psychiatry 132:532–534, 1975

Thara R, Rajkumar S: Gender differences in schizophrenia: results of a follow-up study from India. Schizophr Res 7:65–70, 1992

Tsuang M: Suicide in schizophrenics, manics, depressives and surgical controls: a comparison with general population suicide mortality. Arch Gen Psychiatry 35:153–155, 1978

Wahl OF, Hunter J: Are gender effects being neglected in schizophrenia research? Schizophr Bull 18:313–318, 1992

Walker EF, Lewine RRJ: Sampling biases in studies of gender and schizophrenia. Schizophr Bull 19:1–14, 1993

Warner MD, Peabody CA, Csernansky JG: Olfactory functioning in schizophrenia and depression. Biol Psychiatry 27:457–458, 1990

Wing JK: Epidemiology of schizophrenia. Journal of the Royal Society of Science and Medicine 80:134–135, 1987

Wolyniec PS, Pulver AE, McGrath JA, et al: Schizophrenia: gender and familial risk. J Psychiatr Res 26:17–27, 1992

Yassa R, Jeste DV: Gender differences in tardive dyskinesia: a critical review of the literature. Schizophr Bull 18:701–715, 1992

Young MA, Meltzer HY: The relationship of demographic, clinical, and outcome variables to neuroleptic treatment requirements. Schizophr Bull 6:88–101, 1980

Zigler E, Levine J: Premorbid adjustment and paranoid-nonparanoid status in schizophrenia: a further investigation. J Abnorm Psychol 82:189–199, 1973

SECTION III

Pharmacological Treatments

CHAPTER 12

Standard and Novel Antipsychotic Drugs in Schizophrenia

Richard L. Borison, M.D., Ph.D.;
Ananda Pathiraja, M.D.; Susan Haverstock, M.D.;
Sridhar Gowda, M.D.; and Bruce I. Diamond, Ph.D.

S ince the introduction of antipsychotic drugs in the 1950s, the psychotic disorders, and schizophrenia in particular, have been redefined numerous times, and still today continue to be reconceptualized as new technologies and phenomenological advances are introduced. Despite these radical changes in the clinical understanding of schizophrenia, the therapeutic spectrum of activity and patterns of use of antipsychotic medications have remained relatively stable. In this chapter, we briefly review some areas of current concern in the use of antipsychotic drugs, as well as provide an overview of new trends in the development of antipsychotic agents that may allow future compounds to become "designer" drugs that will more specifically target and treat schizophrenic and psychotic symptomatology.

Antipsychotic Drug Dosing Guidelines

The goal of any pharmacotherapy is to provide maximal therapeutic benefit with minimal side effects; for most chemical compounds, these factors are directly related to the dosing of medication. After the introduction of antipsychotic medications in the early 1950s, many patients were treated with very high dosages, resulting in many extrapyramidal side effects (EPS) and leading to the coining of the term *neuroleptics* to describe this class of drugs because of their propensity to cause EPS. After dosing patterns were moderated in the 1960s and 1970s, the 1980s produced another period of "megadosing" with antipsychotic drugs as a part of a strategy of rapid neuroleptization. Now, in the 1990s, the pendulum has swung back toward the use of lower dosages of antipsychotic medication.

In a review of dosing patterns of neuroleptics, Baldessarini et al. (1984) noted the use of higher dosages (i.e., dosages that exceeded the "equivalent" of 1 g of chlorpromazine) in 40% of prescriptions. Although agreeing with the occasional clinical indications that merit higher dosages, these authors felt that lower dosages were equally effective in the management of the majority of patients.

Although more than 100 clinical studies have measured antipsychotic levels and serum neuroleptic activity (i.e., blood levels), a correlation between dosage and clinical response has not been established. The issue is further complicated by the presence of multiple variables, including patients' metabolism, sex, age, variability, clinical status, pharmacodynamics, pharmacokinetics, and active metabolites. As might be expected, initial findings have shown a wide variation of plasma concentrations of antipsychotics in patients receiving identical dosages (Ortiz and Gershon 1986). Despite these shortcomings, a therapeutic window for chlorpromazine of between 30–35 ng/ml and 300–350 ng/ml was suggested by early investigators (Curry 1985). Similarly, Smith et al. (1982) observed a plasma therapeutic range of 5–15 ng/ml for haloperidol, with patients outside this range having a poor clinical response. Mavroides et al. (1983) came to similar conclusion, but suggested a therapeutic window of 4.2–11 ng/ml for haloperidol and of 2–15 ng/ml for thiothixene. In their review, Davis et al.

(1980) identified a dose-response relationship that showed a plateau in clinical response beyond moderate (600 mg/day) dosages of chlorpromazine.

Baldessarini and Davis (1980), reviewing 23 controlled studies on maintenance neuroleptic therapy, found no significant dose-response relationship between the equivalents of 100 mg and 250 mg of chlorpromazine. They concluded that there were no distinct advantages to using more than a 300-mg chlorpromazine equivalent in the majority of patients. Lehmann et al. (1983), studying the clinical response of chronic schizophrenic patients receiving three different dosages of chlorpromazine equivalents (50 mg, 100 mg, and 600 mg) over a 1-year period, found no difference in the relapse rates in these three groups. Although Kane et al. (1986) described a high relapse rate in a patient population receiving a lower dosage (1.25–5 mg/2 weeks) than the standard regimen (12.5–50 mg/2 weeks) of fluphenazine decanoate, it was felt that this unconventional dosage may have been too low for these patients. Goldberg et al. (1972) compared the clinical efficacy of 60 mg of trifluoperazine with 600 mg of the same medication and concluded that there were no significant differences between the two dosages. Similar results were described by Donlon et al. (1978), who compared dosages of 20 mg and 80 mg of fluphenazine. Van Putten et al. (1988) studied the efficacy of three different dosages of haloperidol (5 mg, 10 mg, and 20 mg) over a 4-week period and found no significant variations between the groups receiving each regimen at the end of treatment. From a clinical perspective, Little et al. (1989) observed the presence of more severe hallucinations as an indication for greater antipsychotic dosing, as such symptoms are suggestive of low serum levels.

In their *neuroleptic threshold hypothesis,* Haase and Janssen (1965) postulated that the onset of antipsychotic action results from drug action on mesolimbic and mesocortical systems, with the first appearance of hypokinesia or rigidity representing the involvement of the nigrostriatal system. Relying on this principle, McEvoy et al. (1991) observed no therapeutic differences between patients who were treated with threshold dosages (4 mg) of haloperidol and those who received higher dosages of this medication. Although there was a decrease in hostility in the patients receiving higher dosages, this was attributed to the tranquilization rather than to the antipsychotic effect.

In summary, although there is no consensus regarding the dosages of antipsychotic drugs to be used, it appears that some clinicians use higher dosages without any scientific rationale. With the potential for long-term adverse experiences such as tardive dyskinesia and acute EPS, clinicians must be cautious about such practices. Fortunately, adherence to lower dosages today appears to be the rule rather than the exception. Vuckovic et al. (1990) were able to document this trend in a retrospective comparison of charts within a 10-year period. In their review, they observed a similar clinical outcome despite changes in prescribing patterns. With the use of supplementary medications such as the benzodiazepines (e.g., in acute psychiatric emergencies), it has become practical to use lower dosages of antipsychotic medications. Unquestionably, individual variations need to be taken into account in any therapeutic regimen; however, it is feasible to reduce the dosage of medications during the maintenance phase of the illness.

Dosage Equivalence: Myth or Fact?

The commercial introduction of various antipsychotic drugs provided clinicians with increased choices among different agents as well as the opportunity to switch from one agent to another. This relatively common clinical practice created the problem of accurately determining the relative dosage equivalencies of antipsychotic drugs when the only data available are those supplied by the pharmaceutical manufacturers of these drugs. As observed by Davis (1974), practitioners could not assume the equipotency of marketed dosages of antipsychotics, because other nonpharmacological factors (e.g., marketing decisions, manufacturing decisions) played a major role in determining recommended dosages for clinical use. This dilemma has highlighted the need for a standard conversion table for different antipsychotics.

Comparisons of antipsychotic dosages were initially done on the basis of clinical experience and animal behavior tests, but with questionable conclusions. Others have tried to rank drugs according to their binding properties to the dopamine D_2 receptors, although these properties did not necessarily reflect the clinical potency of the medications (Snyder et al. 1974).

Davis (1974) reviewed several double-blind studies that had provisions for flexible dosing, and assumed as equipotent those dosages that brought an empirical therapeutic response across a wide range of antipsychotics. Thus, comparisons among different drugs were made by using efficacy studies in which each neuroleptic was compared with a placebo or with chlorpromazine. Using chlorpromazine as the reference drug, dosage equivalence was calculated with the daily dosage of the drug under investigation, which was given a value of 100. Hence, a drug that was twice as potent as chlorpromazine was given a value of 50, with the assumption that it was capable of achieving therapeutic benefit with half the dosage of chlorpromazine on a milligram-to-milligram basis.

Wyatt (1976), in his review of 102 double-blind studies, compared the potencies of 40 neuroleptic drugs and drew conclusions similar to Davis's. However, methodological variation between studies and the resulting margin of error precluded Wyatt's reporting the outcome of his studies in quantitative terms. Furthermore, Wyatt considered his conclusions regarding nonphenothiazines as only tentative, subject to change in the light of further evidence.

In Wyatt's review, when equally effective drugs were classified into groups, dosage data from each study were used to determine the dosage equivalencies of the drugs; furthermore, within each study, the dosage ratio of drugs was calculated in reference to a standard drug such as chlorpromazine. These standardized ratios were averaged across studies for each drug. For those studies that included chlorpromazine, relative potencies were directly calculated. For other studies, indirect calculation was done using an intermediate drug for comparison purposes, provided that it met the following criteria: 1) it had been frequently compared with chlorpromazine, 2) its relationship to chlorpromazine was relatively constant over many studies, and 3) it had been used in many studies not involving chlorpromazine. The data were then reanalyzed to determine the potencies of the drugs in acute versus chronic psychiatric populations. Wyatt (1976) concluded that his results were in reasonable agreement with previously published findings.

In a subsequent study, Wyatt and Torgrow (1976) made an intradiagnostic comparison of clinical potencies of antipsychotic drugs. For this purpose, double-blind studies involving schizophrenic and affective disorder populations were analyzed to determine the "equivalent clinical potency" of drugs. The equal efficacy of each drug was determined for each disorder on a study-by-study basis, founded on each investigator's interpretation of measurements of clinical improvement. An approach similar to the one used in Wyatt's (1976) study was used to calculate potencies. In their conclusion, Wyatt and Torgrow (1976) found equivalent clinical dosages to be equally efficacious across different diagnostic categories.

Unfortunately, because of inherent methodological problems, none of these studies appears to have truly addressed the concept of drug equivalence. From a scientific point of view, it is difficult to make accurate comparisons across different studies. Among other factors, different diagnostic criteria, heterogeneity of patient populations, concurrent medications, and comorbidity states are likely to interfere with reasonable comparisons of drugs. The presence of active metabolites and differences in metabolism in individual patients would further complicate assessment, as there are significant differences between blood levels of antipsychotics in patients who are given identical dosages of medication. In the above reviews, no consideration was given to adverse experiences, because the primary interest was in the therapeutic activity.

In summary, an adequate dosage relationship for antipsychotics has yet to be established, despite the clinical availability of such medications for more than four decades. It is clear that the current conversion tables that are used as the "gold standard" do not adequately address the issue of drug equivalence. Contrary to popular belief, wide variations of clinical potencies are observed when different tables are compared (see Table 12–1).

The only means by which true milligram equivalencies can be determined is in crossover studies of different antipsychotics in a homogeneous schizophrenic population; such studies remain to be conducted. It may thus be recommended that clinicians not slavishly adhere to any one of the dosage conversion tables—as these are inherently flawed and at best are poor approximations—but rather rely on

Table 12–1. Dose equivalents for commonly used antipsychotics by various authors

Generic name	Brand name	Chlorpromazine equivalents (approximate values, mg)				
		Davis (1974)	Wyatt (1976)	Baldessarini (1985)	Hollister (1984)	Schatzberg and Cole (1991)
Phenothiazines						
Chlorpromazine	Thorazine	100	100	100	100	100
Mesoridazine	Serentil	55	45	50	50	55
Thioridazine	Mellaril	95	108	95	100	100
Piperacetazine	Quide	10	19	—	10	10
Perphenazine	Trilafon	9	9	10	10	9
Trifluoperazine	Stelazine	3	4	5	5	3
Fluphenazine	Prolixin	1.2	1.2	2	2.5	1.2
Thioxanthenes						
Thiothixene	Navane	5.2	3.2	4	3	5
Chlorprothixene	Taractan	44	35	75	—	45
Butyrophenones						
Haloperidol	Haldol	1.6	2.4	2.5	2	1.6
Dibenzoxazepines						
Loxapine	Loxitane	—	—	13	10	15
Clozapine	Clozaril	—	—	150	—	60
Indoles						
Molindone	Moban	—	—	9	10	10
Diphenylbutyl- piperidines						
Pimozide	Orap	—	—	1.5	—	—
Rauwolfia						
Reserpine	Serpasil	—	—	4	—	1.5

their clinical knowledge of low-, middle-, and high-dosage ranges for various neuroleptics to determine appropriate conversions of dosages between antipsychotic drugs (i.e., changing from the middle dosage range of one agent to the middle dosage range of another agent).

Oral-to-Depot Conversion of Antipsychotic Drugs

Long-acting, injectable antipsychotics were introduced primarily to facilitate medication compliance, as using them led to less-frequent dosing with medications. From another perspective, injectable antipsychotic medications theoretically reduce the variability in bioavailability seen with oral administration by avoiding first-pass metabolic effects. Thus, depot medications rather than orally administered medications are likely to provide a better correlation of dosages and blood levels, which may be ultimately useful in establishing more precise dosages of antipsychotic drugs. However, contrary to expectations, depot medications have proven to be no more effective than their corresponding oral preparations (Kane 1989). Furthermore, according to Hemstrom et al. (1988), available clinical data do not show any clinical superiority of one depot preparation over another.

Although many long-acting preparations are available worldwide, in the United States, clinicians' experience is limited to haloperidol decanoate, fluphenazine decanoate, and fluphenazine enanthate injections. Haloperidol decanoate is slowly absorbed from the injected site and is hydrolyzed to haloperidol, reaching a steady state in 3–9 days after injection, depending on the administered dosage (Jann et al. 1985). In contrast, fluphenazine decanoate reaches its peak serum level within 24 hours of administration, declining thereafter and maintaining a low plasma level (Hemstrom et al. 1988). The serum concentration of haloperidol decanoate following administration appears to be more stable than that of either of the fluphenazine preparations (Jann et al. 1985).

A simple, pharmacokinetic model–based formula for the conversion of oral to depot preparations (Jann et al. 1985) is given as follows:

$$Dd/Rd = (Do/Ro) \times Td \times F, \text{ where}$$

Dd is the depot dosage in milligrams of neuroleptic base
Rd is the ratio of molecular weight of the depot base to that of its salt
Do is the oral dosage in milligrams of neuroleptic base
Ro is the ratio of molecular weight of the oral base to that of its salt
Td is the dosage interval between depot administration in days
F is the bioavailability of the oral drug form of the neuroleptic as a fraction of 1

Unfortunately, such a formula assumes that there is 1) 100% bioavailability of the drug after intramuscular injection, 2) equipotent dopamine receptor blockage by both oral and depot antipsychotic drugs, 3) a linear relationship between oral and systemic clearance of drugs, and 4) absence of pharmacologically active metabolites. It is clear that none of the available depot medications meet these criteria. Despite these limitations, clinicians may be able to apply this formula as a general guideline in initiating therapy.

In their literature, pharmaceutical companies have provided guidelines for conversion from oral to depot antipsychotic drugs based on bioavailability of the drug. These guidelines are listed in Table 12–2.

Applying the above conversion factor, Deberdt et al. (1980) found "comparable and stable" serum concentrations with both oral and depot haloperidol preparations. In comparison, Nair et al. (1986) found a significantly lower serum concentration with long-acting versus oral haloperidol preparations when a 15-fold conversion factor was used. They demonstrated equivalent serum concentrations using a median conversion factor of 21.4. Kissling et al. (1985), on the other hand, reported similar serum levels of depot and oral haloperidol with a conversion factor of 15. Available data suggest the 20-fold conversion to be optimal for maintaining previously achieved therapeutic responses for the majority of patients, with the exception of those who are elderly (Viukari et al. 1982) and those with hepatic impairment. In these patients, a 15-fold conversion factor may be more appropriate.

In a nonblinded and uncontrolled study, DeCuyper et al. (1986) used twice the dosage of haloperidol decanoate necessary to achieve early steady-state plasma concentrations. Unfortunately, this study resulted in inconsistent clinical improvement at the cost of significant adverse experiences. Both Nair et al. (1986) and Wistedt et al. (1984)

Table 12–2. Guidelines from pharmaceutical companies for converting oral to depot antipsychotic drugs

Compound	Recommendations	Usual dosage
Haldol decanoate	Oral dose × 20 = Depot dose/4 weeks	50–100 mg/4 weeks
Prolixin decanoate	Oral dose × 2.5 = Depot dose/3 weeks	25–37.5 mg/3 weeks
Prolixin enanthate	None	25 mg/2 weeks

found it necessary to supplement depot preparations with oral halo-peridol and levomepromazine, respectively. Because of inadequate data, no further conclusions can be made regarding these methods.

In comparison with haloperidol decanoate, which is converted to relatively nonactive metabolites, fluphenazine decanoate appears to have few similar inactive metabolic products, such as fluphenazine sulfoxide, 7-OH fluphenazine, and fluphenazine N-oxide, although the levels of these metabolites are significantly low in comparison with those of the parent compound. Marder et al. (1989) suggested that drug metabolism was relatively more important for oral fluphenazine than for depot fluphenazine. Although the current conversion guide-lines appear to result in low serum concentrations of fluphenazine (Schulz et al. 1989), this does not appear to affect clinical efficacy. In a patient with a rapid metabolizing rate who would otherwise receive a higher dosage than is usually required, this inherent safety feature may be necessary to avoid unnecessary adverse experiences. Unfortunately, patients who are at their threshold with oral medications may relapse when switched to a depot neuroleptic using this conversion method.

Yadalam and Simpson (1988) questioned the validity of the con-version formulas because they were developed in an era when it was customary to use higher dosages in an inpatient population. In addi-tion, these authors referred to the slow changes in fluphenazine levels observed during periods of dosage initiation and discontinuation. In their regimen, a test dosage of 6.25 mg of fluphenazine decanoate was given to assess sensitivity to the vehicle (sesame oil) and for adverse experiences. This was followed by twice-monthly injections of similar dosages, supplemented by oral fluphenazine on a decreasing schedule, given for up to 8 weeks, depending on the baseline oral dosage (see Table 12–3 for dosage schedule). The basis for Yadalam and Simpson's conversion between intramuscular and oral dosages was the 4-month time period necessary to reach steady-state concentrations with depot fluphenazine when it was given every 2 weeks. Yadalam and Simpson further recommended additional oral therapy rather than higher depot dosages to treat the symptoms of brief clinical decom-pensation. Although the conservative approach followed by Yadalam and Simpson has merit, they themselves noted that the approach was based on clinical experience rather than scientific data.

Table 12–3. Conversion table for fluphenazine decanoate

Baseline oral dosage (mg/day)	Week 0 O	Week 0 IM	Week 2 O	Week 2 IM	Week 4 O	Week 4 IM	Week 6 O	Week 6 IM	Week 8 O	Week 8 IM	Week 10 O	Week 10 IM
5	4.0	6.25	2.5	6.25	1.0	6.25	—	6.25	—	—	—	—
10	7.5	6.25	5.0	6.25	2.5	12.5	—	12.5	—	—	—	—
20	15.0	6.25	10.0	6.25	7.5	12.5	5.0	12.5	2.5	12.5	—	12.5
30	25.0	6.25	20.0	12.5	15.0	25.0	10.0	25.0	5.0	25.0	—	12.5
40	30.0	6.25	25.0	12.5	20.0	25.0	15.0	25.0	10.0	25.0	—	12.5

Note. O = oral dosage; IM = intramuscular dosage.
Source. Yadalam and Simpson (1988).

Goldberg et al. (1972) suggested fluphenazine decanoate and fluphenazine enanthate dosing based on body weight. However, at present, clinical validity and usefulness of such a conversion remains doubtful.

Concomitant Antipsychotic Use

Although it has been 30 years since the first publications concerning the concomitant use of two or more antipsychotic medications came out, there have yet to appear any large-scale, controlled prospective studies regarding this practice. In the 1960s, the use of combinations of antipsychotic medications was widely accepted and recommended. It was felt that combinations of drugs such as chlorpromazine and trifluoperazine or chlorpromazine plus haloperidol enhanced antipsychotic treatment efficacy (Casey et al. 1961; Jones et al. 1968; Swanson et al. 1967; Terrell 1962). In addition, it was argued that the use of a lower dosage of a low-potency agent plus a high-potency agent might minimize the side effects characteristic of each drug while providing additive antipsychotic efficacy. However, Gardos et al. (1968) and Williams et al. (1969) suggested that there was no advantage to this approach with regard either to antipsychotic efficacy or to minimization of side effects. All of the studies either for or against this practice were performed before the appearance of the classification, rating, and laboratory controls currently available. Further, although there have been many clinical caveats and empirically based opinions, there has been very little in the way of systematic studies to produce evidence either for or against the use of dual antipsychotic treatment.

In the 1970s and 1980s, physicians began to look more closely at prescribing patterns. In their survey, Sheppard et al. (1974) examined psychiatrists' prescribing patterns nationally and found the use of multiple antipsychotic medications to be common; in the case of refractory patients, up to six agents were often used concomitantly. Sheppard et al. concluded that "polypharmacy in psychiatry represents an example of legitimate, but unnecessary use of antipsychotic agents" (p. 188). In 1985, Wilson et al. published a study of prescribing practices in eight countries. Of the 739 hospitalized chronic schizophrenic patients involved in this study, 36% were treated with only one neuroleptic, 40% were treated with two neuroleptics simultaneously, 20% were treated with three neuroleptics simultaneously, and 3% were treated with four or five neuroleptics simultaneously.

Despite these practices, many have argued for a simpler, more rational approach toward medication prescribing in general (Edwards and Kumar 1984; Mason 1973; Schatzberg et al. 1974; Thornton and Pray 1975); the use of two medications for the same purpose has been considered redundant, and polypharmacy has been considered less than optimal treatment. These attitudes have been backed by the increasing awareness of the risks of EPS, tardive dyskinesia, and neuroleptic malignant syndrome. A more hostile medicolegal environment has also led to the practice of defensive medicine and the principle of "minimum effective treatment." Also, there is now a focus on nonneuroleptic co-treatments (i.e., combinations of antipsychotics with sedative hypnotics, antidepressants, lithium, and other adjunct medications).

Still, it has been observed clinically that there may be a subgroup of patients who respond better to two or more antipsychotic agents. Godleski et al. (1989) studied 14 chronic schizophrenic patients who were taking more than one antipsychotic agent. They attempted over the course of a year to reduce the regimens to a single agent. Six of the 14 patients successfully adjusted to this conversion, but 8 of the 14 patients decompensated.

In a study involving a group of patients taking a depot neuroleptic plus a different oral antipsychotic agent (Soni et al. 1992), the oral agent was converted to chlorpromazine equivalents, and then to the decanoate, which conversion resulted in an increased decanoate dosage. The subjects were then followed for 12 months. Soni et al. reported a drop in serum neuroleptic levels from baseline over the first 4 months, with 8 of the 13 patients relapsing. They concluded that, although it may be rational to transfer a patient to a single agent, doing so is associated with a high rate of relapse. Both the Godleski et al. (1989) and the Soni et al. (1992) studies point to a need for more work in this area.

There is another study regarding the use of two concomitant antipsychotics that deserves attention. Using animals, Carvey et al. (1986) administered clozapine or thioridazine in combination with haloperidol in an attempt to modify behavioral dopamine hypersensitivity. It was postulated that strongly anticholinergic antipsychotic agents, like other antimuscarinic medications, may have a role in the prevention of tardive dyskinesia. The coadministration of thioridazine was indeed found to attenuate haloperidol-induced behavioral hypersensitivity, whereas clozapine and chlorpromazine did not. The use of anticholinergic agents to prevent the development of tardive dyskinesia remains a controversial topic; further, it must be kept in mind that these animal studies may not reflect human pharmacology.

Rapid Tranquilization

Rapid tranquilization is the use of medication to control the excitatory psychomotor symptoms of highly agitated, potentially dangerous and violent patients. It is typically used for patients who are unable to be verbally redirected when their behavior is out of control, and therefore is used to prevent harm to the patient and others. The patients who warrant such treatment typically present with decompensated psychoses, intoxication, or delirium secondary to medical illness. Rapid tranquilization lessens the need for seclusion and mechanical restraint, and allows the patient to be treated in the least restrictive environment possible. However, core symptoms of schizophrenia are not usually resolved in this process; that is, hallucinations and delusions may persist for weeks after antipsychotic treatment is begun.

Rapid tranquilization should not be confused with *rapid neuroleptization*. Rapid neuroleptization implies the use of very high loading dosages of antipsychotic medication over the first few weeks of treatment in an attempt to produce a more rapid remission of psychosis. Examples of this might include rapidly increased dosages of haloperidol to 60 mg/day (Ericksen et al. 1978) or fluphenazine to 80 mg/day (Donlon et al. 1978). Although this mode of treatment was popular in the early 1980s, researchers have concluded that the procedure is no more efficacious for patients with regard to either rapidity or magnitude of psychotic remission. Escobar et al. (1983) compared patients who received hourly injections of fluphenazine hydrochloride intramuscularly (48.5 mg in 24 hours) with patients who received a total of 7.5 mg of the same medication orally. Both groups demonstrated similar improvement, with the greatest gain occurring between 4 and 8 hours of treatment initiation, when the orally medicated control group had received only a single 2.5-mg oral dose. The only difference between the high- (intramuscular) and low- (oral) dosage group was more reports of EPS with the higher dosages.

With rapid tranquilization, dosing of medication is repeated at frequent intervals until a patient is controllable verbally or is mildly sedated. This procedure once implied the use of only antipsychotic medication, but now may be extended to the use of benzodiazepines or combinations of medications. Medication is typically given orally concurrent with an intramuscular regimen—usually involving one to four doses given at 30- to 60-minute intervals. Intravenous dosing has also been used, although less frequently; this route is mostly used in medical-surgical settings and typically involves administration of benzodiazepines rather than antipsychotics. Although results of studies have demonstrated the efficacy of intravenous haloperidol (Lerner et al. 1979), the U.S. Food and Drug Administration (FDA) has not approved administration via this route.

Both Schaffer et al. (1982) and Dubin et al. (1985) conducted studies in which intramuscular and oral administration of antipsychotic medications in rapid tranquilization were compared. Schaffer et al. (1982) found that intramuscular haloperidol attained peak plasma levels significantly faster than an oral concentrate. Moreover, the total drug availability for each dosage form was not significantly different even when the oral dosage was twice that of the intramuscular dosage. Schaffer et al.'s results suggested that because medication administered intramuscularly attains peak levels more rapidly, intramuscular haloperidol should be used if symptoms are severe enough to warrant establishing immediate control, but that after the first dose, the use of oral medication is equally efficacious. Schaffer et al. cautioned that clinical improvement is not necessarily related to peak plasma levels of drug, however, and that the rate of rise in blood level may be more important in symptom resolution than the actual level attained. Dubin et al. (1985) came to essentially the same conclusion as Schaffer's group. In a study of schizophrenic patients in acutely exacerbated stages of illness, haloperidol (5 or 10 mg/dose) or thiothixene (10 or

12 mg/dose) was administered either orally or intramuscularly at 30-minute intervals, with the intramuscular dosage group receiving a mean total of three doses of medication and the oral dosage group a mean total of four doses. It took only 30 minutes longer for the oral group to be controlled than the intramuscular group.

Coffman et al. (1987), Escobar et al. (1983), and Neborsky et al. (1981) have all supported the use of oral concentrate in rapid tranquilization. They have noted the very low incidence of refusal by patients and suggest that less indignity is imposed on the patient by using the concentrate as opposed to an injection. The use of oral medication may also mitigate later claims regarding the administration of medication by force (Dubin et al. 1986).

Regardless of route, the number of doses of antipsychotic used for rapid tranquilization in most studies is less than six. There is, however, no consensus regarding a ceiling dosage. In the study by Dubin et al. (1985), most patients responded to 15–20 mg of haloperidol, and none required more than 50 mg. The authors also noted that there were no predictor profiles of those who would respond rapidly. "Dose cannot be predicted by body weight, past dose requirements, presence or severity of particular target symptoms, or degree of psychosis; however, the principle of minimum effective dose should be observed" (Dubin et al. 1986, p. 221). Nor are there established guidelines for converting oral or intramuscular dosage used in rapid tranquilization to an oral maintenance dosage (Dubin et al. 1986).

Authors of several studies have also shown that high dosages of antipsychotics have no advantages over low dosages in rapid tranquilization. Several investigators (Davis et al. 1980; Donlon et al. 1980; Eriksen et al. 1978; Quitkin et al. 1975) have demonstrated that 100 mg/day of haloperidol has no increased efficacy over 10 mg/day. It also has been argued by Solano et al. (1989) that hourly dosing with a neuroleptic is not justified by pharmacokinetic data. "Availability of the drug is assured by the first dose; subsequent hourly administration increases accumulation and toxicity without necessarily enhancing therapeutic advantage. After the alpha stage, the drug from the blood reaches the lipid compartment including the lipid-rich brain. At this time, even when the blood level is falling, the brain drug level increases as a result of redistribution" (p. 93).

Because the goal of rapid tranquilization is often mild sedation, drugs other than antipsychotics may be preferable. It is well known that antipsychotic actions generally take much longer to occur than sedative effects, and thus benzodiazepines may be a preferred alternative to antipsychotics. As adjuncts to neuroleptics, benzodiazepines allow lower dosages of both medications (Greenblatt and Raskin 1986). In 1979, Lerner et al. compared the efficacy of intravenous haloperidol (Haldol) and diazepam (Valium) and found no difference in clinical response. In recent years, lorazepam (Ativan) has become the most frequently used and well-studied adjunct for agitated behavior. Lorazepam is well absorbed by oral, intramuscular, or intravenous routes. Dosages of lorazepam are highly variable, depending on patient history and response pattern. In an open trial, Cohen and Khan (1987) demonstrated that patients on greater than 2 mg/day of lorazepam showed more improvement than those on less than 2 mg/day. Precautions are necessary when using benzodiazepines: Diazepam should not be used intramuscularly because of its unpredictable and generally poor absorption, and the FDA has cautioned against the use of midazolam for conscious sedation because it can induce respiratory depression (Physicians' Desk Reference 1991, p. 1860).

One other agent that appears to be a safe and reliable choice for treatment of acute agitation is droperidol. Resnick and Burton (1984) showed this drug to be as effective as haloperidol; indeed, in their study, patients on droperidol required a second injection less often than those on haloperidol (36% as compared with 81%).

Usually, rapid tranquilization is implemented when the knowledge base concerning a patient is incomplete; hence, it is often used early in treatment when a patient presents to the hospital. Results could be disastrous if an undiagnosed physical disorder were to progress in a sedated patient (Ellison et al. 1989). Although it is safe to tranquilize patients who have many medical disorders, the primary medical problems should certainly be addressed first. Overall, the incidence of side effects from rapid tranquilization is very low, at less than 10%. Dubin et al. (1985) cited drowsiness in 16% of his patients, sleep in 11%, hypotension in 4%, and dystonia and akathisia in 6%. Cardiovascular safety of rapid tranquilization is well established, particularly with high-potency agents. Relative contraindications for rapid tranquilization include central nervous system depression, unstable epilepsy, clinically significant hypo- or hypertension, recent head injury, recent drug overdose, or serious hematologic, cardiovascular, renal, or hepatic impairment.

In their review of rapid tranquilization, Lazarus et al. (1989) found that there was no increased mortality associated with rapid tranquilization, and that case reports linking sudden death to rapid tranquilization were associated only with high loading dosages. Lazarus et al. further recommended using intravenous drugs only with cardiac monitoring. A further consideration is that although neuroleptic malignant syndrome is not usually associated with rapid tranquilization, patients with a history of this disorder should be considered high-risk candidates for rapid tranquilization.

Novel Antipsychotic Drugs

The search for new antipsychotic drugs has focused on developing compounds that are less likely to produce EPS and that will improve the therapeutic efficacy of these drugs in schizophrenic patients, particularly in treating the negative symptoms of schizophrenia. This clinical profile represents the idealized *atypical neuroleptic,* the search for which may be likened to the quest for the Holy Grail. It has been a long and frustrating search that sometimes appears to be of mythic proportions, and that, as yet, has not been successful.

Among currently commercially available drugs, clozapine is the compound that most closely conforms to the profile of an atypical neuroleptic, but the clinical utility of clozapine has been hampered by its multitude of nonneurological side effects. Therefore, among the different strategies for developing new antipsychotic drugs, one has been to develop a new generation of safer clozapine-like agents. A second stratagem has been to attempt to improve upon the classic dopamine-blocking antipsychotics, and a third stratagem has been to explore new neurotransmitter systems that may contribute to schizophrenic psychopathology. We now review each of these three strategies in sampling the current state of the art in the development of novel antipsychotic drugs.

Dopamine D₂ Receptor Antagonists: Remoxipride

The benzamide class of antipsychotic medications is familiar to clinicians practicing outside of the United States, with sulpiride being the most widely prescribed of these compounds. A more lipophilic member of this class of drugs is remoxipride, a drug that is highly specific for binding to dopamine D_2 receptors and σ receptors (Hall et al. 1986; Snyder and Largent 1989).

In contrast to most dopamine-blocking agents, remoxipride has negligible action on dopamine D_1, α-adrenergic, serotonergic, histaminic, or muscarinic receptors. Despite its relatively high potency and specificity for dopamine D_2 receptors, in animal studies remoxipride has produced a greater displacement of [^{3}H]spiperone binding in limbic rather than striatal areas, indicating a less-robust action in blocking striatal dopamine D_2 receptors, which would suggest a lower propensity for producing extrapyramidal side effects (Ogren et al. 1984). In human studies using positron-emission tomography, remoxipride occupies greater than 70% of D_2 receptors, well within the range predicted for antipsychotic activity.

Efficacy.   Remoxipride is rapidly absorbed, reaching its peak plasma level in approximately 2 hours, with a half-life of approximately 7 hours. Higher maximal concentrations and increased half-life are seen in patients with either renal or liver disease (von Bahr et al. 1990), whereas in elderly individuals the plasma half-life can be increased by nearly threefold (Movin et al. 1990).

In their review of 12 published controlled studies investigating the clinical efficacy of remoxipride versus that of other antipsychotic agents in schizophrenic patients, Wadworth and Heel (1990) found that when compared with thioridazine (in 2 studies, 58 completed patients, 150–750 mg/day) and haloperidol (9 studies, 840 completed patients, 5–45 mg/day), remoxipride (150–600 mg/day) was equally efficacious. In the only study with a placebo control group (41 completed patients), Chouinard (1990) found that chlorpromazine (300–1200 mg/day) was superior to remoxipride, and that remoxipride could not be therapeutically differentiated from placebo. In a large dosage-ranging trial of 242 schizophrenic patients in an acutely exacerbated stage of illness, Lapierre et al. (1992) compared low-dosage (30–90 mg/day), mid-dosage (120–140 mg/day), and high-dosage (300–600 mg/day) remoxipride with haloperidol (15–45 mg/day). They found that both the mid-range and the high-range dosages produced a statistically significant improvement in psychosis during the 6 weeks of treatment, as evaluated with the Brief Psychiatric Rating Scale (BPRS; Overall and Gorham 1962). This improvement was equivalent to that observed with haloperidol. Although the low-dosage group also showed improvement, it failed to reach statistical significance. Patients showed statistically significant improvement on the positive symptom cluster on the BPRS (i.e., the thought disturbance factor) and on the combined positive and negative symptom clusters with remoxipride at dosages of 120–600 mg/day.

Although placebo-controlled efficacy trials with remoxipride remain to be presented in sufficient numbers in the scientific literature, at this stage of development, remoxipride may combine the efficacy of and lack of autonomic and cardiovascular side effects of a high-potency neuroleptic, such as haloperidol, but with significantly fewer EPS. Remoxipride's lack of sedative side effects may potentially discourage its inpatient use for treating acute exacerbations of schizophrenia, but may likely lead to its use as a more appropriate therapy, with superior patient compliance, in the outpatient setting. Remoxipride has been commercially available in Canada, the United Kingdom, and Scandinavia, where isolated reports of aplastic anemia and death have been noted. These reports have caused the worldwide market removal of remoxipride and its withdrawal from consideration by the FDA.

Another benzamide derivative, amisulpiride, may be the eventual clinical successor to remoxipride; however, additional safety data for all new benzamide antipsychotics are now warranted to rule out their possible association with aplastic anemia.

Side effects.   Although the results from animal studies have predicted that remoxipride would produce antipsychotic actions with minimal EPS, one adverse action of dopamine D_2 receptor blockers is prolactinemia and its attendant side effects of gynecomastia, decreased libido, and galactorrhea in women. Prolactin studies with remoxipride have indicated that it produces a large initial increase in levels of this hormone; however, unlike other typical antipsychotics, this is a relatively transient action, and tolerance develops after 1 month with repeated dosing (Chouinard 1987).

In general, remoxipride has been excellently tolerated by patients. As a relatively specific dopamine D_2 receptor blocker, it would be expected that remoxipride would produce a relatively high incidence of EPS; however, this has not been commonly observed. In a meta-analysis of nine double-blind trials of remoxipride (150–600 mg/day) versus haloperidol (5–45 mg/day), Lewander et al. (1990) observed that remoxipride produced 50% or fewer parkinsonian signs, akathisia, and dystonias than did haloperidol. Moreover, when EPS did occur with remoxipride, it was most likely to be mild in nature; hence, the use of anticholinergic antiparkinsonian agents was more than twofold greater in the patients treated with haloperidol than in those treated with remoxipride. These clinical data appear to corroborate the animal studies suggesting remoxipride's less active blockade of extrapyramidal dopamine receptors.

Although these data on EPS appear to confer an atypical neuroleptic status on remoxipride relative to haloperidol, it remains to be demonstrated whether remoxipride produces fewer EPS than the low-potency neuroleptics. In one study of remoxipride versus thioridazine (McCreadie et al. 1988), remoxipride produced the same degree of EPS as thioridazine, whereas in another study (Phanjoo and Link 1990), remoxipride produced fewer EPS than thioridazine. One confounding factor in attempting to determine the relative propensity of remoxipride to produce EPS is that the incidence of EPS appears to be dosage related (Lapierre et al. 1992), as increasing dosages (30–600 mg/day) of remoxipride are associated with an increased incidence of EPS as well as an increased need for the use of anticholinergic antiparkinsonian agents.

Remoxipride is remarkably free from other common neuroleptic side effects, with hypotension and other cardiovascular side effects being rare, and autonomic side effects (i.e., anticholinergic effects, such as dry mouth) occurring no more frequently than with haloperidol. The incidence of hyperprolactinemic side effects (i.e., breast swelling, galactorrhea, sexual dysfunction, and menstrual disturbance) is similar for remoxipride and haloperidol (Lewander et al. 1990). It would appear not only that remoxipride is relatively nonsedating, but also that its use may be associated with more insomnia as well as the use of more sedative-hypnotic agents than required with haloperidol treatment (Lapierre et al. 1992).

Broad-Spectrum Receptor Antagonists: Zotepine

Zotepine is a dibenzothiepine derivative that has a pharmacological profile similar to a broad-spectrum-blocker antipsychotic agent; that is, it is active in blocking receptors for dopamine, norepinephrine (α_1), serotonin (5-HT$_1$ and 5-HT$_2$), and muscarinic cholinergic receptors.

Efficacy and side effects.   There have been numerous open-label, uncontrolled trials with zotepine that have suggested that this compound is an efficacious agent that produces EPS with a low incidence, similar or less than that seen with the low-potency neuroleptics. Preliminary clinical observations have also suggested that zotepine may have an "activating" action on the negative symptoms of schizophrenia, particularly when used at low dosages (Dieterle et al. 1987).

To test this hypothesis, Barnas et al. (1992) conducted a double-blind study of zotepine (average dosage of 94.4 mg/day) versus haloperidol (average dosage of 4.2 mg/day) in 30 schizophrenic patients who were specifically selected for their preponderance of negative symptoms. After a 1-week placebo washout period, subjects were randomly assigned to a treatment group for a 7-week period. The results indicated that zotepine, but not haloperidol treatment, produced a significant ($P < .05$) improvement in patients on global functioning, as measured by the Clinical Global Impression (CGI) scale (Guy 1976). When measuring psychopathology via the BPRS, Barnas and co-workers found that zotepine outperformed haloperidol treatment by the fifth week of treatment ($P < .05$), and that haloperidol significantly improved performance on only the thought-disorder subscale of the BPRS. In contrast, patients treated with zotepine showed significant improvement on the anxiety-depression and the anergic subscales of the BPRS.

Negative symptoms of schizophrenia were measured using a modification (termed the "Munich version") of the Scale for the Assessment of Negative Symptoms (SANS-M; Dieterle et al. 1986), on which both the haloperidol-treated group ($P < .05$) and the zotepine-treated group ($P < .001$) showed improvement. Although haloperidol lowered the total SANS-M scores, it failed to reach statistical significance in lowering any of the subscale scores, whereas zotepine significantly lowered the subscale scores for affective flattening–blunting ($P < .005$), alogia ($P < .005$), avolition-apathy ($P < .05$), anhedonia-asociality ($P < .01$), and attentional impairment ($P < .001$). Zotepine was most effective (observed after only 1 week of treatment) in improving attentional impairment; it was least effective in improving avolition-apathy (observed after only 5 weeks of treatment). The medications were well tolerated in this study, with EPS being the major side effect reported for both treatments. Five haloperidol-treated patients and only two zotepine-treated patients required anticholinergic antiparkinsonian medication.

In an 8-week, double-blind study, Sarai and Okada (1987) compared zotepine (75–300 mg/day) with thiothixene (15–60 mg/day) in 94 schizophrenic subjects. According to a global rating of patient improvement, zotepine and thiothixene were equivalent in the percentage (53% and 52%, respectively) of patients showing slight to great improvement in psychosis, as well as being equivalent in the percentage of patients demonstrating a worsening of their illness (22% versus 27%, respectively) during the course of the trial. A further analysis of the data revealed that younger patients with undifferentiated or disorganized schizophrenia were the most likely to respond to zotepine, whereas paranoid schizophrenic patients showed the best therapeutic responsiveness to thiothixene treatment. The two treatments were also similar when the BPRS (Overall and Gorham 1962) was used to measure psychopathology. Side effects observed for the two drugs were similar, including EPS, with the only differences being increased insomnia associated with thiothixene and increased dry mouth associated with zotepine.

The data for zotepine are intriguing in that the drug is described clinically as a sedating-activating agent, with sedation—particularly at high dosages—being the major side effect, whereas activation of negative symptom schizophrenic patients can also be observed. This dual action is, of course, also reported for clozapine. At present, the majority of clinical data for zotepine were developed in either uncontrolled or poorly controlled studies, but they suggest a compound that 1) is sedating and moderately anticholinergic without significant cardiovascular side effects, 2) produces a low incidence of EPS, and 3) is effective for both positive and negative symptoms of schizophrenia. This interesting clinical profile warrants further, well-controlled, clinical trials to determine if zotepine use may lead to a safer and better treatment for schizophrenia, particularly for the negative symptoms associated with this illness.

Serotonergic Receptor Antagonists: Ritanserin, Amperozide, and Ondansetron

Although it appears that serotonin may play a critical role in schizophrenia, the role that it plays in the therapeutics of the illness remains uncertain. The latter role can perhaps be best tested by agents that are specific antagonists of serotonergic receptors and that fail to significantly interact with other neurotransmitter receptors. One such agent is ritanserin, a drug that potently blocks serotonin $5\text{-}HT_2$ (and $5\text{-}HT_{1C}$) receptors.

In initial clinical trials in schizophrenic patients (see review by Gerlach 1991), ritanserin was found to have a modest action in ameliorating the symptoms of schizophrenia. Of greater note was that when ritanserin was added to a fixed dosage of haloperidol, there was not only an improvement in the negative symptoms of schizophrenia but also a lessening of haloperidol-induced EPS (Bersani et al. 1986). Therefore, although ritanserin alone demonstrated a modest antipsychotic action in open-label studies, the combination of this potent serotonin $5\text{-}HT_2$ blocker with a potent dopamine D_2 receptor antagonist proved to be the most efficacious treatment.

Serotonin $5\text{-}HT_2$ receptor antagonists: amperozide. The direct role of serotonin $5\text{-}HT_2$ receptor blockade in schizophrenia has been partially tested via the clinical use of amperozide, which is a weak dopamine D_2 receptor blocker but a relatively potent serotonin $5\text{-}HT_2$ antagonist (Bjork et al. 1992). In reviewing four open-label trials with this compound, Bjork and colleagues (1992) found that 75% of patients showed satisfactory improvement in their psychosis, including 75% of a subset of patients known to be treatment resistant to typical neuroleptics. Among those who responded to amperozide treatment, the entire spectrum of schizophrenic psychopathology improved, no EPS were noted, and prolactin levels were not elevated. Results from animal behavior studies (Christensson and Bjork 1990) have suggested that amperozide may more selectively ameliorate the negative symptoms of schizophrenia; further, it appears to have a high selectivity for interacting with the mesolimbic system of the brain. At present, initial double-blind, placebo-controlled trials of amperozide in the United States have not been encouraging, and continued clinical work on amperozide has been suspended.

Serotonin 5-HT$_3$ receptor antagonists: ondansetron. Another strategy for modulating the serotonin system in schizophrenic illness has been via the antagonism of serotonin 5-HT$_3$ receptors. Conceptually, this hypothesis is based upon the data that 5-HT$_3$ receptors are localized in the limbic areas of brain (Kilpatrick et al. 1987), and that the behavioral actions of dopamine injected into the limbic areas of rodent brain are antagonized by 5-HT$_3$ antagonists. In contrast, 5-HT$_3$ antagonists do not affect normal dopamine transmission, nor do they appear to interact with striatal or tuberoinfundibular dopaminergic systems. These data suggest that these drugs would be unique in their ability to normalize schizophrenic behavior, provided that the dopamine hypothesis (Snyder 1976)—which attributes the underlying psychopathology of schizophrenia to a relatively discrete abnormality of limbic area dopamine function—is true.

The actions of serotonin 5-HT$_3$ antagonists in schizophrenia have been studied in a preliminary clinical test (DeVeaugh-Geiss et al. 1992). In a multicenter, 28-day trial of open-label ondansetron in 105 schizophrenic patients, low dosages of the drug (maximum of 16 mg/day) produced a significant lowering of BPRS scores by the second week of treatment. This improvement continued and increased in magnitude during the subsequent 2 weeks of the trial ($P < .005$); for those patients undergoing a placebo washout period at the end of the trial, there was a marked loss of efficacy after the discontinuation of ondansetron. The high-dosage ondansetron group (up to

48 mg/day) showed a less-robust response, with no significant lowering of BPRS scores from baseline by the end of 4 weeks of treatment; however, by the end of the first week of treatment and throughout the trial thereafter, the high-dosage group showed a significant ($P < .001$) improvement in the anxiety-depression subscale of the BPRS. By comparison, the low-dosage group showed less improvement on the anxiety-depression subscale, but showed significant and marked improvement on the thought disturbance and activation BPRS subscales. There were no significant actions of ondansetron at any dosage on the anergia subscale of the BPRS, which is often used as a measure for the negative symptoms of schizophrenia. No EPS were observed during the study, and constipation and headache were the most frequent adverse reactions reported.

These data would suggest that serotonin 5-HT$_3$ antagonists have the potential for correcting states of dopamine dysregulation in schizophrenic subjects, an action that would most specifically and therapeutically target the positive symptoms of schizophrenia, but without producing EPS. At this early point in their development, it remains to be proven whether the 5-HT$_3$ antagonists possess the ability to ameliorate the negative symptoms of schizophrenia.

Currently, further work using ondansetron as an antipsychotic agent has been stopped; however, it is possible that new and more potent 5-HT$_3$ antagonists may be studied in the future for their antipsychotic actions.

Combined Dopamine D$_2$ Receptor and Serotonin 5-HT$_2$ Receptor Antagonists: Risperidone

To date, the clinical trials with the relatively selective serotonergic antagonists have not been particularly successful. This does not, however, negate an important role for serotonin in schizophrenia. It would appear that, just as the neurochemical basis for schizophrenia cannot be reductionistically explained as only a dopaminergic problem, so, too, the therapeutics of schizophrenia cannot be attributed simply to the correction of a serotonergic problem. It is clear, however, from animal studies that serotonergic agents help modulate and regulate dopaminergic function; furthermore, results from clinical studies suggest that serotonergic receptor blockade may reduce EPS and increase the spectrum of therapeutic activity for the negative symptoms of schizophrenia, thus converting a typical to an atypical neuroleptic. It is also undeniable that dopamine D_2 receptor blockade confers antipsychotic potential to a compound. It would therefore appear that the combination of the blockade of serotonin $5-HT_2$ receptors and dopamine D_2 receptors may describe a more desirable biochemical profile for an antipsychotic agent.

Risperidone is a benzisoxazole derivative that combines the strong dopamine D_2 receptor–blocking activity of haloperidol and the potent serotonin $5-HT_2$ receptor antagonistic properties of ritanserin. Furthermore, risperidone is a potent blocker of noradrenergic α_1 and α_2 receptors (Leysen et al. 1992). In animal behavior studies, risperidone has shown a profile similar to that of typical neuroleptics in that it has blocked dopamine-induced abnormal behaviors (Janssen et al. 1988). Like typical neuroleptics, risperidone is capable of producing increases in serum prolactin levels in humans (Bersani et al. 1990). As would be predicted by its potent blockade of α receptors, risperidone has hypotensive potential, but rapid tolerance develops to this side effect with repeated administration; within the usual therapeutic dosage range, significant hypotension is not commonly observed (Claus et al. 1992).

Risperidone is largely metabolized to 9-hydroxy-risperidone, a drug with pharmacological properties similar to those of the parent compound. The maximum plasma concentration of risperidone is achieved within 2 hours of ingestion, and the half-life for risperidone and its active metabolite is approximately 24 hours. The metabolism of risperidone appears to be slowed in elderly individuals and in the presence of renal disease (Grant and Fitton 1994).

Efficacy.   There have been approximately 10 open-label published trials with risperidone in chronic schizophrenic patients (see reviews by Borison et al. [1992a] and Grant and Fitton [1994]). These studies have uniformly shown that risperidone produced its best efficacy at dosages of approximately 4–8 mg/day, and that both positive and negative symptoms of schizophrenia showed an excellent therapeutic response; EPS were relatively uncommon, particularly at the 4- to 8-mg dosage range. In one of these studies (Mertens 1991) involving 111 schizophrenic patients treated for 1 year, the long-term safety and efficacy of risperidone was demonstrated. In this study, although the therapeutic action of risperidone could be observed within the first 1–2 weeks of treatment, gradual improvement continued for up to 7 months of therapy before the patients reached a plateau of beneficial effects.

There have also been five published trials of risperidone in which it was compared with other neuroleptics, with one study using clozapine (Heinrich et al. 1991) and the other four using haloperidol (Borison et al. 1991b; Claus et al. 1992; DeCuyper 1989; Svestka et al. 1990). In Heinrich et al.'s (1991) clozapine trial, 60 acutely psychotic schizophrenic patients were randomized to treatment with fixed dosages of risperidone (4 mg/day or 8 mg/day) or clozapine (400 mg/day) over a 4-week treatment period. The 4-mg dosage of risperidone and the 400-mg dosage of clozapine were equivalent in both their efficacies and their lack of ability to induce EPS; the 8-mg dosage of risperidone proved efficacious but less so than the 4-mg dosage of risperidone or the 400 mg of clozapine treatment.

Results from the four studies comparing risperidone (2–20 mg/day) with haloperidol (2–20 mg/day) in a total of 159 schizophrenic subjects indicated that risperidone was equivalent or therapeutically superior to haloperidol treatment but produced generally fewer EPS. Of these studies, two deserve special comment. One (Claus et al. 1992) involved chronic schizophrenic patients who could be considered to be treatment resistant, as they failed to demonstrate any benefit from haloperidol treatment. This group showed rapid and highly significant improvement when treated with risperidone, including significant improvement in those patients who showed a predominance of negative symptoms. The other study (Borison et al. 1991b) was unique in that it was the first double-blind, placebo-controlled trial comparing risperidone with haloperidol. Both haloperidol and risperidone were found to be superior to placebo treatment, with risperidone being significantly more efficacious than haloperidol. Risperidone treatment in this trial also resulted in far fewer EPS than did haloperidol treatment.

Risperidone was also tested in two large multicenter, double-blind, placebo-controlled trials involving nearly 2,100 schizophrenic patients, as described by Grant and Fitton (1994). In a United States–

Canada multicenter study ($N = 523$; Chouinard et al. 1993; Marder and Meibach 1994), risperidone at fixed dosages (2 mg, 6 mg, 10 mg, and 16 mg) was compared with placebo and with haloperidol (20 mg/day). The results showed that risperidone (at 6 mg/day), but not haloperidol, was significantly superior to placebo ($P < .01$) in the treatment of both positive and negative symptoms of schizophrenia. In addition, risperidone displayed a much quicker onset of therapeutic action than did haloperidol. This multicenter study represents the largest and best-controlled trial demonstrating the efficacy of an antipsychotic agent in the treatment of the negative symptoms of schizophrenia.

Chouinard et al. (1993) reported that in a subsample ($n = 135$) from the larger 523-patient study, the dropout rate for the 6-mg risperidone group was significantly less ($P < .05$) than that for either the placebo or the haloperidol treatment groups. With response assessed as a 20% or greater improvement in rating-scale scores for schizophrenic psychosis, response was achieved in 72.7% of the 6-mg risperidone group ($P < .001$), which was more than that achieved in the haloperidol group (47.6% subjects responding) or the placebo group (13.6% subjects responding). The 6-mg dosage of risperidone also produced a significant ($P < .009$) improvement in the negative symptoms of schizophrenia, whereas haloperidol did not. Moreover, the efficacy of risperidone was manifest at the end of the first week of treatment, and this effect was significantly greater ($P < .05$) and more rapid than the magnitude of therapeutics associated with haloperidol treatment. Risperidone was no different from placebo in the production of EPS or the need for antiparkinsonian drugs; haloperidol, on the other hand, produced significantly more EPS and required more antiparkinsonian agents than did either placebo or risperidone. Patients receiving risperidone showed a greater suppression of tardive dyskinesia movements than did the haloperidol- or the placebo-treated patients.

In a second trial ($N = 1,557$; Müller-Spahn 1992), risperidone at fixed dosages (1 mg/day, 4 mg/day, 8 mg/day, 12 mg/day, and 16 mg/day) was compared with haloperidol (10 mg/day). The 4-mg and 8-mg dosages of risperidone produced the greatest therapeutic response and were more effective than haloperidol. The results of these two studies demonstrate an inverted ∪-shaped curve for the optimal therapeutic dosages of risperidone, with the best dosage being 6 mg/day ± 2 mg/day.

Side effects. Risperidone has been well tolerated in all of the published trials. In clinical trials comparing risperidone at 10 mg/day or less (324 patients) with haloperidol at 20 mg/day or less (140 patients) and with placebo (142 patients), the incidence of EPS with risperidone has been no greater than that with placebo (Grant and Fitton, in press), with insomnia, rhinitis, and constipation being the only complaints associated with risperidone treatment that occurred most frequently above the placebo rate. It does appear, however, that at higher dosages (i.e., dosages greater than 10 mg/day) there is a dosage-related increase in EPS and sedation as side effects. The safety data for risperidone also show that cardiovascular and electrocardiographic changes are relatively rare events. Risperidone does increase plasma prolactin levels, as do typical neuroleptics. A 1- to 2-kg weight increase during short-term treatment with risperidone has been observed; however, weight gain does not persist with long-term therapy. It has also been reported, in a very limited patient sample, that risperidone was superior to haloperidol in the suppression of choreiform movements associated with tardive dyskinesia (Borison et al. 1993).

In summary, it appears that risperidone may be the first antipsychotic drug for which it is possible to provide conclusive evidence of superiority to standard antipsychotics in the treatment of acutely exacerbated schizophrenia. Furthermore, there are data that strongly suggest that, like clozapine, risperidone may also be effective in otherwise treatment-resistant schizophrenic patients. There are stronger data demonstrating risperidone's efficacy in treating the negative symptoms of schizophrenia than for any other antipsychotic agent; also, when used at the appropriate therapeutic dosages, risperidone produces no more EPS than does placebo treatment. Therefore, risperidone may be the agent closest to the ideal atypical neuroleptic, given its therapeutic action with both positive and negative symptoms of schizophrenia, its very low liability for producing EPS, and its excellent safety profile. However, as with all antipsychotic drugs, not all schizophrenic patients respond to risperidone, and the search for new antipsychotic compounds must be continued.

Clozapine-Like, Serotonin 5-HT₂ Receptor Antagonists

One goal in developing novel antipsychotics has been to combine the therapeutic biochemistry of clozapine (Meltzer 1989) in a safer molecule. A number of new agents are currently involved in early development, and all are distinguished not by their potent blockade of dopamine D_2 receptors, but rather by their potent blockade of serotonin 5-HT_2 receptors and their clozapine-like pharmacologies. These agents are briefly reviewed below.

Sertindole. Sertindole is a putative antipsychotic agent that possesses an in vitro–binding profile to dopamine D_1 and D_2 receptors that is essentially identical to that of haloperidol. However, in contrast to haloperidol, sertindole is an extremely potent serotonin 5-HT_2 receptor blocker, possessing a potency approximately 10-fold greater than its dopamine D_2–blocking potency. It is also active on other receptors, possessing a noradrenergic α_1–blocking activity on par with that of dopamine D_2 receptors, and a σ-blocking potency on par with that of haloperidol (Sanchez et al. 1991). These receptor studies have been repeated ex vivo (Hyttel et al. 1992), with the results confirming that the most potent binding for sertindole is on serotonin 5-HT_2 receptors, with a much lower potency for extrapyramidal dopamine D_2 receptors. In electrophysiological studies, sertindole, like clozapine, preferentially blocks the firing of dopaminergically driven cells in the limbic rather than the extrapyramidal system and selectively blocks the behavioral actions of dopamine infused into the limbic system rather than the extrapyramidal system of rodents (Hyttel 1991).

In two studies (both reported in Martin et al. 1993) using a total of 205 subjects, acutely exacerbated inpatient schizophrenic subjects received either sertindole at dosages of 8 mg/day, 12 mg/day, or 20 mg/day or placebo treatment over a 6-week period. Regardless of which of the measures—the BPRS or the Positive and Negative Syndrome Scale (PANSS) for schizophrenia (Kay et al. 1987)—was used to assess frequency, only the 20-mg/day dosage of sertindole was significantly superior ($P < .01$) to placebo treatment (P. T. Martin et al. 1993). Moreover, in assessing a wider range of schizophrenic function using the CGI severity-of-illness scale, sertindole at

20 mg/day again proved superior ($P < .01$) to placebo; this superiority was also manifested in the lesser numbers of patients prematurely terminating study participation because of lack of medication efficacy (sertindole 20 mg/day group, 20%; placebo treatment group, 34%).

The rate of EPS reported for sertindole at 20 mg/day was no different than that observed for placebo, and no sertindole-treated patient required antiparkinsonian medication. The two most common side effects associated with sertindole were nasal congestion and abnormal ejaculation. Less than 5% of the patients receiving sertindole experienced a threefold or greater increase in liver function tests, and a clinically nonsignificant prolongation of QT interval was observed on the electrocardiogram in some patients. Therefore, it would appear that the initial results with sertindole are encouraging and hold the promise that this agent may be an efficacious antipsychotic treatment without associated EPS.

Olanzapine. The thienobenzodiazepine derivative olanzapine is a novel agent with a receptor-binding profile similar to that of clozapine, in that it is most potent in the blockade of serotonin 5-HT$_2$ receptors, with significant H$_1$ antihistaminic, α_1 antiadrenergic, and antimuscarinic cholinergic receptor–binding properties. Its dopamine D$_1$ and D$_2$ receptor–blocking effects are approximately equivalent; these effects are two- to threefold less potent than the antiserotonergic properties of this agent (Tye et al. 1992). In animal behavior tests (Moore et al. 1992), olanzapine showed behavioral activity in the 5-hydroxytryptophan–induced head twitch paradigm, consistent with antiserotonergic activity, and, like clozapine, only poorly induced catalepsy in rodents, suggesting a low propensity for producing EPS. In addition, in drug discrimination tests, animals taught to discriminate to clozapine also responded to olanzapine.

The initial published clinical study with olanzapine (Beasley et al. 1992) was an open-label 4- to 6-week trial in 10 schizophrenic subjects. As a group, the patients showed a dramatic decrease in total BPRS scores after treatment, with very significant improvement in both the positive symptoms (delusions, illogical thinking, paranoia, and hallucinations) and the negative symptoms of schizophrenia (blunted affect, emotional withdrawal, and psychomotor retardation).

No definite EPS were observed, and most patients showed a decrease during olanzapine therapy from their initial positive EPS ratings resulting from their previous neuroleptic therapy. The most frequent side effect experienced was sedation, which occurred in 50% of patients. Thus, these preliminary findings are highly encouraging, suggesting not only that olanzapine's pharmacology is similar to that of clozapine, but also that its clinical profile may perhaps likewise be that of an atypical neuroleptic.

In the first double-blind, placebo-controlled study of olanzapine (Beasley et al. 1993), low (2.5–7.5 mg/day), moderate (7.5–12.5 mg/day), and high (12.5–17.5 mg/day) dosages of olanzapine were compared with haloperidol (10–20 mg/day) and placebo for up to 6 weeks in 335 schizophrenic inpatients in acutely exacerbated stages of the illness. The moderate and high dosages of olanzapine were comparable to haloperidol in the treatment of positive symptoms of schizophrenia, as measured by the BPRS; however, the high-dosage olanzapine showed statistical superiority ($P < .05$) to placebo and haloperidol in treating the negative symptoms of schizophrenia as assessed with the Scale for the Assessment of Negative Symptoms (SANS; Andreasen 1983). The overall efficacy of high-dosage olanzapine treatment was also demonstrated by the relatively low rate of study termination because of lack of efficacy (29.0%) compared with placebo treatment (50.0%). Olanzapine was well tolerated, with the most frequent side effects observed beyond the placebo rate being somnolence and constipation. The somnolence occurred at a rate equivalent to that noted with haloperidol, whereas constipation was noted at approximately twice the incidence seen with haloperidol (14.5% versus 5.8%). Akathisia and drug-induced parkinsonism occurred rarely in the olanzapine-treated patients, and no dystonic reactions were associated with olanzapine. Elevation in transaminase liver enzymes was seen early in treatment in some patients, but these elevations tended to stabilize and decrease with repeated exposure to olanzapine. Increases in serum prolactin were less frequent with olanzapine than with haloperidol. These initial data would therefore suggest that olanzapine may possess the profile of an atypical antipsychotic that produces fewer EPS and less prolactin elevation while successfully treating the negative symptoms of schizophrenia.

Seroquel.   Another clozapine analogue is the dibenzothiazepine derivative, Seroquel (ICI-204636). This compound is also more potent in the blockade of serotonin 5-HT_2 receptors, but, unlike clozapine, is much weaker in its blockade of D_1 and D_2 dopamine receptors, as well as much weaker in its antagonism of cholinergic, muscarinic, and α_1-adrenergic receptors. In electrophysiological studies, Seroquel, like clozapine, preferentially antagonized dopamine's actions in the limbic system as compared with the extrapyramidal system (Goldstein et al. 1990). Moreover, in haloperidol-sensitized cebus monkeys, Seroquel failed to produce EPS (Migler and Warawa 1990), suggesting little or no liability for producing EPS in humans.

In the first clinical trial of this compound (Fabre et al. 1990), 12 schizophrenic subjects received either Seroquel or placebo. There was a prompt and significant decrease in BPRS scores (greater than 35%) in all subjects treated with Seroquel, with no EPS, and with only insomnia and sedation as the most frequent side effects reported. In a larger ($N = 105$) 6-week, open-label trial (Fabre 1993), Seroquel produced a significant ($P < .001$) reduction in psychosis, as measured by the BPRS and the CGI, which was manifest by the end of the first week of treatment and continued for the duration of the trial. Ratings for EPS and abnormal involuntary movements also decreased markedly ($P < .001$) during the course of the study, with no dystonic reactions being observed. The most frequent side effect in this larger study was sedation, observed in 30% of patients.

In its first multicenter, double-blind, placebo-controlled trial in schizophrenic patients, Seroquel appeared efficacious, without producing EPS (L. Arvanitis, personal communication, December 1994). Although still early in its development, Seroquel holds the potential for being a clozapine-like drug, but with fewer physical side effects.

Other Considerations in the Development of New Antipsychotic Drugs

Although the focus in antipsychotic drug development has been on the serotonergic and dopaminergic systems, it should be mentioned that many of the atypical neuroleptics (e.g., clozapine, risperidone) also possess potent noradrenergic-blocking properties. There are biochemical and clinical data that strongly support a noradrenergic pathology in schizophrenia (van Kammen and Gelernter 1987), and it may be that future antipsychotic agents will be synthesized to emphasize the α-noradrenergic contribution to schizophrenia and its therapeutics (Gerlach 1991).

The NMDA-PCP Receptor Complex

Among the difficulties in developing new antipsychotic drugs is finding accurate pharmacological models for the development of more specific therapeutic agents. It does not appear that schizophrenia or psychosis, as now understood in humans, has any true natural analogue in lower animals. Furthermore, the disruption of both human behavior and animal behavior by exogenous agents, such as amphetamine, only poorly approximates the behavior or pharmacology of schizophrenic illness. Despite this caveat, it would appear that, in humans, the closest approximation of a schizophrenic psychosis can be observed in those individuals who have become intoxicated with phencyclidine (PCP). The fact that there is a specific receptor in the human brain for PCP has raised the intriguing hypothesis that endogenous psychotogenic compounds, exerting their actions through the PCP receptor, may in part mediate schizophrenia (Quirion et al. 1984). If true, this would suggest that drugs that antagonize PCP's receptor actions may prove beneficial in the treatment of schizophrenia.

The PCP receptor is a part of a complex receptor mechanism that mediates the actions of the excitatory amino acid neurotransmitter, glutamate. This receptor complex surrounds a cation channel, or ionophore, that regulates the flux of calcium and potassium. The action of glutamate—or of its analog, N-methyl-D-aspartate (NMDA)—on its specific receptor (known as the *NMDA receptor*) is to open the cation channel. Separate receptors for the amino acid glycine and polyamines are also located at the cation channel and work similarly to glutamate to open this ionophore. The PCP receptor is located within the channel and, when activated, causes the ionophore to close. This receptor complex is commonly referred to as the *NMDA-PCP receptor*. Hence, glutamate, through its action on the NMDA receptor, as well as glycine and polyamines exert their actions in direct opposition to PCP. It is of interest to note that the NMDA-PCP receptor complex (Fonnum 1984) is localized in areas of the brain—such as the hippocampus—that are believed to play a role in schizophrenia. Therefore, it is possible that the antagonistic actions of PCP or its congeners on the NMDA-PCP receptor complex may, in part, mediate the schizophrenic psychosis, and that agonists, such as glutamate, would possess palliative actions in treating schizophrenic illness. Because glutamate is neurotoxic, the actions of this neurotransmitter cannot be directly tested as an antipsychotic drug; however, the amino acid neurotransmitter glycine can be safely administered and, similar to glutamate, can block the actions of PCP at the NMDA-PCP receptor complex.

The potentiation of brain glycine as an antipsychotic treatment has been attempted via the administration of the glycine prodrug, milacemide (Tamminga et al. 1992). In a very preliminary report, milacemide was administered to schizophrenic patients using a placebo crossover design. The results of this first report and of subsequent work with milacemide in schizophrenia have been negative and have led to its discontinuation as an antipsychotic in trials (R. Herting, personal communication, April 1993).

An alternative strategy was used by Potkin et al. (1992) in a blinded, 6-week trial of 18 chronic, treatment-resistant schizophrenic patients who received either glycine (15 g/day) or placebo as adjuncts to stabilized dosages of neuroleptics. As a group, the placebo-treated patients showed a worsening, whereas there was a slight improvement or no change in the group receiving glycine. In comparing the glycine and placebo treatments, the patients' scores on the BPRS items of emotional withdrawal, depression, hostility, and uncooperativeness clearly showed an improvement in the glycine-treated group. Despite these encouraging results, questions remain as to whether exogenous glycine treatment can increase the concentration of brain glycine, and whether brain glycine concentrations can be increased at the intended sites of action. Although many questions are currently unanswered, the strategy of developing antipsychotic drugs via their actions on the

NMDA-PCP receptor complex continues to be an area of future research and promise.

The σ Receptor System

A similar strategy in attempting to identify an endogenous psychotogen responsible for schizophrenia has been the consideration of the σ receptor system. The σ receptors were originally identified as a subclass of opiate receptors (W. R. Martin et al. 1976) that appeared to mediate the psychotogenic properties of compounds such as pentazocine. It was further demonstrated that some antipsychotic drugs, such as haloperidol, were potent antagonists at the σ recognition site (Snyder and Largent 1989), and that these sites were altered in the brains of schizophrenic patients (Weissman et al. 1991). Moreover, σ ligands, in part, are also active at PCP receptors (Quirion et al. 1981). These indirect data therefore suggest that σ agonists confer psychotogenic properties, whereas σ antagonists should produce antipsychotic actions. This hypothesis has led to the development of σ antagonists as potential treatments for schizophrenia.

The first σ antagonist to receive clinical trials was rimcazole (BW-234U), a compound with highly specific, albeit weak, σ antagonistic properties. In a series of open-label trials, rimcazole was found to be an effective antipsychotic agent that produced no EPS and few other side effects (see review by Borison et al. 1992b). However, controlled double-blind trials of schizophrenic patients with an acute exacerbation of their illness failed to differentiate the efficacy of rimcazole from placebo treatment (Borison et al. 1991a). Moreover, when rimcazole was tested in the prevention of relapse in stabilized schizophrenic outpatients, it failed to maintain the patients in a disease-remitted state (Munetz et al. 1989). Although the results with rimcazole have been disappointing because of the restriction of the upper dosage of this drug in light of proconvulsant actions and the compound's relatively weak actions on the σ system, it may be assumed that rimcazole did not fairly test the σ hypothesis of antipsychotic action.

The clinical trials with other σ antagonists have provided mixed results as to efficacy. The potent and selective σ antagonist BMY 14802 failed to demonstrate any efficacy in open-label trials in schizophrenic patients in acutely exacerbated stages of illness (Borison et al. 1992b). In contrast, another potent σ antagonist, gevotriline, which also more modestly antagonizes dopamine D_2 and serotonin 5-HT_2 receptors, showed early evidence of efficacy when compared with placebo (Borison et al. 1992b). However, because of several cases of reported pancreatitis associated with this compound, its development has been terminated. Perhaps most disappointing have been the clinical trials with tiospirone, a compound possessing the dopamine D_2–blocking potency of haloperidol, equally strong serotonin 5-HT_2 antagonistic properties, and strong σ-antagonistic properties. Although early double-blind, placebo-controlled trials showed high early dropout rates, schizophrenic patients whose illness was acutely exacerbated and who were able to be maintained for 6 weeks on tiospirone therapy showed an excellent antipsychotic response (Borison et al. 1989). However, in later trials designed to minimize the numbers of early therapeutic dropouts, tiospirone could not be differentiated from placebo treatment (Borison et al. 1992b).

It has been suggested that perhaps there has not, to date, been a fair clinical trial using a selective and specific σ antagonist. Either previous compounds were too weak as σ antagonists, or factors such as poor absorption, rapid metabolism, poor penetration of the blood-brain barrier, or inappropriate dosing were perhaps responsible for the disappointing results. Therefore, the role of σ antagonists remains a potentially important hypothesis in understanding the therapeutics of schizophrenia, but one that still awaits definitive clinical testing.

References

Andreasen NC: The Scale for the Assessment of Negative Symptoms (SANS). Iowa City, IA, University of Iowa, 1983

Baldessarini RJ: Chemotherapy in Psychiatry: Principles and Practice. Cambridge, MA, Harvard University Press, 1985

Baldessarini RJ, Davis JM: What is the best maintenance dose of neuroleptics in schizophrenia? Psychiatry Res 3:115–122, 1980

Baldessarini RJ, Katz B, Cotton P: Dissimilar dosing with high potency and low potency neuroleptics. Am J Psychiatry 141:748–752, 1984

Barnas C, Stuppack CH, Miller C, et al: Zotepine in the treatment of schizophrenic patients with prevailingly negative symptoms: a double-blind trial versus haloperidol. Int Clin Psychopharmacol 7:23–27, 1992

Beasley CM, Montgomery S, Tye NC: Olanzapine: an open-label study in schizophrenia. Paper presented at the 2nd International Conference on Schizophrenia, Vancouver, BC, July 1992

Beasley CM, Tollefson GD, Tye NC, et al: Olanzapine: potential "atypical" antipsychotic. Paper presented at the American College of Neuropsychopharmacology, Honolulu, HI, December 1993

Bersani G, Grispini A, Marini A, et al: Neuroleptic-induced extrapyramidal side-effects: clinical perspectives with ritanserin (R 55667), a new selective 5-HT$_2$ receptor blocking agent. Current Therapeutic Research 40:492–499, 1986

Bersani G, Bresa GM, Meco G, et al: Combined serotonin–5-HT$_2$ and dopamine-D$_2$ antagonism in schizophrenia: clinical, extrapyramidal and neuroendocrine response in a preliminary study with risperidone (R 64766). Human Psychopharmacology 5:225–231, 1990

Bjork A, Bergman L, Gustaversusson LG: Amperozide in the treatment of schizophrenic patients: a preliminary report, in Novel Antipsychotic Drugs. Edited by Meltzer HY. New York, Raven, 1992, pp 47–58

Borison RL, Sinha D, Haverstock S, et al: Efficacy and safety of tiospirone versus haloperidol and thioridazine in a double-blind placebo-controlled trial. Psychopharmacol Bull 25:190–193, 1989

Borison RL, Diamond BI, Dren AT: Does sigma receptor antagonism predict clinical antipsychotic efficacy? Psychopharmacol Bull 27:103–106, 1991a

Borison RL, Diamond BI, Pathiraja AP, et al: Clinical profile of risperidone in chronic schizophrenia, in Risperidone: Major Progress in Antipsychotic Treatment. Edited by Kane JM. Oxford, UK, Oxford Clinical Communications, 1991b, pp 31–36

Borison RL, Diamond BI, Pathiraja AP, et al: Clinical overview of risperidone, in Novel Antipsychotic Drugs. Edited by Meltzer HY. New York, Raven, 1992a, pp 233–239

Borison RL, Pathiraja AP, Diamond BI: Clinical efficacy of sigma antagonists in schizophrenia, in Novel Antipsychotic Drugs. Edited by Meltzer HY. New York, Raven, 1992b, pp 203–210

Borison RL, Pathiraja AP, Diamond BI, et al: Risperidone: clinical safety and efficacy in schizophrenia. Psychopharmacol Bull 29:95–100, 1993

Carvey PM, Kao LC, Tanner CM, et al: The effect of antimuscarinic agents on haloperidol-induced behavioral sensitivity. Eur J Pharmacol 12:193–196, 1986

Casey JLF, Hollister LE, Klett CJ, et al: Combined drug therapy of chronic schizophrenics. Am J Psychiatry 17:997–1003, 1961

Chouinard G: Early phase II clinical trial of remoxipride in treatment of schizophrenia with measurements of prolactin and neuroleptic activity. J Clin Psychopharmacol 7:159–164, 1987

Chouinard G: A placebo-controlled clinical trial of remoxipride and chlorpromazine in newly admitted schizophrenic patients with acute exacerbation. Acta Psychiatr Scand 82 (suppl 358):111–119, 1990

Chouinard G, Jones B, Remington G, et al: A Canadian multicenter placebo-controlled study of fixed doses of risperidone and haloperidol in the treatment of chronic schizophrenic patients. J Clin Psychopharmacol 13:25–40, 1993

Christensson E, Bjork A: Amperozide: a new pharmacological approach in the treatment of schizophrenia. Pharmacol Toxicol 66 (suppl 1):5–7, 1990

Claus A, Bollen J, DeCuyper H, et al: Risperidone versus haloperidol in the treatment of chronic schizophrenic inpatients: a multi-centre double-blind comparative study. Acta Psychiatr Scand 85:295–305, 1992

Coffman JA, Nasrallah H, Lyskowski J, et al: Clinical effectiveness of oral and parenteral rapid neuroleptization. J Clin Psychiatry 48:20–24, 1987

Cohen S, Khan A: Adjunctive benzodiazepines in acute schizophrenia. Neuropsychobiology 18:9–12, 1987

Curry SH: The strategy and value of neuroleptic drug monitoring. J Clin Psychopharmacol 5:263–271, 1985

Davis JM: Dose equivalence of the antipsychotic drugs. J Psychiatr Res 11:65–69, 1974

Davis JM, Schaffer CB, Killian GA, et al: Important issues in the drug treatment of schizophrenia. Schizophr Bull 6:70–87, 1980

Deberdt R, Elens P, Berghmans W, et al: Intramuscular haloperidol decanoate for neuroleptic maintenance therapy: efficacy, dosage schedule and plasma levels. Acta Psychiatr Scand 62:356–363, 1980

DeCuyper HJA: Risperidone in the treatment of chronic psychotic patients: an overview of the double-blind comparative trials, in Thirty Years: Janssen Research in Psychiatry. Edited by Ayd FJ. Baltimore, Ayd Medical Communications, 1989, pp 116–122

DeCuyper H, Bollen J, Van Praag M, et al: Pharmacokinetic and therapeutic efficacy of haloperidol decanoate after loading dose administration. Br J Psychiatry 148:560–566, 1986

DeVeaugh-Geiss J, McBain S, Cooksey P, et al: The effects of a novel 5-HT$_3$ antagonist, ondansetron, in schizophrenia, in Novel Antipsychotic Drugs. Edited by Meltzer HY. New York, Raven, 1992, pp 225–232

Dieterle DM, Albus ML, Eben E, et al: Preliminary experiences and results with the Munich version of the Andreasen scale. Pharmacopsychiatry 19:96–100, 1986

Dieterle DM, Ackenheil M, Muller-Spahn F, et al: Zotepine, a neuroleptic drug with a bipolar therapeutic profile. Pharmacopsychiatry 20:52–57, 1987

Donlon PT, Meadow A, Tupin JP, et al: High versus standard dose of fluphenazine HCL in acute schizophrenia. J Clin Psychiatry 39:800–804, 1978

Donlon PT, Hopkin JT, Tupin JP, et al: Haloperidol for acute schizophrenic patients. Arch Gen Psychiatry 37:691–695, 1980

Dubin WR, Wasman HM, Weiss KJ, et al: Rapid tranquilization: the efficacy of oral concentrate. J Clin Psychiatry 46:475–478, 1985

Dubin WR, Weiss KJ, Dorn JM: Pharmacotherapy of psychiatric emergencies. J Clin Psychopharmacol 6:210–222, 1986

Edwards S, Kumar V: A survey of prescribing of psychotropic drugs in a Birmingham psychiatric hospital. Br J Psychiatry 145:502–507, 1984

Ellison JE, Hughes DH, White KA: An emergency psychiatry update. Hosp Community Psychiatry 40:250–260, 1989

Ericksen SE, Hurt SW, Chang S, et al: Haloperidol dose, plasma levels, and clinical response: a double-blind study. Psychopharmacol Bull 14:15–16, 1978

Escobar JI, Barron A, Kiriakos R: A controlled study of neuroleptization with fluphenazine hydrochloride injections. J Clin Psychopharmacol 3:359–362, 1983

Fabre L: A multicenter, open pilot trial of ICI 204,636 in hospitalized patients with acute psychotic symptomatology. Paper presented at the 3rd International Congress on Schizophrenia Research, Colorado Springs, CO, April 1993

Fabre L, Slotnick V, Jones V, et al: ICI-204,636, a novel antipsychotic: early indication for safety and efficacy in man. Paper presented at the 17th Congress of Collegium Internationale Neuro-Psychopharmacologicum, Kyoto, Japan, July 1990

Fonnum F: Glutamate: a neurotransmitter in mammalian brain. J Neurochem 42:1–11, 1984

Gardos G, Rapkin RM, DiMascio A: Trifluoperazine and chlorpromazine in combinations and individually. Current Therapeutic Research 10:609–612, 1968

Gerlach J: New antipsychotics: classification, efficacy, and adverse effects. Schizophr Bull 17:289–309, 1991

Godleski LS, Kerler R, Barber JW, et al: Multiple versus single antipsychotic drug treatment in chronic psychosis. J Nerv Ment Dis 177:686–689, 1989

Goldberg J, Froch WA, Drossman AK, et al: Prediction of response to phenothiazines in schizophrenia: a cross validation study. Arch Gen Psychiatry 26:367–373, 1972

Goldstein JM, Litwin LC, Sutton EB, et al: Electrophysiological profile of ICI-204,636: a new and novel antipsychotic drug. Society for Neuroscience Abstracts 16:250, 1990

Grant S, Fitton A: Risperidone: a review of its pharmacology and therapeutic potential in schizophrenia. Drugs 48:253–273, 1994

Greenblatt DJ, Raskin A: The use of benzodiazepines for psychotic disorders. Psychopharmacol Bull 22:577–587, 1986

Guy W (ed): ECDEU Assessment Manual for Psychopharmacology, Revised (DHEW Publ No ADM 76-388). Rockville, MD, U.S. Department of Health, Education and Welfare, 1976

Haase HJ, Janssen APJ: The Action of Neuroleptic Drugs. Chicago, IL, Year Book, 1965

Hall H, Sallemark M, Jerning E: Effects of remoxipride and some related substituted salicylamides on rat brain receptors. Acta Pharmacologica et Toxicologica 58:61–70, 1986

Heinrich K, Klieser E, Lehmann E, et al: Experimental comparison of the efficacy and compatibility of risperidone and clozapine in acute schizophrenia, in Risperidone: Major Progress in Antipsychotic Treatment. Edited by Kane JM. Oxford, Oxford Clinical Communications, 1991, pp 7–39

Hemstrom CA, Evans RL, Lobeck FG: Haloperidol decanoate: a depot anti-psychotic. Drug Intelligence and Clinical Pharmacy 22:290–294, 1988

Hollister LE: Drug treatment of schizophrenia. Psychiatr Clin North Am 7:435–452, 1984

Hyttel J: Sertindole—a new concept in neuroleptic research, in Modern Trends in the Treatment of Chronic Schizophrenia. Edited by Johnson DAW. Amsterdam, Netherlands, Excerpta Medica, 1991, pp 3–12

Hyttel J, Nielson JB, Nowack G: The acute effect of sertindole on brain $5\text{-}HT_2$, D_2 and α_1 receptors (ex vivo radioreceptor binding studies). J Neural Transm 89:61–69, 1992

Jann MW, Ereshefsky L, Saklad SR: Clinical pharmacokinetics of the depot antipsychotics. Clin Pharmacokinet 17:238–246, 1985

Janssen PAJ, Niemegeers CJE, Awouters F, et al: Pharmacology of risperidone (R64 766), a new antipsychotic with serotonin-S_2 and dopamine-D_2 antagonistic properties. J Pharmacol Exp Ther 244:685–693, 1988

Jones B, Lehmann HE, Saxena BM, et al: Treatment of chronic schizophrenic patients with haloperidol and chlorpromazine. Current Therapeutic Research 10:276–278, 1968

Kane JM: The current status of neuroleptic therapy. J Clin Psychiatry 50:322–328, 1989

Kane JM, Woerner M, Sarantakos S: Depot neuroleptics: a comparative review of standard, intermediate and low dose regimes. J Clin Psychiatry 47 (suppl 5):30–33, 1986

Kay SR, Fiszbein A, Opler LA: The positive and negative syndrome scale (PANSS) for schizophrenia. Schizophr Bull 13:261–276, 1987

Kilpatrick GJ, Jones BJ, Tyers MB: The identification and distribution of 5-HT$_3$ receptors in rat brains using radioligand binding. Nature 330:746–748, 1987

Kissling W, Moller HJ, Walter L, et al: Double-blind comparison of haloperidol decanoate and fluphenazine decanoate: effectiveness versus side effects, dosage and serum levels during a six month treatment for relapse prevention. Pharmacopsychiatry 18:240–245, 1985

Lapierre YD, Ancill R, Awad G, et al: A dose finding study with remoxipride in the acute treatment of schizophrenic patients. J Psychiatr Neurosci 17:134–145, 1992

Lazarus A, Dubin WR, Jaffe R: Rapid tranquilization with neuroleptic drugs. Clin Neuropharmacol 12:303–311, 1989

Lehmann HE, Wilson H, Deutsch M: Minimal maintenance medication: effects of three dose schedules on relapse rate and symptoms in chronic schizophrenic outpatients. Compr Psychiatry 24:293–303, 1983

Lerner Y, Lwow E, Levitin A, et al: Acute high-dose parenteral haloperidol treatment of psychosis. Am J Psychiatry 36:1061–1064, 1979

Lewander T, Westerbergh SE, Morrison D: Clinical profile of remoxipride—a combined analysis of a comparative double-blind multicentre trial program. Acta Psychiatr Scand 82 (suppl 358):92–98, 1990

Leysen JE, Janssen PMF, Gommeren W, et al: In vitro and in vivo receptor binding and effects on monoamine turnover in rat brain regions of the novel antipsychotics risperidone and ocaperidone. Mol Pharmacol 41:494–508, 1992

Little KY, Gay TL, Vore M: Predictors of response to high dose anti-psychotics in chronic schizophrenics. Psychiatry Res 30:1–9, 1989

Marder SR, Meibach RC: Risperidone in the treatment of schizophrenia. Am J Psychiatry 151:825–835, 1994

Marder SR, Van Putten T, Aravagiri M: Plasma levels of parent drug and reactions in patients receiving oral and depot fluphenazine. Psychopharmacol Bull 25:479–482, 1989

Martin PT, Grebb JA, Schmitz P, et al: Efficacy and safety of sertindole in two double-blind, placebo-controlled trials of schizophrenic patients. Paper presented at the First International Congress on Hormones, Brain and Neuropsychopharmacology, Rhodes, Greece, September 1993

Martin WR, Eades CG, Thompson JA, et al: The effects of morphine- and nalorphine-like drugs in the nondependent and morphine-dependent chronic spinal dog. J Pharmacol Exp Ther 197:517–532, 1976

Mason AS: Basic principles in the use of antipsychotic agents. Hosp Community Psychiatry 18:825–829, 1973

Mavroides ML, Kanter DR, Hirschowitz J: Clinical response and plasma haloperidol levels in schizophrenia. Psychopharmacology (Berl) 81:354–356, 1983

McCreadie RG, Todd N, Livingston M, et al: A double-blind comparative study of remoxipride and thioridazine in the acute phase of schizophrenia. Acta Psychiatr Scand 78:49–56, 1988

McEvoy JP, Hogarty GE, Steingard S: Optimal dose of neuroleptic in acute schizophrenia: a controlled study of the neuroleptic threshold and higher haloperidol dose. Arch Gen Psychiatry 48:739–745, 1991

Meltzer HY: Clinical studies on the mechanism of action of clozapine: the dopamine-serotonin hypothesis of schizophrenia. Psychopharmacology (Berl) 99:S18–S27, 1989

Mertens C: Long-term treatment of chronic schizophrenic patients with risperidone, in Risperidone: Major Progress in Antipsychotic Treatment. Edited by Kane JM. Oxford, UK, Oxford Clinical Communications, 1991, pp 44–48

Migler B, Warawa E: The effect of ICI–204,636, a potential antipsychotic agent, in a battery of behavioral tests predictive of antipsychotic activity and tardive dyskinesia. Society for Neuroscience Abstracts 16:250, 1990

Moore NA, Tye NC, Axton MS, et al: The behavioral pharmacology of olanzapine, a novel "atypical" antipsychotic agent. J Pharmacol Exp Ther 262:545–551, 1992

Movin G, Gustafson L, Franzen G, et al: Pharmacokinetics of remoxipride in elderly psychotic patients. Acta Psychiatr Scand 82 (suppl 358):176–180, 1990

Müller-Spahn F: Risperidone in the treatment of chronic schizophrenic patients: an international double-blind, parallel-group study versus haloperidol. Clin Neuropharmacol 15 (suppl 1, part A):90A–91A, 1992

Munetz MR, Schulz SC, Bellin M, et al: Rimcazole (BW234U) in the maintenance treatment of outpatients with schizophrenia. Drug Development Research 16:79–83, 1989

Nair NPV, Suranyi-Cadotte B, Schwartz G, et al: A clinical trial comparing IM haloperidol decanoate and oral haloperidol in chronic schizophrenic patients: efficacy, safety, and dosage equivalence. J Clin Psychopharmacol 6:30–75, 1986

Neborsky R, Janowsky D, Munson E, et al: Rapid treatment of acute psychotic symptoms with high- and low-dose haloperidol. Arch Gen Psychiatry 38:195–199, 1981

Ogren SO, Hall H, Kohler C, et al: Remoxipride, a new potential antipsychotic compound with selective antidopaminergic actions in the rat brain. Eur J Pharmacol 102:459–474, 1984

Ortiz A, Gershon S: The future of neuroleptic psychopharmacology. J Clin Psychiatry 47 (suppl 5):3–11, 1986

Overall JE, Gorham DR: The Brief Psychiatric Rating Scale. Psychol Rep 10:799–812, 1962

Phanjoo AL, Link C: Remoxipride versus thioridazine in elderly psychotic patients. Acta Psychiatr Scand 82 (suppl 358):181–185, 1990

Physicians' Desk Reference. Oradell, NJ, Medical Economics, 1991

Potkin SG, Costa J, Roy S, et al: Glycine in the treatment of schizophrenia: theory and preliminary results, in Novel Antipsychotic Drugs. Edited by Meltzer HY. New York, Raven, 1992, pp 179–188

Quirion R, Hammer RP, Herkanham M, et al: Phencyclidine (angel dust)/ σ "opiate" receptor: visualization by tritium-sensitive film. Proc Natl Acad Sci U S A 78:5881–5885, 1981

Quirion R, DiMaggio DA, French ED, et al: Evidence for an endogenous pepticle ligand for the phencyclidine receptor. Journal of Peptides 5:967–973, 1984

Quitkin F, Rifkin A, Klein DF: Very high dosage versus standard dosage fluphenazine in schizophrenia. Arch Gen Psychiatry 32:1276–1281, 1975

Resnick M, Burton BT: Droperidol versus haloperidol in the initial management of acutely agitated patients. J Clin Psychiatry 45:298–299, 1984

Sanchez C, Arnt J, Dragsted N, et al: Neurochemical and in vivo pharmacological profile of sertindole, a limbic-selective neuroleptic compound. Drug Development Research 22:239–250, 1991

Sarai K, Okada M: Comparison of efficacy of zotepine and thiothixene in schizophrenia in a double-blind study. Pharmacopsychiatry 20:38–46, 1987

Schaffer CB, Shahid A, Javaid JI, et al: Bioavailability of intra-muscular versus oral haloperidol in schizophrenic patients. J Clin Psychopharmacol 2:274–277, 1982

Schatzberg A, Cole JO: Manual of Clinical Psychopharmacology, 2nd Edition. Washington, DC, American Psychiatric Press, 1991

Schatzberg A, Cole JO, Sheppard C, et al: Polypharmacy in psychiatry: a multi-state comparison of psychotropic drug combinations. Diseases of the Nervous System 35:183–189, 1974

Schulz P, Josephe-Rey M, Dick P, et al: Guidelines for the dosage of neuroleptics changing from daily oral to long acting injectable neuroleptics. Int Clin Psychopharmacol 4:105–114, 1989

Sheppard C, Beyel V, Fracchia J, et al: Polypharmacy in psychiatry: a multi-state comparison of psychotropic drug combinations. Diseases of the Nervous System 35:83–89, 1974

Smith RC, Vraulis G, Shvartsfurd A, et al: RBC and plasma levels of haloperidol and clinical response in schizophrenia. Am J Psychiatry 139:1054–1056, 1982

Snyder SH: The dopamine hypothesis of schizophrenia: focus on the dopamine receptor. Am J Psychiatry 133:197–202, 1976

Snyder SH, Largent BL: Receptor mechanisms in antipsychotic drug action: focus on σ receptors. Journal of Neuropsychiatry 1:7–15, 1989

Snyder SH, Banerjee SP, Yamamura HI, et al: Drugs, neuro-transmitters, and schizophrenia. Science 184:1243–1253, 1974

Solano OA, Sadow T, Ananth J: Rapid tranquilization: a reevaluation. Neuropsychobiology 22:90–96, 1989

Soni SD, Sampath G, Shah A, et al: Rationalizing neuroleptic polypharmacy in chronic schizophrenics: effects of changing to a single depot preparation. Acta Psychiatr Scand 85:354–359, 1992

Svestka J, Ceskova E, Rysanek R, et al: Double-blind clinical comparison of risperidone and haloperidol in acute schizophrenic and schizoaffective psychoses. Activitas Nervosa Superior (Praha) 32:237–238, 1990

Swanson DW, Smith JA, Perez H: A fixed combination of chlorpromazine and trifluoperazine in psychotic patients. Diseases of the Nervous System 28:756, 1967

Tamminga CA, Cascella N, Fakouhi TD, et al: Enhancement of NMDA-mediated transmission in schizophrenia, in Novel Antipsychotic Drugs. Edited by Meltzer HY. New York, Raven, 1992, pp 171–177

Terrell MS: Response to trifluoperazine and chlorpromazine, singly and in combination, in chronic, "back-ward" patients. Dis Nerv Syst 23:41–48, 1962

Thornton WE, Pray BJ: Combination drug therapy in psychopharmacology. J Clin Pharmacol 15:511–517, 1975

Tye NC, Moore NA, Rees G, et al: Preclinical pharmacology of olanzapine: a novel "atypical" antipsychotic agent. Paper presented at the 2nd International Conference on Schizophrenia, Vancouver, BC, Canada, July 1992

van Kammen DP, Gelernter J: Biochemical instability in schizophrenia: the norepinephrine system, in Psychopharmacology: The Third Generation of Progress. Edited by Meltzer HY. New York, Raven, 1987, pp 745–752

Van Putten T, Marder SR, Mintz J, et al: Haloperidol plasma levels and clinical response: a therapeutic window relationship. Psychopharmacol Bull 24:172–175, 1988

Viukari M, Salo O, Lamminsiva U, et al: Tolerance and serum levels of haloperidol during parenteral and oral haloperidol treatment in geriatric patients. Acta Psychiatr Scand 65:301–308, 1982

von Bahr C, Movin G, Yisak W-A, et al: Clinical pharmacokinetics of remoxipride. Acta Psychiatr Scand 82 (suppl 358):41–44, 1990

Vuckovic A, Cohen BM, Keck PE Jr, et al: Neuroleptic dosage regimens in psychotic inpatients: a retrospective comparison. J Clin Psychiatry 51:107–109, 1990

Wadworth AN, Heel RC: Remoxipride: a review of its pharmacodynamic and pharmacokinetic properties and therapeutic potential in schizophrenia. Drugs 40:863–879, 1990

Weissman AD, Casanova MF, Kleinman JE, et al: Selective loss of cerebral cortical σ, but not PCP binding sites in schizophrenia. Biol Psychiatry 29:41–54, 1991

Williams JR, Solecki RT, Puttkammer S: Effects of single, combined, and non-drug treatments on chronic mental patients: preliminary study. Diseases of the Nervous System 30:696–701, 1969

Wilson WH, Ban TA, Guy W: Pharmacotherapy of chronic hospitalized schizophrenics: prescription practices. Neuropsychobiology 14:75–82, 1985

Wistedt B, Persson T, Hellbom E: A clinical double-blind comparison between haloperidol decanoate and fluphenazine decanoate. Current Therapeutic Research 35:804–814, 1984

Wyatt RJ: Biochemistry and schizophrenia, IV: the neuroleptics—their mechanism of action; a review of the biochemical literature. Psychopharmacol Bull 12:5–50, 1976

Wyatt RJ, Torgrow JS : A comparison of equivalent clinical potencies of neuroleptics as used to treat schizophrenia and affective disorders. J Psychiatr Res 13:91–98, 1976

Yadalam KG, Simpson GM: Changing from oral to depot fluphenazine. J Clin Psychiatry 49:346–348, 1988

Dopaminergic and Serotonergic Mechanisms in the Action of Standard and Atypical Neuroleptics

Gary J. Remington, M.D., Ph.D., F.R.C.P.C.

Advances over the last several decades in the fields of physiology, biochemistry, and neuroimaging have considerably shifted psychiatrists' understanding of schizophrenia and its pathophysiology. Of the neurotransmitters implicated in schizophrenia, it is dopamine (DA) that continues to garner the most attention, although more recently there has been an increased focus on serotonin (5-hydroxytryptamine [5-HT]) and its possible interaction with DA. In this chapter I focus on the postulated role of these two neurotransmitters in schizophrenia, with specific reference to the action of typical and atypical neuroleptics.

Dopamine and Schizophrenia

Since the initial trials of chlorpromazine in the 1950s, approximately 20 neuroleptics that reflect the profile of "typical" neuroleptics have been introduced (see Table 13–1). The development of these agents was predicated on the notion that schizophrenia reflects a state of hyperdopaminergic activity, and that neuroleptics manifest their antipsychotic action via an affinity for DA receptors and their blockade.

Five lines of evidence supported this hyperdopaminergic theory of schizophrenia (Seeman 1987):

1. The knowledge that Parkinson's disease is characterized by a DA deficit and the finding that neuroleptics induced parkinsonian symptoms in most patients
2. The psychotomimetic properties of DA agonists
3. Accelerated catecholamine turnover with neuroleptic administration, suggesting a reflex activation of DA release following neuroleptic receptor blockade
4. The identified relationship between antipsychotic efficacy and D_2 blockade by nanomolar concentrations of neuroleptics
5. The finding of elevated numbers of D_2 receptors in postmortem brains of schizophrenic—including unmedicated—individuals

Dopamine Receptors

The distinction between D_1 and D_2 receptor subtypes (i.e., that D_1 receptors stimulate adenylate cyclase whereas D_2 receptors do not; Kebabian et al. 1972) represented a further advance in the dopaminergic theory of schizophrenia. The finding of a linear correlation between neuroleptic affinity for D_2 receptors in vitro and their antipsychotic potency in humans was taken as convincing evidence that D_2 receptors play a critical role in schizophrenia. Positron-emission tomography (PET) data have indicated that clinical effectiveness with neuroleptics occurs when approximately 85%–90% of the D_2 receptors are blocked (Farde et al. 1986). It is not surprising, then, that considerable effort has been directed toward the development of highly selective D_2-blocking agents (e.g., haloperidol, pimozide). These newer agents are much more potent than their earlier counterparts (e.g., chlorpromazine; see comparison of relative binding affinities of these drugs in Figure 13–1; Hyttel et al. 1985). The substituted benzamides (e.g., raclopride, remoxipride) represent a more recent group of antipsychotic agents characterized by selective D_2 antagonism (Ogren and Hall 1992).

The exact involvement of various DA receptor subtypes in schizophrenia has become increasingly complex. More recently, an isoform of the D_2 receptor—D_4—has been identified (Van Tol et al. 1991) that has received increased attention with the finding that clozapine has a particularly high affinity for this specific receptor (Coward 1992; Van Tol et al. 1991).

Renewed interest in the possible role of D_1 receptors in psychosis has occurred with the recognition that clozapine is also more potent in its blockade of central D_1 versus D_2 receptors (Fitton and Heel 1990) and because of reports that D_1 and D_2 receptors may interact in a synergistic fashion (Walters et al. 1987). Seeman et al. (1989) suggested a D_1-D_2 link that was found to be missing in more than half of postmortem brains of schizophrenic individuals. Two isoforms of the D_1 receptor have been identified—specifically, the D_3 and D_5 receptors (Sokoloff et al. 1990; Sunahara et al. 1991). The localization of D_3 receptors to the limbic region and the affinity of most antipsychotics—particularly the newer atypical agents—for this receptor have been taken as evidence that the D_3 receptor may be integrally involved in psychosis (Sokoloff et al. 1990, 1992a, 1992b).

Table 13–1. Standard neuroleptics

Aliphatic phenothiazines	**Thioxanthenes**
Chlorpromazine	Chlorprothixene
Methotrimeprazine	Flupenthixol
Triflupromazine	Thiothixene
Piperidine phenothiazines	**Butyrphenone**
Mesoridazine	Haloperidol
Pericyazine	**Diphenylbutylpiperidines**
Pipotiazine palmitate	Fluspirilene
Thioridazine	Pimozide
Piperazine phenothiazines	**Dibenzoxazepine**
Acetophenazine	Loxapine
Fluphenazine	**Dihydroindolone**
Perphenazine	Molindone
Thioproperazine	
Trifluoperazine	

A further area of interest has been the potential role of DA autoreceptors in the treatment of psychosis. It appears that D_2 and D_3 receptors can act as both autoreceptors and postsynaptic receptors (Sokoloff et al. 1990). Autoreceptors can regulate DA synthesis and release, as well as neuronal firing (Meltzer 1990); at low dosages, DA agonists such as bromocriptine appear capable of decreasing DA neurotransmission via their presynaptic autoreceptor stimulation (Kebabian and Calne 1979; Sitland-Marken et al. 1990; Skirboll et al. 1979). However, at higher dosages they act on DA postsynaptic receptors in the same fashion as DA and can therefore exacerbate psychotic symptomatology. A paucity of autoreceptors in the frontal and prefrontal DA neurons (Ereshefsky et al. 1990) has implications in terms of the use of DA agonists in the treatment of positive and negative symptomatology (see below).

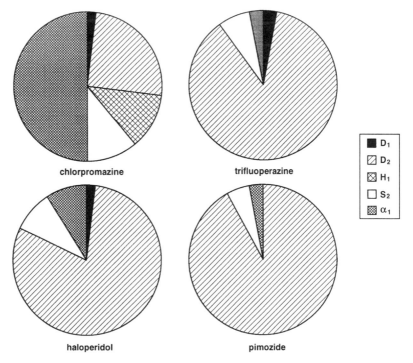

Figure 13–1. Relative binding affinities for typical neuroleptics.
Source. Adapted from Hyttel et al. 1985.

Positive-Negative Symptom Dichotomy: Implications for Dopamine

The focus of neuroleptic development has historically been on agents that would ameliorate the florid symptoms characteristic of schizophrenia (e.g., delusions, hallucinations). Later, Crow's two-dimensional model of schizophrenia (Crow 1980, 1985) encouraged a reevaluation of this position. He defined *type I schizophrenia* as characterized by *positive symptoms,* such as delusions and hallucinations, suggesting that this form of the illness is mediated by biochemical abnormalities and is therefore responsive to neuroleptic treatment. He defined *type II schizophrenia* as representing a predominance of *negative symptomatology* (e.g., affective flattening, poverty of speech, loss of drive) and suggested that this form was more closely associated with structural changes in the brain and thus would respond less well to pharmacotherapy.

Crow's model has been challenged on a number of levels. For example, some patients present with a mixed picture in which both or neither negative and positive syndromes are prominent (Andreasen and Olsen 1982). Moreover, results of neuroimaging studies have not categorically supported the original hypothesis (Marks and Luchins 1990). It has now been suggested that a two-syndrome dichotomy is overly simplistic and that more than two syndromes exist (Liddle 1987; Liddle and Barnes 1990; Peralta et al. 1992).

Regardless of its limitations, Crow's model has had considerable theoretical and clinical implications. Theories of schizophrenia and its pathophysiology now routinely make a distinction between positive and negative symptoms, with the assumption that these may be mediated by different mechanisms (Frith and Done 1988; Kay and Sevy 1990; Reynolds 1989; Strauss 1989; Weinberger 1987). The hypothesis that negative symptoms may be related to biochemical factors has led to a new optimism regarding possible pharmacotherapy, as it has often been assumed that these particular symptoms respond poorly to treatment with typical neuroleptics. Although negative symptoms may, in fact, respond to typical neuroleptics (Brier et al. 1987; S. C. Goldberg 1985; Serban et al. 1992), it appears that other agents may be more effective (Meltzer et al. 1985).

Schizophrenia and Hyperdopaminergic Activity: Theoretical Limitations

Despite the compelling evidence supporting a theory of schizophrenia based on hyperdopaminergic activity and the historical focus on D_2 receptors, this model can be challenged on a number of issues:

1. Even with the highly selective D_2-blocking agents, results from studies have indicated that 5%–25% of schizophrenic patients remain partially or totally unresponsive to existing treatments (Brenner et al. 1990).
2. Clozapine, an atypical neuroleptic with relatively little D_2 in comparison with its D_1 activity, appears efficacious in a significant number of patients nonresponsive to typical neuroleptics (Kane et al. 1988a; Lindstrom 1988; Pickar et al. 1992).
3. There has been a greater focus on distinguishing positive and negative symptomatology in schizophrenia, and clozapine and other novel neuroleptics appear to be more effective than typical neuroleptics in the treatment of negative symptoms (Chouinard et al. 1993; Lindstrom 1988; Meltzer 1992a; Pickar et al. 1992), possibly through involvement of other neurotransmitter systems (e.g., 5-HT) (Bleich et al. 1988; Csernansky et al. 1990; Meltzer 1992b; Pancheri 1991).
4. The finding that clozapine, unlike other typical neuroleptics, demonstrates high binding affinity for the recently cloned D4 receptor (Van Tol et al. 1991) raises the possibility that other receptor subtypes may play an important role in schizophrenia.

Dopamine Dysregulation Hypothesis of Schizophrenia

The notion that DA dysfunction in schizophrenia simply reflects a state of hyperdopaminergic activity has been challenged recently by more complex models. The dopaminergic system can itself be subdivided into a number of pathways: mesolimbic, nigrostriatal, tuberoinfundibular, and mesocortical (Pickar 1986). Mesolimbic dysfunction, represented by hyperdopaminergic activity, has been associated with psychosis and, in particular, positive symptomatology. The nigrostriatal pathway is linked with neuroleptic-induced movement disorders, and the tuberoinfundibular pathway with endocrine side effects (e.g., gynecomastia in males, amenorrhea in females).

In recent years, there has been increased focus on frontal lobe dysfunction in schizophrenia, with parallels drawn between damage to these areas and the deficit or negative symptoms of schizophrenia (Domasio 1979). Impaired performance on the Wisconsin Card Sorting Test (Heaton 1985), for example, has been associated with dysfunction at the level of the prefrontal cortex and negative symptomatology (Davis et al. 1991; T. E. Goldberg and Weinberger 1988). At the same time, there is evidence to link these findings with hypodopaminergic activity. In a review of this topic, Davis et al. (1991) noted studies reporting a negative correlation between cerebrospinal fluid (CSF), homovanillic acid (HVA), and ventricle-to-brain ratio (VBR; Losonczy et al. 1986; Nyback et al. 1983; van Kammen et al. 1983) and a negative correlation between prefrontal brain atrophy and CSF HVA (Doran et al. 1987). Lack of increase in prefrontal blood flow has been associated with low CSF HVA (Weinberger et al. 1988), and DA agonists have been shown to increase prefrontal DA activity and to lead to improvement on the Wisconsin Card Sorting Test (Daniel et al. 1989) as well as improvement in other negative symptomatology (Meltzer et al. 1985).

Weinberger (1987) postulated that mesocortical DA function may be underactive secondary to a lesion that occurred during neurodevelopment, which would adversely affect dopaminergic afferents to the prefrontal cortex. What accounts for this lesion is unclear, but it may be linked to factors such as heredity, infections or immunologic disorders, perinatal trauma, or other environmental assaults. The effect of this lesion, however, is one of impaired prefrontal cortical functioning, reflected in hypodopaminergic activity and negative symptoms. It is speculated that one of the tasks of the prefrontal cortex is modulation of mesolimbic activity. Dysfunction at the prefrontal cortical level results in impaired functioning of this feedback loop (i.e., decreased inhibition), leading to hyperdopaminergic activity at the mesolimbic level.

The implications of such a model are significant, as it suggests that mesolimbic hyperdopaminergic activity is a secondary—rather than primary—process. One might then speculate that changes in mesolimbic activity can be affected by agents acting either directly on this system or indirectly through changes at the prefrontal level. Moreover, other neurotransmitters that influence either of these DA systems (e.g., 5-HT) may play a role in mediating the symptoms of psychosis.

Serotonin and Schizophrenia

As with DA, there have been a number of lines of research suggesting that 5-HT may be of importance in schizophrenia (for reviews, see Bleich et al. 1988; Van Praag 1992):

1. Evidence that hallucinogenic drugs such as lysergic acid diethylamide (LSD) increase central nervous system (CNS) serotonin levels
2. Findings indicating decreased CSF 5-hydroxyindoleacetic acid (5-HIAA) levels in schizophrenic individuals, particularly those belonging to the subgroup characterized by cortical atrophy and ventricular enlargement, as well as patients with a history of suicide attempts
3. Reports of elevated platelet and whole blood 5-HT levels in patients with schizophrenia

Based on the action of hallucinogenic drugs like LSD, it is reasonable to assume that 5-HT agonists should be capable of inducing or exacerbating psychotic symptomatology, whereas 5-HT antagonists should ameliorate such symptoms. A review of the data involving the 5-HT precursors tryptophan and 5-hydroxytryptophan (5-HTP), however, fails to substantiate this assumption (Van Praag 1992). In contrast, results with the more selective direct agonist m-chlorophenylpiperazine (MCPP), which has relatively high binding affinity for 5-HT_{1C} and 5-HT_3 receptors (Glennon et al. 1989; Hoyer 1989), have indicated exacerbation of psychotic symptomatology (Iqbal et al. 1991a, 1991b; Seibyl et al. 1989).

Conversely, agents that decrease or block 5-HT should demonstrate antipsychotic activity. Based on their uncontrolled trial, Cassachia et al. (1975) reported evidence of improvement in three of four acutely psychotic schizophrenic patients with para-chlorophenylalanine (PCPA), a tryptophan hydroxylase inhibitor; however, this finding was not replicated in a placebo-controlled trial with chronic schizophrenic patients (DeLisi et al. 1982). It is interesting that authors of both studies noted improvement in patients' socialization. In one placebo-controlled trial (Shore et al. 1985), fenfluramine, an anorectic agent that leads to 5-HT depletion, failed to produce improvement in a group of schizophrenic patients, but in a second placebo-controlled trial did lead to improvement in negative symptoms (Stahl et al. 1985).

A number of 5-HT receptor-blocking agents have now been tried in the treatment of schizophrenia, with mixed results. In two studies (Gallant et al. 1963; Mendels 1967) involving the treatment of schizophrenic patients with methysergide, which demonstrates primarily 5-HT$_1$–blocking activity as well as some DA agonist and antagonist activity (Hoyer 1988; Sills et al. 1984), no significant improvement was found in psychotic symptoms. In contrast, setoperone, which has 5-HT$_2$- and D$_2$-blocking activity, appeared superior to previous neuroleptic treatment in improving negative symptomatology while inducing fewer extrapyramidal side effects (EPS) (Ceulemans et al. 1985a). Ritanserin, a highly selective 5-HT$_2$–blocking agent lacking significant DA effect, has proven effective in the treatment of psychosis, particularly negative symptomatology, and also appears to have diminished EPS (Ceulemans et al. 1985b; Gelders et al. 1985a, 1985b). Studies evaluating the benefits of adding ritanserin to existing therapy with standard neuroleptics are presently under way.

Several selective 5-HT–blocking agents also have been investigated clinically in the treatment of schizophrenia. Ondansetron, a novel carbazolone and selective antagonist of 5-HT$_3$ receptors, significantly reduced total Brief Psychiatric Rating Scale (BPRS; Overall and Gorham 1962) scores as well as anxiety-depression, thought disturbance, and activation subscale scores at 1 month in a trial of 105 schizophrenic patients (DeVeaugh-Geiss et al. 1992). This agent is currently being used in North America as an antiemetic in cancer chemotherapy (Abramowicz 1991), but there are at present no ongoing clinical trials for its use in schizophrenia. In a single-blind trial, zacopride, also a selective 5-HT$_3$ antagonist, was not found clinically effective in 8 schizophrenic patients who had previously demonstrated a response to standard neuroleptic therapy (Newcomer et al. 1992).

In summary, there is evidence to suggest that 5-HT may be involved in schizophrenia, and results from studies involving 5-HT depletion and $5\text{-}HT_2$ or $5\text{-}HT_3$ antagonism indicate possible efficacy with such agents in the treatment of psychosis, particularly negative symptomatology. In addition, 5-HT antagonism may be associated with improvement in EPS.

Serotonin Receptors

Four main classes of 5-HT receptors have been identified to date: $5\text{-}HT_1$, $5\text{-}HT_2$, $5\text{-}HT_3$, and $5\text{-}HT_4$ (Meltzer and Nash 1991), although there has been some question as to whether there are sufficient formal criteria to designate a $5\text{-}HT_4$ subgroup (Martin 1990). The $5\text{-}HT_1$ receptors may be further subdivided into $5\text{-}HT_{1A}$, $5\text{-}HT_{1B}$, $5\text{-}HT_{1C}$, and $5\text{-}HT_{1D}$ subtypes. It has been suggested that $5\text{-}HT_{1A}$ receptors of the raphe may be important in psychosis because of their role in regulating serotonergic neurotransmission in limbic regions (Palacios et al. 1990). In addition, postmortem studies of patients with schizophrenia have reported increased numbers of $5\text{-}HT_{1A}$ receptors in the frontal cortex (Hashimoto et al. 1991), in contrast to a decrease in $5\text{-}HT_2$ receptors (Arora and Meltzer 1991; Mita et al. 1986). Although $5\text{-}HT_{2A}$ and $5\text{-}HT_{2B}$ receptors have been distinguished, most of the clinical work to date evaluating $5\text{-}HT_2$ receptors has grouped these subtypes together (Gonzalez-Heydrich and Peroutka 1990). Moreover, $5\text{-}HT_{1C}$ receptors are often categorized with $5\text{-}HT_2$ receptors because of their similarities. Originally identified in the periphery, $5\text{-}HT_3$ receptors have since been localized in the CNS (Gonzales-Heydrich and Peroutka 1990). Evidence that selective $5\text{-}HT_3$ antagonists, specifically ondansetron, may have antipsychotic effects suggests that there may be some effect on mesolimbic DA activity (Azmitia and Whitaker-Azmitia 1991). At present, $5\text{-}HT_4$ receptors have not been associated with antipsychotic activity (Meltzer and Nash 1991).

Serotonin-Dopamine Interactions

Whether 5-HT is directly involved in psychotic symptomatology is unclear, in that the serotonergic system can modulate DA functioning and thus may exert its action indirectly. 5-HT cell bodies are found in the brain stem and can be subdivided into superior (caudal linear nucleus, median raphe nucleus, and dorsal raphe nucleus) and inferior (nucleus raphe obscuris, nucleus raphe pallidus, nucleus raphe magnus, and ventral lateral medulla) groups (N. C. Moore and Gershon 1989). Ascending fibers innervate the substantia nigra. Furthermore, Meltzer and Nash (1991), in their review of serotonergic regulation of DA function, summarized evidence suggesting that there is 5-HT inhibition of DA neurotransmission in the nigrostriatal pathway at both cell body and terminal regions, as well as reversal of neuroleptic-induced catalepsy through decreasing 5-HT neurotransmission. Taken together, these lines of evidence would support clinical data indicating that 5-HT–blocking agents may improve or diminish the risk of EPS.

Ascending serotonergic fibers also are abundant in a number of limbic structures (e.g., temporal lobe, amygdaloid nuclei, hippocampus) and can be found in the cortex (N. C. Moore and Gershon 1989). Various reports have indicated that 5-HT may act in a tonic inhibitory fashion on limbic DA activity (Meltzer 1992a), which might account for indications that 5-HT–blocking agents can have some effect on positive psychotic symptoms. Similarly, it has been postulated that 5-HT may have an inhibitory effect on prefrontal cortical DA, and that 5-HT–blocking properties of novel and atypical neuroleptics can lead to increased release of DA from precortical neurons and subsequent improvement in negative symptoms (Ereshefsky et al. 1990).

Novel and Atypical Neuroleptics

Definition

The precise definition of *atypical neuroleptics* is somewhat ambiguous. Generally speaking, these are agents that clinically demonstrate antipsychotic effects without causing significant EPS (e.g., parkinsonism, dystonias, dyskinesias) (Wetzel et al. 1991). In rodents, induction of catalepsy and blockade of stereotyped behaviors via administration of dopamimetic agents (e.g., apomorphine, amphetamine) characterize the action of typical neuroleptics and are thought to represent models of neuroleptic-induced EPS in humans. In contrast, clozapine, the current prototype of atypical neuroleptics, fails to induce catalepsy or reverse the stereotypies. All the compounds thought to have antipsychotic potential, whether typical or atypical, appear to block apomorphine- or amphetamine-induced locomotion and to affect firing in the mesolimbic DA neurons (Wetzel et al. 1991). It is worth noting that atypical neuroleptic response patterns, as defined by animal models, are not necessarily generalizable to humans (Casey 1991).

Like typical neuroleptics, atypical agents may vary along a continuum in terms of side effects. Remoxipride, for example, may be partially atypical in that it has a small but identifiable risk of EPS within its antipsychotic range, while dystonias can occur at higher dosages (Deutch et al. 1991). Similarly, risperidone has been identified as atypical although it still has a risk for EPS, albeit diminished, compared with the typical neuroleptics (Chouinard et al. 1993).

Meltzer (1989) identified lack of increased prolactin response in humans following neuroleptic administration as another characteristic of atypical neuroleptics. This is true for clozapine, although by no means true of all neuroleptics currently designated as atypical. With regard to remoxipride, it has been demonstrated that alterations in prolactin may be dosage dependent (Awad et al. 1991). Risperidone is also associated with increased prolactin levels (Claus et al. 1992).

At present, there appears to be no unitary definition for an atypical antipsychotic (Casey 1992), and even clozapine does not appear to meet all criteria absolutely (Cohen et al. 1991; de Leon et al. 1991; Doepp and Buddeburg 1975; Kane et al. 1991). The term *novel* is perhaps more to the point, as many of these newer compounds appear to meet each criterion to varying degrees.

Novel Neuroleptics With DA–5-HT Activity

In Table 13–2, the comparative binding affinities, including those for DA and 5-HT, are depicted for a number of typical and novel (or atypical) neuroleptics (Meltzer et al. 1989a). As noted, for a number of years, focus turned to the development of agents that were highly selective in blocking D_2 and that had as little involvement as possible in terms of other receptors or neurotransmitter systems. The reintroduction of clozapine, with its apparent efficacy in patients who both were refractory to standard neuroleptic therapy and had negative symptoms, has stimulated the development of new compounds that reflect its more unique biochemical profile.

As an aside, it should be noted that the development of novel agents with combined DA–5-HT activity by no means encompasses all current directions in research. A number of other types of compounds are being investigated, including further selective D_2 antagonists (e.g., remoxipride, raclopride), selective D_1 antagonists (e.g., SCH 31966, NO 756), partial D_2 agonists (e.g., OPC-392, SDZ HDC 912), DA autoreceptor agonists (e.g., PD 128483, B-HT 920), and σ antagonists (e.g., tiospirone) (Deutch et al. 1991; Meltzer 1991).

Clozapine.   In contrast to standard neuroleptics such as haloperidol, clozapine has a relatively low binding affinity for the D_2—as opposed to the D_1—receptor (Coward 1992; see Table 13-3). At the same time, it demonstrates increased binding to the D_3 (Sokoloff et al. 1990) and particularly to the D_4 (Van Tol et al. 1991) receptors, suggesting that these, too, may be critical in its clinical profile. Its

Table 13–2.   pK$_i$ values of D_1, D_2, and 5-HT$_2$ receptor–binding sites and ratios for various typical and atypical neuroleptics

Group	pK$_i$ values D_1	D_2	5-HT$_2$	Ratio of pK$_i$ values (5-HT$_2$/D$_2$)
Typical neuroleptics				
Chlorpromazine	7.5	8.5	8.7	1.02
Haloperidol	7.0	9.0	7.7	0.86
Pimozide	6.1	9.4	8.1	0.86
Fluphenazine	8.3	9.2	8.6	0.94
Atypical neuroleptics				
Clozapine	6.8	7.0	8.3	1.19
Melperone	5.6	6.7	7.5	1.13
Amperozide	6.2	6.3	8.0	1.26
Setoperone	6.0	7.9	9.4	1.29
Tiosperone	6.7	8.8	10.2	1.25

Source. Adapted from Meltzer et al. 1989a.

efficacy also may result from its binding affinity for either the 5-HT_{1C} or the 5-HT_2 receptor (Canton et al. 1990). Findings indicate, however, that the atypical nature of a number of compounds is not related to their binding affinity for the 5-HT_{1C} receptor (Roth et al. 1992).

More recently, it has been suggested that typical and atypical antipsychotics can be differentiated based on the lower D_2 and higher 5-HT_2 pK_i values of the atypical agents (Meltzer 1989, 1992b; Meltzer et al. 1989a, 1989b). In Table 13–2, the $5\text{-HT}_2/D_2$ ratios for a number of typical and atypical agents are presented; it is calculated that a $5\text{-HT}_2/D_2$ ratio greater than or equal to 1.12 defines atypical antipsychotics (Meltzer et al. 1989a). Clozapine's lack of acute blockade of striatal D_2 receptors may account for its decreased risk of EPS, and its failure to suppress striatal DA release with chronic administration, for its decreased risk of tardive dyskinesia (TD; Meltzer and Gudelsky 1992). It also has been postulated that clozapine's decreased risk for TD is related to its combined and balanced D_1-D_2 receptor blockade (Gerlach and Hansen 1992).

First marketed in the 1970s, clozapine was soon associated with a risk for agranulocytosis, which markedly curtailed its use. However, the pivotal multicenter trial carried out in the United States and published in 1988 led to renewed interest in clozapine's clinical use (Kane et al. 1988b). Of particular interest were the findings that, among schizophrenic patients refractory to standard neuroleptic therapy, 30% of those treated with clozapine subsequently responded to it. Moreover, clozapine appeared effective in the treatment of negative— as well as positive—symptomatology, and was associated with a de-

Table 13–3. Relative in vitro binding affinities of clozapine and haloperidol for dopamine and serotonin receptor subtypes[a]

| | | Receptor pK_i | | | | |
	D_1	D_2	5-HT_{1A}	5-HT_{1C}	5-HT_2	5-HT_3
Clozapine	6.6	6.3	6.7	8.2	8.2	7.3
Haloperidol	6.5	8.2	< 6.0	< 6.0	6.6	—

[a]$pK_1 = -\log K_i$, where K_i is inhibition constant nM.
Source. Data generated from S. Urwyler and D. Hoyer, Sandoz Pharmaceuticals Ltd. (adapted from Coward 1992).

creased risk for EPS. A number of reports have since been published supporting these findings (Baldessarini and Frankenburg 1991; Kane 1992; Stephens 1990). However, because of the risk for agranulocytosis, estimated to be 0.6% (Lieberman and Alvir 1992), routine blood monitoring has become a requirement in North America as part of the clinical administration of clozapine.

Risperidone.   Risperidone, a benzisoxazole derivative now released in Canada and the United States, demonstrates particularly high binding affinity for $5\text{-}HT_2$ as well as D_2 receptors (Janssen et al. 1988; Leysen and Janssen 1988; Leysen et al. 1988; see also Figures 13–2 and 13–3). In addition, it displays higher binding affinity than haloperidol for the α_1-adrenergic, α_2-adrenergic, and histamine-H_1 receptors (Leysen et al. 1988). Its binding affinity for the D_4 receptor appears approximately equivalent to its affinity for the D_2 receptor (P. Seeman, personal communication, March 1993).

Results from initial open or single-blind trials have confirmed that risperidone has antipsychotic properties, with a diminished risk for EPS compared with that of standard neuroleptics, as well as possible efficacy in the treatment of both negative and positive symptomatology (Bersani et al. 1990; Bressa et al. 1991; Castelao 1989; Gelders et al. 1990; Meco et al. 1989; Mesotten et al. 1989; Roose et al. 1988).

To date, there have been four published double-blind studies evaluating risperidone in comparison with haloperidol in the treatment of chronic schizophrenia. In one study (Wilms et al. 1992) using computed tomography, it was found that patients with higher VBR showed the greatest improvement in Positive and Negative Syndrome Scale (PANSS; Kay et al. 1987) scores with risperidone or haloperidol, although no difference was noted between treatment groups. In the three remaining investigations (Borison et al. 1992b; Chouinard et al. 1993; Claus et al. 1992), risperidone, particularly within the 4- to 8-mg/day range, appeared superior to haloperidol on objective measures such as the PANSS. More rapid response was reported with risperidone in two studies (Borison et al. 1992b; Chouinard et al. 1993), and greater improvement in total PANSS scores, a combined measure incorporating positive symptom, negative symptom, and general psychopathology subscale scores, was noted in two of the studies

(Chouinard et al. 1993; Claus et al. 1992). In addition, both Claus et al. (1992) and Chouinard et al. (1993) documented greater improvement in negative symptomatology in the risperidone-treated patients. The three studies all reported significantly less EPS with risperidone, as well as a significant reduction in existing dyskinetic movements (Borison et al. 1992b; Chouinard et al. 1993; Claus et al. 1992).

Zotepine. Zotepine, developed in Japan in 1970, is a tricyclic thiepine derivative with combined dopaminergic and serotonergic antagonistic properties and a chemical structure resembling that of the phenothiazines. Although its 5-HT_2 activity is similar to that of chlorpromazine, zotepine demonstrates potent 5-HT_1 activity as well (Harada et al. 1984, 1985, 1986). There appears to be no increase in

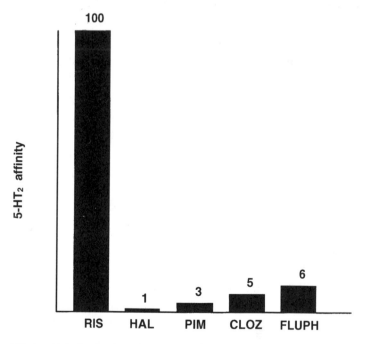

Figure 13–2. Relative in vitro 5-HT_2 receptor–binding affinity, with affinity of risperidone assigned to 100. CLOZ = clozapine; FLUPH = fluphenazine; HAL = haloperidol; PIM = pimozide; RIS = risperidone.
Source. Adapted from Leysen and Janssen 1988; Leysen et al. 1988.

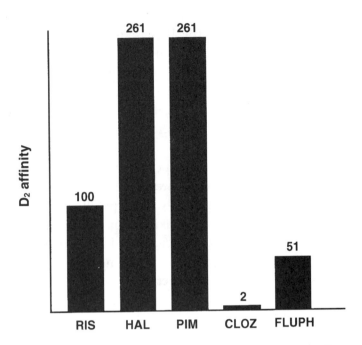

Figure 13–3. Relative in vitro D2 receptor–binding affinity, with affinity of risperidone assigned to 100. CLOZ = clozapine; FLUPH = fluphenazine; HAL = haloperidol; PIM = pimozide; RIS = risperidone.
Source. Adapted from Leysen and Janssen 1988; Leysen et al. 1988.

cortisol or growth hormone with its use, although prolactin levels are increased (von Bardeleben et al. 1987).

In two studies using zotepine alone in the treatment of schizophrenia (Fleischhacker et al. 1987a; von Bardeleben et al. 1987) and one in which zotepine was added to existing neuroleptic therapy (Higashi et al. 1987), improvement was noted in approximately 65%–75% of the patients. A low incidence of EPS was reported in all three studies, and effectiveness was noted by 1–4 weeks. Researchers in three other studies (Barnas et al. 1987; Fleischhacker et al. 1987b, 1987c) reported improvement in negative symptoms within 3–10 weeks after initiation of zotepine treatment, with minimal EPS once again being noted. A relapse rate in 8 of 10 patients over an

8-month interval (Fleischhacker et al. 1987c) may have been related to inadequate dosages of zotepine (i.e., 50–150 mg/day), as no psychotic relapses were reported in the Barnas et al. (1987) study when zotepine at 100 mg/day was added to the existing neuroleptic treatment of 11 residual schizophrenic patients. In their study of treatment-resistant schizophrenic patients with primarily positive symptoms, Harada et al. (1987) indicated minimal improvement in negative symptoms but greater improvement in catatonic and affective symptomatology with zotepine. In an extension of this study, Harada et al. (1991) reported that the best response occurred in patients with catatonic schizophrenia, those with chronic schizophrenia with acute exacerbation, and young patients with a shorter duration of illness. Other researchers (Harada and Otsuki 1986; Otsuki and Harada 1985; Ujike et al. 1983) also have documented zotepine's efficacy in the treatment of mania. Researchers who compared zotepine with propericiazine (Iwanaga et al. 1980), perphenazine (Imai et al. 1980), and thioridazine (Sarai and Okada 1987) have found it to be equal in terms of overall clinical efficacy.

Savoxepine (cipazoxapine, CGP 14986).   Savoxepine is a tetracyclic compound demonstrating a 10-fold higher affinity for D_2 receptors in the hippocampus versus the striatum (Bischoff 1986; Butler and Bech 1987). This, in turn, is associated with a comparative decrease in catalepsy in animals (Bischoff 1992), suggesting effective antipsychotic activity in conjunction with a lower incidence of EPS. In addition to showing a preferential D_2 blockade, savoxepine demonstrates relatively strong 5-HT_2, α_1-adrenergic, and H_1 interaction, as well as moderate 5-HT_1, α_2-adrenergic, H_2, and cholinergic interaction (Waldmeier et al. 1986).

Three open trials testing savoxepine (Butler and Bech 1987; Moller et al. 1989; Wetzel et al. 1991) have produced mixed results. All have demonstrated a moderate or good antipsychotic effect with savoxepine, with one indicating improvement in mainly positive psychotic symptoms (Wetzel et al. 1991). Two of the three reports (Moller et al. 1989; Wetzel et al. 1991), however, noted mild to marked EPS, a finding that was at odds with the preliminary animal data suggesting a low risk for these side effects.

Tiospirone (BMY 13859). Tiospirone represents a novel group of compounds, the benzisothiazoles. In vitro data indicate potent D_2-binding affinity for this drug, although it does not appear that tiospirone causes DA receptor supersensitivity with chronic administration (Cippolina et al. 1991). In addition, tiospirone demonstrates strong interaction with 5-HT_{1A} and 5-HT_2 receptors (Cippolina et al. 1991). It also has been a focus of interest because of its very high affinity for the σ receptor (Taylor and Schlemmer 1992) and the possible action of σ antagonists as antipsychotic agents (Borison et al. 1992a).

In a single-blind crossover study comparing tiospirone with standard neuroleptic therapy, tiospirone was found to have equal antipsychotic efficacy but no evidence of inducing EPS (Jain et al. 1987). In a second single-blind, variable-dosage study (N. C. Moore et al. 1987), significant improvement in BPRS scores was noted, again in the absence of EPS. However, further work with this agent is on hold because of a lack of compelling evidence regarding its efficacy (Taylor and Schlemmer 1992).

Amperozide. Amperozide is chemically related to other neuroleptics by its diphenylbutyl moiety, but also contains a 1-piperazine-carboxamide moiety (Bjork et al. 1992). It has low affinity for striatal D_2 receptors but a strong affinity for cortical 5-HT_2 receptors (Meltzer et al. 1989a, 1992) and a relatively selective affinity for the 5-HT_2 receptor (Albinsson and Andersson 1992). Amperozide demonstrates moderate affinity for the α_1-receptor and low affinity for the 5-HT_{1A}, α_2-adrenergic, D_1, muscarinic M_1 and M_2, opiate σ, and β_2-adrenergic receptors (Svartengren and Simonsson 1990).

Both clozapine and amperozide have been shown to increase basal DA release in the striatum and to decrease D-amphetamine–induced DA release in the nucleus accumbens (Ichikawa and Meltzer 1992a, 1992b). Amperozide may act by blocking DA transport and carrier-mediated release (Yamamoto and Meltzer 1992). It has also been suggested that amperozide's potent effect on the locus coeruleus may be related to a change in the balance between DA and glutamate in favor of glutamate, a hypothesis in keeping with the notion that schizophrenia may reflect a deficient glutamate system (Christensson

1992). Also, like clozapine, amperozide does not cause increased prolactin (Albinsson et al. 1990).

In an open phase II study, Axelsson et al. (1991) reported improvement in BPRS scores for 6 of 10 schizophrenic patients taking amperozide, with the greatest change seen in those with predominantly negative symptoms; a low risk of EPS was also reported. Improvement in both negative and positive symptoms, as well as decreased EPS, were also found in a larger study of amperozide in 53 schizophrenic patients (Bjork et al. 1992). Bjork et al. also noted that marked improvement occurred in 9 of 12 patients refractory to previous standard neuroleptic therapy. Further clinical trials with amperozide are currently ongoing in Europe.

Melperone.   Melperone, a butyrophenone, is similar to clozapine in that its D_2-binding affinity is relatively weak in comparison with its 5-HT_2 binding (Christensson 1989, 1992). This agent demonstrates antiadrenergic properties as well (Christensson 1989). It appears to have a weak effect on striatal DA neurotransmission, as compared with its more potent effects in the cortex and limbic region (Christensson 1989). Melperone's effect on tuberoinfundibular DA neurons and prolactin is similar to that of clozapine (Meltzer et al. 1989c).

In an open study with 20 treatment-resistant schizophrenic patients, Meltzer et al. (1989d) reported that melperone use resulted in slight to moderate improvement in positive and negative symptoms in approximately one-third of the patients, with minimal side effects.

Org 5222 and Org 10490.   Org 5222 is a tetracyclic DA antagonist that is structurally related to mianserin, an antidepressant, and that is capable of inhibiting mesolimbic DA excess (Costall et al. 1988). This compound is unique in comparison with other novel neuroleptics in that it demonstrates a high binding affinity for both D_1 and D_2 receptors in vitro, as well as for 5-HT_2 receptors (Sitsen and Vrijmoed-de Vries 1992). Org 5222 also has a high binding affinity for α_1-adrenergic receptors, with less affinity for H_1 and α_2-adrenergic receptors and negligible affinity for acetylcholine muscarinic receptors.

In a double-blind study of 70 schizophrenic patients in an acutely exacerbated stage of illness, improvement in BPRS scores was similar for Org 5222 when compared with haloperidol (10 mg/day; Vrijmoed-de Vries 1991). Org 5222 was associated with less sedation and EPS, as well as a lower rise in prolactin.

Org 10490 also has demonstrated antidopaminergic and antiserotonergic activity, with weak antiadrenergic and antihistaminergic activity and no anticholinergic activity (Bruin 1992). It, too, is associated with decreased EPS. This drug is currently under investigation.

Olanzapine (LY 170053). Olanzapine belongs to the thiobenzodiazepines, a group of agents with high affinity for D_1, D_2, 5-HT_2, and muscarinic receptors (Chakrabarti et al. 1980). It appears to be more potent than clozapine in its blocking of 5-HT_2 and D_2 receptors, but demonstrates a similar higher affinity for 5-HT_2 than for D_2 receptors (Fuller and Snoddy 1992). In various behavioral measures in animals, olanzapine appears less likely to induce EPS, and it may have anxiolytic as well as potential antipsychotic properties (N. A. Moore et al. 1992). This agent is currently being investigated in the treatment of schizophrenia.

Seroquel (ICI 204,636). Seroquel, a dibenzothiazepine, is similar to clozapine in exhibiting relatively low D_2 affinity and more potent 5-HT_2 antagonism than standard neuroleptics. Unlike clozapine, however, Seroquel has low affinity for both D_1 and muscarinic receptors (Saller and Salama 1993). Both clozapine and Seroquel have been shown to have greater activity in reversing D-amphetamine–induced inhibition of mesolimbic (A10) compared with nigrostriatal (A9) DA neurons, whereas haloperidol demonstrates the opposite selectivity (Goldstein et al. 1993). The notion that Seroquel should have a decreased propensity to induce EPS has been supported in various animal models, demonstrating that it is more like clozapine and not like standard neuroleptics (Migler et al. 1993). Compared with haloperidol and clozapine, Seroquel showed the lowest striatal selectivity in antagonizing behavioral changes induced by DA injections into the corpus striatum (Campbell et al. 1991). Clinical trials with Seroquel are currently under way in both the United States and Canada.

Ocaperidone (R 79 598). Ocaperidone demonstrates pharmacologically equipotent 5-HT_2 and D_2 antagonistic properties and has decreased cataleptogenic activity in comparison with haloperidol (Megens et al. 1992). It appears equipotent to risperidone in terms of $5\text{-}HT_2$ antagonism and is 2.0–8.3 times more potent with respect to D_2 antagonism.

One open pilot study to date (Roose et al. 1990) has found ocaperidone to be effective in dosages of 1–2 mg daily in treatment-resistant psychotic patients in acutely exacerbated stages of illness.

SM-9018.   SM-9018 demonstrates high binding affinity for both $5\text{-}HT_2$ and D_2 receptors, with a $5\text{-}HT_2$–D_2 binding affinity similar to that of zotepine (Hirose et al. 1990). More specifically, its binding affinity for $5\text{-}HT_2$ receptors is 190 times higher than that of haloperidol, and is slightly higher for D_2 receptors as well. SM-9018's binding with the D_1 receptor was approximately 1/30 of that shown for D_2 receptors. Cataleptogenic activity was reduced in comparison with haloperidol, suggesting a decreased risk for EPS. The clinical efficacy of this agent remains to be established.

Conclusions

The potential clinical utility of agents with combined 5-HT and DA antagonism is reflected in the variety of compounds currently under investigation. Taken together, the evidence in favor of their usefulness suggests that they have the following characteristics:

1. Antipsychotic efficacy, with some indication of superiority in patients refractory to standard neuroleptic therapy
2. Efficacy in negative as well as positive symptomatology
3. Decreased risk for EPS and possible antidyskinetic properties

Specific biochemical profiles of individual agents within this group are quite dissimilar, and a number of unanswered questions remain:

1. To what extent does the serotonergic system play a primary role, as compared with a secondary role, through its influence on other systems, such as DA?

2. Is the effect on negative symptoms, at least in part, related to decreased EPS, further improvement in positive symptomatology, or both?
3. Which particular DA receptors are involved (D_1, D_2, D_3, and D_4 have each been implicated)?
4. Which particular 5-HT receptors play a role (with current evidence suggesting $5\text{-}HT_{1A}$ and $5\text{-}HT_2$ receptors)?
5. Is there a ratio for 5-HT/DA that, as suggested by Meltzer et al. (1989a), is critical to the clinical profile of these agents?

This group of compounds represents only one of a number of new directions being taken in the development of novel antipsychotics. However, the unique properties of these agents, in terms of both clinical efficacy and side effects, suggest that they may represent a significant advance in the treatment and understanding of schizophrenia.

References

Abramowicz M (ed): Ondansetron to prevent vomiting after cancer chemotherapy. Med Lett Drugs Ther 33:63 64, 1991

Albinsson A, Andersson G: The effect of amperozide, a new antipsychotic drug, on plasma corticosterone concentration in the rat. Life Sci 51:1535–1544, 1992

Albinsson A, Eriksson E, Andersson G: Amperozide—effect on prolactin release in the rat. Pharmacol Toxicol 66 (suppl 1):49–51, 1990

Andreasen NC, Olsen S: Negative versus positive schizophrenia. Arch Gen Psychiatry 39:789–794, 1982

Arora RC, Meltzer HY: Serotonin$_2$ ($5\text{-}HT_2$) receptor binding in the frontal cortex of schizophrenic patients. J Neural Transm 85:19–29, 1991

Awad AG, Lapierre YD, Jostell K-G, et al: The atypical neuroleptic remoxipride, and prolactin response in the treatment of acute schizophrenia. Schizophr Res 4:311–328, 1991

Axelsson R, Nilsson A, Christensson E, et al: Effects of amperozide in schizophrenia. Psychopharmacology (Berl) 104:287–292, 1991

Azmitia EC, Whitaker-Azmitia PM: Awakening the sleeping giant: anatomy and plasticity of the brain serotonergic system. J Clin Psychiatry 52 (suppl 12):4–16, 1991

Baldessarini RJ, Frankenburg FR: Clozapine: a novel antipsychotic agent. N Engl J Med 324:746–754, 1991

Barnas C, Stuppack C, Unterweger B, et al: Treatment of negative symptoms in schizophrenia with zotepine. J Clin Psychopharmacol 7:370–371, 1987

Bersani G, Bressa GM, Meco G, et al: Combined serotonin–5-HT$_2$ and dopamine-D$_2$ antagonism in schizophrenia: clinical, extrapyramidal and neuroendocrine response in a preliminary study with risperidone (R 64766). Human Psychopharmacology 5:225–231, 1990

Bischoff S: Mesohippocampal dopamine systems: characterization, functional and clinical implications, in The Hippocampus. Edited by Isaacson RL, Pribram KH. New York, Plenum, 1986, pp 1–32

Bischoff S: Towards the understanding of the neuroanatomical substrate of schizophrenia: the contribution of savoxepine, in Novel Antipsychotic Drugs. Edited by Meltzer HY. New York, Raven, 1992, pp 117–134

Bjork A, Bergman I, Gustavsson G: Amperozide in the treatment of schizophrenic patients, in Novel Antipsychotic Drugs. Edited by Meltzer HY. New York, Raven, 1992, pp 47–58

Bleich A, Brown S-L, Kahn R, et al: The role of serotonin in schizophrenia. Schizophr Bull 14:297–315, 1988

Borison RL, Pathiraja AP, Diamond BI: Clinical efficacy of sigma antagonists in schizophrenia, in Novel Antipsychotic Drugs. Edited by Meltzer HY. New York, Raven, 1992a, pp 203–210

Borison LR, Pathiraja AP, Diamond BI, et al: Risperidone: clinical safety and efficacy in schizophrenia. Psychopharmacol Bull 28:213–218, 1992b

Brenner HD, Dencker SJ, Goldstein MJ, et al: Defining treatment refractoriness in schizophrenia. Schizophr Bull 16:551–561, 1990

Bressa GM, Bersani G, Meco G, et al: One year follow-up study with risperidone in chronic schizophrenia. New Trends in Experimental and Clinical Psychiatry 7:169–177, 1991

Brier A, Wolkowitz OM, Doran AR, et al: Neuroleptic responsivity of negative and positive symptoms in schizophrenia. Am J Psychiatry 144:1549–1555, 1987

Bruin RJ: Org 10490: a new antipsychotic drug with 5-HT$_2$ and DA$_2$ antagonistic properties. Schizophr Res 6:111–112, 1992

Butler B, Bech P: Neuroleptic profile of cipazoxapine (savoxepine), a new tetracyclic dopamine antagonist: clinical validation of the hippocampus versus striatum ratio model of dopamine receptors in animals. Pharmacopsychiatry 20:122–126, 1987

Campbell A, Yeghiayan S, Baldessarini RJ, et al: Selective antidopaminergic effects of S(+)N-n-propylnoraporphines in limbic versus extrapyramidal sites in rat brain: comparisons with typical and atypical antipsychotic agents. Psychopharmacology (Berl) 103:323–329, 1991

Canton H, Verriele L, Colpaert FC: Binding of typical and atypical antipsychotics to $5\text{-}HT_{1C}$ and $5\text{-}HT_2$ sites: clozapine potently interacts with $5\text{-}HT_{1C}$ sites. Eur J Pharmacol 191:93–96, 1990

Casey DE: Antipsychotic drugs in schizophrenia: newer compounds and differential outcomes. Psychopharmacol Bull 27:47–50, 1991

Casey DE: What makes a neuroleptic atypical? in Novel Antipsychotic Drugs. Edited by Meltzer HY. New York, Raven, 1992, pp 241–251

Cassachia M, Casati C, Fasio C: P-chlorophenylalanine in schizophrenia. Biol Psychiatry 10:109–110, 1975

Castelao JF, Ferreira L, Gelders YG, et al: The efficacy of the D_2 and the $5\text{-}HT_2$ antagonist risperidone (R 64 766) in the treatment of chronic psychosis. Schizophr Res 2:411–415, 1989

Ceulemans DLS, Gelders Y, Hoppenbrouwers ML, et al: Effect of serotonin antagonism in schizophrenia: a pilot study with setoperone. Psychopharmacology (Berl) 85:329–332, 1985a

Ceulemans DLS, Van Doren J, Nuyts J, et al: Therapeutic efficacy of serotonin and dopamine antagonism on positive and negative symptoms of chronic schizophrenia. Paper presented at the Fourth World Congress of Biological Psychiatry, Philadelphia, PA, September 1985b

Chakrabarti JK, Horsman L, Hotten TM, et al: 4-piperazinyl-10H-thieno[2,3b][1,5]benzodiazepines as potential neuroleptics. J Med Chem 23:878–884, 1980

Chouinard G, Jones B, Remington G, et al: A Canadian multicenter placebo-controlled study of fixed doses of risperidone and haloperidol in the treatment of chronic schizophrenic patients. J Clin Psychopharmacol 13:25–40, 1993

Christensson EG: Pharmacological data of the atypical neuroleptic compound melperone (Buronil). Acta Psychiatr Scand 352:7–15, 1989

Christensson EG: Amperozide and some other atypical compounds with antipsychotic effect, in Novel Antipsychotic Drugs. Edited by Meltzer HY. New York, Raven, 1992, pp 19–32

Cippolina JA, Ruediger EH, New JS, et al: Synthesis and biological activity of the putative metabolite of the atypical antipsychotic agent tiospirone. J Med Chem 34:3316–3328, 1991

Claus A, Bollen J, De Cuyper H, et al: Risperidone versus haloperidol in the treatment of chronic schizophrenic inpatients: a multicentre double-blind comparative study. Acta Psychiatr Scand 85:295–305, 1992

Cohen BM, Keck PE, Satlin A, et al: Prevalence and severity of akathisia in patients on clozapine. Biol Psychiatry 21:1215–1219, 1991

Costall B, Domeney AM, Naylor RJ: Mechanisms of action of novel antipsychotic agents. Schizophr Res 1:2–3, 1988

Coward DM: General pharmacology of clozapine. Br J Psychiatry 160 (suppl 17):5–11, 1992

Crow TJ: Molecular pathology of schizophrenia: more than one disease process? BMJ 280:66–68, 1980

Crow TJ: The two-syndrome concept: origins and current status. Schizophr Bull 11:471–485, 1985

Csernansky J, King RJ, Faustman WO, et al: 5-HIAA in cerebrospinal fluid and deficit schizophrenic characteristics. Br J Psychiatry 156:501–507, 1990

Daniel DG, Berman KF, Weinberger DR: The effect of apomorphine on regional cerebral blood flow during cognitive activation in schizophrenia. J Neuropsychiatry Clin Neurosci 1:377–384, 1989

Davis KL, Kahn RS, Ko G, et al: Dopamine in schizophrenia: a review and reconceptualization. Am J Psychiatry 148:1474–1486, 1991

de Leon J, Moral L, Camunas C: Clozapine and jaw dyskinesia: a case report. J Clin Psychiatry 52:494–495, 1991

DeLisi LE, Freed WI, Gillin JC, et al: P-chlorophenylalanine trial in schizophrenic patients. Biol Psychiatry 17:471–477, 1982

Deutch AY, Moghaddam B, Innis RB, et al: Mechanisms of action of atypical antipsychotic drugs. Schizophr Res 4:121–156, 1991

DeVeaugh-Geiss J, McBain S, Cooksey P, et al: The effects of a novel 5-HT$_3$ antagonist, ondansetron, in schizophrenia, in Novel Antipsychotic Drugs. Edited by Meltzer HY. New York, Raven, 1992, pp 225–232

Doepp S, Buddeburg C: Extrapyramidale symptome unter Clozapin. Nervenarzt 46:589–590, 1975

Domasio A: The frontal lobes, in Clinical Neuropsychology. Edited by Heilman KM, Valenstein E. New York, Oxford University Press, 1979, pp 360–412

Doran AR, Boronow J, Weinberger DR, et al: Structural brain pathology in schizophrenia revisited: prefrontal cortex pathology is inversely correlated with cerebrospinal fluid levels of homovanillic acid. Neuropsychopharmacology 1:25–32, 1987

Ereshefsky L, Tran-Johnson TK, Watanabe MD: Pathophysiologic basis for schizophrenia and the efficacy of antipsychotics. Clin Pharm 9:662–707, 1990

Farde L, Hall H, Ehrin E, et al: Quantitative analysis of D$_2$ dopamine receptor binding in the living human brain by PET. Science 231:258–261, 1986

Fitton A, Heel RC: Clozapine: a review of its pharmacological properties, and therapeutic use in schizophrenia. Drugs 5:722–747, 1990

Fleischhacker WW, Unterweger B, Barnas C, et al: Results of an open phase II study with zotepine—a novel neuroleptic compound. Pharmacopsychiatry 20:64–66, 1987a

Fleischhacker WW, Barnas C, Stuppack C, et al: Zotepine in the treatment of negative symptoms in chronic schizophrenia. Pharmacopsychiatry 20:58–60, 1987b

Fleischhacker WW, Stuppack C, Barnas C, et al: Low-dose zotepine in the maintenance treatment of schizophrenia. Pharmacopsychiatry 20:61–63, 1987c

Frith CD, Done DJ: Towards a neuropsychology of schizophrenia. Br J Psychiatry 153:437–443, 1988

Fuller RW, Snoddy HD: Neuroendocrine evidence for antagonism of serotonin and dopamine by olanzapine (LY 170053), an antipsychotic drug candidate. Res Commun Chem Pathol Pharmacol 77:87–93, 1992

Gallant DM, Bishop MP, Steele CA, et al: The relationship between serotonin antagonism and tranquilizing activity. Am J Psychiatry 119:882, 1963

Gelders Y, Ceulemans DLS, Hoppenbrouwers ML, et al: Ritanserin, a selective serotonin antagonist in chronic schizophrenia. Paper presented at the Fourth World Congress of Biological Psychiatry, Philadelphia, PA, September 1985a

Gelders Y, Ceulemans DLS, Reyntjens A, et al: The influence of selective serotonin antagonism on conventional neuroleptic therapy. Paper presented at the Fourth World Congress of Biological Psychiatry, Philadelphia, PA, September 1985b

Gelders YG, Heylen SLE, Vanden Bussche G, et al: Pilot clinical investigation of risperidone in the treatment of psychotic patients. Pharmacopsychiatry 23:206–211, 1990

Gerlach J, Hansen L: Clozapine and D_1/D_2 antagonism in extrapyramidal functions. Br J Psychiatry 160 (suppl 17):34–37, 1992

Glennon RA, Ismaiel AE-KM, McCarthy BG, et al: Binding of arylpiperazines to $5\text{-}HT_3$ serotonin receptors: results of a structure-affinity study. Eur J Pharmacol 168:387–392, 1989

Goldberg SC: Negative and deficit symptoms in schizophrenia do respond to neuroleptics. Schizophr Bull 11:453–456, 1985

Goldberg TE, Weinberger DR: Probing prefrontal function in schizophrenia with neuropsychological paradigms. Schizophr Bull 14:179–183, 1988

Goldstein JM, Litwin LC, Sutton EB, et al: Seroquel: electrophysiological profile of a potent atypical antipsychotic. Psychopharmacology (Berl) 112:293–298, 1993

Gonzalez-Heydrich J, Peroutka SJ: Serotonin receptor and reuptake sites: pharmacologic significance. J Clin Psychiatry 51 (suppl 4):5–12, 1990

Harada T, Otsuki S: Antimanic effect of zotepine. Clin Ther 8:406–414, 1986

Harada T, Ebara T, Otsuki S: Possible relationship between antimanic effect and activity of zotepine to the $5\text{-}HT_1$ receptor. Folia Psychiatrica et Neurologica Japonica 38:473–480, 1984

Harada T, Sato M, Otsuki S: Neuroleptic drugs and 5-HT₁ receptor: different potencies of various neuroleptic drugs on 5-HT₁ receptors in discrete regions of the rat brain. Folia Psychiatrica et Neurologica Japonica 39:551–558, 1985

Harada T, Fujiwara Y, Otsuki S: The changes of serotonin (5-HT₁, 5-HT₁ₐ, 5-HT₁ᵦ, 5-HT₂) receptor densities in rat brain following chronic zotepine treatment. Jpn J Psychiatry Neurol 40:231–237, 1986

Harada T, Otsuki S, Sato M, et al: Effectivity of zotepine in refractory psychoses: possible relationship between zotepine and non-dopamine psychosis. Pharmacopsychiatry 20:47–51, 1987

Harada T, Otsuki S, Fujiwara Y: Effectiveness of zotepine in therapy-refractive psychoses: an open, multicenter study in eight psychiatric clinics. Fortschr Neurol Psychiatr 59 (suppl 1):41–44, 1991

Hashimoto T, Nishino N, Nakai H, et al: Increase in serotonin 5-HT₁ₐ receptors in prefrontal and temporal cortices of brains from patients with chronic schizophrenia. Life Sci 48:355–363, 1991

Heaton R: Wisconsin Card Sorting Test. Odessa, TX, Psychological Assessment Resources, 1985

Higashi Y, Momotani Y, Suzuki E, et al: Clinical and EEG studies of zotepine, a thiepine neuroleptic, on schizophrenic patients. Pharmacopsychiatry 20:8–11, 1987

Hirose A, Kato T, Ohnao Y, et al: Pharmacological actions of SM-9018, a new neuroleptic drug with both potent 5-hydroxytryptamine₂ and dopamine₂ antagonistic actions. Jpn J Pharmacol 53:321–329, 1990

Hoyer D: Functional correlates of 5-HT₁ recognition sites. J Recept Res 8:59–81 1988

Hoyer D: 5-hydroxytryptamine receptors and effector coupling mechanisms in peripheral tissues, in The Peripheral Actions of 5-hydroxytryptamine. Edited by Fozard JR. Oxford, Oxford University Press, 1989, pp 72–79

Hyttel J et al: Receptor-binding profiles of neuroleptics, in Dyskinesia: Research and Treatment. Edited by Casey DE, Chase TN, Christenssen AV, et al. Berlin, Springer, 1985, pp 9–18

Ichikawa J, Meltzer HY: The effect of chronic atypical antipsychotic drugs and haloperidol on amphetamine-induced dopamine release in vivo. Brain Res 574:98–104, 1992a

Ichikawa J, Meltzer HY: Amperozide, a novel antipsychotic drug, inhibits the ability of d-amphetamine to increase dopamine release in vivo in rat striatum and nucleus accumbens. J Neurochem 58:2285–2291, 1992b

Imai H, Ohtani W, Kondo H, et al: Comparison of efficacy of zotepine and perphenazine in schizophrenia by double-blind, controlled study. Japanese Journal of Neuropsychopharmacology 2:61, 1980

Iqbal N, Asnis GM, Wetzler S, et al: The MCPP challenge test in schizophrenia: hormonal and behavioral response. Biol Psychiatry 30:770–778, 1991a

Iqbal N, Asnis GM, Wetzler S, et al: The role of serotonin in schizophrenia: new findings. Schizophr Res 5:181–182, 1991b

Iwanaga M, Okada I, Ichinomiya Y, et al: Clinical evaluation of zotepine in chronic schizophrenia—a multi-institutional double-blind study in comparison with propericiazine. Japanese Journal of Clinical Psychiatry 9:121, 1980

Jain AK, Kelwala S, Moore N, et al: A controlled clinical trial of tiaspirone in schizophrenia. Int Clin Psychopharmacol 2:129–133, 1987

Janssen PAJ, Niemegeers CJE, Awouters F, et al: Pharmacology of risperidone (R 64 766), a new antipsychotic with serotonin-S_2 and dopamine-D_2 antagonistic properties. J Pharmacol Exp Ther 244:685–693, 1988

Kane JM: Clinical efficacy of clozapine in treatment-refractory schizophrenia: an overview. Br J Psychiatry 160 (suppl 17):41–45, 1992

Kane J, Honigfeld G, Singer J, et al: Clozapine for treatment-resistant schizophrenia. Arch Gen Psychiatry 45:789–796, 1988a

Kane J, Honigfeld G, Singer J, et al: Clozapine for the treatment-resistant schizophrenic: a double-blind comparison with chlorpromazine. Arch Gen Psychiatry 45:789–796, 1988b

Kane JM, Lieberman J, Pollack S, et al: Clozapine and tardive dyskinesia: prospective data. Schizophr Res 4:364–365, 1991

Kay SR, Sevy S: A pyramidal model of schizophrenia. Schizophr Bull 16:537–545, 1990

Kay SR, Fiszbein A, Opler LA: The positive and negative syndrome scale (PANSS) for schizophrenia. Schizophr Bull 13:261–276, 1987

Kebabian JW, Calne DB: Multiple receptors for dopamine. Nature 277:93–96, 1979

Kebabian JW, Petzold GL, Greengard P: Dopamine-sensitive adenylate cyclase in caudate nucleus of rat brain, and its similarity to the "dopamine receptor." Proc Natl Acad Sci U S A 69:2145–2149, 1972

Leysen JE, Janssen PAJ: Specificity of ligands used in psychiatric research, in Intra and Intercellular Communications, Vol 3. Edited by Cinader B. Cambridge, MA, University Press, 1988, pp 526–543

Leysen JE, Gommeren W, Eens A, et al: Biochemical profile of risperidone, a new antipsychotic. J Pharmacol Exp Ther 247:661–670, 1988

Liddle P: The symptoms of schizophrenia: a re-evaluation of the positive-negative dichotomy. Br J Psychiatry 151:145–151, 1987

Liddle PF, Barnes TRE: Syndromes of chronic schizophrenia. Br J Psychiatry 157:558–561, 1990

Lieberman JA, Alvir JMJ: A report of clozapine-induced agranulocytosis in the United States: incidence and risk factors. Drug Saf 7 (suppl 1):49–50, 1992

Lindstrom LH: The effect of long-term treatment with clozapine in schizophrenia: a retrospective study in 96 patients treated with clozapine for up to 13 years. Acta Psychiatr Scand 77:524–529, 1988

Losonczy MF, Song IS, Mohs RC, et al: Correlates of lateral ventricular size in chronic schizophrenia, II: biological measures. Am J Psychiatry 143:1113–1118, 1986

Marks RC, Luchins DJ: Relationship between brain imaging findings in schizophrenia and psychopathology, in Schizophrenia: Positive and Negative Symptoms and Syndromes. Edited by Andreasen NC. Basel, Karger, 1990, pp 89–123

Martin GR: Current problems and future requirements for 5-hydroxytryptamine receptor classification. Neuropsychopharmacology 3:321–333, 1990

Meco G, Bedini L, Bonifati F, et al: Risperidone in the treatment of chronic schizophrenia with tardive dyskinesia. Curr Ther Res 46:876–883, 1989

Megens AAHP, Awouters FHL, Meert TF, et al: Pharmacological profile of the new potent neuroleptic ocaperidone (R 79598). J Pharmacol Exp Ther 260:146–159, 1992

Meltzer HY: Clinical studies on the mechanism of action of clozapine: the dopamine-serotonin hypothesis of schizophrenia. Psychopharmacology 99:S18–S27, 1989

Meltzer HY: The mechanism of action of novel antipsychotic drugs. Schizophr Bull 17:263–287, 1991

Meltzer HY: Presynaptic receptors: relevance to psychotropic drug action in man. Ann N Y Acad Sci 604:353–371, 1990

Meltzer HY: Dimensions of outcome with clozapine. Br J Psychiatry 160 (suppl 17):46–53, 1992a

Meltzer H: The importance of serotonin-dopamine interaction in the action of clozapine. Br J Psychiatry 160 (suppl 17):22–29, 1992b

Meltzer HY, Gudelsky GA: Dopaminergic and serotonergic effects of clozapine: implications for a unique clinical profile. Arzneimittelforschung 42:268–272, 1992

Meltzer HY, Nash JF: Serotonin and neuropsychiatric disorders: implications for the discovery of new psychotherapeutic agents, VII: effects of antipsychotic drugs on serotonin receptors. Pharmacol Rev 43:587–604, 1991

Meltzer HY, Sommers AA, Luchins DJ: The effect of neuroleptics and other psychotropic drugs on negative symptoms in schizophrenia. J Clin Psychopharmacol 6:329–338, 1985

Meltzer HY, Matsubara S, Lee J-C: Classification of typical and atypical antipsychotic drugs on the basis of dopamine D_1, D_2 and serotonin$_2$ pK$_i$ values. J Pharmacol Exp Ther 251:238–251, 1989a

Meltzer HY, Matsubara S, Lee J-C: The ratios of serotonin and dopamine affinities differentiate atypical and typical antipsychotic drugs. Psychopharmacol Bull 25:390–392, 1989b

Meltzer HY, Koenig JI, Nash JF, et al: Melperone and clozapine: neuroendocrine effects of atypical neuroleptic drugs. Acta Psychiatr Scand 352:24–29, 1989c

Meltzer HY, Alphs LD, Bastani B, et al: Effect of melperone in treatment-resistant schizophrenia (abstract), in Psychiatry Today: Accomplishments and Promises. Edited by Stefanis CN, Soldatas CR, Rabavilas AD. New York, Excerptica Medica International Congress Series 899, 1989d, p 502

Meltzer HY, Zhang Y, Stockmeier CA: Effect of amperozide on rat cortical 5-HT$_2$ and striatal and limbic dopamine D_2 receptor occupancy: implications for antipsychotic action. Eur J Pharmacol 216:67–71, 1992

Mendels J: The effect of methysergide (an antiserotonin agent) on schizophrenia: a preliminary report. Br J Psychiatry 124:157–160, 1967

Mesotten F, Suy E, Pietquin M, et al: Therapeutic effect and safety of increasing doses of risperidone (R 64 766) in psychotic patients. Psychopharmacology 99:445–449, 1989

Migler BM, Malick JB, Warawa EJ: Seroquel: behavioral effects in conventional and novel tests for atypical antipsychotic drugs. Psychopharmacology (Berl) 112:299–307, 1993

Mita T, Hanada S, Nishino N, Kuno T, et al: Decreased serotonin (S$_2$) and increased dopamine (D$_2$) receptors in chronic schizophrenics. Biol Psychiatry 21:1407–1414, 1986

Moller HJ, Kissling W, Dietzfelbinger T, et al: Efficacy and tolerability of a new antipsychotic compound (savoxepine): results of a pilot study. Pharmacopsychiatry 22:38–41, 1989

Moore NA, Tye NC, Axton MS, et al: The behavioral pharmacology of olanzapine, a novel "atypical" antipsychotic agent. J Pharmacol Exp Ther 262:545–551, 1992

Moore NC, Gershon S: Which atypical neuroleptics are identified by screening tests? Clin Neuropharmacol 12:167–184, 1989

Moore NC, Meyendorff E, Yeragani V, et al: Tiaspirone in schizophrenia. J Clin Psychopharmacol 7:98–101, 1987

Newcomer JW, Faustman WO, Zipursky RB: Zacopride in schizophrenia: a single-blind serotonin type 3 antagonist trial. Arch Gen Psychiatry 49: 751, 1992

Nyback H, Berggren BM, Hindmarsh T, et al: Cerebroventricular size and cerebrospinal fluid monoamine metabolites in schizophrenic patients and healthy volunteers. Psychiatry Res 9:301–308, 1983

Ogren SO, Hall H: Comparison of the effects of different substituted benzamides on dopamine receptor function in the rat, in Novel Antipsychotic Drugs. Edited by Meltzer HY. New York, Raven, 1992, pp 59–66

Otsuki S, Harada T: Antimanic effect of zotepine. Japanese Journal of Clinical Psychiatry 14:309–321, 1985

Overall JE, Gorham DR: The Brief Psychiatric Rating Scale. Psychol Rep 10:799–812, 1962

Palacios JM, Waeber C, Hoyer D, et al: Distribution of serotonin receptors: the neuropharmacology of serotonin. Ann N Y Acad Sci 600:36–52, 1990

Pancheri P: Neuroleptics and 5-HT receptors: a working hypothesis for antipsychotic effect. New Trends in Experimental and Clinical Psychiatry 7:141–150, 1991

Peralta V, de Leon J, Cuesta MJ: Are there more than two syndromes of schizophrenia? Br J Psychiatry 163:335–343, 1992

Pickar D: Neuroleptics, dopamine, and schizophrenia. Psychiatr Clin North Am 9:35–48, 1986

Pickar D, Owen RR, Litman RE, et al: Clinical and biologic response to clozapine in patients with schizophrenia. Arch Gen Psychiatry 49:345–353, 1992

Reynolds GP: Beyond the dopamine hypothesis: the neurochemical pathology of schizophrenia. Br J Psychiatry 155:305–316, 1989

Roose K, Gelders Y, Heylen S: Risperidone (R 64 766) in psychotic patients. Acta Psychiatr Belg 88:233–241, 1988

Roose KJ, De Wilde M, Dierick M, et al: Pilot study with R 79598 in acute psychotic disorders, in Proceedings of the 17th Congress of Collegium Internationale Neuro-Psychopharmacologium, Abstracts (Vol 2). Kyoto, Japan, September 1990, p 225

Roth BL, Ciaranello RD, Meltzer HY: Binding of typical and atypical antipsychotic agents to transiently expressed 5-HT$_{1C}$ receptors. J Pharmacol Exp Ther 260:1361–1365, 1992

Saller CF, Salama AI: Seroquel: biochemical profile of a potential atypical antipsychotic. Psychopharmacology (Berl) 112:285–292, 1993

Sarai K, Okada M: Comparison of efficacy of zotepine and thiothixene in schizophrenia in a double-blind study. Pharmacopsychiatry 20:38–46, 1987

Seeman P: Dopamine receptors and the dopamine hypothesis of schizophrenia. Synapse 1:133–152, 1987

Seeman P, Niznik HB, Guan H-C, et al: Link between D_1 and D_2 dopamine receptors is reduced in schizophrenia and Huntington diseased brain. Proc Natl Acad Sci U S A 86:10156–10160, 1989

Seibyl JP, Krystal JN, Price LH, et al: Neuroendocrine and behavioral responses to MCPP in unmedicated schizophrenics and healthy subjects. Paper presented at annual meeting of the American College of Neuropsychopharmacology, Maui, HI, December 1989

Serban G, Siegel S, Gaffney M: Response of negative symptoms of schizophrenia to neuroleptic treatment. J Clin Psychiatry 53:229–234, 1992

Shore D, Korpi ER, Bigelow LB, et al: Fenfluramine and chronic schizophrenia. Biol Psychiatry 20:329–352, 1985

Sills MA, Wolf BB, Frazer A: Determination of selective and nonselective compounds for the $5\text{-}HT_{1A}$ and $5\text{-}HT_{1B}$ receptor subtypes in rat frontal cortex. J Pharmacol Exp Ther 231:480–487, 1984

Sitland-Marken PA, Wells BG, Froemming JH, et al: Psychiatric applications of bromocriptine therapy. J Clin Psychiatry 51:68–82, 1990

Sitsen JMA, Vrijmoed-de Vries MC: Org 5222: preliminary clinical results, in Novel Antipsychotic Drugs. Edited By Meltzer HY. New York, Raven, 1992, pp 15–18

Skirboll LR, Grace AA, Bunney BS: Dopamine auto- and postsynaptic receptors: electrophysiologic evidence for differential sensitivity to dopamine agonists. Science 206:80–82, 1979

Sokoloff P, Giros B, Martres M-P, et al: Molecular cloning and characterization of a novel dopamine receptor (D_3) as a target for neuroleptics. Nature 347:146–151, 1990

Sokoloff P, Andrieux M, Besancon R, et al: Pharmacology of human dopamine D_3 receptor expressed in a mammalian cell line: comparison with D_2 receptor. Eur J Pharmacol 225:331–337, 1992a

Sokoloff P, Martres M-P, Giros B, et al: The third dopamine receptor (D_3) as a novel target for antipsychotics. Biochem Pharmacol 43:659–666, 1992b

Stahl SM, Uhr SB, Berger PA: Pilot study on the effects of fenfluramine on negative symptoms in twelve schizophrenic inpatients. Biol Psychiatry 20:1098–1102, 1985

Stephens P: A review of clozapine: an antipsychotic for treatment-resistant schizophrenia. Compr Psychiatry 31:315–326, 1990

Strauss JS: Mediating processes in schizophrenia: towards a new dynamic psychiatry. Br J Psychiatry 155 (suppl 5):22–28, 1989

Sunahara RK, Guan H-C, O'Dowd BF, et al: Cloning of the gene for a human dopamine D_5 receptor with higher affinity for dopamine than D_1. Nature 350:614–619, 1991

Svartengren J, Simonsson P: Receptor binding properties of amperozide. Pharmacol Toxicol 1 (suppl 1):8–11, 1990

Taylor DP, Schlemmer RF Jr: Sigma "antagonists": potential antipsychotics? in Novel Antipsychotic Drugs. Edited by Meltzer HY. New York, Raven, 1992, pp 189–201

Ujike H, Horii S, Ebara T, et al: Efficacy of zotepine in treatment of mania. Japanese Journal of Clinical Psychiatry 12:1575–1586, 1983

van Kammen DP, Mann LS, Sternberg DE, et al: Dopamine-beta-hydroxylase activity and homovanillic acid in spinal fluid of schizophrenics with brain atrophy. Science 220:974–977, 1983

Van Praag HM: Serotonergic mechanisms in the pathogenesis of schizophrenia, in New Biological Vistas on Schizophrenia. Edited by Lindenmayer J-P, Kay SR. New York, Brunner/Mazel, 1992, pp 182–206

Van Tol HMM, Bunzow JR, Guan H-C, et al: Cloning of the gene for a human dopamine D₄ receptor with high affinity for the antipsychotic clozapine. Nature 350:610–614, 1991

von Bardeleben U, Benkert O, Holsboer F: Clinical and neuroendocrine effects of zotepine—a new neuroleptic drug. Pharmacopsychiatry 20:28–34, 1987

Vrijmoed-de Vries MC: Pilot clinical study with a new antipsychotic (abstract of paper presented at the Fifth World Congress of Biological Psychiatry, Florence, Italy). Biol Psychiatry 29 (suppl 11):678S, 1991

Waldmeier PC, Bischoff S, Bittiger H, et al: Pharmacological profiles of four new tetracyclic dopamine antagonists, maroxepine, citatepine, eresepine, and cipazoxepine. Pharmacopsychiatry 19:316–317, 1986

Walters JR, Bergstrom DA, Carlson JH, et al: D₁ dopamine receptor activation required for postsynaptic expression of D₂ agonist effects. American Association for the Advancement of Science 236:719–722, 1987

Weinberger DR: Implications of normal brain development for the pathogenesis of schizophrenia. Arch Gen Psychiatry 44:660–669, 1987

Weinberger DR, Berman KF, Illowsky BP: Physiological dsysfunction of dorsolateral prefrontal cortex in schizophrenia, III: a new cohort and evidence for a monoaminergic mechanism. Arch Gen Psychiatry 45:609–615, 1988

Wetzel H, Wiedemann K, Holsboer F, et al: Savoxepine: invalidation of an "atypical" neuroleptic response pattern predicted by animal models in an open clinical trial with schizophrenic patients. Psychopharmacology 103:280–283, 1991

Wilms G, Van Ongeval C, Baert AL, et al: Ventricular enlargement, clinical correlates and treatment outcome in chronic schizophrenic inpatients. Acta Psychiatr Scand 85:306–312, 1992

Yamamoto BK, Meltzer HY: The effect of the atypical antipsychotic drug, amperozide, on carrier-mediated striatal dopamine release measured in vivo. J Pharmacol Exp Ther 263:180–185, 1992

Clozapine in Treatment-Refractory Schizophrenia

Allan Z. Safferman, M.D.;
Jeffrey A. Lieberman, M.D.; John M. Kane, M.D.;
Sally R. Szymanski, D.O.; and Bruce J. Kinon, M.D.

Although clozapine was first synthesized in 1958, it has taken three decades for it to be commercially marketed in the United States. The development of clozapine was delayed and the conditions for which it is indicated have been limited by its potential for hematologic toxicity. Despite these serious risks, the combination of the tremendous interest generated by clozapine's novel properties and the dearth of other bona fide atypical neuroleptic compounds available for clinical use has fueled efforts to determine the extent of clozapine's clinical utility. Consequently, the

This work was supported by a National Institute of Mental Health (NIMH) Research Scientist Development Award (MH00537) to Dr. Lieberman, by NIMH Grant MH41960 to the Mental Health Clinical Research Center of Hillside Hospital, and by the Sandoz Research Institute.

body of information on clozapine has continued to accumulate from its initial clinical testing and use in Europe and Scandinavia through its U.S. Food and Drug Administration (FDA) approval and introduction to the commercial market in the United States. In this chapter, we provide an overview of current knowledge with regard to the clinical effects of clozapine, both therapeutic and adverse. Although this is a rapidly evolving area of investigation, numerous questions remain unanswered; for example:

- What defines neuroleptic intolerance?
- What is the optimal dosage range for clozapine?
- What is the appropriate duration of a treatment trial of clozapine?

Review of Efficacy

Efficacy in Schizophrenia

Acute treatment studies.   Many of the acute (less than 12 weeks) treatment studies of clozapine used an open-label design and were often uncontrolled (Chouinard and Annable 1976; Matz et al. 1974; Panteleeva et al. 1987; Simpson and Varga 1974). Conclusions that could be drawn from some of these studies were also limited because of a variety of methodological problems, including small sample size, inappropriate dosing, inadequate duration of treatment, and differences in diagnostic criteria. The generally favorable results of these studies, including the relative lack of extrapyramidal side effects (EPS), provided an impetus to conduct double-blind studies.

Double-blind studies.   Four important double-blind studies were reviewed by Honigfeld et al. (1984). In these trials, clozapine was compared with chlorpromazine or haloperidol in various groups of patients (i.e., treatment-refractory and neuroleptic-intolerant patients, patients with tardive dyskinesia, and patients in acute stages of schizophrenia) (Claghorn et al. 1987; Fischer-Cornelssen and Ferner 1976; Sandoz New Drug Application (NDA) [unpublished document]

1987; Shopsin et al. 1979). Investigators in all of these studies used the Brief Psychiatric Rating Scale (BPRS; Overall and Gorham 1962) to quantify improvements in behavioral status, thus allowing more meaningful comparisons across studies. The results of these studies demonstrated that at the endpoint of each study (range 28–56 days), clozapine was generally superior to either haloperidol or chlorpromazine on at least some of the individual BPRS items. These differences were more pronounced when the more severely ill group of patients was analyzed separately.

Investigators in other double-blind studies have evaluated the efficacy of clozapine versus standard agents in acutely ill and not necessarily treatment-refractory or neuroleptic-intolerant schizophrenic patients (Chiu et al. 1976; Guirguis et al. 1977; Van Praag et al. 1976). The results of these studies provided evidence that clozapine's efficacy was essentially comparable to that of other agents. Gelenberg and Doller (1979) prematurely terminated their double-blind comparison of clozapine with chlorpromazine in acutely ill schizophrenic patients (all of whom had a history of drug-induced EPS) because of concerns about clozapine-induced agranulocytosis. Although their small sample size precluded an analysis for statistical significance, the results suggested that clozapine was at least as effective as chlorpromazine.

Efficacy in treatment-refractory patients.   Following reports of agranulocytosis associated with clozapine in Finland, clinical use was generally restricted. However, experience in Europe suggested that deaths associated with clozapine-induced agranulocytosis could largely be prevented by weekly blood count monitoring (Sandoz NDA [unpublished document] 1987). Given clozapine's potential value in treatment-refractory patients, coupled with its risk of producing agranulocytosis, it became clear that this compound could only be marketed in the United States if a carefully designed, well-controlled trial demonstrated statistically significant superiority over a currently available neuroleptic. Such a trial was conducted and reported by Kane et al. (1988).

Patients were eligible for this study if they met the following criteria for treatment refractoriness: 1) they had had at least three periods of treatment in the preceding 5 years with neuroleptic agents (from at least two different chemical classes) at dosages equivalent to or greater than 1,000 mg/day of chlorpromazine for a period of 6 weeks, each without significant symptomatic relief; and 2) they had had no period of good functioning within the previous 5 years. Subjects had to rate at least moderately ill (a score greater than 3) on the Clinical Global Impression (CGI; Guy 1976) scale and at least 45 on the BPRS total score. In addition, item scores of at least 4 (moderate) were required on at least two of the following items: conceptual disorganization, suspiciousness, hallucinations, and unusual thought content. To confirm their drug nonresponsiveness, all patients were treated with (single-blind) haloperidol 60 mg/day for up to 6 weeks prior to entering the double-blind, controlled trial. Improvement criteria were defined in advance as 1) a decrease of BPRS score by at least 20% and 2) either a CGI score less than 4 or a BPRS score less than 36. Only 2% of the patients were considered responsive to the haloperidol trial, confirming the accuracy of historically designating patients as being nonresponsive.

Of the 319 patients initially recruited into the study, 268 were randomized to a double-blind 6-week course of either clozapine or chlorpromazine plus benztropine. Average mean peak dosages were 600 mg/day for clozapine and 1,200 mg/day for chlorpromazine. Using a priori response criteria, 30% of the clozapine-treated patients were judged responsive to treatment, compared with only 4% of the chlorpromazine-treated patients. Total BPRS scores, as well as scores for the four positive-symptom BPRS items mentioned earlier (conceptual disorganization, suspiciousness, hallucinations, and unusual thought content), showed clozapine to be significantly superior to chlorpromazine. In addition, clozapine-treated patients demonstrated superiority on BPRS items that represented negative symptoms of schizophrenia. This study demonstrated that clozapine was clearly superior to chlorpromazine in a well-defined group of severely ill, treatment-refractory schizophrenic patients. It also served as the pivotal study to gain FDA approval to market clozapine in the United States. Some investigators participating in this multicenter trial also reported results separately from their individual study sites (Borison et al. 1988; Conley et al. 1988).

Pickar et al. (1992) conducted a double-blind crossover study without randomization, comparing an initial trial of fluphenazine with clozapine. Twenty-one treatment-refractory schizophrenic patients were initially treated with oral fluphenazine for a mean of 45.8 ± 15.8 days at a daily dosage of 28.9 ± 21.2 mg. This was followed by a placebo washout with a mean duration of 37.1 ± 11.3 days. Clozapine treatment was then initiated (still under double-blind conditions) for a mean of 51.8 ± 14.7 days at a moderate daily dosage (373.8 ± 110.8 mg) and an additional 54.7 days for a total of 106.5 ± 5.1 days' duration of clozapine treatment at an optimal dosage of 542.9 ± 207.4 mg. The response rates as defined by modified Kane et al. (1988) criteria were 38% and 4.8% for clozapine and fluphenazine, respectively. These findings were within expectations based upon shorter (Kane et al. 1988) and longer-term (albeit open-label) studies (Meltzer et al. 1989a).

Follow-up and long-term studies.   Follow-up studies involving clozapine are very important in answering questions such as, Are the therapeutic gains maintained over long periods of time? Is clozapine a safe and well-tolerated agent when taken over extended periods of time? Most of the follow-up studies of clozapine have been retrospective in nature (Kuha and Miettinen 1986; Leon 1979; Leppig et al. 1989; Lindstrom 1988; Naber et al. 1989; Povlsen et al. 1985), whereas others have been prospective (Mattes 1989; Meltzer et al. 1989a; Owen et al. 1989). Investigators in some of these studies looked at various markers of efficacy, including behavioral improvement (e.g., BPRS scores), ability to be discharged from the hospital, and social adjustment (e.g., scores on the Quality of Life Scale [QLS; Heinrichs et al. 1984], patient's ability to work). Although it is beyond the scope of this chapter to describe each of these studies in detail, we note below some of the key results.

Lindstrom (1988) reported on a long-term follow-up study of 96 patients (89 schizophrenic, 7 schizoaffective) treated with clozapine for up to 13 years. Patients were designated as either treatment refractory (85%) or neuroleptic intolerant (15%) prior to clozapine treatment. The results showed that 85% of all patients could be discharged from the hospital following clozapine treatment. Of the

62 patients who were still on clozapine after 2 years, up to 39% were employable on at least a part-time basis. A global evaluation described 43% as significantly improved and 38% as moderately improved.

Povlsen et al. (1985) reported on 216 patients who had received clozapine for up to 12 years. Of this group, 85 had received clozapine alone, and 51% were judged to have benefited from a better therapeutic effect with clozapine than with their previous treatment with standard agents. The group of 131 patients who received clozapine in combination with a typical antipsychotic fared no better than the clozapine-alone group. Povlsen et al. concluded that the overall therapeutic efficacy across all groups ranged between 30% and 50%.

Kuha and Miettinen (1986) studied a group of 108 schizophrenic patients treated with clozapine for up to 7 years. Most of the patients had been designated as treatment resistant. Approximately 33% of the patients were reported to have had a distinct favorable effect with clozapine, and 23% of the patients were able to be discharged from the hospital.

Leon (1979) performed a comparative follow-up study of patients receiving either clozapine ($n = 18$) or chlorpromazine ($n = 19$). He reported that the clozapine group required fewer rehospitalizations and outpatient visits.

Prospective follow-up studies.   Although it may be concluded from the studies cited above that at least 30%–40% of neuroleptic-refractory patients derived sustained, clinically significant long-term benefit from clozapine treatment, those studies did not focus on the time course of response to clozapine. In an attempt to determine the onset of response time beyond 6 weeks in treatment-refractory patients, Meltzer et al. (1989a) conducted an open-label, uncontrolled study involving 51 retrospectively defined treatment-refractory patients for up to 35 months (mean duration of approximately 10 months; see detailed discussion of results in the risk-benefit section, below). Approximately 60% of these patients were considered to be responsive to clozapine after 1 year of treatment, with response being defined as at least a 20% decrease in BPRS scores from baseline.

Mattes (1989) reported results in a small group of patients who received clozapine for up to 2 years. Of the 14 patients who started the study, 6 were still taking clozapine after 2 years and had statistically significant improvement as measured by BPRS scores compared with baseline ratings. Of interest was that only about 50% of the eventual BPRS improvement was noted after 12 weeks of treatment.

Owen et al. (1989) followed a group of schizoaffective or schizophrenic patients who received ongoing open-label clozapine treatment for up to 4 years. Of the treatment-refractory patients in this study, 50% had improved significantly at 12 weeks. Although the therapeutic effects were maintained for the duration of the study, there was no additional improvement in the BPRS ratings beyond this point.

All of the follow-up studies had significant flaws in their design and methodology. A partial list of problems of the studies just mentioned includes reliance on incomplete or inaccurate medical records, lack of a control group, use of an open-label design, lack of dosage standardization, small sample size, lack of a precise definition of what constituted an adequate response to treatment, and lack of standardization of treatments (e.g., differences in efforts at adjunctive nonpharmacological treatment [e.g., psychosocial rehabilitation] or use of concomitant antipsychotic medication).

Efficacy in Other Disorders

Clozapine has been reported to be efficacious in patients diagnosed with schizoaffective disorder (Lindstrom 1988; McElroy et al. 1991; Owen et al. 1989; Wood and Rubinstein 1990) and bipolar disorder with psychosis (McElroy et al. 1991). Although this limited evidence suggests that clozapine appears to be an effective agent for these disorders, more research needs to be done. Little can be said for what role clozapine may have in the long-term treatment of neuroleptic-resistant psychotic patients with major depression, delusional disorder, or psychosis not otherwise specified (e.g., mental retardation with psychosis, borderline personality disorder with psychosis) because there is insufficient literature to draw any meaningful conclusions.

Clozapine has also been successfully used for patients who were determined to be neuroleptic intolerant because of severe EPS (including akathisia) and tardive dyskinesia (Claghorn et al. 1987; Levin et al. 1992; Lindstrom 1988; Small et al. 1987a). Some of these patients were not treatment refractory and therefore could be expected to respond at least as well as they did with typical antipsychotic agents. Indeed, clozapine is indicated for those schizophrenic patients with neuroleptic intolerance (in this instance, "intolerance" is defined as experiencing EPS that cannot be adequately managed with antipsychotic dosage reduction, antiparkinsonian drugs, or agents to control akathisia).

Several investigators have studied clozapine's effects on preexisting tardive dyskinesia (TD; Caine et al. 1979; Gerbino et al. 1980; Lieberman et al. 1989a, 1991; Simpson and Varga 1974; Small et al. 1987a). Although these studies were small or uncontrolled, did not have effects on TD as a primary focus (Cole et al. 1980; Kane et al. 1988), or were just case reports (Blake et al. 1991; Van Putten et al. 1990), results from some indicated a therapeutic effect in reducing TD when at least moderate dosages of clozapine were given. The extent to which clozapine suppresses TD, corrects the underlying pathophysiology, or spares the striatum of chronic D_2 dopamine blockade (thereby allowing a spontaneous remission) needs to be determined by carefully designed studies.

Clozapine has been evaluated for its effects in treating tremor or L-dopa–induced psychosis. Pakkenberg and Pakkenberg (1986) evaluated the efficacy of low-dosage clozapine in the treatment of benign essential tremor, tremor of idiopathic Parkinson's disease (IPD), alcohol tremor, and tremor of multiple sclerosis. They concluded that clozapine in dosages of 75 mg or less was effective in reducing tremor in all of these disorders. Similarly, Friedman and Lannon (1990), Fischer et al. (1990), and Kahn et al. (1991) found low-dosage clozapine to be effective in reducing tremor of IPD. Factor and Brown (1992) reported that clozapine dosages as low as 6.25 mg every other day up to 75 mg/day were effective in treating and preventing the recurrence of drug-induced psychosis in IPD. Wolters et al. (1989) stated that although low-dosage (25–50 mg/day) clozapine might be effective in treating L-dopa–induced psychosis in IPD, higher dosages (100–250 mg) might exacerbate the parkinsonism or cause delirium. This caution contrasts with the case report by Friedman et al. (1987), who described the successful treatment of a patient with coexistent schizophrenia and IPD who took both L-dopa + carbidopa (Sinemet) and clozapine (300 mg/day) with good effect. There have been other case reports in which clozapine has been used to treat tremor in IPD (Pfeiffer et al. 1990; Roberts et al. 1989). Clearly, more work is needed to determine clozapine's place in these and other neurological or neuropsychiatric disorders.

Review of Adverse Effects

Were it not for its relatively high propensity to cause agranulocytosis, clozapine could likely be a first or second choice rather than a last resort, in the treatment of schizophrenia and other psychotic disorders. Many of the side effects that have been observed with clozapine could be predicted from its pharmacological properties. Other side effects (i.e., agranulocytosis) could not have been predicted or observed until clozapine was administered to large numbers of patients for extended periods of time.

In addition to its effects on dopamine neuronal systems, clozapine exhibits actions on multiple neurotransmitters, including antimuscarinic, antiserotonergic ($5\text{-}HT_2$, $5\text{-}HT_3$, $5\text{-}HT_{1A}$, $5\text{-}HT_{1B}$, and $5\text{-}HT_{1C}$), antiadrenergic (especially α_1, α_2, and β), and antihistaminic (H_1) activity (Coward 1992; Meltzer et al. 1989b). In addition, compared with most classical neuroleptics, clozapine has a weaker affinity for D_2 dopamine receptors (Richelson 1985) and a stronger affinity for D_1 (Andersen and Braestrup 1986) as well as D_4 receptors (Seeman 1992; Van Tol et al. 1991). Its affinity for D_1 relative to D_2 receptors is proportionally greater than that of typical neuroleptics (Farde et al. 1989). These pharmacodynamic properties may be partially responsible for clozapine's clinical efficacy as well as its adverse effects (Meltzer 1990).

The incidence of side effects reported with the use of clozapine varies widely in some cases because of differences in reporting methods, study design and duration (i.e., whether retrospective or prospective), dosing and titration strategies, definitions for a particular adverse reaction, frequency of monitoring for a particular side effect, and concomitant medications. Keeping this in mind, we list in Table 14–1 some of the more frequently observed side effects observed during clozapine treatment in premarketing studies in the United States.

Agranulocytosis

The most serious adverse effect of clozapine is *agranulocytosis,* which is often defined as a granulocyte count greater than $500/mm^3$. *Neutropenia* can also occur during treatment with clozapine and is defined as a neutrophil count greater than $1,000/mm^3$, with *leukopenia* being defined as a white blood cell (WBC) count of less than $3,500/mm^3$.

During clinical trials in Europe from 1962–1972, four cases of clozapine-induced agranulocytosis were reported. This translated into

Table 14–1. Selected adverse reactions reported with clozapine during premarketing studies by manufacturer[a]

Reaction[b]	Percentage of patients
Drowsiness or sedation	39
Salivation	31
Tachycardia	25 (1,700 patients)
Dizziness	19
Constipation	14
Nausea, vomiting	11
Hypotension	9
Sweating	6
Dry mouth	6
Tremor	6
Urinary problems	6
Visual disturbance	5
Fever	5
Hypertension	4
Weight gain	4
Seizures	3
Akathisia	3
Rigidity	3
Agranulocytosis	1 (1,700 patients)

[a]Data from premarketing studies by Sandoz ($N = 842$).
[b]Not reported: acute dystonic reactions, tardive dyskinesia, menstrual dysfunction, galactorrhea.
Source. Sandoz 1990.

a frequency of 4 cases per 2,900 patients, or 1.38 per 1,000 (Griffith and Saameli 1975), a figure that was comparable to the agranulocytosis rates reported with the phenothiazines (1/1,300) (Pisciotta 1973). However, 16 cases of agranulocytosis (out of an estimated 2,500–3,200 patients) were reported in the first 6 months of 1975 in the southern and western regions of Finland (Idanpaan-Heikkila et al. 1977). Despite the uneven geographic distribution and apparently higher rate of clozapine-induced agranulocytosis in Finland than elsewhere, no genetic or environmental risk factors could be determined (De la Chapelle et al. 1977). These events prompted Sandoz, the manufacturer of the drug, to withdraw clozapine from the market in some countries and to limit its use in others to treatment-resistant or neuroleptic-intolerant schizophrenic patients (provided that regular WBC monitoring was performed). Following that action, close hematologic monitoring significantly reduced the mortality rate.

Krupp and Barnes (1989) reviewed 185 cases of clozapine-induced agranulocytosis or neutropenia and made the following observations:

- The greatest risk of clozapine agranulocytosis is between weeks 4 and 18 after starting clozapine (77% of the cases occurred within the first 18 weeks of treatment).
- The rate of agranulocytosis among patients treated for 6 weeks or longer is 1%; however, if cumulative incidence is calculated after 1 year of treatment, the rate is 1.6%.
- The mean onset of agranulocytosis occurred after 67 days of exposure (range 2–1,065 days).
- The ratio of female to male cases was 1:0.56.

Krupp and Barnes concluded that 1) the mortality rate is significantly decreased in cases in which clozapine is immediately discontinued when agranulocytosis occurs, and if agranulocytosis is detected before signs of infection develop, and 2) regular WBC monitoring is essential in preventing fatalities. In a follow-up report involving 366 cases of clozapine-induced granulocytopenia, Krupp and Barnes (1992) did not revise their earlier findings.

Lieberman and Alvir (1992) reported on 11,555 patients who had received clozapine for at least 3 weeks. They found 73 cases of agranulocytosis, with a cumulative incidence rate of 0.8% and 0.91% after 1 and 1.5 years of treatment, respectively. Older and female patients were at significantly greater risk for agranulocytosis. A higher clozapine dosage (or cumulative dosage) did not appear to increase the risk. Incidence rates reported by Lieberman and Alvir were slightly lower than those in the Krupp and Barnes (1989) report, possibly because of early discontinuation of clozapine in those patients who may not have gone on to develop agranulocytosis (e.g., those with transient or benign neutropenia; Hummer et al. 1992). As in the Krupp and Barnes reports (1989, 1992), Lieberman and Alvir reported that the period of greatest risk was within the first 6 months of treatment (over 95% of cases), and that females were at greater risk for developing this side effect. The risk of agranulocytosis drops significantly beyond the 6-month point but is not entirely eliminated (Alvir et al. 1993).

In premarketing studies (up until September 1989) in the United States, the number of cases of agranulocytosis was 16 out of 1,743 patients. From February 6, 1990, to December 31, 1992, there were a total of 45,788 patients in the United States who had received clozapine (including those who continued on the drug from the premarketing period). During that period, there were 1,041 cases of leukopenia or granulocytopenia, and 198 reported cases of agranulocytosis in the United States (J. Schwimmer, Sandoz, personal communication, 1993). It would not be accurate to calculate an agranulocytosis incidence rate of 198 + 16/45,788, as these patients had been on clozapine for varying intervals and many had not yet entered or completed the full period of maximum risk for agranulocytosis. Accurate estimates of risk require a cumulative incidence that takes into account the length of exposure of those receiving the drug. The United States (premarketing) experience with clozapine-induced agranulocytosis is similar to that in Europe, with an estimated cumulative incidence of 2% after 1 year of treatment (Lieberman et al. 1988). There have been 12 deaths in the United States as a consequence of clozapine-induced agranulocytosis through October 1992 (Sandoz, personal communication, December 1994).

Lieberman et al. (1988) described the natural history of the clozapine-induced agranulocytosis that developed in five patients, all of whom were of Jewish descent. This provided evidence that there might be a genetically determined, selective vulnerability to this adverse effect. Onset of agranulocytosis was usually gradual and in all cases reversible over a period of about 2 weeks. A selective loss of granulocyte stem cells was found in bone marrow aspirates but other cell lines were unaffected. Because these patients were treated with numerous psychotropic medications before clozapine and after recovery without return of agranulocytosis, it was suggested that there was no cross-reactivity between clozapine and other drugs. In a follow-up study, Lieberman et al. (1990) examined the human leukocyte antigen (HLA) haplotype of patients who developed clozapine-induced agranulocytosis and found that the incidence of HLA-B38, -DR4, and -DQw3 (5 of 5 patients) was significantly increased in Jewish patients who developed clozapine-induced agranulocytosis compared with those who did not (only 2 of 17 patients). This was an important finding because it provided evidence for genetic vulnerability to developing clozapine-induced agranulocytosis that could lead to more efficient methods to reduce the risk (e.g., genetic screening). Pfister et al. (1992) described a case of clozapine-induced agranulocytosis in a native American Indian who had haplotypes HLA B-16 (variant B39, DR4, DqW3), thereby lending support to Lieberman et al.'s (1990) findings.

Claas et al. (1992) performed an HLA study in non-Jewish patients, comparing 103 patients with clozapine-induced granulocytopenia with 95 matched control subjects. There was no statistically significant association between HLA alleles and clozapine-induced granulocytopenia. Further studies are under way in the United States to resolve the issue of whether HLA typing can be a useful tool for reliably predicting agranulocytosis in at least certain populations (e.g., Ashkenazi Jews).

Guidelines and parameters for the management of a drop in the WBC count have been published by the manufacturer of clozapine (Sandoz 1990). Any fever or sign of infection (e.g., pharyngitis) is an immediate indication for a WBC count, especially within weeks 4 to 8 of beginning treatment. If the patient has a WBC count below 2,000 or a granulocyte count below 1,000, clozapine must be permanently discontinued. In addition, a drop in the WBC count to between 3,000 and 3,500 requires at least twice-weekly WBC counts with differential. A WBC count of 2,000–3,000 or neutrophil count of 1,000–1,500 requires clozapine treatment to be suspended and daily WBC counts with differential performed until the WBC count normalizes. Weekly blood counts should include the differential because of the possibility of severe neutropenia occurring in the absence of leukopenia (Cates et al. 1992).

The mechanism of clozapine-induced agranulocytosis remains unclear, but evidence favors an immune-mediated mechanism. Pisciotta et al. (1992) identified a cytotoxic factor in serum from patients with clozapine agranulocytosis that can be neutralized by complement-dependent anti-IgM. In a review by Safferman et al. (1992a), nine patients who developed agranulocytosis on clozapine were subsequently rechallenged with clozapine following their hematologic recovery. Eight of the nine patients redeveloped agranulocytosis in approximately 50% less time than with their initial exposure, lending further support to an immune-mediated mechanism. Gerson and Meltzer (1992) proposed that a toxic mechanism might be responsible for agranulocytosis. They suggested that some patients might have heightened sensitivity to the cytotoxic effects of *N*-desmethylclozapine, a common metabolite of clozapine. They suggested that, alternatively, some patients have elevated levels of *N*-desmethylclozapine because of different patterns of clozapine metabolism, thereby achieving toxic concentrations.

Another interesting hypothesis is that neutrophils and their committed stem cell precursors can metabolize clozapine into metabolites that are free radicals—and, as such, cytotoxic (Mason and Fischer 1992). This has led some to suggest that (clozapine-induced) agranulocytosis might be prevented by administering vitamin C (Mason and Fischer 1992) and other antioxidants (vitamin E) or by augmenting the activity of free-radical–scavenging enzymes with trace element enzyme cofactors such as selenium, zinc, and copper (Pippenger et al. 1991).

Although low WBC counts are not proven to be a risk factor, it is suggested that patients with WBC levels below 3,500 not receive clozapine because of the difficulty that would be involved in the early identification of agranulocytosis. In addition, drugs that have a relatively high likelihood of causing neutropenia (e.g., carbamazepine) should not be coadministered with clozapine because of the potential additive risk of agranulocytosis (Gerson et al. 1991) or the difficulties involved in following patients with a benign drug-induced (e.g., carbamazepine) neutropenia.

Other hematologic changes that have been described with clozapine include leukocytosis (Lieberman et al. 1988), eosinophilia, the leukopenia-neutropenia–decreased-WBC syndrome (Sandoz 1990), thrombocytopenia (Panteleeva et al. 1987), and mild anemia (Gerson et al. 1991). Eosinophilia may occur with leukocytosis (Stricker and Tielens 1991; Tiihonen and Paanila 1992) and may be more prevalent than is widely believed (Banov et al. 1993; Battegay et al. 1977). Eosinophilia induced by clozapine is usually of no clinical significance and in most cases will not require discontinuation; however, it could mask a decline in the neutrophil fraction if only a WBC count without a differential is obtained.

Clozapine-induced agranulocytosis is time limited once clozapine is discontinued, with uncomplicated cases lasting 2–3 weeks. Although most often gradual in onset, there have been cases in which the onset of agranulocytosis has been precipitous (e.g., within days of a previously normal neutrophil count). Identification of affected patients prior to the onset of sepsis results in less morbidity and mortality. Some investigators have shortened bone marrow recovery time in clozapine-induced agranulocytosis by administering granulocyte-macrophage colony stimulating factor (Barnas et al. 1992) and granulocyte colony stimulating factor (Weide et al. 1992). Although experience is still limited for this use, it appears to be well tolerated and effective in at least some cases.

Seizures and Other Central Nervous System Effects

Like other antipsychotic medications, clozapine has been found to produce electroencephalographic changes (Koukkou et al. 1979; Schmauss et al. 1989; Small et al. 1987b; Tiihonen et al. 1991) that are dosage related (Leppig et al. 1989), and it also causes a relatively greater incidence of grand mal seizures than do standard neuroleptic agents (Baker and Conley 1991; Devinsky et al. 1991; Haller and

Binder 1990; Lieberman et al. 1989b; Povlsen et al. 1985; Simpson and Cooper 1978). The risk of seizures is dosage related: dosages up to 300 mg/day carry a risk of 1%–2%; 300–600 mg/day, 3%–4%; and 600–900 mg/day, 5% (Sandoz 1990). A preexisting seizure disorder or history of head trauma places the patient at even higher risk for seizures (Haller and Binder 1990; Povlsen et al. 1985). Devinsky et al. (1991) reported that the cumulative seizure rate with clozapine treatment for up to 3 years approaches 9%.

Various guidelines have been suggested to minimize or manage this risk, including obtaining an electroencephalogram (EEG) prior to raising the dosage above 600 mg/day, combining clozapine with an anticonvulsant at dosages at which a seizure previously occurred (Haller and Binder 1990), monitoring clozapine blood levels (Simpson and Cooper 1978), and reducing the dosage to 50% of the dosage at which a seizure occurred and obtaining a neurological consultation (Lieberman et al. 1989b). Tiihonen et al. (1991) suggested that there is no need to alter clozapine treatment as long as there are no epileptiform changes on EEGs.

As a general rule, it is important to look for other causes of seizures and to avoid combining clozapine with other drugs that lower the seizure threshold. If the clinician decides to taper any medications that raise the seizure threshold (e.g., benzodiazepines, anticonvulsants), this should be done very slowly if the patient is receiving clozapine to avoid precipitating seizures. Avoidance of other drugs known to reduce the seizure threshold (e.g., tricyclics, bupropion, lithium), adhering to slow titration rates, and using the minimum effective dosage of clozapine (Baker and Conley 1991) should reduce the incidence of seizures.

Combining anticonvulsants with clozapine, although sometimes necessary, can significantly alter blood levels of each drug. For example, phenytoin has been reported to significantly lower clozapine blood levels because of its effects in inducing hepatic microsomal P-450 enzymes (D. D. Miller 1991). Carbamazepine may also reduce clozapine blood levels through induction of hepatic microsomal enzymes (Raitasuo et al. 1992). The use of carbamazepine is to be avoided, given the relatively high incidence of benign neutropenia as well as a possibly additive risk of agranulocytosis associated with it.

Although it has not been systematically investigated for potential pharmacokinetic interactions, valproic acid appears to be the anticonvulsant of choice, as it may be less likely to affect clozapine blood levels and is usually well tolerated. A clozapine-induced seizure is not usually a contraindication to restarting clozapine if some of the suggestions outlined above are implemented.

There have also been reports of myoclonic movements—and, rarely, cataplectic-like events (Lieberman et al. 1989b; Lindstrom 1988) in which the patient described a sudden loss of muscle tone in a part of the body without loss of consciousness—with clozapine treatment. Some investigators have contended that this side effect is often subtle and, hence, underreported (Chiles et al. 1990). Berman et al. (1992) suggested that clozapine-induced cataplexy and myoclonus are themselves seizures and are an indication that the patient is at a very high risk of developing a grand mal seizure. This problem can usually be eliminated by reducing the clozapine dosage, adding valproic acid, or both.

Sedation is the most common side effect seen with clozapine and is experienced by most patients. It is prominent early in treatment, but at least partial tolerance develops over the first few weeks (Lieberman et al. 1989b; Lindstrom 1988). Sedation may be minimized by giving either the larger portion or the entire dosage at bedtime and by avoiding coadministration of other central nervous system (CNS) depressants. The sedative effects associated with clozapine may be related to its antihistaminic (H_1) and antiadrenergic (α_1) properties.

Other CNS effects reported include dizziness, syncope, and confusion (Sandoz 1990). Dizziness and syncope are most likely caused by orthostatic hypotension. As with sedation, tolerance may occur with continued treatment. Patients beginning treatment should be instructed to avoid rising suddenly from a seated or supine position.

Confusion or toxic delirium may occur with clozapine (Banki and Vojnik 1978; Grohmann et al. 1989; Naber et al. 1989; Szymanski et al. 1991a). This effect has been successfully—albeit transiently—reversed by intravenous physostigmine (Gerbino et al. 1980; Schuster et al. 1977), thereby providing evidence that the delirious states associated with clozapine may in some cases be a manifestation of CNS anticholinergic toxicity.

Transient emergence of obsessive-compulsive symptoms during clozapine treatment have been reported (Patil 1992). This phenomenon may be related to clozapine's potent central antiserotonergic activity.

Hypersalivation

Sialorrhea is a commonly reported side effect that develops early in the course of treatment (Sandoz 1990). This is an unexpected adverse reaction because clozapine is anticholinergic and has a low incidence of EPS. Hypersalivation is most pronounced during sleep and may be voluminous. Patients can be told to cover their pillow with a towel or cloth. Treating this problem with anticholinergic agents may be effective (Ereshefsky et al. 1989) but will heighten the risk of toxicity (Lieberman et al. 1989b). This side effect is an infrequent cause of discontinuing treatment and, although some tolerance occurs, the effect is often persistent even after several years of treatment. Different receptors located on salivary glands, including adrenergic (α and β) (Mandel et al. 1975), muscarinic (Ukai et al. 1989), and the tachykinin substance P (Kaniucki et al. 1984), can alter salivary flow or composition. It is conceivable that the contribution of alterations in peripheral adrenergic tone and substance P can override the antimuscarinic effects of clozapine at the level of the salivary glands. Clonidine (an α_2 agonist) is sometimes effective in reducing this adverse effect (Grabowski 1992). Sweating, dry mouth, and visual disturbances (e.g., blurred vision) have also been observed.

Cardiovascular and Respiratory Effects

Cardiovascular side effects frequently encountered are tachycardia and postural hypotension. The tachycardia may be related to clozapine's direct vagolytic effects, increases in plasma norepinephrine, or both (Pickar et al. 1992). It can be found when the patient is resting in a supine position and therefore is not simply attributable to orthostatic changes. Increased pulse rates of between 20 and 25 beats per minute were found when clozapine was titrated to 300 mg/day over a 7-day period (Sandoz NDA [unpublished document] 1987). Although some tolerance may occur, in many cases the tachycardia will persist unless the dosage is reduced. As an alternative, adding a beta-blocker such as atenolol may be helpful (Lieberman et al. 1989b) if the patient's blood pressure permits it. Postural hypotension is related to clozapine's antiadrenergic properties. Early studies using initial dosages of greater than 75 mg/day resulted in a very high incidence of orthostatic collapse (Sandoz NDA [unpublished document] 1987). Tolerance often develops over time and this problem may be avoided when the initial dosage is low (e.g., 25 mg/day) and the titration schedule is gradual. It can usually be managed by a dosage reduction or adjunctive treatment (e.g., support stockings, increased sodium intake, fludrocortisone) (Lieberman et al. 1989b). Sinus tachycardia is the most commonly encountered abnormal electrocardiogram (ECG) finding. Reversible, nonspecific ST–T wave changes or T wave flattening or inversions (repolarization effects) are seen infrequently but in most instances are of no clinical significance. Clozapine-induced arrhythmias have been observed but occur rarely at therapeutic dosages. These ECG findings are comparable to those seen with other antipsychotics (Sandoz NDA [unpublished document] 1987) and are dosage dependent.

Sudden-death events have not been seen more frequently with clozapine than with other available antipsychotic agents. Hypertension has also been reported to occur. Because clozapine frequently produces clinically relevant hemodynamic changes, it should be used with great caution in patients with preexisting cardiovascular disease (e.g, history of myocardial infarction, history of arrhythmias). Close monitoring of vital signs is advised in all patients during the first few weeks of treatment.

There have been a small number of cases of respiratory depression associated with initiation of clozapine treatment, especially in those patients who are also taking benzodiazepines. Although this event is rather uncommon, it is suggested that use of benzodiazepines and other CNS depressants be minimized or avoided altogether when initiating clozapine.

Gastrointestinal Effects

The most common gastrointestinal side effect is constipation. Nausea, heartburn, and vomiting occur less frequently. The antimuscarinic effects of clozapine are believed to be largely responsible for causing constipation. This should be treated symptomatically with stool softeners, laxatives, fiber supplements, and adequate fluid intake. Failure to treat this symptom could result in intestinal obstruction. Nausea—and, less frequently, vomiting—may be managed by dosage reduction, antacids, or both. H_2 blockers such as ranitidine may be effective in relieving these gastrointestinal disturbances, but cimetidine should be avoided, as it may elevate clozapine blood levels through its inhibition of hepatic microsomal cytochrome P-450 enzymes (Szymanski et al. 1991b). Metoclopramide has been suggested (Lieberman et al. 1989b) to manage these effects, but others recommend avoiding this and other dopamine D_2 blockers because of their EPS (Jenkins and Metzer 1990).

Liver function abnormalities have been reported (Kane et al. 1988; Kirkegaard and Jensen 1979; Leppig et al. 1989; Naber et al. 1989). These changes have been relatively mild, transient, and of no clinical consequence. However, at least one case report of cholestatic jaundice has been reported (Dorta et al. 1989). It is prudent to obtain a baseline liver enzyme profile and to periodically monitor this, especially during the initial stages of treatment and after dosage increases. Pancreatitis has rarely been observed during clozapine treatment (Frankenburg and Kando 1992; Martin 1992).

Urogenital Effects

Urogenital effects seen with clozapine have included incontinence (enuresis), frequency or urgency difficulties, hesitancy problems, urinary retention, retrograde ejaculation, priapism, and impotence. Because these symptoms may be embarrassing for patients and not readily volunteered, it behooves the physician to inquire about them, as failure to do so may result in medical complications, noncompliance, and a further deterioration in the quality of life for these patients. Clozapine may produce these effects through alterations in muscarinic and adrenergic transmission. Because clozapine may produce urinary retention, it is suggested that the drug should be avoided in patients with symptomatic prostatic hypertrophy and other preexisting conditions that involve an incomplete voiding of urine from the bladder.

It is difficult to accurately quantify the incidence of sexual dysfunction (i.e., decreased libido, impotence, ejaculatory dysfunction, or anorgasmia) in chronically psychotic patients (Sullivan and Lukoff 1990), and it is not clear to what extent clozapine differs from typical neuroleptics in this regard. Clozapine's weak D_2 dopamine receptor–blocking effects coupled with an increased activity of tuberoinfundibular dopamine neurons (Gudelsky and Meltzer 1989) may explain its inability to produce sustained hyperprolactinemia (Kane et al. 1981; Meltzer et al. 1979). The loosely bound clozapine on the D_2 receptors of the lactotrophs would be displaced by endogenously released dopamine. Therefore, the secondary effects of hyperprolactinemia, such as amenorrhea, galactorrhea, and gynecomastia, are not observed. One consequence of this is the increased fertility attributable to the absence of hyperprolactinemia. Priapism has rarely been associated with clozapine treatment (Rosen and Hanno 1992; Seftel et al. 1992; Ziegler and Behar 1992).

Thermoregulation

When it occurs, benign hyperthermia is seen within the first 3 weeks of starting clozapine, with a peak incidence on the tenth day (Sandoz NDA [unpublished document] 1987). It usually involves an increase of 1–2°F, spontaneously resolves over a few days with continued clozapine treatment, and is of no clinical significance. However, in some cases, temperature elevations well above 101°F can be seen. When this occurs, clozapine should be temporarily withheld and frequent hematologic monitoring performed. Differential diagnoses can include drug fever, intercurrent infection, infection secondary to agranulocytosis, dehydration, heat stroke, "lethal" catatonia, and neuroleptic malignant syndrome (NMS). Patients who have developed a high fever may be offered clozapine a second time, but the dosage titration schedule should be more gradual. If this strategy is not successful, clozapine may need to be avoided.

Mild hypothermia is observed in a large proportion of patients (87%) on clozapine. This effect is seen just as frequently with chlorpromazine and presumably by extension with other classical neuroleptics. The precise mechanism by which clozapine causes temperature dysregulation is not known but is believed to be mediated by the hypothalamus (Heh et al. 1988).

Weight Changes

Weight gain has been reported to occur with clozapine (Carson and Forbes 1990; S. Cohen et al. 1990; Leadbetter and Viewig 1990; Povlsen et al. 1985; Schmauss et al. 1989). Clozapine appears no less likely to cause weight gain than other neuroleptics and may have a greater weight-increasing effect (Lamberti et al. 1992; Leadbetter et al. 1992; Lieberman et al. 1989b; Sandoz NDA [unpublished document] 1987). This side effect may be related, in part, to clozapine's antiserotonergic and antihistaminic (H_1) activity.

Extrapyramidal System Effects

Acute extrapyramidal effects.   Unlike typical neuroleptic drugs, clozapine causes a very low incidence of EPS (Claghorn et al. 1987; Kane et al. 1988; Lindstrom 1988; Matz et al. 1974; Povlsen et al. 1985). It is widely known that noncompliance with antipsychotic medication is an all too common problem. One important reason given for neuroleptic medication noncompliance is the occurrence of EPS, particularly akathisia (Van Putten 1974). Consistent with the reported low incidence of EPS with clozapine, Claghorn et al. (1987) found that only 1 of 75 patients treated with clozapine had to be withdrawn from their study because of EPS, compared with 11 of 76 chlorpromazine-treated patients. If hypersalivation is excluded as an extrapyramidal effect (Casey 1989), the frequency of EPS such as tremor, akathisia, and rigidity is significantly lower with clozapine than with standard antipsychotic agents (Ayd 1961). B. M. Cohen et al. (1991) reported that the frequency of akathisia with clozapine is similar to that seen with typical antipsychotic agents. This has been questioned by others who have suggested that B. M. Cohen et al. (1991) compared dissimilar patient populations, nonequivalent dosages, and dissimilar durations of treatment and overlooked the possibility of persistent or tardive akathisia (Safferman et al. 1992b). In addition, there is evidence of a decrease in persistent or tardive akathisia with chronic treatment and higher dosages of clozapine (Safferman et al. 1993). There are no published reports of acute dystonic reactions with clozapine. On this basis alone, one can expect that patients will be more compliant with clozapine than with typical agents. At the same time, it might be suggested that there is an inherent bias toward selecting more compliant patients for clozapine, as they all must accept weekly phlebotomy in order to receive the drug.

Tardive dyskinesia. In one large prospective study, it was determined that the overall incidence of TD after cumulative exposure to typical neuroleptics is 18.5% after 4 years, 40% after 8 years (Kane et al. 1986), and 44% after 10 years (Kane et al. 1994). The TD incidence is even higher in patients over the age of 55 years, with rates reported as high as 31% after only 43 weeks of cumulative neuroleptic exposure (Saltz et al. 1991). Thus, it is striking that, to date, there have been only three cases of TD attributed to clozapine treatment (de Leon et al. 1991; Kane et al. 1993). Attributing TD to clozapine is open to question in these cases because all three patients were exposed to typical neuroleptics prior to receiving clozapine, and two had questionable dyskinesia ratings prior to clozapine treatment. Even if clozapine can produce TD, the incidence is certain to be substantially lower than that seen with typical antipsychotics.

Neuroleptic malignant syndrome. In keeping with clozapine's weak D_2 dopamine-blocking effects in the striatum, clozapine would not be expected to produce NMS. However, there are at least two case reports of apparent NMS when clozapine was combined with lithium (Pope et al. 1986) and with carbamazepine (Muller et al. 1988). In both cases, the patients had previously experienced NMS with typical neuroleptic agents. In addition, cases of classic NMS in which clozapine was the sole agent have now been reported (Anderson and Powers 1991; DasGupta and Young 1991; D. M. Miller et al. 1991). Stoudemire and Clayton (1989) reported that clozapine was safely used in one patient with a prior history of NMS after treatment with typical neuroleptics. Anderson and Powers's (1991) patient had a history of NMS with typical neuroleptics and also redeveloped it with clozapine. However, they were able to successfully rechallenge the patient with clozapine without recurrence of NMS. It is therefore suggested that the best approach is to avoid giving clozapine in combination with lithium or carbamazepine (carbamazepine should be avoided for other reasons, as well) in patients with a history of NMS. In addition, because clozapine can induce signs that overlap with those seen in NMS (e.g., hyperthermia, cardiovascular effects, delirium, diaphoresis, elevations in creatine phosphokinase, leukocytosis [Levenson 1985]), increased vigilance is warranted in the identification and diagnosis of NMS in patients being treated with clozapine. Indeed, some investigators have described cases of atypical NMS in which patients receiving clozapine developed all the characteristic signs of the syndrome with the exception of rigidity (Goates and Escobar 1992; Nopoulos et al. 1990). Controversy exists as to whether NMS without muscular rigidity is really a valid subtype of NMS (Roth et al. 1986).

Rebound Psychosis

There have been a few reports of rapid return of psychotic symptoms after abrupt discontinuation of clozapine (Borison et al. 1988; Ekblom et al. 1984; Eklund 1987; Perenyi et al. 1985). Although these investigators have linked this return to a "supersensitivity psychosis" (supersensitivity of the mesolimbic system), as described by Chouinard et al. (1978), others question its existence (Singh et al. 1990). We have observed seven patients abruptly withdrawn from clozapine following the development of agranulocytosis and did not see a rebound psychosis. However, we have also observed three patients whose psychosis worsened or reemerged within 1–3 weeks after clozapine was withdrawn. It is more likely that what is being observed in these cases is the rapid elimination of the pharmacodynamic effects of clozapine because of its relatively weak affinity for central dopamine receptors rather than a supersensitivity psychosis. It is also important to consider the nature of the patient population receiving clozapine before assuming a specific drug effect. When clinical circumstances permit, clozapine should be tapered gradually to avoid withdrawal symptoms such as diaphoresis, diarrhea, restlessness, and insomnia.

Discussion

The decision to use clozapine represents a challenge to the clinician because of the complexities involved in accurately assessing its risks and benefits. In the previous section, we reviewed the two most important variables of the benefit-risk equation: clinical efficacy and adverse effects of clozapine. We now discuss these in greater detail.

Benefits and Advantages

Our review suggests that there is compelling evidence of clozapine's superior efficacy over typical antipsychotic agents in the treatment of severely ill, neuroleptic-refractory schizophrenic patients. The claim that clozapine is superior in reducing the negative symptoms of schizophrenia requires further investigation. This advantage in treating negative symptoms has been conclusively demonstrated only within the context of coexisting positive symptomatology. Others have concluded that clozapine is comparable in efficacy to haloperidol in treating negative symptoms (Angst et al. 1989). To our knowledge, there is no direct proof that clozapine is superior to other antipsychotics when negative symptoms are the sole or predominant psychopathology. In addition, when evaluating clozapine's effects on negative symptoms in the context of a comparative trial between clozapine and a classical neuroleptic, the potentially confounding effects of acute EPS (e.g., akinesia) must be considered. Thus, the question of whether clozapine has therapeutic effects on negative symptoms remains to be answered.

Another major advantage of clozapine is its favorable acute EPS profile, even in those patients with a known sensitivity to this side effect. Very few patients who were treated with clozapine in both short-term prospective and long-term retrospective studies discontinued treatment because of EPS. Because the occurrence of EPS is a major reason that patients do not comply with treatment with neuroleptic medications, clozapine has another distinct advantage over typical antipsychotic agents in terms of its tolerability. Another aspect of its favorable acute EPS profile is that clozapine may not produce TD.

The claim that clozapine does not cause TD will be put to the test as its use in large numbers of patients is extended over very long periods of time (Casey 1989). A small number of studies have demonstrated that clozapine may actually be an effective treatment for some TD patients, especially those with severe variants such as tardive dystonia (Lieberman et al. 1991). Further studies will determine if this is another advantage that clozapine can offer.

Unlike typical agents, clozapine also offers the advantage of not causing a sustained hyperprolactinemic state and its attendant secondary adverse effects. This may also serve to enhance medication compliance in some patients, particularly women with oligomenorrhea or amenorrhea from classical neuroleptic treatment. It may increase the likelihood of pregnancy in those women because they are no longer hyperprolactinemic. There have been a small number of women who have taken clozapine throughout pregnancy with no known adverse effects to their newborns (M. Krassner, personal communication, 1993; Waldman and Safferman 1992).

Risks and Disadvantages

The most frequent adverse effects seen with clozapine are sedation, hypersalivation, dizziness, tachycardia, hypotension, and constipation. These are usually manageable or tolerated, and in some cases may disappear with continued treatment. Most side effects can be minimized or avoided by a gradual dosage titration and by using the lowest effective dosage. A recommended dosage titration schedule has been published by Sandoz (1990). Titrating the clozapine dosage more quickly than the guidelines suggest may be problematic because the incidence and intensity of some side effects associated with its use rise dramatically. Sandoz now suggests an initial clozapine dosage of 12.5 mg once or twice a day (W. Westlin, Sandoz, personal communication, 1992) to minimize risk of orthostasis and syncope.

The adverse effects of primary concern include agranulocytosis and, to a lesser extent, seizures. The period of maximum risk of clozapine-induced agranulocytosis is the first 4–18 weeks. However, it should be emphasized that although the risk of agranulocytosis appears to decline after this period, it does not fall to zero. Therefore, the risk-benefit ratio may change over time. Fatalities can be prevented only if regular hematologic monitoring is strictly maintained. Clearly, patients must be willing to comply with this requirement on an ongoing basis; this requirement may preclude clozapine's use in some patients.

Despite the controversy that has surrounded it, the Clozaril Patient Monitoring System (CPMS) has largely succeeded in preventing fatalities, thereby demonstrating that the risk associated with clozapine-induced agranulocytosis is a manageable one. Alternatives to CPMS (Caremark Homecare and Sandoz) have been developed and thus far have achieved the same high level of patient safety standards. However, there continues to be a very small number of deaths reported each year in Europe and the United States associated with clozapine-induced agranulocytosis. Most of these deaths have occurred within the first 18 weeks of treatment. Seven deaths attributable to clozapine-induced agranulocytosis have occurred despite the fact that the patients in question had their blood counts monitored weekly. The persistence of fatalities, albeit in small numbers, emphasizes the need for continued careful surveillance and prompt intervention at any sign of fever or infection.

Indications

There remain numerous questions as to who should receive a trial of clozapine. At present, the indications approved by the FDA are for severely ill schizophrenic patients who have failed to respond adequately to treatment with appropriate courses of standard antipsychotic drugs because of either insufficient effectiveness or inability to achieve an effective dosage as the result of intolerable adverse effects from these drugs. Clearly, a variety of issues require clinical judgment (e.g., how adequate response or intolerable adverse effects should be defined or measured). In addition, it is well recognized that drug labeling is only one of several sources of prescribing information on which a physician must base a judgment regarding the treatment of an individual patient.

No clearly established, well-validated criteria are available for defining treatment refractoriness; however, the criteria in the Kane et al.

(1988) study did lead to the selection of individuals who had failed to respond to trials of haloperidol and chlorpromazine but among whom 30% benefited from clozapine. It should be kept in mind, however, as emphasized by Marder and Van Putten (1988), that these patients were severely ill, with a mean BPRS total score of 61 at baseline.

Whether or not these criteria are too stringent remains to be determined, and as Marder and Van Putten noted, there is a very large population of inpatients and outpatients with schizophrenia who have had a suboptimal response to neuroleptics, but who would not necessarily meet the Kane et al. (1988) criteria for refractoriness. The indications for clozapine in these patients remain to be determined, but some earlier trials with clozapine seem to support its value among inpatients who respond below optimal levels (Claghorn et al. 1987; Fischer-Cornelssen and Ferner 1976).

Questions also remain as how many trials of how many different drugs and at what dosages should be implemented before considering a patient a candidate for clozapine. Clinicians should also consider the possibility that patients are noncompliant or idiosyncratic metabolizers with resulting low blood levels despite what would generally be considered an adequate oral dosage. The measurement of neuroleptic blood levels and the use of parenterally administered medication (to ensure compliance, increase bioavailability, and reduce first-pass hepatic metabolism) are approaches to be considered in those nonresponsive to treatment, perhaps prior to using clozapine.

It is important to emphasize that not all patients will benefit from clozapine, but for the subgroup that does, the effects may be very positive, not just in terms of reducing psychopathology but also in terms of making the patient more amenable and responsive to renewed efforts at psychosocial and vocational therapies. Obviously, any improvement in psychopathology in a patient who has been chronically ill is only one step toward overcoming disabilities in a variety of areas.

Another question that often arises is how to approach patients who have not shown a response after receiving clozapine for 12 weeks. Treatment strategies for those nonresponsive to clozapine could include continuing clozapine up to an additional 12 weeks at the same or greater dosages; increasing the dosage of clozapine to achieve a plasma level of at least 350 ng/ml (Perry et al. 1991); and instituting adjunctive treatments, including typical neuroleptics, lithium, anticonvulsants, antidepressants, and electroconvulsive therapy (Safferman and Munne 1992). These approaches have not been systematically investigated but have been helpful in some cases.

Ideally, we would like to have predictors of clozapine response to help clinicians identify those patients most likely to benefit from the medication. Attempts at identifying such predictors have not been very rewarding to date (Honigfeld and Patin 1989), but further research is necessary. Pickar et al. (1992) have provided some evidence that high levels of EPS with fluphenazine predicted a good response to clozapine.

Other Considerations in Clozapine Treatment

There also continues to be debate and uncertainty as to what represents an adequate trial of clozapine. To date, there have been no well-designed, dosage-ranging studies to determine what the optimal dosage of clozapine should be. Toward this end, it is apparent that significantly different dosing practices have developed throughout the world. For example, clinicians in the United States have thus far tended to use higher dosages than have clinicians in most European countries (e.g., Germany). By extension, a related issue potentially affecting clozapine's efficacy has been the question of clozapine blood levels. Although some studies examined variables that may affect clozapine blood levels (Haring et al. 1990), there is little guidance from the literature as to what constitutes a therapeutic range or minimum threshold (Perry et al. 1991).

Investigators have attempted to determine the appropriate duration of a treatment trial. As was mentioned earlier, Meltzer et al. (1989a) conducted an open, uncontrolled prospective study of 51 treatment-resistant patients with an average treatment duration of over 10 months. Only 45% of patients who ultimately responded could be identified within the first 6 weeks. In the end, about 60% of the patients responded when clozapine treatment was extended up to 1 year. Meltzer et al. therefore suggested that a 6- to 12-month trial of clozapine be given to identify all who might respond to the drug. Doing this, however, would subject patients to the period of maximum risk for developing clozapine-induced agranulocytosis. Nearly

75% of the patients in Meltzer et al.'s study were identified as responsive to the medication by the third month of treatment. In addition, all of the improvement in QLS (Heinrichs et al. 1984) scores was seen by week 12 of clozapine treatment. Owen et al. (1989) also suggested that the largest amount of improvement in BPRS scores occurred within the first 12 weeks of treatment. In open, uncontrolled trials taking place in the context of high expectations and intensive psychosocial therapy, it is difficult to know to what those gains occurring over a period of many months should be attributed. Therefore, given clozapine's risks (and current cost), we believe that more justification exists for a 3-month trial of clozapine.

It is essential that clinicians identify and assess target signs and symptoms in order to make a considered judgment as to whether clozapine should be continued beyond the initial acute treatment trial. No guidelines have been suggested for this decision, and each case should be viewed individually, weighing all benefits and risks. Patients and their families should be involved in the decision to use clozapine. The potential benefits and risks as well as the monitoring required should be clearly explained, and this educational process should be documented in the medical record.

It is hoped that the availability of clozapine will stimulate further research to help evaluate other potential indications for its use. In the meantime, clinicians who use this compound for indications not currently included in the labeling should have compelling and carefully documented reasons for doing so as well as informed consent.

It is hoped that ongoing research will help to clarify the most appropriate dosage range for acute treatment, the appropriate length of trial, and the predictive factors that might help identify those who will potentially respond to the drug. With more extensive experience, it may be possible to clarify the time course of agranulocytosis risk. If, for example, the risk of agranulocytosis occurring after 1 year is no greater than that associated with phenothiazines, the frequency of required WBC monitoring could be reduced. At the same time, if further progress is made in identifying risk factors for or the pathophysiologic mechanism of agranulocytosis, strategies might be developed to reduce overall incidence of this adverse reaction. Any increase that can be achieved in the benefit-risk ratio will in all likelihood expand the indications for and utilization of clozapine. Clearly, this compound continues to present both opportunity and challenge to the field.

References

Alvir JMJ, Lieberman JA, Safferman AZ, et al: Clozapine-induced agranulocytosis. N Engl J Med 329:162–167, 1993

Andersen PH, Braestrup C: Evidence for different states of the dopamine D₁ receptor: clozapine and fluperlapine may preferentially label an adenylate cyclase-coupled state of the D₁ receptor. J Neurochem 47:1822–1831, 1986

Anderson ES, Powers PS: Neuroleptic malignant syndrome associated with clozapine use. J Clin Psychiatry 52:102–104, 1991

Angst J, Stassen HH, Woggon B: Effect of neuroleptics on positive and negative symptoms and the deficit state. Psychopharmacology (Berl) S41–S46, 1989

Ayd FJ: A survey of drug-induced extrapyramidal reactions. JAMA 175:1054–1060, 1961

Baker RW, Conley RR: Seizures during clozapine therapy (letter). Am J Psychiatry 148:1265–1266, 1991

Banki CM, Vojnik M: Cooperative simultaneous measurement of cerebrospinal fluid 5-hydroxyindoleacetic acid and blood serotonin levels in delirium tremens and clozapine-induced delirious reaction. J Neurol Neurosurg Psychiatry 41:420–424, 1978

Banov MD, Tohen M, Friedburg J: High risk of eosinophilia in women treated with clozapine. J Clin Psychiatry 54:466–469, 1993

Barnas C, Zwierzina H, Hummer M, et al: Granulocyte-macrophage colony stimulating factor (GM-CSF) treatment of clozapine-induced agranulocytosis: a case report. J Clin Psychiatry 53:245–247, 1992

Battegay R, Cotar B, Fleischhauer J, et al: Results and side effects of treatment with clozapine (Leponex R). Compr Psychiatry 18:423–428, 1977

Berman I, Zalma A, DuRand CJ, et al: Clozapine-induced myoclonic jerks and drop attacks. J Clin Psychiatry 53:329–330, 1992

Blake LM, Marks RC, Nierman P, et al: Clozapine and clonazepam in tardive dystonia (letter). J Clin Psychopharmacol 11:268–269, 1991

Borison RL, Diamond BI, Sinha D, et al: Clozapine withdrawal rebound psychosis. Psychopharmacol Bull 24:260–263, 1988

Caine ED, Polinsky RJ, Kartzinel R, et al: The trial use of clozapine for abnormal involuntary movement disorders. Am J Psychiatry 136:317–320, 1979

Carson WH, Forbes RA: Clozapine-induced weight gain (letter). Am J Psychiatry 147:1694, 1990

Casey DE: Clozapine: neuroleptic-induced EPS and tardive dyskinesia. Psychopharmacology (Berl) 99:S47–S53, 1989

Cates M, Lusk K, Wells BG: Nonleukopenic neutropenia in a patient treated with clozapine. N Engl J Med 326:840–841, 1992

Chiles JA, Cohen S, McNaughton A: Dropping objects: possible mild cataplexy associated with clozapine. J Nerv Ment Dis 175:663–664, 1990

Chiu E, Burrows G, Stevenson J: Double-blind comparison of clozapine in acute schizophrenic illness. Aust N Z J Med 10:343, 1976

Chouinard G, Annable L: Clozapine in the treatment of newly admitted schizophrenic patients: a pilot study. J Clin Pharmacol 16:289–297, 1976

Chouinard G, Jones BD, Annable L: Neuroleptic-induced supersensitivity psychosis. Am J Psychiatry 135:1409–1410, 1978

Claas FHJ, Abbott PA, Witvliet MD, et al: No direct clinical relevance of the human leukocyte antigen (HLA) system in clozapine-induced agranulocytosis. Drug Saf 7 (suppl 1):3–6, 1992

Claghorn J, Honigfeld G, Abuzzahab F, et al: The risks and benefits of clozapine versus chlorpromazine. J Clin Psychopharmacol 7:377–384, 1987

Cohen BM, Keck PE, Satlin A, et al: Prevalence and severity of akathisia in patients on clozapine. Biol Psychiatry 29:1215–1219, 1991

Cohen S, Chiles J, McNaughton A: Weight gain associated with clozapine. Am J Psychiatry 147:503–504, 1990

Cole JO, Gardos G, Tavsy D, et al: Drug trials in persistent dyskinesia, in Tardive Dyskinesia: Research and Treatment. Edited by Fann WE, Smith RC, Davis JM, et al. New York, SP Medical & Scientific Books, 1980, pp 419–427

Conley RR, Schulz SC, Baker RW, et al: Clozapine efficacy in schizophrenic nonresponders. Psychopharmacol Bull 24:269–274, 1988

Coward DM: General pharmacology of clozapine. Br J Psychiatry 160 (suppl 17):5–11, 1992

DasGupta K, Young A: Clozapine-induced neuroleptic malignant syndrome. J Clin Psychiatry 52:105–107, 1991

De la Chapelle A, Kari C, Nurminen M, et al: Clozapine-induced agranulocytosis: a genetic and epidemiologic study. Hum Genet 37:183–194, 1977

de Leon J, Moral L, Camunas C: Clozapine and jaw dyskinesia: a case report. J Clin Psychiatry 52:494–495, 1991

Devinsky O, Honigfeld G, Patin J: Clozapine-related seizures. Neurology 41:369–371, 1991

Dorta G, Siebenmann R, Frohli P, et al: Clozapin-induzierter cholestatischer ikterus: ein fallbericht. Z Gastroenterol 27:388–390, 1989

Ekblom B, Eriksson K, Lindstrom LH: Supersensitivity psychosis in schizophrenic patients after sudden clozapine withdrawal. Psychopharmacology (Berl) 83:293–294, 1984

Eklund K: Supersensitivity and clozapine withdrawal (letter). Psychopharmacology (Berl) 91:135, 1987

Ereshefsky L, Watanabe MD, Tran-Johnson TK: Clozapine: an atypical antipsychotic agent. Clin Pharmacol 8:691–709, 1989

Factor SA, Brown D: Clozapine prevents recurrence of psychosis in Parkinson's disease. Mov Disord 7:125–131, 1992

Farde L, Wiesel FA, Nordstrom AL, et al: D_1 and D_2 dopamine receptor occupancy during treatment with conventional and atypical neuroleptics. Psychopharmacology (Berl) 99:S28–S31, 1989

Fischer PA, Baas H, Hefner R: Treatment of parkinsonian tremor with clozapine. J Neural Transm 2:233–238, 1990

Fischer-Cornelssen KA, Ferner UJ: An example of European multicenter trials: multispectral analysis of clozapine. Psychopharmacol Bull 12:34–39, 1976

Frankenburg F, Kando J: Clozapine-related pancreatitis (letter). Lancet 340:251, 1992

Friedman JH, Lannon MC: Clozapine-responsive tremor in Parkinson's disease. Mov Disord 5:225–229, 1990

Friedman JH, Max J, Swift R: Idiopathic Parkinson's disease in a chronic schizophrenic patient: long-term treatment with clozapine and L-dopa. Clin Neuropharmacol 10:470–475, 1987

Gelenberg AJ, Doller JC: Clozapine versus chlorpromazine for the treatment of schizophrenia: preliminary results from a double-blind study. J Clin Psychiatry 40:238–240, 1979

Gerbino L, Shopsin B, Collora M: Clozapine in the treatment of tardive dyskinesia: an interim report, in Tardive Dyskinesia, Research and Treatment. Edited by Fann WE, Smith RC, Davis JM, et al. New York, SP Medical & Scientific Books, 1980, pp 475–489

Gerson SL, Meltzer H: Mechanisms of clozapine-induced agranulocytosis. Drug Saf 7 (suppl 1):17–25, 1992

Gerson SL, Lieberman JA, Friedenberg WR, et al: Polypharmacy in fatal clozapine-associated agranulocytosis. Lancet 338:262, 1991

Goates MG, Escobar JI: An apparent neuroleptic malignant syndrome without extrapyramidal symptoms upon initiation of clozapine therapy: report of a case and results of a clozapine rechallenge (letter). J Clin Psychopharmacol 12:139–140, 1992

Grabowski J: Clonidine treatment of clozapine-induced hypersalivation (letter). J Clin Psychopharmacol 12:69–70, 1992

Griffith RW, Saameli K: Clozapine and agranulocytosis. Lancet 2:657, 1975

Grohmann R, Ruther E, Sassim N, et al: Adverse effects of clozapine. Psychopharmacology (Berl) 99:S101–S104, 1989

Gudelsky GA, Meltzer HY: Activation of tubero-infundibular dopamine neurons following the acute administration of atypical antipsychotics. Neuropsychopharmacology 2:45–51, 1989

Guirguis E, Voineskos G, Gray J, et al: Clozapine (Leponex) vs chlorpromazine (Largactil) in acute schizophrenia. Current Therapeutic Research: Clinical and Experimental 21:707–719, 1977

Guy W (ed): ECDEU Assessment Manual for Psychopharmacology, Revised (DHEW Publ No ADM 76-388). Rockville, MD, U.S. Department of Health, Education and Welfare, 1976

Haller E, Binder RL: Clozapine and seizures. Am J Psychiatry 147:1069–1071, 1990

Haring C, Fleischhacker WW, Schett P, et al: Influence of patient-related variables on clozapine plasma levels. Am J Psychiatry 147:1471–1475, 1990

Heh CW, Herrara J, DeMet E, et al: Neuroleptic-induced hypothermia associated with amelioration of psychosis in schizophrenia. Neuropsychopharmacology 1:149–156, 1988

Heinrichs DW, Hanlon ET, Carpenter WT Jr: The Quality of Life scale: an instrument for rating the schizophrenic deficit syndrome. Schizophr Bull 10:388–398, 1984

Honigfeld G, Patin J: Predictors of response to clozapine therapy. Psychopharmacology (Berl) 99:S64–S67, 1989

Honigfeld G, Patin J, Singer J: Clozapine: antipsychotic activity in treatment-resistant schizophrenics. Advances in Therapy 1:77–97, 1984

Hummer M, Kurz M, Barnas C, et al: Transient neutropenia induced by clozapine. Psychopharmacol Bull 28:287–290, 1992

Idanpaan-Heikkila J, Alhava E, Olkinuera M, et al: Agranulocytosis during treatment with clozapine. Eur J Clin Pharmacol 11:193–198, 1977

Jenkins M, Metzer SW: Avoidance of metoclopramide for the treatment of clozapine-induced nausea (letter). J Clin Psychiatry 51:S210, 1990

Kahn N, Freeman A, Juncos JL, et al: Clozapine is beneficial for psychosis in Parkinson's disease. Neurology 41:1699–1700, 1991

Kane JM, Cooper TB, Sacher EJ, et al: Clozapine: plasma levels and prolactin response. Psychopharmacology (Berl) 73:184–187, 1981

Kane JM, Woerner M, Borenstein M, et al: Integrating incidence and prevalence of tardive dyskinesia. Psychopharmacol Bull 22:254–258, 1986

Kane J, Honigfeld G, Singer J, et al: Clozapine for the treatment-resistant schizophrenic: a double-blind comparison with chlorpromazine/benztropine. Arch Gen Psychiatry 45:789–796, 1988

Kane JM, Woerner MG, Pollack S, et al: Does clozapine cause tardive dyskinesia? J Clin Psychopharmacol 13:286–287, 1993

Kane JM, Woerner MG, Borenstein M, et al: The Hillside Hospital prospective study of TD development: incidence and risk factors. Paper presented at the NCDEU Annual Meeting, Marco Island, FL, May 1994

Kaniucki MD, Stefano FJG, Pevec CJ: Clonidine inhibits salivary secretion by activation of postsynaptic α_2-receptors. Naunynschmiedebergs Arch Pharmacol 326:313–316, 1984

Kirkegaard A, Jensen A: An investigation of some side effects in 47 psychotic patients during treatment with clozapine and discontinuing of the treatment. Arztliche-Forschung/Drug Research 29:851–858, 1979

Koukkou M, Angst J, Zimmer D: Paroxysmal EEG activity and psychopathology during treatment with clozapine. Pharmacopsychiatry 12:173–183, 1979

Krupp P, Barnes P: Leponex-associated granulocytopenia: a review of the situation. Psychopharmacology (Berl) 99:S118–S121, 1989

Krupp P, Barnes P: Clozapine-associated agranulocytosis: Risk and aetiology. Br J Psychiatry 160 (suppl 17):38–40 1992

Kuha S, Miettinen E: Long term effect of clozapine in schizophrenia: a retrospective study of 108 chronic schizophrenics treated with clozapine for up to seven years. Nordisk Psykiatrisk Tidsskrift 40:225–230, 1986

Lamberti JS, Bellnier T, Schwarzkopf SB: Weight gain among schizophrenic patients treated with clozapine. Am J Psychiatry 149:689–690, 1992

Leadbetter RA, Viewig V: Clozapine-induced weight gain (letter). Am J Psychiatry 147:1693–1694, 1990

Leadbetter R, Shutty M, Pavalonis D, et al: Clozapine-induced weight gain: prevalence and clinical relevance. Am J Psychiatry 149:68–72, 1992

Leon CA: Therapeutic effects of clozapine: a four year follow-up of a controlled clinical trial. Acta Psychiatr Scand 60:471–480, 1979

Leppig M, Bosch B, Naber D, et al: Clozapine in the treatment of 121 outpatients. Psychopharmacology (Berl) 99:S77–S79, 1989

Levenson J: Neuroleptic malignant syndrome. Am J Psychiatry 142:1137–1145, 1985

Levin H, Chengappa KNR, Kambhampati RK, et al: Should chronic treatment-refractory akathisia be an indication for the use of clozapine in schizophrenic patients? J Clin Psychiatry 53:248–251, 1992

Lieberman JA, Alvir JMJ: A report of clozapine-induced agranulocytosis. Drug Saf 7 (suppl 1):1–2, 1992

Lieberman JA, Johns C, Kane JM, et al: Clozapine induced agranulocytosis: non-cross reactivity with other psychotropic drugs. J Clin Psychiatry 49:271–277, 1988

Lieberman JA, Saltz BL, Johns CA, et al: Clozapine effects on tardive dyskinesia. Psychopharmacol Bull 25:57–62, 1989a

Lieberman J, Kane J, Johns C: Clozapine: guidelines for clinical management. J Clin Psychiatry 50:329–338, 1989b

Lieberman JA, Yunis J, Egea E, et al: HLA-B38, DR4, DQw3 and clozapine-induced agranulocytosis in Jewish patients with schizophrenia. Arch Gen Psychiatry 47:945–948, 1990

Lieberman JA, Saltz BL, Johns CA, et al: The effects of clozapine on tardive dyskinesia. Br J Psychiatry 158:503–510, 1991

Lindstrom LH: The effect of long term treatment of clozapine in schizophrenia: a retrospective study of 96 patients treated with clozapine for up to 13 years. Acta Psychiatr Scand 77:524–529, 1988

Mandel JD, Zengo A, Katz R, et al: Effect of adrenergic agents on salivary composition. J Dent Res 54 (special issue B):B27–B33, 1975

Marder SR, Van Putten T: Who should receive clozapine? Arch Gen Psychiatry 45:865–867, 1988

Martin A: Acute pancreatitis associated with clozapine use (letter). Am J Psychiatry 149:714, 1992

Mason RP, Fischer V: Possible role of free radical formation in drug-induced agranulocytosis. Drug Saf 7 (suppl 1):45–50, 1992

Mattes JA: Clozapine for refractory schizophrenia: an open study of 14 patients treated up to 2 years. J Clin Psychiatry 50:389–391, 1989

Matz R, Rick W, Oh D, et al: Clozapine—a potential antipsychotic agent without extrapyramidal manifestations. Current Therapeutic Research, Clinical and Experimental 16:687–695, 1974

McElroy SL, Dessain EC, Pope HG, et al: Clozapine in the treatment of psychotic mood disorders, schizoaffective disorder, and schizophrenia. J Clin Psychiatry 52:411–414, 1991

Meltzer HY: Clozapine: mechanism of action in relation to its clinical advantages, in Recent Advances in Schizophrenia. Edited by Kales A, Stefanis CN, Talbott J. New York, Springer-Verlag, 1990, pp 237–256

Meltzer HY, Goode DJ, Schyve PM, et al: Effect of clozapine on human serum prolactin levels. Am J Psychiatry 136:1550–1555, 1979

Meltzer HY, Bastani B, Youngkwon K, et al: A prospective study of clozapine in treatment-resistant schizophrenic patients, I: preliminary report. Psychopharmacology (Berl) 99:S68–S72, 1989a

Meltzer HY, Matsubara S, Lee JC: The ratios of serotonin$_2$ and dopamine$_2$ affinities differentiate atypical and typical antipsychotic drugs. Psychopharmacol Bull 25:390–392, 1989b

Miller DD: Effect of phenytoin on plasma clozapine concentrations in two patients. J Clin Psychiatry 52:23–25, 1991

Miller DM, Sharafuddin MJA, Kathol RG: A case of clozapine-induced neuroleptic malignant syndrome. J Clin Psychiatry 52:99–101, 1991

Muller T, Becker T, Fritze J: Neuroleptic malignant syndrome after clozapine plus carbamazepine. Lancet 2:1500, 1988

Naber D, Leppig M, Grohmann R, et al: Efficacy and adverse effects in the treatment of schizophrenia and tardive dyskinesia—a retrospective study of 387 patients. Psychopharmacology (Berl) 99:S73–S76, 1989

Nopoulos P, Flaum M, Miller DD: Atypical neuroleptic malignant syndrome (NMS) with an atypical neuroleptic. Annals of Clinical Psychiatry 2:251–253, 1990

Overall JE, Gorham DR: The Brief Psychiatric Rating Scale. Psychol Rep 10:799–812, 1962

Owen RR, Beake BJ, Marby D, et al: Response to clozapine in chronic psychotic patients. Psychopharmacol Bull 25:253–256, 1989

Pakkenberg H, Pakkenberg B: Clozapine in the treatment of tremor. Acta Neurol Scand 73:295–297, 1986

Panteleeva GP, Tsutsulkovskaya MY, Belyaev BS et al: Clozapine in the treatment of schizophrenic patients: an international multicenter trial. Clin Ther 10:57–68, 1987

Patil VJ: Development of transient obsessive-compulsive symptoms during treatment with clozapine (letter). Am J Psychiatry 149:272, 1992

Perenyi A, Kuncz E, Bagdy G: Early relapse after sudden withdrawal or dose reduction of clozapine. Psychopharmacology (Berl) 86:244, 1985

Perry PJ, Miller DD, Arndt SV, et al: Clozapine and norclozapine plasma concentrations and clinical response of treatment-refractory schizophrenic patients. Am J Psychiatry 148:231–235, 1991

Pfeiffer RF, Kang J, Graber B, et al: Clozapine for psychosis in Parkinson's disease. Mov Disord 5:239–242, 1990

Pfister GM, Hanson DR, Roerig JL, et al: Clozapine-induced agranulocytosis in a native American: HLA typing and further support for an immune-mediated mechanism. J Clin Psychiatry 53:242–244, 1992

Pickar D, Owen RR, Litman RE, et al: Clinical and biologic response to clozapine in patients with schizophrenia: crossover comparison with fluphenazine. Arch Gen Psychiatry 49:345–353, 1992

Pippenger CE, Xianzhong M, Rothner AD, et al: Free radical enzyme scavenging activity profiles in risk assessment of idiosyncratic drug reactions, in Idiosyncratic Reactions to Valproate: Clinical Risk Patterns and Mechanisims of Toxicity. Edited by Levy RH, Penry JK. New York, Raven, 1991, pp 75–88

Pisciotta AV: Immune and toxic mechanisms in drug-induced agranulocytosis. Semin Hematol 10:279–310, 1973

Pisciotta AV, Konigs SA, Ciesemier LL, et al: Cytotoxic activity in serum of patients with clozapine-induced agranulocytosis. J Lab Clin Med 119:254–266, 1992

Pope GH, Cole JO, Chopas PT, et al: Apparent neuroleptic malignant syndrome with clozapine and lithium. J Nerv Ment Dis 174:493–495, 1986

Povlsen UJ, Noring U, Fog R, et al: Tolerability and therapeutic effect of clozapine: a retrospective investigation of 216 patients treated with clozapine for up to 12 years. Acta Psychiatr Scand 71:176–185, 1985

Raitasuo V, Lehtovaara R, Huttunen MO: Carbamazepine and plasma levels of clozapine. Am J Psychiatry 150:169, 1992

Richelson E: Pharmacology of neuroleptics in use in the United States. J Clin Psychiatry 46:8–14, 1985

Roberts HE, Dean RC, Stoudmire A: Clozapine treatment of psychosis in Parkinson's disease. J Neuropsychiatry Clin Neurosci 1:190–192, 1989

Rosen S, Hanno P: Clozapine-induced priapism. J Urol 148:876–877, 1992

Roth SD, Addonizio G, Susman VL: Diagnosing and treating neuroleptic malignant syndrome. Am J Psychiatry 143:673, 1986

Safferman AZ, Munne R: Combining clozapine with ECT. Convulsive Therapy 8:141–143, 1992

Safferman AZ, Lieberman JA, Alvir JMJ, et al: Rechallenge in clozapine induced agranulocytosis (letter). Lancet 339:1296–1297, 1992a

Safferman AZ, Lieberman JL, Pollack S, et al: Clozapine and akathisia (letter). Biol Psychiatry 31:753–754, 1992b

Safferman AZ, Lieberman JL, Pollack S, et al: Akathisia and clozapine treatment. J Clin Psychopharmacol 13:286–287, 1993

Saltz BL, Woerner MG, Kane JM, et al: Prospective study of tardive dyskinesia, incidence in the elderly. JAMA 266:2402–2406, 1991

Sandoz Pharmaceuticals Corp: Clozaril (Clozapine): The Atypical Antipsychotic. East Hanover, NJ, Sandoz Pharmaceuticals Corp, 1990

Schmauss M, Erfurth A, Ruther E: Tolerability of long term clozapine treatment. Psychopharmacology (Berl) 99:S105–S108, 1989

Schuster P, Gabriel E, Kufferle B, et al: Reversal by physostigmine of clozapine-induced delirium. Clinical Toxicology 10:437–441, 1977

Seeman P: Dopamine receptor sequences. Neuropsychopharmacology (Berl) 7:261–284, 1992

Seftel AD, Saenz de Tejada I, Szetela B, et al: Clozapine-associated priapism: a case report. J Urol 147:146–148, 1992

Shopsin B, Klein H, Aaronsom M, et al: Clozapine, chlorpromazine and placebo in newly hospitalized, acutely schizophrenic patients: a controlled, double-blind comparison. Arch Gen Psychiatry 36:657–664, 1979

Simpson GM, Cooper TA: Clozapine plasma levels and convulsions. Am J Psychiatry 135:99–100, 1978

Simpson GM, Varga E: Clozapine—a new antipsychotic agent. Current Therapeutic Research: Clinical and Experimental 16:679–686, 1974

Singh H, Hunt JI, Vitiello B, et al: Neuroleptic withdrawal in patients meeting criteria for supersensitivity psychosis. J Clin Psychiatry 135:319–321, 1990

Small JG, Milstein V, Marhenke JD, et al: Treatment outcome with clozapine in tardive dyskinesia, neuroleptic sensitivity, and treatment-resistant psychosis. J Clin Psychiatry 48:263–267, 1987a

Small JG, Milstein V, Small IF, et al: Computerized EEG profiles of haloperidol, chlorpromazine, clozapine, and placebo in treatment resistant schizophrenia. Clin Electroencephalogr 18:124–135, 1987b

Stoudemire A, Clayton L: Successful use of clozapine in a patient with a history of neuroleptic malignant syndrome. J Neuropsychiatry Clin Neurosci 1:303–305, 1989

Stricker BHC, Tielens JAE: Eosinophilia with clozapine. Lancet 338:1520–1521, 1991

Sullivan G, Lukoff D: Sexual side effects of antipsychotic medication: evaluation and interventions. Hosp Community Psychiatry 41:1238–1241, 1990

Szymanski S, Jody D, Liepizig R, et al: Anticholinergic delirium caused by retreatment with clozapine (letter). Am J Psychiatry 148:1752, 1991a

Szymanski S, Lieberman JA, Picou D, et al: A case report of cimetidine-induced clozapine toxicity. J Clin Psychiatry 52:21–22, 1991b

Tiihonen J, Paanila J: Eosinophilia associated with clozapine (letter). Lancet 339:488, 1992

Tiihonen J, Nousiainen U, Hakola P, et al: EEG abnormalities associated with clozapine treatment (letter). Am J Psychiatry 148:1406, 1991

Ukai Y, Taniguchi TI, Kimura K: Muscarinic supersensitivity and subsensitivity induced by chronic treatment with atropine and diisopropylfluorophosphonate in rat submaxillary glands. Arch Int Pharmacodyn Ther 297:148–157, 1989

Van Praag HM, Korf J, Dols LCW: Clozapine versus perphenazine: the value of the biochemical mode of action of neuroleptics in predicting their therapeutic activity. Br J Psychiatry 129:547–555, 1976

Van Putten T: Why do schizophrenic patients refuse to take their drugs? Arch Gen Psychiatry 31:67–72, 1974

Van Putten T, Wirshing WC, Marder SR: Tardive Meige syndrome responsive to clozapine (letter). J Clin Psychopharmacol 10:381–382, 1990

Van Tol HHM, Bunzow JR, Guan HC, et al: Cloning of a human dopamine D_4 receptor gene with high affinity for the antipsychotic clozapine. Nature 350:614–619, 1991

Waldman MD, Safferman AZ: Pregnancy and clozapine (letter). Am J Psychiatry 150:168–169, 1992

Weide R, Koppler H, Heymans J, et al: Successful treatment of clozapine induced agranulocytosis with granulocyte-colony stimulating factor (G-CSF). Br J Haematol 80:557–559, 1992

Wolters EC, Hurvitz TA, Peppard RF, et al: Clozapine: an antipsychotic agent in Parkinson's disease? Clin Neuropharmacol 12:83–90, 1989

Wood MJ, Rubinstein M: An atypical responder to clozapine (letter). Am J Psychiatry 147:369, 1990

Ziegler J, Behar D: Clozapine-induced priapism (letter). Am J Psychiatry 149:272–273, 1992

CHAPTER 15

Drug Treatment of Negative Schizophrenic Symptoms

Yvon D. Lapierre, M.D., F.R.C.P.C., and
Barry D. Jones, M.D., F.R.C.P.C.

For many years, the treatment of schizophrenia has focused primarily on the positive symptoms of the illness, such as hallucinations, delusions, and behavioral disorders. These symptoms attracted the most attention in terms of the need for treatment and frequently served as the end point for the evaluation of neuroleptic medications. Once the hallucinations and delusions had subsided and behavior was controlled, it was felt that the illness was under control.

However, clinicians were still confronted with patients who remained disabled from what was considered to be the deficit side of schizophrenia. These deficit symptoms are now recognized as *negative symptoms*. Although they had been described by many authors over the years, only recently have they been more intensively described and categorized (Andreasen 1988; Andreasen et al. 1990; Siris et al. 1988; Tandon and Greden 1991; Tandon et al. 1990a). They include emotional components—such as blunted affect, poverty of speech, anhedonia, and loss of energy, drive, and interest—and cognitive deficits—such as poor attention span, concentration difficulties, thought blocking, and psychomotor retardation. Socially, patients displaying these symptoms become withdrawn, are inattentive to their grooming and personal hygiene, and are unable to establish relationships.

For documentation purposes, these negative symptoms have been divided into various subtypes or clusters. However, it is generally recognized that there are three clusters of negative symptoms: 1) cognitive impairment and inappropriate affect, 2) anhedonia and anergia, and 3) retardation and flattening of affect (Barnes and Liddle 1990).

Prior to embarking on a psychopharmacological regimen of treatment directed toward negative symptoms, it is essential that clinicians determine whether the negative symptoms are primary or secondary to another condition that may contribute to the appearance and prolongation of the symptoms (Whiteford and Peabody 1989).

Secondary Negative Symptoms

The most important consideration should be directed toward the recognition of depression (Lewine 1990; see also Chapter 7). It is now generally accepted that depression can occur in schizophrenic patients de novo, totally independent of the schizophrenic disorder (Glick et al. 1989). In this situation, treatment may be directed toward the depression itself. On the other hand, depression may form part of the course of schizophrenia, particularly after an acute episode, in which case it is generally referred to as *postpsychotic depression*. This form of depression can be variously explained as stress-induced depression brought on by the stressful events of an acute psychotic break; as the appearance of depression in the form of "insight" when viewed from a psychodynamic perspective; or as depression secondary to the losses incurred either from the illness or during recovery from the illness. In these situations, the combination of rehabilitative and adaptive psychotherapeutic interventions with or without pharmacological agents may be considered.

Depression may also occur secondary to a medication regimen. It is well recognized that beta-blockers, particularly propranolol, can be associated with symptoms of depression. Beta-blockers are occasionally used for the treatment of akathisia in schizophrenic patients. Benzodiazepine therapy, which is often used as adjunctive medication in acute schizophrenic episodes, has also been associated with symptoms suggestive of depression. Finally, injectable neuroleptics such as fluphenazine decanoate or fluphenazine enanthate have been associated with depression. One further consideration, however, is that the specificity of these cases of depression as being attributable to schizophrenia or to the treatment of schizophrenia remains to be determined in comparison with the incidence of depression observed in other chronic medical conditions.

Extrapyramidal side effects may mimic the negative symptoms of schizophrenia (Merriam et al. 1990). Neuroleptic-induced parkinsonism may present with a decrease in facial expressiveness and emotional reactivity. Part of the parkinsonian syndrome is akinesia, which may present either as part of the syndrome or as a separate entity. Given that drug-induced akinesia is worse in the morning, the resulting diurnal rhythm may be falsely attributed to depression. Akinesia may, however, also be part of a depressive syndrome. Decreased mobility may thus be a presenting feature of the psychomotor retardation of depression or of the motor retardation of parkinsonism, and the two may be very difficult to differentiate clinically. In a similar vein, there may also be a relationship between tardive dyskinesia and the negative syndrome (Waddington et al. 1987).

Environmental stimulation is often not fully appreciated by clinicians. Schizophrenic patients in general tend to withdraw from stress and stimulation. Eventually, this understimulation from their environment compounds an illness that by nature leads those affected by it to become isolated. This isolation becomes all the more obvious when the patient's withdrawal and apparent lack of drive are secondary to a psychotic symptom complex of a paranoid nature. The suspicious paranoid schizophrenic patient will understandably avoid social contact and interactions with people.

The relationship between schizoid personality type and schizophrenia is controversial. However, it is well recognized that a number of patients who eventually become schizophrenic had an initial premorbid schizoid personality and were not involved with other people.

Once the acute schizophrenic episode subsides, the reemergence of this premorbid personality may lead the clinician to misdiagnose negative symptomatology. Of course, the premorbid schizoid personality may also be conceptualized as being the forerunner of early negative symptoms, particularly in the social sphere.

Concurrent physical illness may also contribute to the development of symptoms that may be considered part of the negative syndrome. Such illnesses include endocrine disorders affecting the thyroid and adrenal systems, malignancies with their resulting debilitating effects, and cerebrovascular diseases. Finally, in older schizophrenic patients, early symptoms of senile dementia of the Alzheimer's type may present with an increase in negative symptoms.

Substance abuse, particularly the long-term, heavy use of cannabis, may lead to a syndrome that in a number of ways is suggestive of negative symptoms of schizophrenia. Also, water intoxication, present in as many as 7% of chronic schizophrenic patients, may give rise to cognitive decline and associated symptoms resembling the negative syndrome (Jose and Perez-Cruet 1979).

It is essential to address these differential diagnoses in the evaluation of any subsequent psychopharmacological intervention, as any attempts at treating this aspect of the schizophrenic syndrome will not be successful in the presence of one of these complicating conditions.

Primary Negative Symptoms: Research and Clinical Implications

The identification of negative symptoms in the schizophrenic patient has heuristic value and clinical importance. From the research perspective, attempts have been made at determining clinical-pathological correlations between the presence of negative symptoms and neurophysiology and neuropathology. Results from Crow's (1980) studies have suggested that type I schizophrenia, characterized by a predominance of positive symptoms, is not usually associated with neuropathological abnormalities, whereas type II schizophrenia is characterized by a predominance of negative symptoms and is associated with increased neuropathological abnormalities. Andreasen et al. (1990) have suggested a bipolarity in the presentation of schizophrenia with an overlap of the positive and negative symptoms, whereas others (Ciccone 1988; Keefe et al. 1991) have considered the negative and positive symptomatology as different dimensions of a common psychopathology of the illness. Neural circuits linking regions such as the limbic system, hippocampus, and frontal cortex could, if disturbed, lead to varying expressions of both positive and negative symptoms. Negative symptoms would generally emanate from frontal lobe dysfunction, whereas positive symptoms would be linked to limbic overactivity (Weinberger et al. 1988).

Looking from the clinical perspective, Kay and Opler (1987) paid particular attention to the positive and negative symptom dimensions of schizophrenia. In their patient cohort, they were able to demonstrate that both groups of symptoms correlate with the severity of the illness, and that the positive and negative symptom groups had a partial inverse correlation to each other. In the acute phase, negative symptoms suggested a favorable genetic background and symptom profile, whereas positive symptoms indicated a poor prognosis. In the chronic phase of the illness, the persistence of negative symptoms suggested a poor prognosis.

Another perspective is that of Liddle (1987), who suggested that positive and negative symptoms represent discrete processes of the same illness, that these symptom constellations are independent dimensions of a common psychopathology, and that their change over the course of time is an unpredictable sequence unrelated to the severity or the profile of the illness in a specific patient.

On the other hand, Keefe et al. (1991) suggested that the positive and negative symptoms are state dependent. In the acute phase, there would be an increased loss of attention, a more pronounced flattening of affect, alogia, and avolitional apathy, whereas symptoms such as anhedonia and social withdrawal would be stable in patients throughout the course of the illness, whether it be in the acute or the remission phase.

Although drug-induced parkinsonism, especially akinesia, may be confused with negative symptoms, one does not seem to predict the other. On the other hand, the presence of negative symptoms seems to put the patient at a greater risk for developing tardive dyskinesia (Barnes et al. 1989). Once tardive dyskinesia has developed, it has been suggested that the severity of the oral-facial movement abnormalities is associated with a more marked cognitive dysfunction in chronic schizophrenic patients (Waddington et al. 1987).

The presence of negative symptoms has generally been considered a bad prognostic omen in the pharmacological treatment of schizophrenia. However, Harvey et al. (1991) reported that, in drug-free schizophrenic patients presenting with low levels of anergia, the response to haloperidol was quicker than in those with more pronounced anergia. Moreover, in the patients treated with high dosages of haloperidol, there was a greater induction of anergic symptoms.

The debate on the efficacy of treatment of positive and negative symptoms of schizophrenia with neuroleptics was addressed by Angst et al. (1989), who concluded that the administration of neuroleptics (clozapine, haloperidol, and fluperlapine) resulted in a reduction of both positive and negative symptoms. Meltzer and Zureick (1989) also concluded that treatment with typical or standard neuroleptics resulted in the improvement of both negative and positive symptoms.

The reviews and conclusions noted above suggest a commonality of substrate between the negative and positive symptom groupings. However, in general, there is a consensus that atypical antipsychotics may have a greater propensity to be more effective in the treatment of negative symptoms than do the typical neuroleptics (Breier et al. 1987). We now examine the evidence in favor of the psychopharmacological approach in the treatment of primary negative symptoms, including recent treatment strategies.

Psychopharmacological Strategies in the Treatment of Negative Symptoms

Typical Neuroleptics

As mentioned earlier, Meltzer and colleagues' (Meltzer and Zureick 1989; Meltzer et al. 1986) and Angst et al.'s (1989) reviews suggested that standard neuroleptics can be effective not only in controlling positive symptoms but also in improving negative symptomatology. It should be noted that standard neuroleptics have a typical receptor-blocking profile at normal dosage ranges. However, at very low or high dosages, they may convey a different pharmacological profile that could allow them to improve negative symptoms. This dosage-atypicality relationship is, however, supported only by case reports.

Diphenylbutylpiperidines

Diphenylbutylpiperidines are currently represented by pimozide and fluspirilene. Another drug in this group, penfluridol, was withdrawn a number of years ago for toxicological reasons. Diphenylbutyl-piperidines are highly specific dopamine D_2 receptor blockers that have an additional pharmacological action on calcium channel blockade. They are considered to be superior to standard neuroleptics in the alleviation of negative symptoms (Kane and Mayerhoff 1989; Meltzer et al. 1986).

Results of an open study by Feinberg et al. (1988) suggested that pimozide is more effective on negative symptoms than on positive symptoms. Lapierre and colleagues (Lapierre 1975; Lapierre and Lavallée 1976) demonstrated that pimozide is superior to fluphenazine in improving social interactions in chronic schizophrenic patients, both for patients treated individually and for those undergoing group psychotherapy. This superiority rests in the improvement of certain features of the negative syndrome (e.g., interpersonal interactions, participation in group psychotherapy), with more appropriate affective involvement and socialization than that generated by fluphenazine. Penfluridol was also superior to fluphenazine in the improvement of anergia and emotional withdrawal of schizophrenic patients treated in an outpatient setting over a 1-year period (Lapierre 1978). Results from another study by Lapierre et al. (1981)—on the treatment of chronically ill, long-term institutionalized schizophrenic patients using fluspirilene—suggested a similar improvement over a 1-year period. Whether this improvement is attributable to a positive action of diphenylbutylpiperidines on negative symptoms or to the absence of blockade of other neurotransmitter systems by phenothiazines is not clear. The role of calcium channel blockade of diphenylbutyl-piperidines in these patients remains unclear.

Dibenzodiazepines

Angst et al. (1989) compared the two dibenzodiazepines clozapine and fluperlapine with haloperidol in acute and chronic schizophrenic patients. Their findings supported the superiority of dibenzodiazepines over haloperidol in the improvement of the negative symptoms of both acute and chronic schizophrenic patients. Kane and Mayerhoff (1989) demonstrated the superiority of clozapine over chlorpromazine, a phenothiazine, in the improvement of negative symptoms. This improvement occurred with or without similar improvements of positive symptoms. Fluperlapine and another dibenzodiazepine, zotepine, were also found to be effective in the improvement of negative symptoms in chronic residual schizophrenic patients after 10 weeks of treatment (Barnas et al. 1987).

Benzamides

Amisulpiride has been studied extensively in Europe. Boyer et al. (1990) found this benzamide to be superior to fluphenazine in rapidly reducing the negative symptomatology of schizophrenic patients, whereas it was not different from the phenothiazine in improving positive symptoms. Berner et al. (1989) observed that, in small dosages, amisulpiride was highly effective in activating patients and that the improvement in the negative symptoms was directly related to the patients' global improvement.

Most of the studies on benzamides included schizophrenic patients who were in the acute phase of their illness, without consideration of the predominance of negative over positive symptoms. Remoxipride, studied in a large multicenter trial (Lapierre et al. 1992), showed a stronger tendency to improve negative symptoms than did haloperidol in acute schizophrenic patients treated over a 6-week period. The fact that the degree of improvement in negative symptoms was more pronounced with the higher dosage levels of the medication in Lapierre et al.'s study suggests that this therapeutic benefit could be explained as a specific positive pharmacological effect of benzamides rather than being attributable to the absence of sedation or anergia-like extrapyramidal side effects with lower dosages. Although remoxipride was recently withdrawn from general use because of its toxicity to blood formation, these findings may be of relevance to the understanding of the negative-symptom aspect of schizophrenia.

Calcium Channel Blockers

One question arising from earlier studies on pimozide was, What is the role of calcium channel blockade in the clinical effect of pimozide? This question was addressed in a number of studies with drugs that are primarily calcium channel blockers. Verapamil was examined in two studies by Uhr et al. (1988), who also reviewed the literature available at that time. In none of the studies they reviewed did they find any therapeutic benefits for verapamil on negative symptoms of schizophrenia. Under double-blind conditions, Price and Pascari (1987) compared verapamil with placebo in a small number of patients being simultaneously treated with haloperidol. They concluded that verapamil may contribute to a superior improvement in the negative symptoms of schizophrenia when administered in conjunction with haloperidol.

Dopamine Agonists

Patients with Parkinson's disease present many of the signs and symptoms found in schizophrenic patients with predominantly negative symptomatology. Although the use of L-dopa is controversial because of its propensity to produce psychotic symptoms such as hallucinations and delusions, there have been suggestions that this agent may be useful in improving negative symptomatology (Kane and Mayerhoff 1989; Meltzer et al. 1986). In fact, L-dopa seems to be most effective when used in patients showing predominantly negative symptoms, as well as when used in conjunction with neuroleptic therapy to prevent psychotic exacerbation (Berry 1988; Gerlach and Lubdorf 1975; Inanaga et al. 1972).

Amphetamines in combination with neuroleptics have also been studied. Their use may result in an improvement of anergia symptoms. This benefit, however, as is the case with L-dopa, is accompanied by an increased risk of the emergence of positive symptoms and subsequent relapse (Cesarec and Nyman 1985).

Bromocriptine was studied in a small number of patients by Levi-Minzi et al. (1991), with some favorable responses in some patients. This approach may well merit further investigation.

Partial Dopamine Agonists–Antagonists

Partial dopamine agonists–antagonists are agonistic to dopamine in the presence of a supersensitive postsynaptic dopamine receptor and antagonistic in the presence of receptor subsensitivity. These agents have been used on the rationale that negative symptoms may be caused by a decrease in dopamine release or a decrease in postsynaptic receptor reactivity. Olbrich and Schanz (1988) studied terguride in a small open study and observed a slight reduction in negative symptoms of schizophrenia. Gerbaldo et al. (1988) studied OPC-4392, a 3-(3-hydroxyphenyl)-N-n-propylpiperidine (3-PPP)–related substance and partial dopamine agonist, in 11 patients. Although there was an improvement in negative symptoms in 7 patients, 4 patients had to be withdrawn because of psychotic relapse.

Norepinephrine Mechanisms

The rationale for exploring norepinephrine (NE) mechanisms in the treatment of negative symptoms (van Kammen et al. 1987, 1990) relates to 1) the fact that increased NE activity has been associated with relapses of schizophrenia and 2) the suggestion that there is a relationship between NE metabolite levels and negative symptoms. Kane and Mayerhoff (1989) found the beta-blocker propranolol to be slightly effective in improving negative symptoms.

Mizuki et al. (1990) studied treatment of schizophrenic patients with mianserin, an α_2 antagonist, in conjunction with neuroleptics, and reported an improvement of negative symptoms over a period of 6 weeks. Imipramine has also been studied because of its inhibition of

NE reuptake (Siris et al. 1990). Imipramine use resulted in an improvement of negative symptoms in those schizophrenic patients presenting with depressive symptomatology. This finding was also observed with desipramine, a more specific NE reuptake inhibitor (Kane and Mayerhoff 1989).

Gamma-Aminobutyric Acid Mechanisms

In a preliminary study by Wolkowitz et al. (1986), two patients treated with the benzodiazepine alprazolam, in combination with a neuroleptic, showed an improvement in both negative and positive symptoms. The improvement was short-lived, however, and the initial symptomatology worsened upon cessation of the benzodiazepine. Csernansky et al. (1988) observed an initial improvement in negative symptoms in patients treated with alprazolam when compared with treatment with diazepam. However, at an end point of 6 weeks, the patients treated with alprazolam and with diazepam did not differ from those treated with placebo.

Anticholinergic Mechanisms

There are suggestions that cholinergic overactivity may contribute to the presence of negative symptoms (Tandon et al. 1991). This possibility is supported by clinical observations that anticholinergic medications taken for the improvement of a mood state or drug-induced parkinsonism have resulted in associated secondary negative symptomatology. In a preliminary study on trihexyphenidyl, 4 of the 5 patients treated showed improvement (Tandon et al. 1988). A short-term trial with biperiden in medication-free schizophrenic patients resulted in an increase in patients' positive symptoms and a decrease in their negative symptoms after 2 days. Results from studies conducted by Tandon et al. (1990b, 1991) have indicated that cholinergic overactivity may be operative in the negative symptoms of schizophrenia, and that blockade by anticholinergic medications may contribute to improvement in those symptoms. However, the efficacy of anticholinergic agents in the treatment of negative schizophrenic symptoms still remains to be demonstrated.

Conclusion

Because studies of psychosocial interventions have not been successful in demonstrating the value of psychosocial rehabilitation in the improvement of primary negative schizophrenic symptoms (McGlashan et al. 1990), the search must continue along biological lines. The biological substratum of schizophrenia must be addressed on the premise that negative symptoms, whether they are at the core of the schizophrenic syndrome or one specific dimension of the disorder, may be treated directly with specific compounds or through the use of compounds that have a broader spectrum of activity that addresses negative symptoms as well as symptoms considered positive and more acute. Only in this manner will psychiatry move forward from the present anti*psychotic* drugs to more comprehensive anti*schizophrenic* treatments.

References

Andreasen NC: Dr. Andreasen comments. Am J Psychiatry 145:1181, 1988

Andreasen NC, Flaum M, Swayze VW II, et al: Positive and negative symptoms in schizophrenia: a critical reappraisal. Arch Gen Psychiatry 47:615–621, 1990

Angst J, Stassen HH, Woggon B: Effect of neuroleptics on positive and negative symptoms and the deficit state. Psychopharmacology 99:S41–S46, 1989

Barnas C, Stuppack C, Unterweger B, et al: Treatment of negative symptoms in schizophrenia with zotepine. J Clin Psychopharmacol 7:370–371, 1987

Barnes TRE, Liddle PF: Evidence of the validity of negative symptoms, in Modern Problems of Pharmacopsychiatry, Vol 24: Schizophrenia: Positive and Negative Symptoms and Syndromes. Edited by Andreasen NC. Basel, Switzerland, Karger, 1990, pp 43–72

Barnes TRE, Liddle PF, Curson DA, et al: Negative symptoms, tardive dyskinesia and chronic schizophrenia. Br J Psychiatry 155 (suppl 7):99–103, 1989

Berner P, Kuefferle B, Friedmann A, et al: Traitement des symptômes déficitaires de la schizophrénie par les neuroleptiques. Encephale 15:457–463, 1989

Berry T: L-dopa for the negative symptoms of schizophrenia. Am J Psychiatry 145:1180–1181, 1988

Boyer P, Lecrubier Y, Puech AJ: Treatment of positive and negative symptoms: pharmacologic approaches, in Modern Problems of Pharmacopsychiatry, Vol 24: Schizophrenia: Positive and Negative Symptoms and Syndromes. Edited by Andreasen NC. Basel, Switzerland, Karger, 1990, pp 152–174

Breier A, Wolkowitz OM, Doran A, et al: Neuroleptic responsivity of negative and positive symptoms of schizophrenia. Am J Psychiatry 144:1549–1555, 1987

Cesarec Z, Nyman AK: Differential response to amphetamine in schizophrenia. Acta Psychiatr Scand 71:523–528, 1985

Ciccone P: Debate on the two-syndrome hypothesis of schizophrenia (letter). Am J Psychiatry 145:1180, 1988

Crow TJ: Molecular pathology of schizophrenia: more than one disease process. BMJ 280:66–68, 1980.

Csernansky JG, Riney SJ, Lombrozo L, et al: Double-blind comparison of alprazolam, diazepam, and placebo for the treatment of negative schizophrenic symptoms. Arch Gen Psychiatry 45:655–659, 1988

Feinberg SS, Kay SR, Elijovich LR, et al: Pimozide treatment of negative schizophrenic syndrome: an open trial. J Clin Psychiatry 49:235–238, 1988

Gerbaldo H, Demisch L, Lehmann CO, et al: The effect of OPC-4392, a partial dopamine receptor agonist, on negative symptoms: results of an open study. Pharmacopsychiatry 21:387–388, 1988

Gerlach J, Lubdorf K: The effect of L-dopa on young patients with simple schizophrenia treated with neuroleptic drugs. Psychopharmacologia 44:105–110, 1975

Glick ID, Jacobs M, Lieberman J, et al: Prediction of short term outcome in schizophrenia: depressive symptoms, negative symptoms and extrapyramidal signs. Psychopharmacol Bull 25:344–347, 1989

Harvey PD, Davidson M, Powchik P, et al: Time course and clinical predictors of treatment response in schizophrenia. Schizophr Res 5:161–166, 1991

Inanaga K, Inoue K, Tachibana H, et al: Effect of L-dopa in schizophrenia. Folia Psychiatrica et Neurologica Japonica 26:145–157, 1972

Jose CJ, Perez-Cruet J: Incidence and morbidity of self-induced water intoxication in state mental hospital patients. Am J Psychiatry 136:221–222, 1979

Kane JM, Mayerhoff D: Do negative symptoms respond to pharmacological treatment? Br J Psychiatry 155 (suppl 7):115–118, 1989

Kay SR, Opler LA: The positive-negative dimension in schizophrenia: its validity and significance. Psychiatric Developments 5:79–103, 1987

Keefe RSE, Lobel DS, Mohs RC, et al: Diagnostic issues in chronic schizophrenia: Kraepelinian schizophrenia, undifferentiated schizophrenia, and state-independent symptoms. Schizophr Res 4:71–79, 1991

Lapierre YD: Pimozide and the social behaviour of schizophrenics. Current Therapeutic Research 18:181–188, 1975

Lapierre YD: A controlled study of penfluridol in the treatment of schizophrenia. Am J Psychiatry 135:956–959, 1978

Lapierre YD, Lavallée J: A controlled pimozide, fluphenazine and group psychotherapy study of chronic schizophrenics. Revue de Psychiatie de l'Université d'Ottawa 1:8–13, 1976

Lapierre YD, Chaudry R, Sipos V: A long-term efficacy and toxicity study of fluspirilene in chronic schizophrenia. Current Therapeutic Research 30:793–802, 1981

Lapierre YD, Ancill R, Awad G, et al: A dose-finding study with remoxipride in the acute treatment of schizophrenic patients. J Psychiatry Neurosci 17:134–145, 1992

Levi-Minzi S, Bermanzohn PC, Siris SG: Bromocriptine for "negative" schizophrenia. Compr Psychiatry 32:210–216, 1991

Lewine RRJ: A discriminate validity study of negative symptoms with a special focus on depression and antipsychotic medication. Am J Psychiatry 147:1463–1466, 1990

Liddle PF: The symptoms of chronic schizophrenia: a re-examination of the positive-negative dichotomy. Br J Psychiatry 151:145–151, 1987

McGlashan TH, Heinssen RK, Fenton WS: Psychosocial treatment of negative symptoms in schizophrenia, in Modern Problems of Pharmacopsychiatry, Vol 24: Schizophrenia: Positive and Negative Symptoms and Syndromes. Edited by Andreasen NC. Basel, Switzerland, Karger, 1990, pp 174–200

Meltzer HY, Zureick J: Negative symptoms in schizophrenia: a target for new drug development. Psychopharmacol Ser 7:68–77, 1989

Meltzer HY, Sommers AA, Luchins DJ: The effect of neuroleptics and other psychotropic drugs on negative symptoms in schizophrenia. J Clin Psychopharmacol 6:329–338, 1986

Merriam AE, Kay SR, Opler LA, et al: Neurological signs and the positive-negative dimension in schizophrenia. Biol Psychiatry 28:191–192, 1990

Mizuki Y, Kajimura N, Imai T, et al: Effects of mianserin on negative symptoms in schizophrenia. Int Clin Psychopharmacol 5:83–95, 1990

Olbrich R, Schanz H: The effect of the partial dopamine agonist terguride on negative symptoms in schizophrenics. Pharmacopsychiatry 21:389–390, 1988

Price WA, Pascarzi GA: Use of verapamil to treat negative symptoms in schizophrenia (letter). Journal of Psychopharmacology 7:357, 1987

Siris SG, Adan F, Cohen M, et al: Postpsychotic depression and negative symptoms: an investigation of syndromal overlap. Am J Psychiatry 145:1532–1537, 1988

Siris SG, Mason SE, Bermanzohn PC, et al: Adjunctive imipramine maintenance in post-psychotic depression/negative symptoms. Psychopharmacol Bull 26:91–94, 1990

Tandon R, Greden JF: Negative symptoms of schizophrenia: the need for conceptual clarity. Biol Psychiatry 30:321–325, 1991

Tandon R, Greden JF, Silk KR: Treatment of negative schizophrenic symptoms with trihexyphenidyl. J Clin Psychopharmacol 8:212–215, 1988

Tandon R, Goldman RS, Gordon JA, et al: Mutability and relationship between positive and negative symptoms during neuroleptic treatment in schizophrenia. Biol Psychiatry 27:1323–1326, 1990a

Tandon R, Mann NA, Eisner WH, et al: Effect of anticholinergic medication on positive and negative symptoms in medication-free schizophrenic patients. Psychiatry Res 31:235–241, 1990b

Tandon R, Shipley JE, Greden JF, et al: Muscarinic cholinergic negative symptoms. Schizophr Res 4:23–30, 1991

Uhr SB, Jackson K, Berger PA, et al: Effects of verapamil administration on negative symptoms in chronic schizophrenia (letter). Psychiatry Res 23:351–352, 1988

van Kammen DP, Hommer DW, Malas KL: Effect of pimozide on positive and negative symptoms in schizophrenic patients: are negative symptoms state dependent? Neuropsychobiology 18:113–117, 1987

van Kammen DP, Peters J, Yao J, et al: Norepinephrine in acute exacerbations of chronic schizophrenia: negative symptoms revisited. Arch Gen Psychiatry 47:161–168, 1990

Waddington J, Youssef HA, Dolphin C, et al: Cognitive dysfunction, negative symptoms, and tardive dyskinesia in schizophrenia: their association in relation to topography of involuntary movements and criterion of their abnormality. Arch Gen Psychiatry 44:907–912, 1987

Weinberger DR, Berman KF, Illowsky BP: Physiological dysfunction of dorsolateral prefrontal cortex in schizophrenia. Arch Gen Psychiatry 45:609–615, 1988

Whiteford HA, Peabody CA: The differential diagnosis of negative symptoms in chronic schizophrenia. Aust N Z J Psychiatry 23:491–496, 1989

Wolkowitz OM, Pickar D, Doran AR, et al: Combination alprazolam/neuroleptic treatment of the positive and negative symptoms of schizophrenia. Am J Psychiatry 143:85–87, 1986

CHAPTER 16

Antipsychotic Medication and the Long-Term Course of Schizophrenia

Richard Jed Wyatt, M.D.

C ommonly held tenets about schizophrenia suggest that its course is predetermined, and that its treatments are capable of diminishing symptoms and improving quality of life only while they are being applied. In practice, this view is probably held most firmly by those who believe that the roots of schizophrenia are biological; psychodynamic and some other psychological explanations of schizophrenia imply that treatment can improve the long-term course of the illness.

The concept that antipsychotic intervention might affect the long-term course of schizophrenia has been largely forgotten (Davis 1985; Miller 1989; Wyatt 1991a). Although early investigators were optimistic that antipsychotic medications could improve the course of schizophrenia, they soon discovered that most patients relapsed after their

I wish to thank Ioline Henter for her invaluable editing and organizational skills.

medication was discontinued. This in turn fostered the view that the long-term course of the illness was independent of the use of antipsychotic medications. Today, despite the recognized risks involved with maintenance therapy (Jeste and Wyatt 1982), maintenance treatment has been widely accepted and, when medications are taken, they vastly increase the quality of life for millions of patients.

In this chapter, I briefly review some of the studies that can be used to test this concept and tentatively conclude that, when appropriately applied, antipsychotic medications do improve the course of schizophrenia. Based on this conclusion, I then discuss issues of clinical care and pathophysiologic processes.

Studies of Antipsychotic Medication and the Long-Term Course of Schizophrenia

Mirror-image studies.   In a previous review (Wyatt 1991b), I examined studies that addressed the effects of early intervention with antipsychotic medications; this review encompassed nine published mirror-image studies comparing similar patients before and after the introduction of antipsychotic medications. In Table 16–1, I provide a summary of the analyses of these studies done either by myself or by the original authors. The majority of these studies showed that the administration of antipsychotic medication to first-break schizophrenic patients improved their long-term outcome. Because these and many of the other studies that are described in the literature were performed before the widespread use of maintenance antipsychotic medication, maintenance use of medication probably would not explain the differences.

Delayed-intervention studies.   A second group of studies compared first-break schizophrenic patients who received early intervention with antipsychotic medications with patients for whom intervention was delayed. The results of these delayed-intervention studies are presented in Table 16–2. Results from two of the three studies (Anzai et al. 1988; Crow et al. 1986) showed that the use of

Table 16–1. Results of mirror-image studies comparing the long-term outcome of first-break schizophrenic patients before and after the introduction of antipsychotic medication

Study	Improvement between pre- and postantipsychotic periods
McWalter et al. (1961)	$P = .003$
Ødegård (1964)	$P < .06$
Peterson and Olson (1964)	$P < .001$
Astrup and Noreik (1966)	$P = .003$
Pritchard (1967a, 1967b)	Nonsignificant
Murakami (1971)	$P = .22$
Shimazono (1973)	$P = .03$
Huber et al. (1979, 1980)	$P < .001$
Watt et al. (1983)	Nonsignificant

antipsychotic medications early in the course of the illness had a positive influence on the long-term outcome.

In 1992, Loebel et al. published the results of a 3-year follow-up study of 70 first-break patients with predominately schizophrenic and schizoaffective disorders. The patients received a standardized treatment of fluphenazine, with other medications ultimately being prescribed for those who were nonresponsive. Duration of illness prior to treatment was defined in two ways: from prodromal symptoms and from the onset of psychotic symptoms. An association was reported between the duration of prodromal and psychotic symptoms and the length of treatment prior to response; the longer the duration of symptoms, the longer it took the patient to respond to treatment. In addition, the duration of prodromal and psychotic symptoms was

Table 16–2. Results of studies of early and delayed intervention with antipsychotic medication in first-break schizophrenic patients

Study	Improvement of outcome between early and delayed intervention
Aritome (1978)	Inconclusive
Crow et al. (1986)	$P = .03–.003$
Anzai et al. (1988)	$P = .03$

negatively associated with the degree of remission. In other words, the longer the time until treatment response, the poorer the response was. Moreover, because the mode of onset (defined as the time between the onset of prodromal and psychotic symptoms) was not associated with the time until treatment response, it was suggested that the difference could not explained by the older concepts of process and reactive schizophrenia (i.e., slow versus acute development).

Retrospective studies.   There have also been a number of retrospective studies, the results of which support the value of early intervention; however, these studies were not as well controlled as the previous studies. In a 10-year follow-up study, for example, Lo and Lo (1977) found that Chinese schizophrenic patients who had a shorter duration of illness or an acute onset before their treatment began had a more favorable outcome than those with a longer duration of illness before treatment. Inoue et al. (1986) evaluated a group of patients with schizophrenic and schizoaffective disorders who were followed for at least 3 years, and noted a less favorable outcome for those who were ill for longer periods before the initiation of treatment.

Rabiner et al. (1986) followed 36 first-break schizophrenic patients for 1 year after they began treatment. These researchers found that patients who did not respond to treatment had had pretreatment behavioral changes about three times longer than those patients who did respond but had relapsed at 1 year, and approximately four times longer than patients who responded and were still in remission at 1 year. Angrist and Schulz (1990) reviewed 10 studies from the 1950s and noted findings similar to those of Rabiner et al. It should be pointed out, however, that although the vast majority of investigators have observed a relationship among the time when symptoms or psychosis appear, the time when treatment begins, and the final outcome, there is at least one study that did not replicate these findings (Kolakowska et al. 1985).

Contemporaneous control-group studies.   The most useful design for testing the value of early intervention comes from contemporaneous control-group studies. There have been eight such studies, the results of which were mixed (see Table 16–3). The results of the largest and most carefully controlled of these studies (May et al. 1976b) showed, not unexpectedly, that first-break schizophrenic patients treated with antipsychotic medications improved much more rapidly than those not treated with antipsychotic medications. Surprisingly, however, the patients initially treated with antipsychotic medication continued to do better than the nontreated group for at least 3 years after their initial discharge from the hospital.

Results from a number of studies have indicated that some first-break schizophrenic individuals do well regardless of whether they have been given antipsychotic medications. These responsive patients might be expected to have a more benign course than those patients who took longer to improve or those who required antipsychotic medications to improve. To test this concept, records were obtained (Wyatt 1991a) from the May et al. (1976a, 1976b) studies. Although these records were incomplete, we were able to examine most of them for the participating patients who were discharged from the hospital within 6 months of their admission. Eighty-nine patients had received antipsychotic medication with or without psychotherapy, and nearly 100 had received milieu or psychotherapy without medication. Fourteen of the patients who had been in the milieu and the psychotherapy groups without medication and 64 patients who had been given antipsychotic medication, either alone or in combination with psychother-

Table 16–3. Results of contemporaneous control group studies examining the effects of early intervention with antipsychotic medication on the long-term outcome of schizophrenia

Study	Improvement of outcome between early and normal intervention
Wirt and Simon (1959)	$P < .01$
Pritchard (1967a, 1967b)	$P = .1$
Schooler et al. (1967)	Inconclusive
May et al. (1976a, 1976b)	$P < .05$
Carpenter et al. (1977)	Inconclusive
M. Rappaport et al. (1978)	Inconclusive
Matthews et al. (1979)	Inconclusive
Karon and Vandenbos (1981)	Inconclusive

apy, were discharged within 6 months of admission. During the 3-year follow-up period, the 14 patients who had not required antipsychotic medication to be discharged within 6 months of their admission required a mean of 160.6 days of rehospitalization compared with a mean of 73.2 days for the patients who were initially treated with medication ($P < .04$). Even more surprising is that during the third year of follow-up, the patients who were initially treated without antipsychotic medications were using the same amount or slightly more medication than those who were initially treated with antipsychotic medications (Wyatt 1991a).

One study (Karon and Vandenbos 1981) that was not covered in the original review shared some of the difficulties associated with studies that attempt to compare patients treated with psychotherapy with those treated with antipsychotic medication. In their study, Karon and Vandenbos stressed the quality of the psychotherapy and of the psychotherapist. They intended to include only first-break patients who had experienced less than 3 months of psychosis but who could not be discharged within 2 weeks of admission (this was the time that was required for working up the patients to determine if they qualified for the study). Because the study took place in the mid-1960s, it is likely that these patients were treated with antipsychotic medications during this workup period. After their workups, patients were randomly assigned to one of three groups. The first group was a psychoanalytic psychotherapy group in which patients received five sessions per week until discharge, and one session per week thereafter as outpatients. Although the investigators did not intend to give antipsychotic medications to this group, antipsychotics were administered for up to 2 weeks if the ward staff felt it was necessary, with the result that this group probably received antipsychotic medication prior to the study and some of the patients received medication again during the study. The second group received between one and three weekly sessions of ego-analytic psychotherapy and up to 600 mg of chlorpromazine equivalents per day. The third group received phenothiazines as their primary treatment and were under the supervision of a resident. Patients in the third group who did not respond after 2 weeks were transferred to a state hospital. These patients changed psychiatrists when the transfer from hospitals took place and again when they became outpatients. Neither the first nor the second group experienced such a disruption in their environment. Results of the study showed that, depending on the period of follow-up, the psychoanalytic and ego-analytic groups (with and without medication) were doing better than the medication-alone group.

Unfortunately, after the patients had entered the study, a number of them were found to have had previous hospitalizations. For the medication-only group, 5 of 13 patients had been previously hospitalized, and in the two psychotherapy groups, 6 of 21 patients had been previously hospitalized. These patients therefore represented a more chronic population than the authors had intended.

Trying to make sense out of the Karon and Vandenbos study in relationship to the substantial body of literature that indicates that intensive psychotherapy has little value for schizophrenic individuals is a complicated task. Karon and Vandenbos argued that their extensive experience in providing psychoanalytic psychotherapy to schizophrenic patients accounts for the difference between their study's results and those of other studies. There have been, however, several other controlled studies that have used well-trained, psychodynamically oriented psychotherapists. Results from the most recent of these, the Boston Psychotherapy Study (Katz and Gunderson 1990), showed little difference between the schizophrenic patients who received exploratory, insight-oriented psychotherapy and those who did not. It is interesting to note that the benefit that was gained from insight-oriented psychotherapy in the Katz and Gunderson study appeared to be in those patients who had the greatest amount of negative symptoms.

After reading Karon and Vandenbos' account of their study, my personal experience led me to suspect that their enthusiasm and caring were responsible for their results, but this hypothesis probably cannot be tested. The results of the study should not affect the notion that antipsychotic medication can change the course of the illness. The most obvious confounding factor in this study was that, on average, the group that was treated with antipsychotic medication was reported to have received approximately 400 mg/day of chlorpromazine or its equivalent, with some patients receiving greater or lesser amounts (the range was 100–1,400 mg per day of chlorpromazine equivalents). However, there is considerable evidence suggesting that a daily dosage of chlorpromazine equivalents of 400 mg or less is not much better than placebo (American Psychiatric Association 1992). In contrast, patients in the ego-analytic psychotherapy group received up to 600 mg of chlorpromazine equivalents, which may have been, on average, a higher dosage than that received by those in the medication-alone group. Furthermore, the psychoanalytic and the psychotherapy plus medication groups were being carefully followed by virtue of the continuous nature of the psychotherapy. In contrast, if the patients in the medication-alone group were treated like most patients in the 1960s, follow-up would have been uneven at best. In summary, the results from the Karon and Vandenbos study imply only that the combination of psychotherapy—provided by enthusiastic, caring therapists—with some antipsychotic medication is better than a poorly administered placebo.

Discontinuation studies. It is also important to know what happens to patients when they are taken off antipsychotic medications, as both patients and their physicians often express the natural desire to stop these medications. Although it is well recognized that such patients relapse, only a few studies have examined what contribution, if any, the relapse makes to the long-term course of the illness. Curson et al. (1985) studied a group of chronic schizophrenic patients after their stabilization for 8 weeks on depot antipsychotic medication. Patients who did not comply with their medication and therefore had more relapses (although it is possible that they did not comply because of a relapse) had a worse social adjustment at the end of 7 years than those who did not relapse.

D. A. W. Johnson et al. (1983) demonstrated a similar phenomenon in a more deliberately designed study. Stabilized chronic schizophrenic patients who relapsed because their antipsychotic medication had been discontinued had poorer social adjustment than a similar group of patients who were maintained on antipsychotic medication. The poorer social adjustment was still present after those patients who had relapsed had been given the opportunity to recover. Furthermore, after their relapse had been acutely treated, these patients required more antipsychotic medication than they had before being taken off their medication.

Discussion

Clinical Considerations With Antipsychotic Medications

The evidence reviewed here indicates that early and sustained intervention has a beneficial effect on schizophrenia that can last for 8 (Wirt and Simon 1959) and perhaps 12 years (Ey et al. 1957). One of these benefits is the prevention of the recurrence of those symptoms that would cause rehospitalization. It is important to point out that this benefit is in addition to preventing the recurrence of symptoms, because the patients are receiving maintenance antipsychotic treatment. Benefits might also include an improvement in the patient's level of functioning, as indicated by his or her ability to be gainfully employed (May et al. 1981).

Other evidence that antipsychotic medication (and perhaps other somatic treatments) can change the course of schizophrenia comes from long-term follow-up studies. Results from these studies (M. Bleuler 1978; Der et al. 1990; Eagles and Whalley 1985; Munk-Jorgensen 1987) have suggested that there has been an improvement in the course of schizophrenia since the early part of the century. It is also possible that at least some of this improvement is related to the success of somatic treatments (first convulsive treatments, then antipsychotic medications) in decreasing the time and severity of psychosis.

It is unclear whether nonsomatic treatments aimed at decreasing the length and severity of psychosis can produce the same benefits. In a retrospective study in which he examined the records of patients admitted to Worchester State Hospital from 1833 to 1852 (dates that fall within the era of "moral treatment"), Bockoven (1956) found that 71% of the patients who had been ill for less than 1 year were discharged as recovered, compared with 45% of the patients whose illness had been present for more than 1 year at the time of admission. Although uncertainty of diagnosis in this population clouds any interpretation, it is interesting that a substantial percentage of the patients did not require subsequent hospitalization.

Perhaps Bockoven's findings support recent studies in which it is indicated that there is something about gentle care of schizophrenic patients that may be important (Ciompi et al. 1992; Karon and Vandenbos 1981; Matthews et al. 1979). Unfortunately, it has proven difficult to consistently provide such treatment without using medication (Ciompi et al. 1992), and there is a dearth of replicated experimental studies that show that caring, without the simultaneous administration of medications, is sufficient to treat schizophrenia. In fact, there is evidence that overly ambitious psychotherapy, particularly in patients who are not stabilized with antipsychotic medications, is harmful (Herz 1990).

Until it can be established that other methods do as well, the evidence indicates that early and sustained intervention with antipsychotic medications in schizophrenia is important, not only for decreasing the immediate symptoms of the illness—thereby decreasing the risk of patients harming themselves and others—but also for improving the long-term outcome. This is not a wholesale endorsement for using these medications without monitoring or without developing an alliance with the patient. In fact, all patients need to be given the opportunity to weigh the potential benefits and risks of antipsychotic medication (i.e., to give their informed consent) (Wyatt 1994). On the other hand, informed consent cannot simply consist of explaining the side and adverse effects of these medications; any informed consent must also provide weighted information about the considerable benefits that these medications provide (Wyatt 1987).

The issue of when to introduce antipsychotic medications into the treatment of an individual who is believed to be schizophrenic or who is experiencing prodromal symptoms has not yet been addressed. This is largely an uncharted area that requires considerable research. Perhaps the most interesting study has been the one by Falloon (1992), in which he provided preliminary evidence that early intervention—employing a variety of techniques—with patients presenting prodromal symptoms consistent with those of schizophrenia decreases the incidence of schizophrenia. It may be of some importance that antipsychotic medications played a very small role in preventing psychosis in Falloon's (1992) study. Certainly, these primary findings need to be followed by a carefully controlled study.

Another uncharted area is how long a schizophrenic individual should be kept on antipsychotic medications before those medications are discontinued. Again, although there are no experimental data to indicate exactly when to discontinue medication, or which patients can have their antipsychotic medication safely discontinued, the relapse rates of patients 6 months to 2 years after they have been stabilized on antipsychotic medications is very high (ranging from 65% to 100% in patients followed for 12 months or more [American Psychiatric Association 1992]). In practice, it seems prudent to gradually reduce the dosage of antipsychotic medication after the patient has undergone a period of stabilization. For example, a patient who has recovered from a psychotic episode and has been maintained on a stable 10-mg/day dosage of haloperidol for a period of 6 months to 1 year might have the dosage reduced by 1 mg/month while being watched for signs of prodromal symptoms or relapse. When the dosage becomes smaller than 2 mg/day, a more gradual taper might be indicated instead of a halving of the dosage. During this time, there is ample evidence that it is important to teach the patient ways of decreasing stress and coping with his or her environment (Falloon 1990).

In addition to experimental clinical studies, there are other theoretical reasons to believe that early intervention might decrease the morbidity of the illness. Tienari (1992), in an ongoing adoption study, has demonstrated that individuals who are genetically at risk for developing schizophrenia are more likely to express the illness if their family members have schizophrenia or suffer from "soft spectrum" disorders.

Theoretical Issues

Development of symptoms.   How do antipsychotic medications interact with the putative pathophysiologic changes that take place during the first few years of a psychotic illness such as schizophrenia? In answering this question, it must be taken into account that the symptoms of schizophrenia usually remain relatively unobtrusive until adolescence or later. Because of the physical, social, and psychological changes an individual undergoes during adolescence and early adulthood, symptoms might then develop that are recognized as schizophrenia. If the psychological, social, and possibly physical scars do not become too great during this activation, there is a chance for the brain to partially (Drake and Sederer 1986) or completely heal itself (Carone et al. 1991). Another way to state this is that, in addition to suppressing symptoms, antipsychotic medications also prevent secondary handicaps (i.e., social and psychological [D. A. W. Johnson 1979]).

Substrate for symptom development.   Results from twin and recent adoption studies (e.g., Gottesman 1991; Kety and Ingraham 1992; Kety et al. 1994) continue to support the view that at least some individuals have a genetic predisposition for developing schizophrenia. However, although the evidence for genetic contribution is strong, it is far less clear exactly what is being transmitted. The strongest evidence suggests that it is those characteristics that typically accompany schizotypal personality disorder that are inherited, such as social isolation, magical thinking, self-referential ideation, perceptual distortions, peculiar use of language, and disturbances in psychological measures of attention (Parnas et al. 1990; Siever 1991). Together with this genetic predisposition, perinatal complications or early stress (e.g., in the form of institutional rearing) might be sufficient to produce schizophrenia (Parnas et al. 1990)

In fact, there is increasing evidence that prenatal changes (Bracha et al. 1992; Susser and Lin 1992; Weinberger et al. 1980), perinatal changes (O'Callaghan et al. 1992), or both, either in combination with genetic alterations or by themselves, can lead to subsequent episodes of schizophrenia.

The dormant years.   Prior to the onset of schizophrenia, there are a number of years during which the individual, unless carefully tested (Cornblatt et al. 1992), does not appear to be obviously abnormal. Although some preschizophrenic individuals are thought to have slightly lower-than-average functioning (Aylward et al. 1984), the differences are not striking. During this time, the illness appears to be dormant.

Onset of symptoms.   Although researchers are still far from understanding the pathophysiological process associated with the initial psychotic episode of a schizophrenic patient, it has often been noted that individuals seem to be more likely to have psychotic symptoms when they move away from home (e.g., to attend college, to serve in the armed services). It is possible that these ordinary, but stressful, events are the last straw for a vulnerable person.

A number of pathophysiologic mechanisms have been proposed for what might be taking place during the onset of symptoms. Feinberg (1982) suggested that synaptic pruning, which normally is a very active process during early adolescence, may be less active in individuals who will develop schizophrenia. If the wrong synapses are eliminated, or if too many or too few are pruned, this could lead to defects in neuronal integration and eventually to the symptoms of schizophrenia. Friedhoff (1986) espoused the theory that the dopamine system is restitutive. Normally, the dopamine system attempts to accommodate stress. But when it cannot adequately compensate, psychopathology (e.g., a schizophrenic psychosis) develops. Others (Murry et al. 1985; Weinberger 1987) have proposed that a brain that is damaged early in life develops normally until new brain systems are engaged. These new systems are not capable of functioning normally alongside the previously compromised brain, and the result of the increased demands on this lesioned brain is psychopathology. Certainly, hormonal changes that occur from puberty into adolescence produce a substantial physical and psychological disruption that is mildly stressful to an otherwise healthy individual and perhaps overly stressful to a more vulnerable individual (see Figure 16–1) (Mason et al. 1988; Mendleson et al. 1977; Seeman 1989). Finally, it is of interest that a number of psychiatric illnesses first manifest themselves during late adolescence and early adulthood; the average age at onset of manic-depressive illness, for example, is 28 years (Goodwin and Jamison 1990).

The course of the illness. Results from long-term follow-up studies have indicated that schizophrenic individuals tend to improve later in life (Harding 1988; Harding et al. 1992), although the exact nature of the improvement has not been well defined. In a short follow-up study, Carone et al. 1991) found that, 5 years after their initial hospitalization, first-break schizophrenic patients required fewer hospitalizations, a finding that was consistent with the results of a recent review by Ram et al. (1992). In the Carone et al. (1991) follow-up

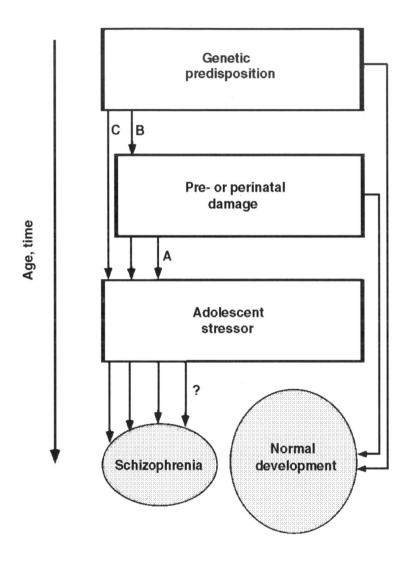

Figure 16–1. Pathways toward developing schizophrenia in late adolescence and early adulthood. *Pathway A* assumes that there is pre- or perinatal damage, followed by either an external or an internal stressor during adolescence. Internal stressors could range from neurodevelopmental changes within the brain to hormonal changes. *Pathway B* makes the same assumption as pathway A, except that there is also a genetic predisposition. *Pathway C* assumes a genetic predisposition and an adolescent stressor, but no pre- or perinatal damage.

study, however, only 17% of the patients had a complete remission after 5 years. It appears that the concept of the course of schizophrenia has advanced only slightly since E. Bleuler wrote in 1911:

> By the term "dementia praecox" or "schizophrenia" we designate a group of psychoses, whose course is at times chronic, at times marked by intermittent attacks, and which can stop or retrograde at any stage, but does not permit a restitutio ad integrum. (E. Bleuler 1911/1950)

Presumably, a vulnerable individual could decrease both the risk of developing the illness and the potential severity of that illness by decreasing stressors during adolescence. One of the stressors, however, may be the illness itself; thus, the length of time a person is psychotic and the severity of the person's symptoms determine, in part, that person's long-term morbidity. In turn, the severity and length of psychosis are influenced by the treatment received. As the individual passes into middle age, the driving force behind the psychosis seems to lose its power, and the individual is left with whatever residual defects he or she had prior to the psychosis as well as those that developed during the course of the illness (Figure 16–2).

During psychosis.   What are the processes that occur while individuals are psychotic, resulting in their decrease in functioning, and that are subsequently affected by antipsychotic medications and other treatments? Although in a number of studies (Bilder et al. 1991; Crawford et al. 1992; Lubin et al. 1962; Nelson et al. 1990; S. Rappaport and Webb 1950; Schwartzman and Douglas 1962a, 1962b), the presence of psychosis has been associated with intellectual deficits, the concomitant physiological changes have been difficult to document. Only a few brain-scan studies have shown some change associated with psychosis (Woods et al. 1990). Also, only a few histological studies have interpreted changes in the brains of schizophrenic patients as being of recent origin (Bruton et al. 1990; Nieto and Escobar 1972; Stevens 1991). Whereas Meltzer and others (Meltzer et al. 1980; reviewed by El-Mallakh et al. 1992) found evidence of leakage of enzymes from *muscles* into the bloodstream during psychosis, only one study (Vale et al. 1974) has demonstrated that enzymes may also leak from the *brain* during psychosis. G. Johnson et al. (1992) have indicated that the phase reactant α_2-FS-haptoglobin may be elevated in the cerebrospinal fluid of schizophrenic individuals. Although the hypothesis put forth here assumes that there are physiological changes during psychosis, evidence for those changes has been only sporadic.

Developing a Model of Schizophrenia

Because there is no widespread agreement on which specific brain changes are associated with schizophrenia, it is difficult to build a conceptual model of what takes place in the brain that leads to psychosis or to model the changes that take place in the brain during psychosis. Nevertheless, such hypotheses can lead to empirical tests

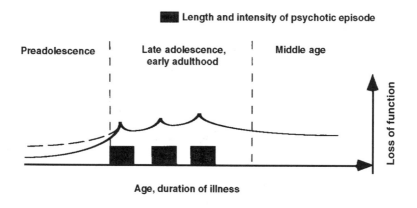

Figure 16–2. The contribution of multiple or severe psychotic episodes to a poorer long-term outcome in schizophrenia. The dashed line indicates poorer premorbid functioning. The horizontal axis represents the age of the individual and the direction of the illness; the vertical axis represents loss of function. With each psychotic episode, there is an increased loss of function that depends on both the length and the degree of the psychosis. Some of these changes may not, however, be permanent. There is evidence that, with enough time, some functions may return. This implies that some natural healing of the brain may occur in the absence of psychosis.

that can be used to accept or reject various theories (Wyatt et al. 1989).

My general thesis in this chapter is that during psychosis, there are brain changes that add to a schizophrenic individual's long-term burden. By decreasing the length or severity of the psychosis, the long-term course of schizophrenia is improved. There are at least two concepts involved in this hypothesis: first, that something takes place during psychosis that is physiologically detrimental; and second, that when the length of time or the severity of the psychosis is decreased, the pathophysiological process is diminished.

To model these notions, we (Wyatt et al. 1989) assumed that during acute psychosis the individual is under great stress. Stress is associated with a number of bodily changes, one of which is an increase in intrasynaptic dopamine, particularly in the prefrontal cortex (Abercrombie et al. 1989). Because the antipsychotic medications are thought to exert their function, at least in part, by blocking dopamine receptors, and because high concentrations of catecholamines are thought to be toxic (Cadet 1988), it seemed reasonable to develop an animal model in which there would be high concentrations of extraneuronal dopamine in the prefrontal cortex.

This model was based on cocaine, a drug that increases extraneuronal dopamine by blocking dopamine's reentry into the presynaptic neuron. Furthermore, although a cocaine-induced psychosis is thought to look phenomenologically very different from a schizophrenic psychosis, certain aspects of depression following cocaine use are similar to some of the negative symptoms seen in schizophrenia (Wyatt et al. 1989).

To determine if cocaine could produce biochemical changes in animals similar to what is expected in schizophrenic individuals, rats were given 10 mg/kg of cocaine intraperitoneally, twice a day, for 1 week. Results from this trial indicated that dopamine and one of its metabolites, dihydroxyphenylacetic acid (DOPAC), were reduced in the prefrontal cortex for at least 6 weeks following cocaine withdrawal (Karoum et al. 1990). When we looked at the autopsied brains of schizophrenic patients, we found similar decreases in dopamine and DOPAC (Table 16–4). The urine of chronic schizophrenic patients (Karoum et al. 1987) and the urine collected from rats given cocaine both exhibited a similar decrease in dopamine and DOPAC (Karoum et al. 1990). In Table 16–4, these and other changes found after cocaine was administered to rats and to humans, as well as the similarities between the rats and the schizophrenic individuals, are described. Efforts are under way to develop methods of preventing these changes in cocaine-fed animals. If such methods prove to be nontoxic, they could be tried early in the course of schizophrenia.

A further parallel can be seen between a cocaine-induced brain

Table 16–4. Biochemical similarities between animals and humans during cocaine withdrawal and chronic schizophrenia

Chronic schizophrenia	Change	Cocaine withdrawal	Change
Postmortem test results			
Cortex		Cortex	
Cingulate		Rat frontal	
Dihydroxyphenylacetic acid	Down		Down
Homovanillic acid	Down		Down
Dopamine	No change		Down
Prefrontal			
[^{3}H] GBR 12935	Down as age (duration of illness) increases	Rat	Down
Serotonin	Not known		Down
Neuropeptide Y	Not known		Down
Positron-emission tomography results			
Prefrontal cortex		Human prefrontal cortex	
Metabolism	Down	Metabolism	Down
Urine test results			
Human		Rat	
Sum molar dopamine/ sum molar norepinephrine	Down	Sum molar dopamine/ sum molar norepinephrine	Down

Sources. Hitri and Wyatt 1993; Hitri et al., in press; Karoum et al. 1987, 1990; Wahlestedt et al. 1991; Wyatt et al., in press.

change and a postmortem finding from schizophrenic individuals. GBR 12935 is an agent that binds to the dopamine transporter site and that can be used as a measure of the number of dopamine transporters in a given brain region (Hitri et al. 1991). Presumably, the number of transporters present is a reflection of the number of dopamine terminals that are present. Rats given cocaine for 1 week were followed for up to 12 weeks after drug withdrawal (Hitri and Wyatt 1993). Frontal cortex [^{3}H]GBR 12935 binding in the cocaine-fed rats was found to be decreased in comparison with that in the saline-injected control rats when the animals were sacrificed at weeks 2–6 from the time of cocaine withdrawal. At 12 weeks after withdrawal, the number of sites was still decreased compared with that in the controls, but the decrease appeared to be related to a rise in [^{3}H]GBR 12935 binding in the controls over time (the binding sites increased with age in both the control animals and the cocaine-treated animals, but the increase in the treated animals lagged behind that in the untreated animals). This finding was similar to the results of a postmortem study that found that [^{3}H]GBR 12935 binding appeared to decrease with age in the prefrontal cortex of schizophrenic individuals, whereas there was no change over the same age range in control subjects (Hitri et al., in press). To date, however, there have not been enough data to determine whether schizophrenic individuals initially have low [^{3}H]GBR 12935 binding or whether they lose these receptor sites later in the illness. If the older group is indeed different (i.e., if long-term schizophrenic patients do lose their reuptake sites), this implies that a process takes place over time that changes the brains of schizophrenic individuals. Again, the nature of the process and how it is associated with the change of symptoms over time are not known.

References

Abercrombie ED, Keefe KA, DiFrischia DS, et al: Differential effect of stress on in vivo dopamine release in striatum, nucleus accumbens, and medial frontal cortex. J Neurochem 52:1655–1658, 1989

American Psychiatric Association: Tardive Dyskinesia: A Task Force Report of the American Psychiatric Association. Edited by Kane JM, Jeste DV, Barnes TRE, et al. Washington, DC, American Psychiatric Association, 1992

Angrist BM, Schulz SC (eds): The Neuroleptic-Nonresponsive Patient: Characterization and Treatment. Progress in Psychiatry Series. Series edited by Spiegel D. Washington DC, American Psychiatric Press, 1990

Anzai N, Okazaki Y, Miyauchi M, et al: Early neuroleptic medication within one year after onset can reduce risk of later relapses in schizophrenic patients, in Annual Report of the Pharmacopsychiatric Research Foundation, Vol 19. Pharmacopsychiatric Research Foundation, 1988, pp 258–265

Aritome T: A study on the long-term prognosis of schizophrenia under psychotropic drug medication. Jikeikai Medical Journal 25:269–286, 1978

Astrup C, Noreik K: Functional Psychoses: Diagnostic and Prognostic Models. Springfield, IL, Charles C Thomas, 1966

Aylward E, Walker E, Bettes B: Intelligence in schizophrenia: meta-analysis of the research. Schizophr Bull 10:430–459, 1984

Bilder RM, Lipschutz-Broch L, Reiter G, et al: Neuropsychological deficits in the early course of first episode schizophrenia. Schizophr Res 5:198–199, 1991

Bleuler E: Dementia Praecox or The Group of Schizophrenias (1911). Translated by Zinkin J. New York, International Universities Press, 1950

Bleuler M: The Schizophrenic Disorders: Long-Term Patient and Family Studies. Translated by Clemens SM. New Haven, CT, Yale University Press, 1978

Bockoven JS: Moral treatment in American psychiatry. J Nerv Ment Dis 124:292–321, 1956

Bracha H, Torrey E, Gottesman I, et al: Second-trimester markers of fetal size in schizophrenia: a study of monozygotic twins. Am J Psychiatry 149:1355–1361, 1992

Bruton CJ, Crow TJ, Frith CD, et al: Schizophrenia and the brain: a prospective clinico-neuropathological study. Psychol Med 20:285–304, 1990

Cadet J: Free radical mechanisms in the central nervous system: an overview. Int J Neurosci 40:13–18, 1988

Carone BJ, Harrow M, Westermeyer JF: Posthospital course and outcome in schizophrenia. Arch Gen Psychiatry 48:247–258, 1991

Carpenter WT Jr, McGlashan TH, Strauss JS: The treatment of acute schizophrenia without drugs: an investigation of some current assumptions. Am J Psychiatry 134:14–20, 1977

Ciompi L, Dauwalder H-P, Maier C, et al: The pilot project 'Soteria Berne': clinical experiences and results. Br J Psychiatry 161:145–153, 1992

Cornblatt BA, Lenzenweger MF, Dworkin RH, et al: Childhood attentional dysfunctions predict social deficits in unaffected adults at risk for schizophrenia. Br J Psychiatry 161:59–64, 1992

Crawford J, Besson J, Bremner M, et al: Estimation of premorbid intelligence in schizophrenia. Br J Psychiatry 161:69–74, 1992

Crow T, MacMillan J, Johnson A, et al: The Northwick Park Study of first episodes of schizophrenia, II: a randomized controlled trial of prophylactic neuroleptic treatment. Br J Psychiatry 148:120–127, 1986

Curson DA, Barnes TRE, Bamber RW, et al: Long-term depot maintenance of chronic schizophrenic out-patients: the seven year follow-up of the Medical Research Council fluphenazine/placebo trial. Br J Psychiatry 146:464–480, 1985

Davis J: Maintenance therapy and the natural course of schizophrenia. J Clin Psychiatry 11:18–21, 1985

Der G, Gupta S, Murray RM: Is schizophrenia disappearing? Lancet 335:513–516, 1990

Drake RE, Sederer LI: The adverse effects of intensive treatment of chronic schizophrenia. Compr Psychiatry 27:313–326, 1986

Eagles JM, Whalley LJ: Decline in the diagnosis of schizophrenia among first admissions to Scottish mental hospitals from 1969 to 1978. Br J Psychiatry 146:151–154, 1985

El-Mallakh R, Egan M, Wyatt R: Creatine kinase and enolase: intracellular enzymes serving as markers of central nervous system damage in neuropsychiatric disorders. Psychiatry 55:392–402, 1992

Ey H, Igert C, Rappard P: Psychoses aigues et évolutions schizophréniques dans un service de 1930 à 1956. Ann Med Psychol (Paris) 115:231–240, 1957

Falloon IRH: Behavioral family therapy with schizophrenic disorders, in Handbook of Schizophrenia, Vol 4: Psychosocial Treatment of Schizophrenia. Edited by Herz MI, Keith SJ, Docherty JP. New York, Elsevier, 1990, pp 135–151

Falloon IRH: Early intervention for first episodes of schizophrenia: a preliminary exploration. Psychiatry 55:4–15, 1992

Feinberg I: Schizophrenia: caused by a fault in programmed synaptic elimination during adolescence? J Psychiatr Res 17:319–334, 1982

Friedhoff AJ: A dopamine-dependent restitutive system for the maintenance of mental normalcy. Ann N Y Acad Sci 463:47–52, 1986

Goodwin FK, Jamison KR: Manic-Depressive Illness. New York, Oxford University Press, 1990

Gottesman II: Schizophrenia Genesis: The Origins of Madness. New York, WH Freeman, 1991

Harding CM: Course types in schizophrenia. Schizophr Bull 14:633–644, 1988

Harding CM, Zubin J, Strauss JS: Chronicity in schizophrenia: revisited. Br J Psychiatry 161:27–37, 1992

Herz MI: Early intervention in schizophrenia, in Handbook of Schizophrenia, Vol 4: Psychosocial Treatment of Schizophrenia. Edited by Herz MI, Keith SJ, Docherty JP. New York, Elsevier, 1990, pp 25–44

Hitri A, Wyatt R: Regional differences in rat brain dopamine transporter binding: function of time after chronic cocaine. Clin Neuropharmacol 16:525–539, 1993

Hitri A, Venable D, Nguyen H, et al: Characteristics of [^{3}H]GBR 12935 binding in the human and rat frontal cortex. J Neurochem 56:1663–1672, 1991

Hitri A, Casanova MF, Kleinman JE, et al: Age-related changes in [^{3}H]GBR 12935 binding site density in the prefrontal cortex of controls and schizophrenics. Biol Psychiatry (in press)

Huber G, Gross G, Schuttler R: Schizophrenie, Verlaufs- und soczialpsychiatrische Langzeituntersuchungen an den 1945 bis 1959 in Bonn hospitalisierten schizophrenen Kranken. Monographien aus dem Gesamtgebiete der Psychiatrie. Berlin, Springer/Verlag, 1979

Huber G, Gross G, Schuttler R: Longitudinal studies of schizophrenic patients. Translated by Clemens SM. Schizophr Bull 6:592–605, 1980

Inoue K, Nakajima T, Kato N: A longitudinal study of schizophrenia in adolescence, I: the one- to three-year outcome. Jpn J Psychiatry Neurol 40:143–151, 1986

Jeste DV, Wyatt RJ: Understanding and Treating Tardive Dyskinesia. New York, Guilford, 1982

Johnson DAW: Further observations on the duration of depot neuroleptic maintenance therapy in schizophrenia. Br J Psychiatry 135:524–530, 1979

Johnson DAW, Pasterski G, Ludlow JM, et al: The discontinuance of maintenance neuroleptic therapy in chronic schizophrenic patients: drug and social consequences. Acta Psychiatr Scand 67:339–352, 1983

Johnson G, Brane D, Block W, et al: Cerebrospinal fluid protein variations common to Alzheimer's disease and schizophrenia. Appl Theor Electrophor 3:47–53, 1992

Karon BP, Vandenbos GR: Psychotherapy of Schizophrenia: The Treatment of Choice. Northvale, NJ, Jason Aronson, 1981

Karoum F, Karson D, Bigelow L, et al: Preliminary evidence of reduced combined output of dopamine and its metabolites in chronic schizophrenia. Arch Gen Psychiatry 44:604–607, 1987

Karoum F, Suddath R, Wyatt R: Chronic cocaine and rat brain catecholamines: long-term reduction in hypothalamic and frontal cortex dopamine metabolism. Eur J Pharmacol 186:1–8, 1990

Katz HM, Gunderson JG: Individual psychodynamically oriented psychotherapy for schizophrenic patients, in Handbook of Schizophrenia, Vol 4: Psychosocial Treatment of Schizophrenia. Edited by Herz MI, Keith SJ, Docherty JP. New York, Elsevier, 1990, pp 69–90

Kety SS, Ingraham LJ: Genetic transmission and improved diagnosis of schizophrenia from pedigrees of adoptees. J Psychiatr Res 26:247–255, 1992

Kety SS, Wender PH, Jacobsen B, et al: Mental illness in the biological and adoptive relatives of schizophrenic adoptees: replication of the Copenhagen Study in the rest of Denmark. Arch Gen Psychiatry 51:442–455, 1994

Kolakowska T, Williams AO, Ardern M: Schizophrenia with good and poor outcome, I: early clinical features, response to neuroleptics and signs of organic dysfunction. Br J Psychiatry 146:229–246, 1985

Lo W, Lo T: A ten-year follow-up study of Chinese schizophrenics in Hong Kong. Br J Psychiatry 131:63–66, 1977

Loebel AD, Lieberman JA, Alvir JMJ, et al: Duration of psychosis and outcome in first-episode schizophrenia. Am J Psychiatry 149:1183–1188, 1992

Lubin A, Gieseking C, Williams H: Direct measurement of cognitive deficit in schizophrenia. Journal of Consulting Psychiatry 26:139–143, 1962

Mason J, Giller E, Kosten T: Serum testosterone differences between patients with schizophrenia and those with affective disorder. Biol Psychiatry 23:357–366, 1988

Matthews SM, Roper MT, Mosher LR, et al: A non-neuroleptic treatment for schizophrenia: analysis of the two-year post-discharge risk of relapse. Schizophr Bull 5:322–333, 1979

May PRA, Tuma AH, Dixon WJ: Schizophrenia: a follow-up study of results of treatment, I: design and other problems. Arch Gen Psychiatry 33:474–478, 1976a

May PRA, Tuma AH, Yale C, et al: Schizophrenia: a follow-up study of results of treatment, II: hospital stay over two to five years. Arch Gen Psychiatry 33:481–486, 1976b

May PRA, Tuma AH, Dixon WJ: Schizophrenia: a follow-up study of results of five forms of treatment. Arch Gen Psychiatry 38:776–784, 1981

McWalter HS, Mercer R, Sutherland MM, et al: Outcomes of treatment of schizophrenia in a north-east Scottish mental hospital. Am J Psychiatry 118:529–533, 1961

Meltzer HY, Ross-Stanton J, Schlessinger S: Mean serum creatine kinase activity in patients with functional psychoses. Arch Gen Psych 37:650–655, 1980

Mendleson W, Gillin J, Wyatt R: Sexual physiology and schizophrenia. Acta Cient Venez 28:417–425, 1977

Miller R: Schizophrenia as a progressive disorder: relations to EEG, CT, neuropathological and other evidence. Neurobiology 33:17–43, 1989

Munk-Jorgensen P: Why has the incidence of schizophrenia in Danish psychiatric institutions decreased since 1970? Acta Psychiatr Scand 75:62–68, 1987

Murakami K: Changes in clinical course and symptomatology of schizophrenia following introduction of pharmacotherapy (in Japanese). Psychiatrie et Neurologia Japonica 73:635–649, 1971

Murry RM, Lewis SW, Revely AM: Towards an aetiological classification of schizophrenia. Lancet 1:1023–1026, 1985

Nelson HE, Pantelis C, Carruthers K, et al: Cognitive functioning and symptomatology in chronic schizophrenia. Psychol Med 20:357–365, 1990

Nieto D, Escobar A: Major psychoses, in Pathology of the Nervous System. Edited by Minkler J. New York, McGraw-Hill, 1972, pp 2654–2665

Nuechterlein KH, Snyder KS, Mintz J: Paths to relapse: possible transactional processes connecting patient illness onset, expressed emotion, and psychotic relapse. Br J Psychiatry 161:88–96, 1992

O'Callaghan E, Gibson T, Colohan H, et al: Risk of schizophrenia in adults born after obstetric complications and their association with early onset of illness: a controlled study. BMJ 305:1256–1259, 1992

Ødegård O: Pattern of discharge from Norwegian psychiatric hospitals before and after the introduction of psychotropic drugs. Am J Psychiatry 120:772–778, 1964

Parnas J, Schulsinger F, Mednick A: The Copenhagen high-risk study: major psychopathological and etiological findings, in Schizophrenia: Concepts, Vulnerability, and Intervention. Edited by Straube E, Hahlweg K. New York, Springer-Verlag, 1990, pp 45–56

Peterson DB, Olson GW: First admitted schizophrenics in drug era. Arch Gen Psychiatry 11:137–144, 1964

Pritchard DM: Prognosis of schizophrenia before and after pharmacotherapy, I: short term outcome. Br J Psychiatry 113:1345–1352, 1967a

Pritchard DM: Prognosis of schizophrenia before and after pharmacotherapy, II: three-year follow-up. Br J Psychiatry 113:1353–1359, 1967b

Rabiner CJ, Wegner JT, Kane JM: Outcome study of first-episode psychosis, I: relapse rates after 1 year. Am J Psychiatry 143:1155–1158, 1986

Ram R, Bromet EJ, Eaton WW, et al: The natural course of schizophrenia: a review of first-admission studies. Schizophr Bull 18:185–207, 1992

Rappaport M, Hopkins HK, Hall K, et al: Are there schizophrenics for whom drugs may be unnecessary or contraindicated? International Pharmacopsychiatry 13:100–111, 1978

Rappaport S, Webb W: An attempt to study intellectual deterioration by premorbid and psychotic testing. Journal of Consulting Psychiatry 14:95–98, 1950

Schooler NR, Goldberg SC, Boothe H, et al: One year after discharge: community adjustment of schizophrenic patients. Am J Psychiatry 123:986–995, 1967

Schwartzman A, Douglas V: Intellectual loss in schizophrenia, part 1. Can J Psychology 16:1–10, 1962a

Schwartzman A, Douglas V: Intellectual loss in schizophrenia, part 2. Can J Psychology 16:161–168, 1962b

Seeman M: Prenatal gonadal hormones and schizophrenia in men and women. Psychiatric Journal of the University of Ottawa 14:473–475, 1989

Shimazono Y: Comment and discussion, in Biological Mechanisms of Schizophrenia and Schizophrenia-Like Psychosis. Edited by Mitsuda H, Fukada T. Tokyo, Igaku Shoin, 1973, pp 126–128

Siever L: The biology of the boundaries of schizophrenia, in Advances in Neuropsychiatry and Psychopharmacology, Vol 1: Schizophrenia Research. Edited by Tamminga CA, Schulz SC. New York, Raven, 1991, pp 181–191

Stevens JR: Schizophrenia: static or progressive pathophysiology? Schizophr Res 3:184–186, 1991

Susser E, Lin S: Schizophrenia after prenatal exposure to the Dutch hunger winter of 1944–1945. Arch Gen Psychiatry 49:983–988, 1992

Tienari P: Implications of adoption studies of schizophrenia. Br J Psychiatry 161:52–58, 1992

Vale S, Espejel M, Calcaneo F, et al: Creatine phosphokinase: increased activity of the spinal fluid in psychotic patients. Arch Neurology 30:103–104, 1974

Wahlestedt C, Karoum F, Jaskiw G, et al: Cocaine-induced reduction of brain neuropeptide Y synthesis dependent on medial prefrontal cortex. Proceedings of the National Academy of Sciences 88:2078–2082, 1991

Watt DC, Katz K, Shepherd M: The natural history of schizophrenia: a 5-year prospective follow-up of a representative sample of schizophrenics by means of standardized clinical and social assessment. Psychol Med 13:663–670, 1983

Weinberger DR: Implications of normal brain development for the pathogenesis of schizophrenia. Arch Gen Psychiatry 44:660–669, 1987

Weinberger DR, Cannon-Spoor E, Potkin SG, et al: Poor premorbid adjustment and CT scan abnormalities in chronic schizophrenia. Am J Psychiatry 137:1410–1413, 1980

Wirt RD, Simon W: Differential Treatment and Prognosis in Schizophrenia. Springfield, IL, Charles C Thomas, 1959

Woods B, Yurgelen-Todd D, Benes F, et al: Progressive ventricular enlargement in schizophrenia: comparison to bipolar affective disorder and correlation with clinical course. Biol Psychiatry 27:341–352, 1990

Wyatt RJ: Side effects: introduction, in Psychopharmacology: The Third Generation of Progress. Edited by Meltzer HY. New York, Raven, 1987, pp 1407–1409

Wyatt RJ: The effect of early neuroleptic intervention on the course of schizophrenia (abstract). Schizophr Res 4:297, 1991a

Wyatt RJ: Neuroleptics and the natural course of schizophrenia. Schizophr Bull 17:235–280, 1991b

Wyatt RJ: Practical Psychiatric Practice: Clinical Interview Forms, Rating Scales, and Patient Handouts. Washington, DC, American Psychiatric Press, 1994

Wyatt RJ, Fawcett R, Kirch D: A possible animal model of defect state schizophrenia, in Schizophrenia: Scientific Progress. Edited by Schulz SC, Tamminga CA. New York, Oxford University Press, 1989, 184–189

Wyatt RJ, Karoum F, Casanova H: Decreased DOPAC in the anterior cingulate gyrus of individuals with schizophrenia. Biol Psychiatry (in press)

CHAPTER 17

Recognition and Management of Neuroleptic Noncompliance

Peter J. Weiden, M.D.;
Tasha Mott, M.A.; and Nancy Curcio, Psy.D.

D uring the 1960s, the proposal that neuroleptic agents could alter the course of schizophrenia was greeted with much optimism. However, this initial optimism was tempered by persistently high rates of noncompliance with neuroleptic medication. Despite continued advances in drug development and treatment, noncompliance remains a major public health problem. In fact, Weiden et al. (1991) found that, within 2 years of discharge, 74% of neuroleptic-responsive schizophrenic outpatients become noncompliant with their neuroleptic regimen. Similar noncompliance rates have been found in other longitudinal studies (Allgulander 1989; Serban and Thomas 1974) in a wide variety of clinical and geographic settings.

This work was supported by National Institute of Mental Health Grant R29 MH43635.

In this chapter, we focus on neuroleptic noncompliance during the outpatient phase of treatment in schizophrenia. Unless otherwise specified, we are referring specifically to patients with a clearly established diagnosis of schizophrenic, schizoaffective, or schizophreniform disorder and with a known neuroleptic-responsive treatment history.

The unreferenced data cited in this chapter are from a National Institutes of Health/National Institute of Mental Health–funded prospective study of rates and risk factors for noncompliance in schizophrenia ("Neuroleptic Noncompliance in Schizophrenia," MH 43635; P. Weiden, principal investigator; B. Rapkin, A. Zygmunt, T. Mott, D. Goldman, and A. Frances, co-investigators). The study was designed to identify and follow consecutive neuroleptic-responsive schizophrenic inpatients discharged to the community from one of three greater New York City area hospital sites. Symptom, side effect, and compliance measures were obtained by an independent rater not involved with the subjects' treatment. Major assessments were performed at discharge, and were repeated at 1, 6, and 12 months postdischarge. Patients, families, and clinicians each received a separate battery of compliance interviews that measured quantitative compliance behavior and perceptions and attitudes regarding medication therapy. The study followed a total of 124 subjects recruited between 1988 and 1991.

Scope of the Problem

Although noncompliance leads to relapse in many cases, investigators of early studies in which noncompliance was identified as the predominant cause of relapse (Mason et al. 1963; Raskin and Dyson 1968) did not recognize that noncompliance is sometimes a symptom, rather than a cause, of relapse (Lin et al. 1979; McEvoy et al. 1989). Therefore, longitudinal studies comparing the course of illness of compliant and noncompliant patients provide the best determination of how noncompliance and relapse are related. In one such study, Curson et al. (1985) found that, over a 7-year period, compliant patients had a 50% chance of rehospitalization, compared with a 100%

rehospitalization rate for intermittently or completely noncompliant patients ($P < .001$). Similarly, Serban and Thomas (1974) found that noncompliance was highly associated ($\chi^2 = 18.3$; $df = 1$; $P < .001$) with rehospitalization in a cohort of 516 chronic schizophrenic patients that were followed for 2 years. From a meta-analysis of the compliance and maintenance literature, Weiden and Olfson (in press) have estimated that noncompliance accounts for at least 40% of all relapse.

Relapse secondary to neuroleptic noncompliance may be more dangerous than relapse occurring in the context of compliance. Johnson et al. (1983) followed 60 schizophrenic patients with a remitted course of illness who stopped their medication over the course of 2 years. Compared with the relapses of medicated schizophrenic control subjects, relapses among the noncompliant patients were more common, severe, and disruptive and took longer to resolve. The effects were most prominent in the second follow-up year, suggesting that the negative impact of neuroleptic noncompliance increases over time. Neuroleptic noncompliance has also been associated with increased rates of completed suicide (Cohen et al. 1964; Planansky and Johnston 1973), assault (Virkkunen 1974), and homicide (Tanay 1987). Finally, as discussed in depth in Chapter 16 of this book, longitudinal studies support the notion that, in addition to preventing relapse, maintenance neuroleptic therapy improves the long-term prognosis of schizophrenia.

Defining Noncompliance

Most patients do not adhere strictly to their physicians' advice. Deviation from medication regimens, referred to as *dosage deviation,* and irregularity in following prescription routines are typical in all chronic diseases (Gordis et al. 1969). Therefore, it is essential to determine what the specific cutoffs are for a patient's behavior to qualify as true noncompliance with neuroleptic medication. We define noncompliance along two behavioral dimensions: complete versus partial and continuous versus transient.

Complete versus partial noncompliance. This behavioral dimension is addressed by the following question: How much of the recommended neuroleptic medication must be refused for the patient to be considered noncompliant? Some schizophrenic patients are obviously noncompliant, refusing all medication and voicing their opposition loudly and clearly. A more common—and problematic—situation occurs when the patient is intermittently compliant or is reluctant to divulge information regarding the true nature of his or her compliance. It would be overinclusive to label all patients who deviate from the neuroleptic regimen as noncompliant, because deviations occur along a continuum.

The term *noncompliant* is most meaningful when it is related to prognostic implications, management implications, or both. One important consideration is that, according to analyses of the dose-response curve for maintenance neuroleptic therapy (Kane et al. 1983; Marder et al. 1984), the minimal effective dosage is often lower than the prescribed dosage. Therefore, the dosages of many of those who deviate from the prescribed dosage may still fall within therapeutic range. Based on all of the above information, we conclude that only the complete cessation of all prescribed neuroleptic medication accurately captures true noncompliance.

Continuous versus transient noncompliance. This behavioral dimension is addressed by the following question: How much time must pass following cessation of neuroleptic medication before a patient is considered noncompliant? Establishing the minimum time criterion for medication cessation presents a more difficult task than differentiating dosage deviation from true noncompliance. In our own data analysis, we examined 36 cases of complete medication cessation. Our analysis revealed that patients who stopped medication for less than 1 week were likely to restart medication and to maintain compliance (11 out of 14 [79%]). In contrast, those patients who discontinued medication for more than 1 week were much less likely to resume maintenance medication (20 out of 22 [91%] stayed off all neuroleptic regimen until relapse; $\chi^2 = 23.6$; $df = 1$; $P < .001$). Therefore, we have determined that medication cessation for more than 1 week (8 days) is the minimum time criterion to establish true noncompliance.

Measuring Noncompliance

When measuring neuroleptic noncompliance, it is important to consider both the patient's attitude toward medication and his or her actual medication-taking behavior. Compliance behavior, by itself, does not tell the whole story. Samuel Butler *(Hubridas,* 1663) wrote, "He that complies against his will is of the same opinion still." Consequently, it is recommended that distinct and separate quantitative and qualitative noncompliance assessments be used. In this section, we outline our methods and rationale for the quantitative and qualitative assessments of noncompliance.

Quantitative Assessment

Measurement techniques.   As documented in several reviews of noncompliance (Dunbar 1981; May et al. 1976; Weintraub et al. 1973), all known methods of quantifying compliance have major limitations. For example, many of the more invasive measurement approaches cannot be used for the most noncompliant patients, as such patients will not tolerate these techniques. Other limitations include the difficulty of establishing test validity and the time-limited nature of cross-sectional assessments. A discussion of the most commonly used techniques follows.

Clinician interviews consistently underestimate the magnitude of noncompliance. Kapur et al. (1992) reported this finding in a study of schizophrenic patients on maintenance neuroleptic treatment in which clinician judgment was compared with a urine riboflavin marker. Our research also supports this finding, as is discussed below.

Appointment compliance is straightforward and relatively easy to measure. Unfortunately, like clinician interviews, appointment compliance leads to overestimations of compliance with oral regimens (Gordis et al. 1969). However, in the case of long-acting depot preparations for the maintenance neuroleptic treatment of schizophrenia, appointment compliance is an ideal tracking method provided that several conditions exist: documentation is fastidious (e.g., accurate clinical records are kept), the patient is geographically stable, and the patient does not receive treatment at an alternate site (e.g., walk-in clinic, emergency room).

Clinical outcome (e.g., relapse rate) is considered to be one of the weakest measures of compliance (Gordis 1979). Although relapse and noncompliance are both common, they are not the same. Noncompliance is sometimes a symptom of relapse, and relapse frequently occurs in the context of compliance.

Direct tracking methods (e.g., videotaping, electronic pill containers) are costly and intrusive. Of the "low-tech" tracking techniques, pill counts and patient diaries are the most practical. Although pill counts may be adequate for detecting minor dosage deviations, the accuracy of pill counts is limited by patient carelessness and "fudging" (e.g., dumping the pills out of the container before the appointment [Rudd et al. 1989]). Pill counts are not as useful as focused interviews for identifying major episodes of noncompliance (Rickels and Briscoe 1970). Patient diaries that potentially track medication schedules may be most appropriate for motivated patients who struggle with a complex drug regimen (e.g., a medically ill person on multiple medications [Hulka et al. 1975]). However, such a demanding tracking method is not feasible for many schizophrenic individuals.

Plasma and urine neuroleptic levels, which measure medication-taking events within a relatively short time frame, are limited by the large variations in interindividual steady state (Dahl 1986; Ko et al. 1985) and changes in patient metabolism over time (Currey 1985). Therefore, bioassays do not detect dosage deviation and are most effective for identifying recent cessation of an oral neuroleptic regimen (Cooper 1978; Dahl 1990).

Multisource interviewing.   Because the approaches reviewed above are either too cumbersome or too imprecise to identify most of the noncompliant schizophrenic outpatients, we have determined that noncompliance is best assessed by multisource clinical interviewing. Relying solely on patient report is not recommended. Patients tend to overstate their compliance because of their desire to display socially acceptable behaviors (Svarstad 1974). In addition, we have found that thought disorder and distorted reporting of events obscure compliance assessments. Thus, patient reports need to be supplemented with family and clinician interviews, and all of the information should be considered for a final global assessment.

Until recently, no standardized psychometric measures to quantitatively assess medication compliance in schizophrenia have been available. To address this need for compliance interview measures, our research group developed a multisource quantitative instrument named the Treatment Compliance Interview (TCI; P. J. Weiden, unpublished data, available on request). The TCI is a semistructured clinical interview, separate versions of which are given to patients, families, and clinicians. This measure reviews every dose taken for the previous 3 days (or, for depot-administered medications, the last three injections) and provides an estimate of the overall percentage of medication taken since the last visit. It also documents whether medication was stopped at any time during the interval and, if so, for how long. In addition, information is obtained about the patient's knowledge of the regimen and any changes in the patient's attitude toward compliance. Finally, there is a "truthfulness of report" estimate based on rater global impression. For research purposes, we use the source reporting the greatest amount of noncompliance.

Qualitative Assessment

Approach to the compliance interview. The interview needs to be conducted in a relaxed and nonjudgmental fashion. Although the prescribing physician is presumably most familiar with the patient and the prescribed neuroleptic regimen, the major drawback to the physician's conducting the compliance interview is that many patients are reluctant to disclose information regarding noncompliance to their prescribing physician. It is preferable, if at all possible, to have someone who is not directly treating the patient conduct the interview. In this case, the interviewer should spend some time establishing rapport with the patient. The interviewer may begin by explaining that he or she wishes to understand the patient's experience and attitude toward medication. We have found that the assessment is more accurate if the interviewer first obtains background information from the patient or an outside source. Such background information includes the specific recommended medication, dosage, route of administration, and daily schedule; who prescribed the medication and where it is obtained; recent changes in medication or treatment system; the patient's current living situation; and the degree of medication supervision. Once this information has been gathered, the interview proceeds to ascertain the patient's general attitude toward medication and potential reasons for compliance and noncompliance.

Interview problems.   One difficulty in conducting an attitudinal interview about medication is that it requires conditional thinking on the part of the patient. Even a patient who is 100% compliant is asked to give reasons why he or she might prefer not to take the medicine. Similarly, a patient who is noncompliant is asked to give reasons why he or she might be inclined to take the medicine. In these cases, we have found it useful to say something like the following:

> I understand that you take the medicine regularly and that you want to; but still, lots of people have mixed feelings about medicine. There must be times when you think to yourself, "I would really rather not take it or I wish I did not have to take it." I understand this does not cause you to actually stop taking the medication, but I am interested in what you think.

Other difficulties in assessing neuroleptic noncompliance (e.g., the patient's schizophrenia-related ambivalence, thought disorder, or hostility) may result in inconsistent responses to the interviewer's questions. In these cases, it is necessary for the interviewer to use his or her judgment in assessing what best reflects the patient's basic attitude.

Subjective measures of compliance.   As part of a longitudinal study of neuroleptic noncompliance among schizophrenic patients, Weiden et al. (1994) developed a scale for the qualitative assessment of noncompliance, named the Rating of Medication Influences (ROMI) scale. The ROMI assesses attitudinal and behavioral factors that influence compliance with neuroleptic treatment.

In addition to the ROMI, two other subjective scales of neuroleptic effect have been psychometrically tested and found to correlate with compliance behavior: the Drug Attitude Inventory (DAI; Hogan et al. 1983) and the Neuroleptic Dysphoria Scale (ND; Van Putten and May 1978). Our results (Weiden et al. 1994) showed that these measures strongly correlate on simultaneously obtained compliance summary scores and are all reasonable measures of global attitude toward medication. Therefore, we recommend that the choice of measure be based on other criteria, such as the purpose of the measure, the patient's hospital status, the need for a multidimensional measure, and training and resource constraints. In Table 17–1, we summarize the advantages and disadvantages of these measures. Use of the ROMI is indicated when assessment of psychosocial and environmental factors is considered the primary measurement goal. Of the three measures, the DAI is the most appropriate for ascertaining specific subjective responses to drug effects. Finally, the ND is superior to the ROMI and the DAI for use with acutely psychotic inpatients.

Recognizing Noncompliance

Noncompliance is a pervasive and persistent problem. Even those patients who have been completely compliant for a number of years may be at risk for stopping their medication. The contrary is also true: many seemingly hopeless patients whose lives are negatively impacted by persistent neuroleptic noncompliance can change their behavior with time or when the proper therapeutic "angle" is found. Therefore, continued surveillance and repeated psychoeducation about the effectiveness of medication remain indicated for all schizophrenic patients.

Clinician Recognition

Our research group compared compliance assessments reported by patients with those reported by physicians and primary family members in a sample of patients who deviated from their neuroleptic regimen. Of the compliance assessments reported for the 61 patients in the sample, 23 (38%) were obtained from family report alone; 12 (20%), from patient report alone; and the remaining 26 (42%), from multiple sources. The physicians did not detect any cases of noncompliance that otherwise would not have been picked up by other sources. This finding demonstrated that prescribing physicians frequently do not recognize patients' dosage deviations and may not detect noncompliance. Therefore, we conclude that the report of neuroleptic noncompliance is best obtained from as many separate sources as possible (e.g., family members, case workers, members of the patient's community, pharmacists).

Table 17–1.   Advantages and disadvantages of subjective measures of neuroleptic effects

---

Rating of Medication Influences (ROMI) Scale[a]
Advantages
1.   Directly inquires about influences leading to compliance and noncompliance.
2.   Covers more domains than other measures.
3.   Has been validated across other information sources.
4.   Has been successfully field tested with a variety of patient populations and in a variety of clinical settings.
Disadvantages
1.   Requires a trained rater familiar with outpatient schizophrenia.
2.   Rater judgment items are not reliable.
3.   Often is not appropriate for acutely psychotic patients.
Drug Attitude Inventory (DAI)[b]
Advantages
1.   Can be used as a self-report measure.
2.   Has forced-choice response format, not affected by rater bias.
3.   Requires minimal rater training.
4.   Has a brief administration time.
Disadvantages
1.   Has not been prospectively tested for patients whose compliance is not known.
2.   Does not include certain domains that are known to be important in compliance (e.g., stigma, environment).
Neuroleptic Dysphoria (ND) Scale[c]
Advantages
1.   Is the most global subjective measure.
2.   Requires minimal rater training.
3.   Has a brief administration time.
Disadvantages
1.   Psychometric properties have not been established for an outpatient population.
2.   Items may be too broad to separate dysphoria from side effects from other effects.

---

[a]Weiden et al. 1994b. [b]Hogan et al. 1983. [c]Van Putten and May 1978.

Multiple information sources are particularly useful for clinicians beginning treatment with a new patient. A patient's self-reported compliance history is not always reliable. Patients sometimes claim to have stopped medication based on a professional's recommendation. Although this assertion may be true in some cases, such reports are frequently distorted. In reality, one of the following may have occurred:

- The patient may have received contrasting advice about medication (e.g., one clinician was in favor of medication whereas another was opposed).
- The patient may have wanted to stop medication despite the advice of the doctor and consequently changed doctors or treatment systems until he or she found someone who did not recommend medication.
- The patient may have insisted on stopping medication, and the physician's reluctant acquiescence may then have been interpreted as a recommendation.

Clinical Indicators of Noncompliance

The association between noncompliance and relapse has already been discussed (see above); to summarize, although noncompliance can lead to relapse, noncompliance could also be a secondary symptom of relapse. In addition to the reemergence of psychotic symptoms, professionals working with schizophrenic patients should routinely screen for various clinical indicators of noncompliance, including physical, attitudinal or cognitive, environmental, interpersonal, and psychological indicators.

Physical signs suggestive of neuroleptic noncompliance can be observed during the clinical interview. For example, increased dyskinetic movements or decreased parkinsonian movements are characteristic of cessation of medication (Gardos et al. 1978). Laboratory testing may also reveal signs of noncompliance, such as a normal prolactin level or the absence of neuroleptics in urine drug-screening tests (Dahl 1986).

Attitudinal and cognitive signs of noncompliance are more difficult to discern than the physical signs. The clinician should be wary if a patient suddenly becomes less concerned about side effects or less resistant to neuroleptic medication. Indifference to logistical issues involved in obtaining medication (e.g., patient does not spontaneously ask about refilling prescriptions) may also signal noncompliance. Similarly, it is highly probable that a patient with little or no knowledge of the details of the drug regimen (e.g., the color or shape of the pill, the frequency of doses)—especially when that patient's medication regimen is unsupervised—is noncompliant. In addition, a patient with erroneous beliefs about neuroleptics (e.g., that the medication is addictive, that the medication is the cause of the voices the patient hears) is unlikely to adhere to the regimen.

Episodes of noncompliance are frequently precipitated by *environmental factors* (Blackwell 1976). Such situations include the patient's going away on a trip; the absence of the family member who usually supervises the medication regimen; a therapist's vacation; the change of therapist, physician, or treatment setting; or a transient financial obstacle (e.g., the loss of a Medicaid card, a pending application for medical financial assistance). Another environmental factor is the availability of illicit drugs. Obviously a major problem in its own right, substance abuse may precipitate noncompliance (Drake and Wallach 1989). Patients often stop their medicine to "get high," believing that the combination of proscribed and prescribed drugs is dangerous (see Chapter 32).

Interpersonal factors often impact compliance. Noncompliant behavior can be influenced by significant others (e.g. friends, family members, a nonprescribing therapist) who are opposed to medication. In addition, changes in the patient's living situation or in the composition of the patient's household can be disruptive and trigger noncompliant episodes.

Episodes of noncompliance are frequently associated with *psychological factors* (Corrigan et al. 1990). Clinicians should be sensitive to the patient's expression of feelings of embarrassment regarding illness. Often, the medication acts as a concrete and painful reminder of the stigma surrounding mental illness. A related patient concern involves the perception that taking medication reflects moral weakness. Some patients are uncomfortable with the fact that they are dependent on medication to function. In addition, a patient's mental status may impact his or her willingness to take medication (Lin et al. 1979). Frequently, after a period of improved functioning, a patient may believe that he or she is cured and no longer needs medication. Or, in extreme cases, a patient may deny that he or she ever had the illness. This denial can sometimes be an expression of psychotic processes. In either situation, the patient does not feel that the neuroleptic medication is necessary.

Research Findings

Our analysis (Weiden et al. 1994) of the ROMI scale supports the presence of a number of the above clinical indicators as impacting on the schizophrenic patient's compliance to medication.

Reluctance domains.   We have identified five domains related to reluctance to take medication.

- *Denial of mental illness*—The patient's perceptions that he or she is not ill, does not need medication, and is distressed by side effects.
- *Lack of benefit from treatment*—The patient's perceptions of a poor therapeutic alliance and a lack of ongoing benefit from medication
- *Environmental obstacles*—The patient's difficulty accessing treatment or the patient's report of a lack of family support
- *Rejection of mental illness label*—The patient's report of feeling embarrassed about his or her mental illness
- *Financial obstacles*—Monetary issues that impede the patient's continued use of neuroleptic medication.

Willingness domains.   Using the ROMI, we have also identified three domains related to willingness to take medication. These domains are good prognostic indicators for compliance.

- *Influence of significant others*—The patient's perception of a positive relationship with the prescribing doctor or therapist, and of family members' or friends' endorsement of the medication.
- *Prevention of illness*—The patient's belief that medication will keep the illness from returning and, thus, prevent him or her from having to be rehospitalized
- *Daily benefit from medication*—The patient's perception of a benefit from the medication and feeling that there is no pressure to comply

Familiarity with the above-identified domains can be useful in determining how much attention needs to be focused on compliance issues in treatment. Patients who report several items or at least one reluctance domain are at high risk for noncompliance. Conversely, patients who report several items or at least one willingness domain may not be at imminent risk. These factors can aid the clinician in managing noncompliance.

Managing Noncompliance

All mental health service providers should be actively involved in managing neuroleptic noncompliance. Many concrete approaches to management are available that are effective in promoting compliance. The following recommendations are divided into psychopharmacologic and psychosocial management; in practice, however, these approaches often overlap. The techniques discussed below may supplement the clinical treatment strategies outlined in other chapters.

Psychopharmacological Management

Minimizing extrapyramidal side effects.   Untreated or unrecognized side effects are very distressing and contribute to medication resistance. Weiden et al. (1989) found akinesia and akathisia to be the most commonly reported side effects related to noncompliance. Extrapyramidal side effects (EPS) should be aggressively managed through adjustment of neuroleptic dosage, addition of antiparkinsonian agents, or a combination of these strategies. There is considerable variability in patient response to antiparkinsonian agents; therefore, it can be useful to try several different agents sequentially for patients with persistent parkinsonian symptoms. Clinicians should treat suspected akathisia aggressively; akathisia is associated with both noncompliance and neuroleptic nonresponse (Levinson et al. 1990). The risk-benefit ratio for treating akathisia is strongly in favor of treating equivocal cases. Risperidone is less likely to induce acute EPS than are other high-potency neuroleptic agents (Marder and Meibach 1994).

For this reason, risperidone should be considered when minimizing acute EPS is the primary pharmacological goal. One situation in which this goal is particularly important is that in which a family member stops supporting a patient's medication treatment with a standard neuroleptic because of concern over neuroleptic-induced akinesia (Weiden 1994).

The prophylactic use of anticholinergic medications is controversial; however, for patients with unknown EPS histories who are prescribed high-potency neuroleptics, anticholinergic drugs can prevent an acute dystonic reaction that may result in long-term conditioned avoidance of neuroleptic medication. Another approach to minimizing EPS is to start the neuroleptic medication at a daily dosage lower than the eventual target dosage and to reach the final target dosage within 3–4 days.

Preventing relapse.   Aggressive treatment of early signs of relapse (e.g., positive symptoms) may circumvent noncompliance or relapse secondary to noncompliance (Herz and Melville 1980). Recommended strategies include finding the most effective drug for the individual patient and considering risperidone or clozapine for outpatients whose noncompliance seems driven by refractory psychotic symptoms despite compliance. When dosage lowering is indicated for outpatients on maintenance therapy, it is important to lower the dosage gradually to prevent relapse. Such a technique involves a maximum reduction of 10%–20% per month.

Using depot drug delivery.   Converting from an oral to a long-acting form of neuroleptic medication may improve compliance. In a preliminary study of the effects of depot conversion on future compliance (Weiden et al., in press), inpatients converted to depot medication had significantly better compliance at the 1-month postdischarge point. Demographic, hospital site, or baseline medical attitudes or symptom differences at discharge did not account for this finding. The initial beneficial compliance effect of depot medication subsided; no significant differences between depot and oral medication compliance were found at 6 and 12 months postdischarge. Converting schizophrenic inpatients from an oral to a depot neuroleptic regimen while still in the hospital facilitates the transition to outpatient treatment; however, other interventions are needed to maintain compliance over time. Although it has not yet been established that depot administration improves long-term compliance, switching patients to depot medication facilitates the early identification of noncompliant patients. In addition, when depot patients relapse, it is much easier to determine whether the decompensation occurred in the context of noncompliance than it is for patients maintained on an oral regimen.

We strongly advise initiating depot medication during inpatient hospitalization rather than after discharge. Many patients are fearful of injections or resist changes in their drug regimen, and a hospitalization may be the only opportunity to make the switch from oral to depot medication. In our experience, approximately two-thirds of inpatients who initially resisted a depot delivery were eventually persuaded to accept the recommendation; the majority of those patients received at least one further depot injection as an outpatient. When initiating depot therapy for the first time, we suggest starting with a low dosage (e.g., 6.25 mg of fluphenazine decanoate or 50 mg of haloperidol decanoate) and gradually increasing the dosage over 4–6 weeks while continuing the oral medication. Although this technique is more cumbersome than administering a loading dosage, it prevents overshooting and subsequent toxicity (Weiden et al. 1993).

Prescribing atypical neuroleptics and other adjunctive treatments. Risperidone and clozapine are the currently available antipsychotic medications in North America. Both of these agents are less likely than standard neuroleptics to induce acute extrapyramidal symptoms. The hope that atypical antipsychotics will, in the long run, improve outpatient compliance makes intuitive sense but has yet to be proven. One report has implied that crossover to risperidone improved outpatient compliance (Addington et al. 1993), but methodologic limitations prevent drawing any firm conclusions. Similarly, Meltzer (1992) reported that 32 of 155 clozapine-tolerant patients were noncompliant after a median follow-up duration of 31 months. Again, this finding is potentially limited by selection-bias issues and nonspecific compliance improvements that might occur from the increased services that clozapine patients require (e.g., weekly blood count monitoring). For clinicians wishing to improve medication compliance with atypical agents, risperidone, because of its relative ease of use, is preferable over clozapine.

Usually, clinicians hesitate to prescribe clozapine to patients who have a prominent history of noncompliance. There are situations, however, in which an atypical neuroleptic such as clozapine may be indicated despite noncompliance. The first indication for use of atypical neuroleptics is when the patient's noncompliance is deemed to be secondary to noncooperation that is a symptom of a refractory psychosis. The goal of clozapine treatment would be to break the "catch-22" noncooperation-noncompliance cycle. Kane et al. (1988) found that, compared with chlorpromazine-treated patients, clozapine-treated patients were significantly more cooperative by the end of the first week of treatment. An appropriate candidate for an atypical neuroleptic would be a patient who remains severely symptomatic and non-cooperative even after a 6-week trial of standard neuroleptic in which compliance is confirmed by plasma neuroleptic or depot delivery. A second indication for an atypical neuroleptic is when the patient's noncompliance is secondary to EPS-related neuroleptic intolerance. A third set of patients who are appropriate for a trial of atypical neuroleptics are those who are cooperative in taking medication and acknowledge their illness, but who have stopped standard neuroleptic medications because of severe EPS-induced distress.

Prospective compliance studies comparing newer drugs with the more conventional drugs, and comparing the depot route of drug delivery with the oral route, are urgently needed.

Simplifying the drug regimen. Complex medication regimens have been consistently shown to represent a strong risk factor for noncompliance (Haynes 1979). During inpatient hospitalization, complicated multidrug regimens are frequently prescribed and then continued postdischarge. For example, a schizoaffective patient might be discharged on multiple medications—for instance, oral haloperidol, lithium, carbamazepine, lorazepam, and benztropine—with a follow-up clinic appointment for 1 month later. It is unlikely that, without adequate social supports, such a patient would be able to follow this regimen.

Schizophrenia, in particular, poses special challenges to patients in following complicated regimens. Psychotic symptoms or concrete thinking often interfere with a patient's ability to follow a prescribed regimen. For example, one patient took only half the prescribed dosage when the pharmacist substituted two 5-mg tablets for his usual one 10-mg tablet. In another case, a patient refused to take the pills when her green capsules were switched to generic white pills. Careful attention must be paid to the specifics of the regimen, as seemingly innocuous changes can cause major compliance problems. The regimen should be thoroughly reviewed with the patient. Often, enlisting the help of a family member or pharmacist can further assist the patient in understanding his or her medication regimen.

Psychosocial Management

Arranging the logistical aspects of treatment.   Many opportunities to minimize the likelihood of noncompliance arise during inpatient treatment. Highly disorganized or less-motivated patients may abandon their medication soon after discharge if a treatment system is not in place (Zygmunt et al. 1992). Therefore, it is important to arrange for outpatient medication benefits (e.g., Medicaid), an appropriate living situation, and psychiatric aftercare. Compliance among chronic schizophrenic outpatients is very vulnerable to changes in medication reimbursement systems (Soumerai et al. 1994). Such issues also need to be addressed during the outpatient phase of treatment, given that even minor transportation difficulties can prevent access to treatment. In some cases, simply providing concrete medication directions and reviewing them with the patient, or enlisting the help of a pharmacist, can be an effective solution.

Addressing psychological factors.   The clinician's recognition of each patient's specific psychological factors can help promote adherence to the treatment regimen. Such factors may include denial of illness, sensitivity to the stigma associated with mental illness, and psychotic symptoms. For patients who deny their illness, it is helpful to find a mutually agreed-upon symptom (e.g., anxiety, insomnia) that will allow the patient to justify the use of the neuroleptic. This approach is also indicated for patients who feel stigmatized by schizophrenia. With these patients, drawing a parallel between their disorder and medical illnesses (e.g., diabetes, tuberculosis) may ameliorate feelings of embarrassment. In addition, emphasizing the patient's perception of daily benefit from and feelings of well-being while on the neuroleptic can decrease the patient's resistance to medication. As previously noted, it is critical to minimize acute EPS, particularly the movement disorders. These disorders are readily visible to others and, therefore, often embarrassing to the patient.

Fostering the therapeutic alliance. An additional advantage to addressing the above psychological factors is that the clinician may be fostering the therapeutic alliance. Our research group has found that a strong patient-clinician relationship is a primary reason for compliance in a substantial number of schizophrenic patients (Weiden et al. 1994). For these patients, exclusive emphasis on medication is not sufficient. Instead, some aspect of a strong clinical relationship (e.g., stability, nurturance, authority) provides a more powerful incentive to maintain compliance.

Individualizing the level of medication supervision. Careful assessment is required to determine the level of structure and supervision appropriate for each patient. For example, a highly structured and supervised setting is most effective in the treatment of patients experiencing negative symptoms or disorganization. Conversely, this type of setting may be ineffective for paranoid patients, who often require solitude, or for patients who keenly feel the stigma associated with mental illness; these latter patients may need to distance themselves from formal psychiatric settings. A low-key, low-frequency treatment approach may be more beneficial for such patients. In extreme circumstances, such as during suicidal or psychotic exacerbations, more structure may be indicated. Families or treatment systems may need to use pressure techniques (e.g., threatened eviction, loss of privileges) in response to a patient's noncompliance. However, these techniques are generally not effective as a long-term solution, and may in fact be detrimental.

Offering psychoeducation.   Psychoeducation actively involves the patient and family in the treatment system. Keith et al. (1991) found an association between attendance at psychoeducation groups and subsequent patient compliance. Prescribing physicians or other treatment staff should encourage participation in psychoeducation. Early on in treatment it is necessary to dispel misperceptions about the illness, discuss the need for maintenance neuroleptic treatment, and review the early warning signs of relapse. Later, patient and family concerns related to side effects, stigma, and logistical issues need to be addressed. Eckman et al. (1990) developed a focused medication management module with videotape for patients. This module has been shown to improve patient compliance on short-term follow-up.

Conclusions

Although a majority of schizophrenic patients can benefit from neuroleptic treatment, many do not adhere to their prescribed regimen. These patients function below their capacity, at great cost both to themselves and to society. On an individual basis, clinicians can address this problem through the timely recognition and effective management of noncompliance. However, management at this level does not sufficiently address the pervasive nature of the problem. Instead, neuroleptic compliance needs to be a public health priority. Systematic changes within the public health system could facilitate treatment delivery to noncompliant patients (e.g., outreach, education, drop-in centers). Finally, more research needs to be done to test the efficacy of depot drug delivery and recently developed antipsychotic agents as pharmacological methods to promote compliance.

References

Addington DE, Jones BD, Bloom D, et al: Reduction in hospital days in chronic schizophrenic patients treated with risperidone: a retrospective study. Clin Ther 15:917–925, 1993

Allgulander C: Psychoactive drug use in a general population sample, Sweden: correlates with perceived health, psychiatric diagnoses, and mortality in an automated record. Am J Public Health 79:1006–1009, 1989

Blackwell B: Treatment adherence. Br J Psychiatry 129:513–531, 1976

Cohen S, Leonard CV, Faberbrow AC, et al: Tranquilizers and suicide in schizophrenic patients. Arch Gen Psychiatry 11:312–321, 1964

Cooper TB: Plasma level monitoring of antipsychotic drugs. Clin Pharmacokinet 3:14–38, 1978

Corrigan PW, Liberman RP, Engel JD: From noncompliance to collaboration in the treatment of schizophrenia. Hosp Community Psychiatry 41:1203–1211, 1990

Currey SH: Commentary: the strategy and value of neuroleptic drug monitoring. J Clin Psychopharmacol 5:263–271, 1985

Curson DA, Barnes TR, Bamber RW, et al: Long-term depot maintenance of chronic schizophrenic outpatients: the 7-year follow-up of the Medical Research Council fluphenazine placebo trial, III: relapse postponement or relapse prevention? the implications for long-term outcome. Br J Psychiatry 146:474–480, 1985

Dahl SG: Plasma level monitoring of antipsychotic drugs: clinical utility. Clin Pharmacokinet 11:36–61, 1986

Dahl SG: Pharmacokinetics of antipsychotic drugs in man. Acta Psychiatr Scand Suppl 358:37–40, 1990

Drake RE, Wallach MA: Substance abuse among the chronically mentally ill. Hosp Community Psychiatry 40:1041–1046, 1989

Dunbar J: Adhering to medical advice, a review. International Journal of Mental Health 9:70–87, 1981

Eckman TA, Liberman RP, Phipps CC, et al: Teaching medication management skills to schizophrenic patients. J Clin Psychopharmacol 10:33–38, 1990.

Gardos G, Cole JO, Tarsy D: Withdrawal syndromes associated with antipsychotic drugs. Am J Psychiatry 135:1321–1324, 1978

Gordis L: Conceptual and methodologic problems in measuring patient compliance, in Compliance in Health Care. Edited by Haynes RB, Taylor DW, Sackett DL. Baltimore, John Hopkins University Press, 1979, pp 23–48

Gordis L, Mankowitz M, Lilienfeld AM: Studies in the epidemiology and preventability of rheumatic fever, IV: a quantitative determination of compliance in children on oral penicillin prophylaxis. Pediatrics 43:173–182, 1969

Haynes RB: Determinants of compliance: the disease and the mechanics of treatment, in Compliance in Health Care. Edited by Haynes RB, Taylor DW, Sackett DL. Baltimore, John Hopkins University Press, 1979, pp 49–62

Herz MI, Melville C: Relapse in schizophrenia. Am J Psychiatry 137:801–805, 1980

Hogan TD, Awad AG, Eastwood R: A self-report scale predictive of drug compliance in schizophrenics: reliability and discriminative validity. Psychol Med 13:177–183, 1983

Hulka B, Kupper L, Cassel J, et al: Medication use and misuse: physician-patient discrepancies. Journal of Chronic Disease 28:7–21, 1975

Johnson DAW, Pasterski G, Ludlow JM, et al: The discontinuation of maintenance neuroleptic therapy in chronic schizophrenic patients: drug and social consequences. Acta Psychiatr Scand 67:339–352, 1983

Kane JM, Rifkin A, Woerner M, et al: Low-dose neuroleptic treatment of outpatient schizophrenics. Arch Gen Psychiatry 40:893–896, 1983

Kane J, Honigfeld G, Singer J, et al: Clozapine for the treatment-resistant schizophrenic: a double-blind comparison with chlorpromazine. Arch Gen Psychiatry 45:789–796, 1988

Kapur S, Ganguli R, Ulrich R, et al: Use of random-sequence riboflavin as a marker of medication compliance in chronic schizophrenics. Schizophr Res 6:49–53 1992

Keith SJ, Bellack A, Frances A, et al: The influence of diagnosis and family treatment on acute treatment response and the short-term outcome in schizophrenia. Psychopharmacol Bull 25:336–339, 1991

Ko GN, Korpi E, Linnoila M: On the clinical relevance and methods of quantification of plasma concentration of neuroleptics. J Clin Psychopharmacol 5:253–262, 1985

Levinson DF, Simpson GM, Singh H, et al: Fluphenazine dose, clinical response, and extrapyramidal symptoms during acute treatment. Arch Gen Psychiatry 47:761–768, 1990.

Lin IF, Spiga R, Fortsch W: Insight and adherence to medication in chronic schizophrenics. J Clin Psychiatry 40:430–432, 1979

Marder SR, Meibach R: Risperidone in the treatment of schizophrenia. Am J Psychiatry 151:825–835, 1994

Marder SR, Van Putten T, Mintz J, et al: Costs and benefits of two doses of fluphenazine. Arch Gen Psychiatry 41:1025–1029, 1984

Mason AS, Forrest I, Forrest F, et al: Adherence to maintenance therapy and rehospitalization. Diseases of the Nervous System 24:103–104, 1963

May PRA, Tuma AH, Yale C, et al: Schizophrenia: a follow-up study of results of treatment. Arch Gen Psychiatry 33:481–486, 1976

McEvoy JP, Appelbaum PS, Apperson LJ, et al: Why must some schizophrenic patients be involuntarily committed? the role of insight. Compr Psychiatry 30:13–17, 1989

Meltzer H: Treatment of the neuroleptic-nonresponsive schizophrenic patient. Schizophr Bull 18:515–542, 1992

Planansky K, Johnston R: Clinical setting and motivation in suicide attempts of schizophrenics. Acta Psychiatr Scand 49:680–690, 1973

Raskin M, Dyson WL: Treatment problems leading to readmission of schizophrenic patients. Arch Gen Psychiatry 19:356–360, 1968

Rickels K, Briscoe E: Assessment of dosage deviation in outpatient drug research. J Clin Pharmacol 10:153–161, 1970

Rudd P, Byyny RL, Zachary V, et al: The natural history of medication compliance in a drug trial: limitations of pill counts. Clin Pharmacol Ther 46:169–176, 1989

Serban G, Thomas A: Attitudes and behaviors of acute and chronic schizophrenic patients regarding ambulatory treatment. Am J Psychiatry 136:991–995, 1974

Soumerai S, McLaughlin TJ, Ross-Degnan D, et al: Effects of limiting Medicaid drug-reimbursement benefits on the use of psychotropic agents and acute mental health services by patients with schizophrenia. N Engl J Med 331:650–655, 1994

Svarstad BL: Physician-patient communication and patient conformity with medical advice, in The Growth of Bureaucratic Medicine. Edited by Mechanic D. New York, Wiley, 1974

Tanay E: Homicidal behavior in schizophrenics. J Forensic Sci 32:1382–1388, 1987

Van Putten T, May PRA: Subjective response as a predictor of outcome in pharmacotherapy: the consumer has a point. Arch Gen Psychiatry 35:477–480, 1978

Virkkunen M: Observations on violence in schizophrenia. Acta Psychiatr Scand 50:145–151, 1974

Weiden PJ: Neuroleptics and quality of life: the patient and family perspectives (abstract). Neuropsychopharmacology 10 (suppl 3):241, 1994

Weiden PJ, Olfson M: Costs of relapse in schizophrenia. Schizophr Bull (in press)

Weiden PJ, Mann JJ, Dixon L, et al: Is neuroleptic dysphoria a healthy response? Compr Psychiatry 30:546–552, 1989

Weiden PJ, Dixon L, Frances A, et al: Neuroleptic noncompliance in schizophrenia, in Advances in Neuropsychiatry and Psychopharmacology, Vol 1: Schizophrenia Research. Edited by Tamminga C, Schulz C. New York, Raven, 1991, pp 285–296

Weiden PJ, Schooler N, Severe J, et al: Stabilization and depot neuroleptic dosages. Psychopharmacol Bull 29:269–275, 1993

Weiden PJ, Rapkin B, Mott T, et al: Rating of Medication Influences (ROMI) scale in schizophrenia. Schizophr Bull 20:297–310, 1994

Weiden PJ, Rapkin B, Mott T, et al: Converting schizophrenic inpatients from an oral to a depot neuroleptic regimen during acute hospitalization: effects on outpatient compliance. Psychiatric Services (in press)

Weintraub M, Au W, Lasagna L: Compliance as a determinant of serum digitoxin concentration. JAMA 224:481–484, 1973

Zygmunt A, Weiden P, Goldman D, et al: Predictors of noncompliance in schizophrenia. Paper presented at the annual meeting of the American Psychiatric Association, Washington, DC, May 1992

CHAPTER 18

Clinical Use of Neuroleptic Plasma Levels

Theodore Van Putten, M.D.,[†] and
Stephen R. Marder, M.D.

For the past two decades, it has been known that there is enormous (up to a 100-fold) variation in plasma levels of most neuroleptics in patients on the same dosage (Dahl 1986; Midha et al. 1988). On this basis, it was hoped that aberrant plasma levels could explain some cases of treatment resistance. Much of the research on the relationship between plasma levels of antipsychotic drug and clinical change, however, has been difficult to interpret because of assay shortcomings or design deficiencies (e.g., lack of fixed-dosage design, contamination of pharmacotherapy with other treatments, inclusion of treatment-resistant patients) (Davis et al. 1978; P. R. A. May and Van Putten 1978). One important question that remains to be adequately addressed is whether the drug is biologically available to the patient.

This manuscript was supported by a Department of Veterans Affairs Merit Review Grant to Theodore Van Putten, M.D.

[†]Deceased.

Bioavailability as a Cause of Treatment Failure

Although *hypermetabolism, decreased absorption,* and *decreased bioavailability* are terms used to justify high dosages of neuroleptics, there are few examples in the literature that support decreased bioavailability as the cause of treatment failure (Van Putten et al. 1991). Because most treatment-refractory patients, at least in public institutions, have been given a trial of treatment with fluphenazine decanoate (thereby avoiding the first-pass metabolism that could lead to aberrantly low plasma levels), it is very unlikely that decreased bioavailability is an adequate explanation for treatment failure, except in an occasional patient. To confirm this, Van Putten et al. (1985) examined the plasma levels in 12 treatment-refractory schizophrenic patients who had been in a state hospital for many years. Over the years, these patients had been on high dosages of haloperidol (40–420 mg/day) because of the prescribing clinician's assumption that they were "hypermetabolizers" or "poor absorbers." Van Putten et al. (1985) found that in only two patients was the plasma haloperidol level low relative to the dosage, but not so low as to explain those patients' resistance to medication treatment. Since that study, we have consulted on the cases of at least 30 other treatment-refractory patients on high dosages of neuroleptics (greater than 30 mg/day of haloperidol); in none of these cases was the plasma level of haloperidol greater than 15 ng/ml.

Although plasma levels of neuroleptics (at least in the case of haloperidol) in treatment-resistant patients are usually adequate, there remains the possibility that the drug is not available to the central nervous system because of excessive protein binding. It is well known that drugs such as chlorpromazine, trifluoperazine, thioridazine, and haloperidol are extensively bound to plasma proteins (Cohen et al. 1976; Forsman and Ohman 1977; Nyberg et al. 1978; Verbeeck et al. 1983). Consequently, only a small portion of the total drug in the plasma remains free from binding, although it is the "free fraction" that is responsible for therapeutic activity. Therefore, it may be important to establish the protein-binding status of a refractory patient who appears to have adequate total levels of neuroleptic medication in his or her plasma. To date, this has not been investigated.

Identification of Behavioral Toxicity

If there is a therapeutic window relationship between neuroleptic plasma levels and clinical response, then some patients, at least in theory, could be refractory (or exhibit behavioral toxicity) because of excessively high plasma levels. Behavioral toxicity secondary to neuroleptics is well documented. For example, the administration of phenothiazines can lead to the development of a catatonic-like state (Gelenberg 1976; R. H. May 1959). Akathisia is often difficult to differentiate from psychotic excitement and can be associated with psychotic exacerbation (Van Putten and Marder 1987). Akinesia is very difficult (if not impossible) to differentiate from schizophrenic blunting, apathy, and withdrawal; in fact, a syndrome named *akinetic depression* has been described (Van Putten and Marder 1987). An unsettled question is whether behavioral toxicity is associated with unusually high plasma levels.

High Plasma Level and Behavioral Toxicity

Investigators in several studies have described therapeutic window relationships between neuroleptic plasma levels and clinical response (see review in Dahl 1986). There have been only a few reports, however, of improvement in patients who manifest psychotic symptoms concomitant with high plasma neuroleptic levels once their neuroleptic dosage is reduced.

Van Putten et al. (1981) observed that four of six patients who became worse after a dosage increase had chlorpromazine plasma concentrations well above 95 ng/ml. Three of these patients (with plasma chlorpromazine concentrations of 270 ng/ml, 120 ng/ml, and 110 mg/ml) developed an agitated excitement and became assaultive. When their plasma chlorpromazine levels were lowered, those behaviors disappeared. Curry et al. (1970) published their findings on a patient with a high (605 ng/ml) plasma level of chlorpromazine who remained "uncooperative, assaultive, fearful and hostile" (p. 293).

Reduction of this patient's dosage by one-third (to 600 mg/day) resulted in a corresponding reduction in plasma level concentrations and in considerable and sustained improvement, characterized by a reduction of fear and hostility and an absence of assaultive behavior.

Extein et al. (1983) also reported on a single patient in whom the initial antipsychotic effect of haloperidol was lost but then regained, as plasma levels went above (27.5 ng/ml) and then were brought back into the therapeutic window (10 ng/ml). Schulz et al. (1984) published data on a patient who improved on haloperidol at a dosage of 5 mg/day; at this dosage, the patient had a surprisingly high plasma haloperidol level (22 ng/ml). When the dosage of haloperidol was increased to 15 mg/day, the patient showed a plasma level of 64 ng/ml and developed increased psychotic symptomatology. When the dosage (and thereby the plasma level) was lowered, the psychotic symptomatology improved.

Bjorndal et al. (1980) compared standard versus high dosages of haloperidol in 22 male, relatively treatment-resistant, chronic schizophrenic inpatients. These patients were randomly assigned to receive either 2-mg tablets (standard dosage) or 20-mg tablets (high dosage) of haloperidol. At the end of the trial, the dosage of haloperidol in the standard-dosage group was 12–36 mg/day (mean = 15 mg/day) and that in the high-dosage group was 10–240 mg/day (mean = 103 mg/day). Three of the high-dosage patients with plasma levels above 100 ng/ml exhibited attacks of violent aggression during which they struck fellow patients and staff and damaged furniture. These attacks disappeared after a 50% reduction in their plasma level concentrations. Further, Bjorndal et al. noted that depressive symptomatology (e.g., somatic concern, anxiety, guilt, depressive mood) increased significantly in those treated with high dosages.

Results from the aforementioned cases indicate that, at least for some patients, there is behavioral toxicity at higher plasma levels. Furthermore, these high plasma levels in some cases occurred at very ordinary dosages. Because treatment-refractory patients are usually on high dosages of neuroleptics, it is likely that some would improve if their dosages (and thereby their plasma levels) were lowered. In clinical settings, patients who have been resistant to treatment have shown marked improvement after the dosage of their medication has been reduced. The extent of this phenomenon is unknown; systematic research in which high plasma levels are systematically lowered in treatment-resistant patients is only now beginning (Van Putten et al. 1993).

Assays

Since 1981, high-performance liquid chromatography (HPLC) methods for nearly all neuroleptics have been available (Dahl 1986). Radioimmunoassays tend to be less precise but more sensitive than HPLC methods and are available for haloperidol (Poland and Rubin 1981) and fluphenazine (Midha et al. 1980). The radio-receptor assay (RRA) is a new biological technique in which a neuroleptic drug and its dopamine-blocking metabolites compete with tritiated spiroperidol (or tritiated haloperidol) for dopamine D_2-binding sites on preparations of membranes from rat striatum. Theoretically, RRA measures the total dopamine D_2 receptor–blocking activity of drug and metabolites in the plasma or serum. Although attractive in theory, the utility of the RRA is unknown; it does hold the promise of becoming useful to practicing psychiatrists (Midha et al. 1987). At this time, the state of the art for measuring neuroleptic plasma levels is the HPLC.

Fixed-Dosage Plasma Level Studies With Neuroleptics

To detect a relationship between plasma levels of a neuroleptic and clinical response, patients need to be treated with a fixed dosage of neuroleptic medication. It is preferable for patients to be randomly assigned to low-, average-, and high-dosage groups so that both ends of the therapeutic window (if such exists) are represented. Variable-dosage studies tend to produce artifactual therapeutic windows (Van Putten and Marder 1986).

Most of the work on the relation between plasma levels of neuroleptics and clinical response has been done with haloperidol and fluphenazine.

Haloperidol

In Table 18–1, we summarize the results of the 12 fixed-dosage studies with haloperidol performed to date. Results from 6 of these studies have indicated a therapeutic window relationship between plasma haloperidol and clinical response: 4.2–11 ng/ml (Mavroidis et al. 1983); 4–26 ng/ml (Potkin et al. 1985); 5–12 ng/ml (Van Putten et al. 1992); 6–14.4 ng/ml (Bernardo et al. 1993); 7–17 ng/ml (Smith et al. 1984); and 12–55 ng/ml (Santos et al. 1989). The therapeutic range reported by Santos et al. (1989) of 12–55 ng/ml was higher than and out of line with the therapeutic ranges of the aforementioned studies. Inspection of Santos et al.'s data indicates a positive linear relationship between about 2 ng/ml and 20 ng/ml, with a plateau relationship starting at 20 ng/ml. A recalculation of Santos et al.'s data using two sigmoidal dosage-effect functions (see section, "A new mathematical analysis," below) indicates a plateau relationship starting approximately at 19 ng/ml, and a logarithmic conversion of plasma haloperidol levels suggests a plateau relationship starting around 18 ng/ml.

Results from 6 of the fixed-dosage studies listed in Table 18–1 did not indicate a therapeutic window relationship, but these studies were designed in such a way that detection of a therapeutic window relationship (if such exists) was unlikely: investigators in 3 of the studies (Bigelow et al. 1985; Itoh et al. 1984; Rimon et al. 1981) used patients who had shown poor response to neuroleptics. In addition, in 3 of the 6 studies, the dosages used were so low (5 or 10 mg [Bleeker et al. 1984]; 6 mg [Itoh et al. 1984]; 0.2 mg/kg [Wistedt et al. 1984]) that detection of an upper toxic limit was unlikely, whereas in the other 3 studies the dosages used were too high (60 and 120 mg [Rimon et al. 1981]; 0.4 mg/kg [Bigelow et al. 1985]; 30 mg [Linkowski et al. 1984]) to result in plasma levels in the subtherapeutic range. Thus, of the 12 fixed-dosage studies with haloperidol, the 6 that appear, in retrospect, to have been designed properly found a therapeutic window relationship.

In 5 of the 6 studies in which a therapeutic range was suggested (Bernardo et al. 1993; Mavroidis et al. 1983; Potkin et al. 1985; Santos et al. 1989; Smith et al. 1984), there were only 28 cases that

Table 18–1. Results of fixed-dosage studies with haloperidol

Study	N	Haloperidol dosage (mg/day)	Duration of treatment (weeks)	Patient type	Proposed haloperidol window (ng/ml) or other relationship
Rimon et al. (1981)	12	60 and 120	8	Institutionalized patients with poor response to medication	None
Mavroidis et al. (1983)	14	6, 12, or 24	2	Newly admitted DSM-III[a] schizophrenic patients in psychotic exacerbation	4.2–11.0
Bleeker et al. (1984)	29	5 or 10	2	Patients with atypical and brief reactive psychosis	None
Itoh et al. (1984)	11	6	4	Institutionalized chronic schizophrenic patients	None
Linkowski et al. (1984)	20	30	6	6 acute, 8 subacute, and 6 subchronic newly admitted schizophrenic patients	None
Smith et al. (1984)	27	10, 20, or 25	3	Newly admitted schizophrenic patients; patients with poor response to medication were excluded	7.0–17.0
Wistedt et al. (1984)	10	0.2/kg	4	Acute schizophrenic patients	Linear
Bigelow et al. (1985)	19	0.40/kg	6	Institutionalized patients with poor response to medication	None
Potkin et al. (1985)	43	0.40 or 0.15/kg	6	Chinese schizophrenic patients	4.0–26.0
Santos et al. (1989)	30	10, 15, or 30	3	Excluded patients nonresponsive to medication and patients with schizophreniform and schizoaffective disorders	12.0–55.0
Van Putten et al. (1992)	69	5, 10, or 20	4	Newly admitted DSM-III[a] schizophrenic patients; patients with poor response to medication were excluded	5.0–12.0
Bernardo et al. (1993)	20	10, 20, or 30	3	Schizophrenic inpatients with acute exacerbation (DSM III-R[b]); patients with poor response to medication were excluded	6.0–14.4

[a]American Psychiatric Association 1980. [b]American Psychiatric Association 1987.

defined the proposed toxic range; 17 of these cases were from Potkin et al.'s (1985) investigation of Chinese schizophrenic patients, in which the curvilinear fit explained only 8% of the variance of clinical improvement. Furthermore, investigators in these studies failed to address the clinically obvious question: What was the clinical state of patients with toxic haloperidol levels? and, more compelling, Do patients with toxic plasma levels improve when their plasma levels of medication are lowered and, conversely, do their toxic plasma levels worsen when the plasma levels of medication are raised? Only Mavroidis et al. (1983) noted that when they halved the dosage in the patient with the highest plasma level (18.5 ng/ml) and smallest clinical improvement, the patient improved dramatically.

In our study (Van Putten et al. 1992), 13 patients had mean haloperidol plasma levels greater than 12 ng/ml at the end of the fixed-dosage period. Three patients insisted on leaving the hospital before a dosage adjustment was possible (at the fixed dosage, all had become more paranoid and two had become extremely dysphoric) and 2 patients refused dosage reduction. The remaining 8 patients, when their plasma levels were reduced to below the 12-ng/ml level (range = 4.0–10.8 ng/ml; mean = 7.8 ng/ml), experienced lesser side effects (i.e., decreases in their subjective sense of sedation, objective akinesia, or both), became less psychotic (5 out of 8) or less dysphoric (3 out of 8), or showed less motor retardation (8 out 8). No patient's condition deteriorated. In summary, in the fixed-dosage studies, higher (possibly toxic) plasma levels were reduced in only 9 patients (1 in the Mavroidis et al. [1983] study and 8 in our study).

A new mathematical analysis.   The data from our study (Van Putten et al. 1992) were fit to a theoretical model that proposed the presence of two sigmoidal dosage-effect functions, one resulting in a positive treatment response and the other resulting in toxicity or other negative effects, as suggested by Teicher and Baldessarini (1985). In this two-component model, the predicted Brief Psychiatric Rating Scale (BPRS; Overall and Gorham 1962) change score is obtained by subtracting the negative or toxic component from the positive or therapeutic component. We believe that this method is better than the more usual quadratic analysis that tests for the therapeutic window.

In Figure 18–1, we illustrate this two-component model superimposed on the scatterplot of improvement on BPRS psychosis cluster versus mean plasma haloperidol (multiple $r = .46$; $P = .001$). By inspection, it appears reasonable to divide the data into the following ranges: less than 2 ng/ml = ineffective range; 2–5 ng/ml = threshold range; 5–12 ng/ml = optimal range; and greater than 12 ng/ml = suboptimal (toxic) range. Mean improvement on BPRS psychosis cluster was significantly greater, as measured by t test, in the optimal than in the toxic ($P = .004$) or the threshold range ($P = .004$) (see Table 18–2). Mean improvement in the optimal range was roughly twice that in the threshold and toxic ranges. The standardized effect sizes were both large (.95 and .90, respectively).

Assignment to predetermined plasma levels. In two studies (Coryell et al. 1990; Volavka et al. 1992), patients were randomly assigned

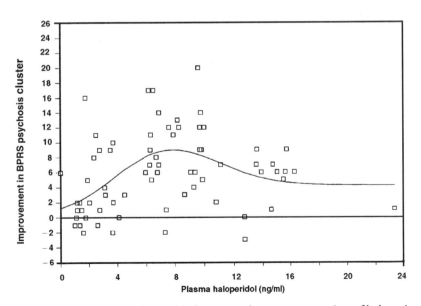

Figure 18–1. Curvilinear relationship between plasma concentration of haloperidol and change in psychosis cluster on the Brief Psychiatric Rating Scale (BPRS; Overall and Gorham 1962).
Source. Van Putten et al. 1992.

Table 18–2. Psychosis cluster score on the Brief Psychiatric Rating Scale (Overall and Gorham 1962)

Haloperidol plasma level range (ng/ml)	Mean	Standard deviation	N
Ineffective (less than 2)	2.4	4.9	12
Threshold (2–5)	4.2	4.4	14
Optimal (5–12)	8.8	5.0	30
Suboptimal/toxic (greater than 12)	4.6	3.7	13

Source. Van Putten et al. 1992.

to predetermined plasma haloperidol ranges. Volavka et al. (1992) assigned 152 schizophrenic inpatients to three fixed haloperidol plasma level ranges: low (2–13 ng/ml), medium (13.1–24 ng/ml), and high (24.1–35 ng/ml). Raters were blind to the patients' plasma levels. Patients were then rated on the BPRS and the Simpson-Angus Scale (Simpson and Angus 1970) for side effects. No significant differences were detected among any of the three groups in side effects, dropout rates, BPRS raw score, or categorical improvement. It is difficult to reconcile the results of this well-designed study with the results of the aforementioned studies. Possible explanations for Volavka et al.'s findings may include the selection of patients who were relatively less responsive to haloperidol, a large dropout rate, a failure to adequately distinguish side effects on the basis of their severity, or the selection of a setting in which a dropoff in antipsychotic effect at higher plasma levels either did not occur or was not detectable.

In the second study, Coryell et al. (1990) assigned 25 newly admitted psychotic patients (17 with schizophrenia, 4 with schizoaffective disorder, and 4 with unspecified functional psychosis) to one of two plasma level ranges: a high plasma level group (20–35 ng/ml) or a medium plasma level group (8–18 ng/ml). During the 4 weeks of treatment, patients with plasma levels less than 18 ng/ml had a better outcome in terms of total BPRS score as well as positive and negative symptom scores. The relationship between plasma level and outcome was most powerful for the first week of treatment. With a BPRS total score of 40 or less as the indicator of global improvement, 45% of the patients in the medium plasma level range improved, as compared with none of the patients in the high plasma level range ($P = .005$).

On balance, there is evidence for a therapeutic window type of relationship with haloperidol in the acutely exacerbated patient. In our opinion, response drops off but does not disappear at higher haloperidol plasma levels (e.g., levels greater than 12 ng/ml), probably because of the stress of side effects (Van Putten et al. 1991). There certainly is no evidence that higher plasma levels (e.g., levels greater than 12 ng/ml) are associated with superior response. The lower limit appears to be around 5 ng/ml. Because the correlation between dosage and plasma level was rather high ($r = .76$) in ours and other studies, a plasma level usually does not provide much extra information. On a dosage of 10–15 mg/day, nearly all patients would be in the therapeutic window. Recent work from the Karolinska Institute (Llerena et al. 1992), however, has indicated that about 7% of Caucasians may be at risk for developing side effects because of aberrantly high plasma haloperidol levels. Specifically, Llerena et al. found that 7% of Caucasians have a decreased capacity to hydroxylate debrisoquin, and that those patients who poorly metabolized debrisoquin eliminated a 4-gm haloperidol dosage significantly more slowly than those who metabolized debrisoquin normally. Furthermore, those who poorly metabolized debrisoquin developed severe extrapyramidal side effects.

Otherwise, plasma haloperidol level may be most informative with drug interactions. For example, carbamazepine is known to reduce plasma haloperidol levels by 50% or more through microsomal enzyme induction (Ereshefsky et al. 1984; Fast et al. 1986; Jann et al. 1985). Other drug interactions are likely to be discovered.

Fluphenazine

Investigators in four fixed-dosage studies (Dysken et al. 1981; Levinson et al. 1988; Mavroidis et al. 1983; Van Putten et al. 1991) have examined the relationship between plasma fluphenazine and clinical response in newly admitted schizophrenic patients (see summary of results in Table 18–3).

Table 18–3. Results of plasma level studies with fluphenazine

Study	N	Fluphenazine dosage (ng/day)	Duration of treatment (weeks)	Patient type	Proposed fluphenazine treatment therapeutic range (ng/ml) or other relationship
Dysken et al. (1981)	29	5, 10, or 20	2	Newly admitted schizophrenic patients	0.2–2.8
Mavroidis et al. (1983)	19	5, 10, or 20	2	Newly admitted schizophrenic patients	0.13–0.7
Levinson et al. (1988)	22	10 or 20	3 1/2	Newly admitted schizophrenic patients	Linear relationship ($r = .43$) between plasma fluphenazine and improvement over the entire 0.2–4.5 range
Van Putten et al. (1991)	72	5, 10, or 20	4	Newly admitted schizophrenic patients (patients with history of nonresponse excluded)	Linear relationship between global improvement and plasma fluphenazine over the entire 0.1–4.2 range (however, 90% of patients had disabling side effects at 2.7)

The findings from our study (Van Putten et al. 1991) are illustrated in Figures 18–2 through 18–4. In Figure 18–2, we show the logistic regression for patient improvement as a function of plasma levels of fluphenazine, which was significant at the $P = .015$ level. In Figure 18–3, the logistic regression for disabling side effects as a function of plasma levels of fluphenazine, which was significant at the $P = .0008$ level, is illustrated. Disabling side effects experienced by patients consisted of some admixture of fatigue, sedation, akathisia, or a feeling of being slowed down (akinesia) that—at least from the patient's point of view—interfered with functioning or even outweighed the therapeutic effect of the drug. (We emphasize that although some of these patients did not appear fatigued, akathisic, or functionally hindered, they subjectively felt that way.) In Figure 18–4, the patient improvement and plasma level data from Figures 18–2 and 18–3 are combined into a single graph.

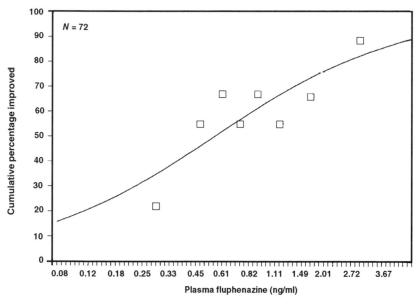

Figure 18–2. Patient improvement as a function of plasma fluphenazine levels. — = Logistic regression model ($P = .0154$). ❑ = Actual percentage of patients improved, with data divided into eight equal portions (displayed at midpoint for each portion).
Source. Van Putten et al. 1991.

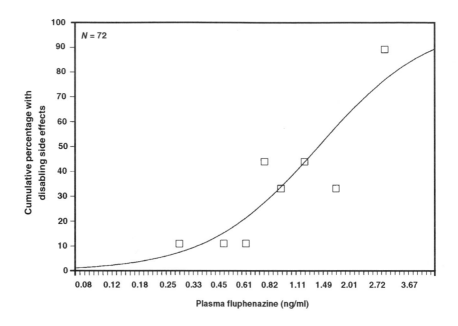

Figure 18–3.   Disabling side effects as a function of plasma fluphenazine levels. — = Logistic regression model (P = .0008). ☐ = Actual percentage of patients showing disabling side effects, with data divided into eight equal portions (displayed at midpoint for each portion).
Source.   Van Putten et al. 1991.

In Figure 18–5, we show the percentage of schizophrenic patients who improved without experiencing disabling side effects (the figure should not be construed as a therapeutic window). As shown, at a plasma fluphenazine level of 0.67 ng/ml, the maximum percentage of patients (around 48%) improved without experiencing disabling side effects. Above this plasma fluphenazine level, an increasing percentage of patients improved with regard to psychotic symptomatology but at the same time experienced a progressive increase in disabling side effects. From the patient's viewpoint, the disabling side effects negated or compromised the improvement in psychotic symptoms. We believe that such a risk-benefit assessment may be the most appropriate way of analyzing neuroleptic plasma level and clinical response data.

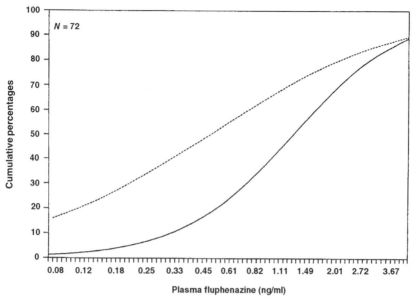

Figure 18–4. Patient improvement and disabling side effects as a function of plasma fluphenazine. — = Logistic regression model for improvement (*P* = .0154). ... = Logistic regression model for disabling side effects (*P* = .0008). *Source.* Van Putten et al. 1991.

Fluphenazine Decanoate

There have been few controlled studies that have focused on the relationship between drug plasma levels and relapse rates for schizophrenic patients treated with depot fluphenazine. Wistedt et al. (1982) studied levels of fluphenazine and a metabolite, 7-hydroxyfluphenazine, in patients who received depot fluphenazine (mean dosage = 21.4 mg every 2 weeks). Patients who relapsed had lower plasma levels of fluphenazine (mean = 0.92 ng/ml) than those who did not relapse (mean = 1.36 ng/ml).

We (Marder et al. 1990) monitored plasma levels of fluphenazine in schizophrenic patients randomly assigned to a double-blind comparison of 5 mg and 25 mg of depot fluphenazine administered every 2 weeks. We measured plasma levels at 3, 6, and 9 months (it takes 3 months to reach steady state with fluphenazine decanoate) and evaluated the relationship between these levels and the patients' rates of psychotic exacerbation over the following year. As illustrated in Figure 18–6, the patients' rates of psychotic exacerbation were relatively low above fluphenazine levels of 0.8 or 0.9 ng/ml, suggesting that this may be a reasonable plasma level for maintenance. On the other hand, very few patients with fluphenazine plasma levels above 1.2 ng/ml experienced an exacerbation of their illness, suggesting that if a clinician has given priority to preventing relapse and is less concerned about side effects, then this higher level might be preferable. Our findings indicated that patients with fluphenazine plasma levels lower than 0.9 ng ml may be on the linear part of the curve and might benefit from a dosage increase. Patients who received 25 mg of depot fluphenazine every 2 weeks had mean drug plasma levels of about 1.4 ng/ml, with nearly all of these patients measuring on the flatter part of the curve. Patients receiving a 5-mg dosage in our study had mean fluphenazine plasma levels of 0.6–0.7 ng/ml, with standard deviations of 0.5–0.6, indicating that this medication dosage caused a

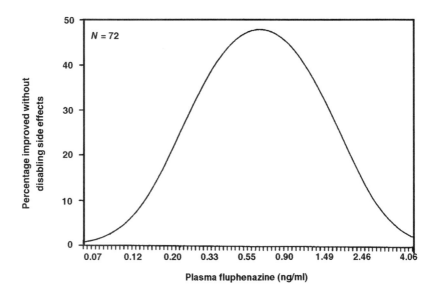

Figure 18–5.   Risk-benefit assessment as a function of plasma fluphenazine level. *Source.* Van Putten et al. 1991.

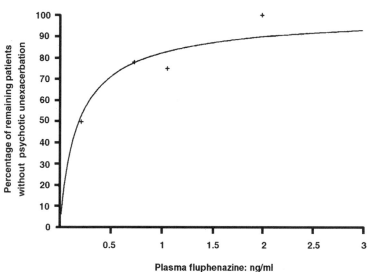

Figure 18–6. Relationship between risk of psychotic exacerbations over the following year and plasma fluphenazine levels at 6 months ($n = 35$), showing logistic regression functions (—) computed from the actual data, and the actual data points (+) computed by ordering the plasma specimens from lowest to highest plasma level. For each quartile of the sample, the percentage of patients remaining unexacerbated over the following year was computed and the data point (+) placed at the midpoint of the plasma range for each quartile (e.g., for 6 months: $\chi = 4.38$; $P = .04$). *Source.* Marder et al. 1990.

substantial number of patients to have drug plasma levels that rendered them vulnerable to psychotic exacerbations.

Conclusions

At this time, a patient's neuroleptic plasma level is useful in demonstrating decreased bioavailability or surreptitious noncompliance (Van Putten et al. 1990). A nondetectable or aberrantly low plasma level, after noncompliance has been ruled out, should dictate a dosage increase or a switch to a depot form of neuroleptic. Because most treatment-resistant patients, in public institutions at least, have had a trial of depot neuroleptics (which overcomes absorption problems and first-pass metabolism), it is unlikely that decreased bioavailability explains much treatment resistance. Decreased bioavailability is more likely to occur with concomitant administration of known enzyme inducers (e.g., carbamazepine can lower neuroleptic levels by 50% or more); other drug interactions are also likely to be discovered.

Aberrantly high plasma levels are more problematic. Only in the case of haloperidol (and, to a lesser degree, chlorpromazine) is there a suggestion of an upper limit beyond which therapeutic response seems to diminish in at least some patients. In the case of chlorpromazine, plasma levels above 100 ng/ml may be associated with behavioral toxicity, but the evidence for this effect is confined to only four patients (Van Putten et al. 1981). In the case of haloperidol, a plasma level above 12 ng/ml in a nonresponsive patient should at least raise the possibility of reducing that patient's dosage. With fluphenazine (Marder et al. 1990), perphenazine (Bolvig Hansen and Larsen 1985; Bolvig Hansen et al. 1982), and haloperidol (Van Putten et al. 1991), side effects—particularly those that are subjectively experienced—are related to plasma levels. In the case of fluphenazine, a plasma level greater than 2 ng/ml in a nonresponsive patient should alert the clinician to the possibility of subjective disabling side effects that might compromise improvement. In the case of perphenazine, optimal antipsychotic effect with minimal extrapyramidal side effects appears to be in the range of 0.8–2.4 ng/ml. Above this range, patients experience extrapyramidal side effects with no gain (and possibly a loss) in antipsychotic effect (Bolvig Hansen et al. 1982). It may be that a plasma level is most useful when the distinction between side effects and worsening psychosis is difficult.

In Table 18–4, we summarize reported therapeutic plasma concentrations for some antipsychotic drugs. These "therapeutic" plasma levels cannot be regarded as having been established by any means, but may help to identify aberrant plasma levels.

The utility of high neuroleptic plasma levels in treatment-resistant patients has not been investigated. Further, the relationship between plasma level and clinical state in chronic treatment-refractory patients is likely to be complicated. The setting and the psychological requirements of a patient may affect plasma level requirements. Thus, in some treatment-resistant patients, particularly those in poorly staffed institu-

Table 18–4. Reported therapeutic plasma concentration ranges for antipsychotic
drugs

Drug	Therapeutic plasma concentration (ng/ml)
Chlorpromazine	30.0–100.0[a]
Fluphenazine	0.2–2.0[b]
Haloperidol	5.0–12.0[a]
Perphenazine	0.8–2.4[b]

[a]Consider dosage reduction in patients with plasma level above upper limit. [b]Range of concentrations in which good response without debilitating side effects has been found; no evidence that reduction of plasma levels above the upper limit improves antipsychotic effect. *Source.* Chlorpromazine range—Van Putten et al. 1981; fluphenazine range—Marder et al. 1990; haloperidol range—Van Putten et al. 1991; perphenazine range—Bolvig Hansen et al. 1982.

tions, high plasma levels are actually used for chemical restraint, which is conceptualized as a combination of akinesia and sedation. Chemical restraint can also be the least restrictive form of treatment for patients who are aggressive in response to intractable hallucinations or delusions. Also, some treatment-resistant patients actually prefer sedation and akinesia to dampen their misery or to help contain their destructive impulses. Studies are needed in which treatment-refractory patients with high plasma levels are randomly assigned to plasma level reduction or to a control group in which plasma level remains the same.

References

American Psychiatric Association: Diagnostic and Statistical Manual of Mental Disorders, 3rd Edition. Washington, DC, American Psychiatric Association, 1980

American Psychiatric Association: Diagnostic and Statistical Manual of Mental Disorders, 3rd Edition, Revised. Washington, DC, American Psychiatric Association, 1987

Bernardo M, Palao DJ, Arauxo A, et al: Monitoring plasma level of haloperidol in schizophrenia. Hosp Community Psychiatry 44:115–118, 1993

Bigelow LB, Kirch DG, Braun T, et al: Absence of relationship of serum haloperidol concentration and clinical response in chronic schizophrenia: a fixed-dose study. Psychopharmacol Bull 21:66–68, 1985

Bjorndal N, Bjerre M, Gerlach J, et al: High dosage haloperidol therapy in chronic schizophrenic patients: a double-blind study of clinical response, side effects, serum haloperidol, and serum prolactin. Psychopharmacology (Berl) 67:17–23, 1980

Bleeker JAC, Dingemans PM, Frohn-De Winder ML: Plasma level and effect of low-dose haloperidol in acute psychosis. Psychopharmacol Bull 20:317–319, 1984

Bolvig Hansen L, Larsen NE: Therapeutic advantages of monitoring plasma concentrations of perphenazine in clinical practice. Psychopharmacology (Berl) 87:16–19, 1985

Bolvig Hansen L, Larsen NE, Gulmann N: Dose-response relationships of perphenazine in the treatment of acute psychoses. Psychopharmacology (Berl) 78:112–115, 1982

Cohen BM, Herschel M, Aoba A: Neuroleptic, antimuscarinic and anti-adrenergic activity of chlorpromazine, thioridazine and their metabolites. Psychiatry Res 1:199–208, 1976

Coryell W, Kelly M, Perry PJ, et al: Haloperidol plasma levels and acute clinical change in schizophrenia. J Clin Psychopharmacol 10:397–402, 1990

Curry SH, Marshall JHL, Davis JM, et al: Chlorpromazine plasma levels and effects. Arch Gen Psychiatry 22:289–296, 1970

Dahl SG: Plasma level monitoring of antipsychotic drugs: clinical utility. Clin Pharmacokinet 11:36–61, 1986

Davis JM, Erikson S, Dekirmenjian H: Plasma levels of antipsychotic drugs and clinical response, in Psychopharmacology: A Generation of Progress. Edited by Lipton MA, DiMascio A, Killam KF. New York, Raven, 1978, pp 905–915

Dysken MW, Javaid JI, Chang SS, et al: Fluphenazine pharmacokinetics and therapeutic response. Psychopharmacology (Berl) 73:205–210, 1981

Ereshefsky L, Davis CM, Harrington CA: Haloperidol and reduced haloperidol plasma levels in selected schizophrenic patients. J Clin Psychopharmacol 4:138–142, 1984

Extein I, Pottash AL, Gold MS: Therapeutic window for plasma haloperidol in acute schizophrenic psychosis (letter). Lancet 1:1048–1049, 1983

Fast DK, Jones BD, Kusalic M, et al: Effect of carbamazepine on neuroleptic plasma level and efficacy (letter). Am J Psychiatry 143:117–118, 1986

Forsman A, Ohman R: Studies on serum protein binding of haloperidol. Current Therapeutic Research 21:245–255, 1977

Gelenberg AJ: The catatonic syndrome. Lancet 1:1339–1341, 1976

Itoh H, Yagi G, Fuji Y, et al: The relationship between haloperidol blood levels and clinical responses. Prog Neuropsychopharmacol Biol Psychiatry 8:285–292, 1984

Jann MW, Ereshefsky L, Saklad SR: Effects of carbamazepine on plasma haloperidol levels. J Clin Psychopharmacol 5:106–109, 1985

Levinson DF, Simpson GM, Singh H, et al: Neuroleptic plasma level may predict response in patients who meet a criterion for improvement (letter). Arch Gen Psychiatry 45:877–879, 1988

Linkowski P, Hubain P, von Frenckell R, et al: Haloperidol plasma levels and clinical response in paranoid schizophrenics. Eur Arch Psychiatry Neurosci 234:231–236, 1984

Llerena A, Alm C, Dahl ML, et al: Haloperidol disposition is dependent on debrisoquine hydroxylation phenotype. Ther Drug Monit 14:92–97, 1992

Marder SR, Van Putten T, Aravagiri M, et al: Fluphenazine plasma levels and clinical response. Psychopharmacol Bull 26:256–259, 1990

Mavroidis ML, Kanter DR, Hirschowitz J, et al: Clinical response and plasma haloperidol levels in schizophrenia. Psychopharmacology 81:354–356, 1983

May PRA, Van Putten T: Plasma and saliva levels of chlorpromazine in schizophrenia: a critical view of the literature. Arch Gen Psychiatry 35:1081–1087, 1978

May RH: Catatonic-like states following phenothiazine therapy. Am J Psychiatry 115:1119–1120, 1959

Midha KK, Cooper JK, Hubbard JW: Radioimmunoassay for fluphenazine in human plasma. Communications in Psychopharmacology 4:107–114, 1980

Midha KK, Hawes EM, Hubbard JW, et al: The search for correlations between neuroleptic plasma levels and clinical outcome: a critical review, in Psychopharmacology: The Third Generation of Progress. Edited by Meltzer HY. New York, Raven, 1987, pp 1341–1351

Midha KK, Hubbard JW, May PRA: The role of the analytical biochemist in resistant schizophrenia, in Treatment Resistance in Schizophrenia. Edited by Dencker SJ, Kulhanek F. Braunschweig/Wiesbaden, Vieweg, 1988, pp 56–64

Nyberg G, Axelson R, Martenson E: Binding of thioridazine and thioridazine metabolites to serum proteins in psychiatric patients. Eur J Clin Pharmacol 14:341–350, 1978

Overall JE, Gorham DR: The Brief Psychiatric Rating Scale. Psychol Rep 10:799–812, 1962

Poland RE, Rubin RT: Radioimmunoassay of haloperidol in human serum: correlation of serum haloperidol with serum prolactin. Life Sci 29:1837–1845, 1981

Potkin SG, Shen Y, Zhou D, et al: Does a therapeutic window for plasma haloperidol exist? preliminary Chinese data. Psychopharmacol Bull 21:59–61, 1985

Rimon R, Averbuch I, Rozick P, et al: Serum and CSF levels of haloperidol by radioimmunoassay and radioreceptor assay during high-dose therapy of resistant schizophrenic patients. Psychopharmacology 73:197–199, 1981

Santos JL, Cabranes JA, Almoguera I, et al: Clinical implications of determining plasma haloperidol levels. Acta Psychiatr Scand 79:348–354, 1989

Schulz SC, Butterfield L, Garicano M, et al: Beyond the therapeutic window: a case presentation. J Clin Psychiatry 45:223–225, 1984

Simpson GM, Angus JSW: Rating scale for extrapyramidal side effects. Acta Psychiatr Scand 212:11–19, 1970

Smith RC, Baumgartner R, Misra CH, et al: Haloperidol plasma levels and prolactin response as predictors of clinical improvement in schizophrenia: chemical versus radioreceptor plasma level assay. Arch Gen Psychiatry 41:1044–1049, 1984

Teicher MH, Baldessarini RJ: Selection of neuroleptic dosage. Arch Gen Psychiatry 42:636–637, 1985

Van Putten T, Marder SR: Variable dose studies provide misleading therapeutic windows. J Clin Psychopharmacol 6:55–56, 1986

Van Putten T, Marder SR: Behavioral toxicity of antipsychotic drugs. J Clin Psychiatry 48 (suppl 9):13–19, 1987

Van Putten T, May PRA, Jenden DJ: Does a plasma level of chlorpromazine help? Psychol Med 11:729–734, 1981

Van Putten T, Marder SR, May PRA, et al: Plasma levels of haloperidol and clinical response. Psychopharmacol Bull 21:69–72, 1985

Van Putten T, Marder SR, Wirshing WC, et al: Surreptitious noncompliance with oral fluphenazine in a voluntary inpatient population (letter). Arch Gen Psychiatry 47:786, 1990

Van Putten T, Marder SR, Wirshing WC, et al: Neuroleptic plasma levels. Schizophr Bull 17:197–216, 1991

Van Putten T, Marder SR, Mintz J, et al: Haloperidol plasma levels and clinical response: a therapeutic window relationship. Am J Psychiatry 149:500–505, 1992

Van Putten T, Marshall BD, Liberman RP, et al: Systematic dose reduction in treatment-resistant schizophrenic patients. Psychopharmacol Bull 29:315–320, 1993

Verbeeck RK, Cardinal JA, Hill AG, et al: Binding of phenothiazine neuroleptics to plasma proteins. Biochem Pharmacol 32:2565–2570, 1983

Volavka J, Cooper T, Czobor P, et al: Haloperidol blood levels and clinical effects. Arch Gen Psychiatry 49:354–361, 1992

Wistedt B, Jorgensen A, Wiles D: A depot neuroleptic withdrawal study: plasma concentration of fluphenazine and flupenthixol and relapse frequency. Psychopharmacology (Berl) 78:301–304, 1982

Wistedt B, Johanidesz G, Omerhodzic M, et al: Plasma haloperidol levels and clinical response in acute schizophrenia. Nordisk Psychiatrik Tidsskrift 1:9–13, 1984

Do Neuroleptic-Responsive and Neuroleptic-Resistant Patients Have Different Illnesses?

Walter A. Brown, M.D.

Auseful nosology of schizophrenia continues to elude psychiatric researchers and clinicians. Current classification schemes, based on patterns of signs and symptoms, have failed to identify meaningful schizophrenic subtypes—subtypes associated with family history, biological variables, treatment response, or prognosis.

Since the 1950s, when neuroleptics became available in clinical practice, schizophrenic patients have been routinely treated with these agents—including patients who did not seem to benefit from them. One reason for the indiscriminate use of neuroleptics has been a practical one: they are the only clearly effective treatment. But another explanation for their routine use in schizophrenia has been the assumption that this syndrome is pathophysiologically homogeneous and that neuroleptic drugs address this singular pathophysiology (Schulz et al. 1989).

In fact, schizophrenic patients vary markedly in their response to neuroleptic treatment. Some patients are extremely responsive to neuroleptic medication; when their neuroleptic treatment is stopped or their neuroleptic dosage reduced, they quickly develop psychotic symptoms. With renewed or increased neuroleptic treatment, these symptoms rapidly subside. Other schizophrenic patients (about 25% of all schizophrenic patients) are clearly resistant to neuroleptics. Even with apparently adequate or high neuroleptic dosages and neuroleptic blood levels, these treatment-refractory patients remain flagrantly psychotic (Hollister and Kim 1982; Rimon et al. 1981). Still other schizophrenic patients improve somewhat but not completely with neuroleptic treatment, and others show a waxing and waning of schizophrenic symptoms, entering episodes of remission or psychosis independently of neuroleptic treatment.

The data gathered over the last two decades have consistently shown that neuroleptic-refractory patients either do not differ from neuroleptic-responsive patients in their neuroleptic dosage and blood levels, or have higher neuroleptic dosages and blood levels than neuroleptic-responsive patients (Faraone et al. 1987). Furthermore, neuroleptic-refractory patients rarely improve with substantial dosage increases (Little et al. 1989). Thus, patients' varying responses to neuroleptics do not appear to be accounted for simply by differences in peripheral pharmacokinetics. But it has been thought possible that these differences in neuroleptic response occur as a result of variations in the degree to which neuroleptics cross the blood-brain barrier. That explanation became untenable when Wolkin et al. (1989), using positron-emission tomography (PET) scan technology, demonstrated that neuroleptic-responsive and neuroleptic-refractory patients do not differ in the extent to which neuroleptics block their brain dopamine receptors. Accordingly, differences in neuroleptic response cannot be accounted for by differences in either peripheral or central neuroleptic bioavailability. Neuroleptic-responsive and neuroleptic-refractory patients do appear to differ pharmacodynamically; their brains respond differently to neuroleptics.

Can the diversity in neuroleptic response among schizophrenic patients provide some information about the heterogeneity and pathophysiology of schizophrenia? The idea that patients' responses to pharmacological treatment can shed light on the pathophysiology of psychiatric illness and should be used to classify psychiatric disorders has surfaced repeatedly. This concept, more often than not, is rejected on the grounds that diverse conditions can respond symptomatically to the same treatment (e.g., "headaches, bruises, and rheumatism all respond to aspirin" [Kendell 1975, p. 43]) or that patients with the same condition can respond to different treatments.

Nonetheless, patients with similar clinical presentations but different pathophysiologies—such as can occur with pneumonia, hypertension, and, in all likelihood, schizophrenia—can be expected to differ in their response to treatments directed at one specific etiology or pathophysiological process.

Do neuroleptic-responsive and neuroleptic-refractory schizophrenic patients, grossly similar in clinical presentation, have different illnesses at the pathophysiological or etiologic level? Crow (1980) explicitly suggested that neuroleptic responsiveness and resistance were associated with pathophysiologically and symptomatically discrete subtypes of schizophrenia. And his idea has been implicit in studies in which the symptomatic, cognitive, biochemical, and neuroanatomical features of schizophrenia have been examined, with neuroleptic responsiveness as the dependent or independent variable (Awad 1989; Friedman et al. 1992; Garver et al. 1987; Losonczy et al. 1986; Marder et al. 1984). Furthermore, it has been suggested that the search for genetic and biochemical underpinnings of schizophrenia might be expedited by subtyping the illness based on neuroleptic response (Bersani et al. 1989). Nonetheless, the concept that variability in neuroleptic response has nosological and pathophysiologic pertinence has yet to be fully scrutinized or subjected to empirical study. I feel that the validity of this concept deserves careful examination.

Several conditions must be met for the variability of response to a treatment to be nosologically useful and pertinent to the pathophysiology of an illness:

1. It must be possible to reliably and accurately identify patients as responsive or nonresponsive to the treatment.
2. For recurrent or chronic illnesses, individuals should be consistent in their response to treatment.

3. Differences in response to treatment should be associated with pathophysiologically meaningful variables (e.g., symptoms, signs, prognosis, family history, genes, tissue or humoral changes) and, when discovered, should be linked to the fundamental pathophysiology and etiology.
4. The treatment in question should affect some feature of the fundamental pathophysiology, not merely nonspecific symptoms or phenomena entirely peripheral to the disorder's pathogenesis.

Identification of Neuroleptic Responsiveness

Can schizophrenic patients be reliably and accurately identified along the neuroleptic-response dimension? It can be difficult, particularly in the acute treatment context, to isolate the effects of neuroleptic treatment from those of the treatment milieu, the passage of time, and shifts in family behavior, to name just a few confounding variables. Apparent nonresponse can result from an inadequate dosage and/or too high a dosage. Neuroleptic toxicity or side effects can be misidentified as nonresponse (Bishop et al. 1965; Van Putten and Marder 1986). Uncertain compliance, placebo effects, the natural course of the illness, and pharmacokinetic differences among patients further complicate assessment of response to neuroleptic treatment.

Despite these difficulties, Brown and Herz (1988) and Csernansky et al. (1983) found that independent ratings of neuroleptic responsiveness based on chart reviews agree reasonably well, with greater than 85% agreement found. Such retrospective assessments would be expected to yield lower agreement rates than prospective assessments.

Definitive research on neuroleptic responsiveness awaits innovative methods for accurately identifying neuroleptic-induced clinical effects. Any proposed method should eliminate or control for other therapeutic interventions, differentiate drug-related from other symptomatic changes, attend to pharmacokinetic variables, and consider the confounding influence of side effects. Using serum prolactin concentration as an index of pharmacological effect, Gelder and Kolakowaska (1979) proposed an approach to classifying patients as those whose symptoms remit spontaneously (i.e., patients who, with little pharmacological effect, improve during neuroleptic treatment), those who respond to neuroleptics (i.e., patients who improve in the face of a clear pharmacological effect and who, with little pharmacological effect, relapse or fail to improve), and those who do not respond to neuroleptics (i.e., patients who, despite a clear pharmacological effect, fail to improve). In this approach, both pharmacological and clinical response variables are considered.

In a series of studies examining serum neuroleptic concentrations, serum prolactin, neuroleptic dosage reduction, and clinical outcome, my colleagues and I (Brown et al. 1982; Faraone et al. 1987) classified patients who, during maintenance neuroleptic treatment, had positive schizophrenic symptoms at 50% or more of their outpatient visits as persistently psychotic or neuroleptic-refractory patients, and those who displayed positive schizophrenic symptoms on fewer than 50% of their outpatient visits as remitted or neuroleptic-responsive patients. These criteria, although admittedly arbitrary, consistently yielded two groups of patients that differ in ways reasonably related to neuroleptic responsiveness. Neuroleptic-responsive patients defined in this manner regularly showed relationships in the predicted direction between serum neuroleptic and prolactin levels and clinical outcome (i.e., lower serum levels lead to higher rates of relapse), whereas neuroleptic-refractory patients consistently failed to show such relationships (Faraone et al. 1987). Furthermore, the patients classified as responsive to neuroleptics showed a higher rate of "relapse" (defined as the necessity for dosage increase) with rapid—as opposed to slow—dosage reduction, whereas the nonresponsive patients showed similar rates of relapse with rapid and slow reduction (Green et al. 1992). When neuroleptic dosages were substantially reduced (e.g., by 80%), the incidence of relapse in both those who were neuroleptic responsive and those who were not was similar (about 50% require a dosage increase within 6 months), but the quality of relapse differed: relapse in the neuroleptic-responsive patients involved the emergence of positive symptoms, whereas relapse in the neuroleptic-refractory patients involved behavioral changes such as activation and restlessness (A. Green, personal communication, December 1992; Green et al. 1992).

Thus, our approach to classifying patients as neuroleptic responsive or neuroleptic resistant appeared to reveal meaningful and reproducible differences between these patients. In addition, retrospective classification of neuroleptic responsiveness based on chart review and global clinical impression appears to be fairly reliable (Csernansky et al. 1983) and even predictive of future responsiveness (Duncan et al. 1992). Nevertheless, valid, clearly operationalized methods for assessing neuroleptic response would expedite further inquiry. Particularly important is the development of methods for disentangling drug-related from other clinical effects. Relapse with dosage reduction or cessation and subsequent improvement with neuroleptic medication in the maintenance neuroleptic treatment setting may more clearly indicate a neuroleptic response per se than does the improvement that occurs during hospitalization for an acute episode.

Consistency of Neuroleptic Response

Is neuroleptic responsiveness consistent over time? The assessment of this variable is confounded by the assumed rhythmicity in the responsiveness of relevant brain cells to neuroleptics, changes in the density of neuronal receptors with age (Severson et al. 1982), and the possibility that neuroleptic treatment alters neuroleptic responsiveness. Naber et al. (1981, 1982) found circadian and circannual changes in dopamine receptor density in untreated rats; these rhythms were altered with chronic fluphenazine administration. The clinical import of these short- and long-term receptor changes remains to be explored. It is clear that some schizophrenic patients vary from episode to episode in their response to the same neuroleptic (Van der Velde 1976). Notwithstanding the above, clinical impression, case reports (Knobler et al. 1986), and two studies offering data on neuroleptic response over time (Duncan et al. 1992; Kolakowska et al. 1985) have suggested a noteworthy degree of response consistency.

Kolakowska et al. (1985) studied neuroleptic response over multiple treatment episodes. They classified 61 schizophrenic patients with regard to their response to neuroleptic treatment during their most recent psychotic episode: 21 were classified as very responsive, 15 as partially responsive, and 25 as poorly responsive. The 21 who responded well had two to seven previous psychotic episodes and, in all episodes, improvement occurred within a few weeks of initiating neuroleptic treatment. Among the 15 who responded only partially, 12 showed consistently incomplete responses to neuroleptic treatment and 3 changed from an initial good response to a partial response. Among the 25 who responded poorly, 14 had never responded to neuroleptic treatment and 11 had experienced a partial response in earlier episodes. On the basis of this trichotomous classification, 77% of the patients had consistent responses to neuroleptics over time.

Duncan et al. (1992), in their study of plasma homovanillic acid (pHVA) levels in neuroleptic-responsive and neuroleptic-refractory patients, selected patients for a prospective haloperidol treatment trial who, on the basis of previous treatment, were classified as presumptively responsive or nonresponsive to neuroleptics. Those who were considered nonresponsive both had failed to respond to adequate neuroleptic treatment in the past and had been persistently psychotic for more than 2 years. Nine patients were classified as nonresponsive, 7 as responsive, and 3 had never been treated with neuroleptics. These 19 patients were treated with haloperidol to a target plasma level of 15 ng/ml for 6 weeks. All those presumed to be nonresponsive did in fact fail to meet the criteria for response (35% or greater change from baseline on the Brief Psychiatric Rating Scale [BPRS; Overall and Gorham 1962] schizophrenia symptoms subscale); all of the other patients met the criteria for response.

Results from these studies and clinical experience have therefore suggested that, more often than not, patients are consistent in their neuroleptic responsiveness over time. Replication of the findings to date in a rigorously designed prospective or even retrospective study involving multiple independent ratings and ensuring the independence of one episode's rating from another's would substantiate this apparent consistency in neuroleptic response.

The Search for Predictors of Neuroleptic Response

Are neuroleptic responsiveness and neuroleptic resistance selectively associated with pathophysiologically meaningful symptoms or signs?

The best-articulated model dealing with the pathophysiological implications of treatment responsiveness is Crow's (1980) two-disease proposition. According to this model, type I patients display positive symptoms—hallucinations, bizarre behavior, and thought disorder—in the context of acute episodes. The symptoms of these patients respond to neuroleptics, their illness remits, and intellectual impairment is absent. The putative pathology is an increase in dopamine receptors. Type II patients display negative symptoms—blunted affect, loss of drive, withdrawal, and poverty of speech—in the context of chronic illness. Their response to neuroleptics is poor, their illness seems irreversible, and intellectual impairment is sometimes present. Cell loss and structural brain changes are proposed as the cause. Although Crow's model has had clear heuristic value and is theoretically appealing, it has not been supported on empirical grounds. Types of symptoms, structural brain abnormalities, and intellectual impairment have not been consistently or robustly associated with response to neuroleptics.

The distribution in schizophrenic patients of positive and negative symptoms and their pathophysiological implications are reviewed in detail in Chapters 5 and 6 in this book. The positive symptom–negative symptom dichotomy has not held up well to empirical scrutiny; most schizophrenic patients have—in varying degrees of intensity—both positive and negative symptoms at different times during the course of their illness. In addition, the intensity and number of positive and negative symptoms have not been consistently associated with neuroleptic response. For example, Kolakowska et al. (1980, 1985) found a higher frequency of negative symptoms in neuroleptic-refractory patients than in neuroleptic-responsive patients, but Goldberg (1985), in a review of early studies in which symptoms and response to neuroleptics were examined, found ample evidence that negative symptoms are associated with a good response. Goldberg observed that placebo-controlled studies revealed the responsiveness of negative symptoms, noting that positive symptoms may respond to placebo more than negative symptoms do. Keefe et al. (1987) reported that the most seriously impaired (i.e., "Kraepelinian") schizophrenic patients have severe positive as well as negative symptoms and are relatively nonresponsive to haloperidol.

The search for other symptoms or symptom clusters that might predict response to neuroleptic treatment continues, largely unsuccessfully. Investigators in early studies of neuroleptic treatment—in which the superiority of neuroleptic treatment over phenobarbital and placebo was established—were unable to identify consistent symptomatic predictors of treatment response (Hollister et al. 1974). Some investigators have found symptoms or symptom clusters predictive of treatment response: confusion, autism, hebephrenia, social participation, self-care, tension, activity, social isolation, and high and low activation (Casey et al. 1960; Klein 1967; National Institute of Mental Health Psychopharmacology Research Branch [PRB] Collaborative Study Group 1967). Other investigators, however, have found no symptom predictors (Galbrecht and Klett 1968; Goldberg et al. 1972). In several large-scale studies, opposite results with respect to paranoia have been found; some investigators have reported that these patients fared relatively well with neuroleptics, whereas others reported that paranoid patients fared relatively poorly (Galbrecht and Klett 1968; Goldberg et al. 1977; Goldstein 1970; Hollister et al. 1974; National Institute of Mental Health PRB Collaborative Study Group 1967). More recently, investigators have also failed to find robust or consistent symptom predictors of treatment response (Kay and Singh 1989).

It would be hard to say that the book is closed on the possibility that those patients who are responsive and those who are nonresponsive to neuroleptics have different symptoms. The assessment of symptoms and neuroleptic response in the studies to date has been obscured by methodological limitations. Standard clinical rating scales, most commonly the BPRS, are widely used to assess pretreatment symptoms and symptom change. But it is not clear if total scores on such scales—the most frequently applied measure—are ideally sensitive to neuroleptic effects. Furthermore, as noted above, when a patient's clinical state improves during neuroleptic treatment, it is extraordinarily difficult to isolate the effects of the neuroleptic from other influences. If, as one would expect on intuitive grounds, patients responsive and nonresponsive to neuroleptics differ clinically, we do not yet have the methodology to detect such differences.

The development of noninvasive techniques for visualizing the brain has reawakened interest in the structural brain pathology of schizophrenic patients. Crow (1980) and others have hypothesized that schizophrenic patients with evidence of cerebral atrophy, primarily a high ventricle-to-brain ratio (VBR), are relatively nonresponsive to neuroleptic treatment. This suggestion makes sense; if schizophrenic symptoms arise from structural brain abnormalities, such abnormalities and the symptoms they produce are not likely to be reversed by drugs. Reasoning along similar lines, one might also assume that if any schizophrenic patients have a "dopamine disease" responsive to the dopamine-blocking neuroleptic agents, it would be those with normal-appearing brains.

This idea has been far more compelling on theoretical grounds than on empirical ones. In a separate chapter in this book (Chapter 10), Nasrallah reviews this issue. Briefly stated, about half the studies examining the relationship between structural brain abnormalities and neuroleptic response have found a relationship in the predicted direction and the other half have not. In their review of 33 studies examining the relationship between structural brain pathology and neuroleptic response, Friedman et al. (1992) found a trivial effect size. These researchers concluded that structural brain pathology does not predict treatment response. It is of interest that the studies with the largest effect size in the predicted direction included patients with the most extreme structural abnormalities, suggesting that there might be a subgroup of schizophrenic patients with marked cerebral atrophy who are in fact relatively nonresponsive to neuroleptic treatment.

The studies to date have differed in brain-imaging technology and methods for assessing treatment, and the possibility of a Type II (beta) error looms. The weight of current evidence, however, suggests that differences in structural brain pathology do not account for much, if any, of the variance in neuroleptic response.

Several investigators have pursued the notion that symptoms of brain dysfunction, such as neurological soft signs and cognitive impairment, are associated with a relatively poor response to neuroleptic treatment. This notion, like the structural brain pathology idea to which it is related, has also been more compelling on theoretical than on empirical grounds.

Although the small subject numbers and methodological limitations of the existing studies render both the negative and the positive findings far less than definitive, the results to date are notably inconsistent and, when an effect has been found in the predicted direction, it is a small one. For example, Whelton et al. (1992) observed modest correlations between postnatal and current neurological impairment and persistent positive symptoms during neuroleptic treatment. Bartko et al. (1989) found no relationship between either neurological soft signs or cognitive impairment and neuroleptic response. Smith et al. (1992) reported that improvement with neuroleptic treatment was negatively correlated with performance on 2 of 10 tests of neuropsychological function. (See a detailed review of this matter in Chapter 9 of this book.)

Implicit in several and explicit in a few of the studies in which correlates of neuroleptic responsiveness have been examined has been the notion that only those who are responsive to neuroleptics have a "dopamine disease." The most direct test of this suggestion has been the pretreatment assessment of pHVA levels. Arguably a reliable indicator of brain dopamine turnover, pHVA levels have correlated with the severity of schizophrenic symptoms in some, but not all, studies (Davidson et al. 1991a; Pickar et al. 1986). pHVA levels do undergo predictable shifts with neuroleptic treatment. Bowers et al. (1987) found that, in a group of patients with mixed psychotic disorders, relatively high pHVA levels before treatment were associated with rapid improvement during neuroleptic treatment; furthermore, both Van Putten et al. (1989) and Davidson et al. (1991b) found that pretreatment pHVA levels were higher in neuroleptic-responsive patients than in neuroleptic-refractory patients, but not significantly so. Duncan et al. (1992), however, found that patients who were responsive to neuroleptics had slightly (although not significantly) lower pHVA than those who were nonresponsive.

The hypothesis that neuroleptic-responsive patients have enhanced brain dopamine activity reflected in relatively high pHVA levels has received only a smattering of support from the studies to date. Nonetheless, one should hesitate before abandoning such an attractive hypothesis. The heterogeneity of the condition under study and the rudimentary nature of the measurement technology renders these studies highly vulnerable to Type II (beta) errors. If those responsive and those nonresponsive to neuroleptics do, in fact, differ in brain dopamine activity or on some other dimension of brain neurochemistry, the detection of such differences will require a substantial advance in our methods for assessing both clinical phenomena and brain neurochemistry.

A handful of other findings—preliminary, fragmentary, and yet to be substantiated—suggest differences of possible pathophysiological relevance between those responsive to neuroleptics and those non-responsive. In light of the preliminary nature of these findings and the propensity to report positive but not negative findings, the implications of these results need to be evaluated cautiously. Marder et al. (1984) observed that schizophrenic patients with the greatest impairment in information processing responded relatively poorly to neuroleptic treatment. Some investigators (Pandurangi et al. 1987) have found that exacerbation of psychotic symptoms with stimulants (amphetamines or methylphenidate) portends a good response to neuroleptic treatment, whereas others (Little et al. 1989) have reported the opposite finding—that improvement in psychotic symptoms with stimulants portends a good response to treatment. Noting that the previous literature on this matter was inconclusive, Lindstrom et al. (1992) reported that a low degree of electrodermal activity predicts a relatively poor response to neuroleptic treatment.

Investigators using electroencephalograms (EEGs) in their studies have found that schizophrenic patients with relatively frequent alpha activity respond poorly to neuroleptics (Czobor and Volavka 1991; Itil et al. 1981). As for negative findings, Bartko et al. (1990) reported that the spontaneous blink rate, which is at least in part a function of central dopamine activity and which decreases with neuroleptic treatment, does not predict neuroleptic response.

Factors That Covary With Clinical Response to Neuroleptics

Supporting the concept that differences in neuroleptic responsiveness among patients reflect differences not in pharmacokinetics but in the substrate on which the neuroleptics act has been the identification of several variables that in a fairly consistent and robust fashion covary with the clinical response to neuroleptics. Itil et al. (1975) observed distinct EEG power spectra for those responsive and nonresponsive to neuroleptics. Itil et al. (1981) investigated computerized EEG recordings in neuroleptic-resistant patients before and after challenge dosages of neuroleptic drugs. They found few of the frequency changes characteristic of neuroleptics; instead, they found changes typical of stimulants. The most consistent effect of neuroleptics on the EEG is an increase in theta activity (Czobor and Volavka 1992). Czobor and Volavka found a relationship between haloperidol blood levels and theta activity in patients responsive to neuroleptics, but not in those who were nonresponsive. They concluded that patients who are responsive and nonresponsive to neuroleptics differ in their physiologic response to neuroleptics.

Karson et al. (1982) found that blink-rate reduction correlated with positive symptom response. In a related finding, Bartko et al. (1990) observed that patients who failed to decrease their blink rate with a test dose of haloperidol showed little clinical improvement with haloperidol.

One of the more compelling observations supporting the notion that patients responsive and nonresponsive to neuroleptics differ in their brain response to neuroleptic drugs is that patients who experience dysphoria with their initial doses of neuroleptic ultimately have a poor clinical response (May et al. 1980). Hogan and Awad (1992) noted that such patients also have a relatively high incidence of extrapyramidal side effects, particularly rigidity, after 3 weeks of treatment. Most (Hogan and Awad 1992; Hogan et al. 1985; Nedopil and Ruther 1981) although not all (Ayers et al. 1984) investigators examining this issue have confirmed the relationship between early dysphoric response and poor clinical outcome.

Recent interest in the physiological covariates of neuroleptic response has centered on pHVA measurements. In general, pHVA levels rise at the onset of neuroleptic treatment and drop with continued neuroleptic treatment (Pickar et al. 1986). Both the degree of pHVA increase at the onset of neuroleptic treatment (Davila et al. 1988; Duncan et al. 1992) and the degree of pHVA decrease after several weeks of treatment (Davidson et al. 1991b; Davila et al. 1988; Pickar et al. 1986) have been correlated with the degree of clinical response. These data suggest that schizophrenic patients who respond to neuroleptics undergo shifts in central dopamine activity to a greater extent than those who do not.

Therapeutic Mechanism of Neuroleptics

Do neuroleptics influence some fundamental pathophysiological component of schizophrenia? The relative ineffectiveness of barbiturates and other sedative and tranquilizing drugs in schizophrenia as compared with neuroleptics suggests that the beneficial effect of neuroleptics on schizophrenic symptoms cannot be attributed to their general tranquilizing or sedating properties. Moreover, when they are effective, neuroleptics alleviate not just one or two schizophrenic symptoms but multiple and diverse schizophrenic symptoms, such as thought disorganization, withdrawal, delusions, hallucinations, sleep disruption, agitation, deteriorated social and occupational functioning, and self-neglect. This syndromal effect would be expected when a drug corrects the underlying pathophysiology. Neuroleptic drugs, to be sure, also correct the agitation and psychotic symptoms associated with other disorders, such as mania and dementia. However, neuroleptics' overall therapeutic profile seems to fit schizophrenia or some schizophrenias better than other syndromes.

Diverse dopamine agonists can mimic or exacerbate schizophrenic symptoms, and the clinical potency of neuroleptics correlates highly with their affinity for dopamine receptors (Peroutka and Snyder 1980). These observations suggest a role for enhanced dopamine activity in the expression of schizophrenic symptoms and for reduced dopamine activity in the alleviation of such symptoms. Notwithstanding the likely role of other neuronal systems in the pathophysiology of schizophrenia and the likelihood that neuroleptic drugs—perhaps in particular the atypical neuroleptics—exert their therapeutic effects through nondopamine mechanisms, the weight of the evidence supports some involvement of dopamine in the therapeutic activity of these agents. Whether enhanced dopaminergic activity contributes to the pathogenesis of schizophrenia and whether neuroleptics affect the pathogenetic process remain to be seen.

Discussion

Models of schizophrenia, schemes for subtyping it, and etiologic theories explaining it are not in short supply. What they all have in common is an absence of empirical support. Given the heterogeneity of schizophrenia with respect to family history, symptomatic presentation, treatment response, and prognosis, as well as the current poor understanding of its pathophysiology, the hypothesis that neuroleptic responsiveness and resistance are associated with clinically and pathophysiologically meaningful subtypes warrants systematic study.

Current evidence indicates that differences among patients in neuroleptic response cannot be accounted for by differences in pharmacokinetics. Neuroleptics appear to have different effects on the brain tissue of neuroleptic-responsive patients than on that of neuroleptic-refractory patients. The processes mediating these differences and the level of biological organization at which they work remain to be determined. The fact that some of the most appealing hypotheses as to differences between those responsive and nonresponsive to neuroleptics (e.g., structural brain pathology, neurological soft signs, cognitive impairment) have not as yet been supported does not mean that neuroleptic-responsive and neuroleptic-refractory patients do not differ pathophysiologically. It is more likely that investigators have not yet looked in the right places. Recent data, for example, suggest that the dopamine D_4 receptor, to which clozapine binds with high affinity, exists in several polymorphic variations (Van Tol et al. 1992). These types of receptor variations may underlie the observed differences in responsiveness to neuroleptic drugs.

Zubin (1985) provided a cautionary note about using treatment response to shape nosology. He pointed to the short life of the idea that psychiatric patients who respond to insulin treatment be classified as dysglycolic and those who respond to electroconvulsive therapy be classified as dysoxic, with these terms signifying separate illnesses.

Notwithstanding the above, in the case of a syndrome generally responsive to a drug, as is the case with schizophrenia, the failure of some patients to respond has often proven informative. As Murray and Murphy (1978) pointed out, "the existence of renal rickets and nephrogenic diabetes insipidus was only suspected after patients were unexpectedly found resistant to vitamin D and antidiuretic hormone respectively" (p. 675). And one should not ignore other lessons of history: in 1785, William Withering wrote his classic treatise introducing the purple foxglove (digitalis) as a treatment for dropsy (edema). At that time, edema was considered a primary disease, and digitalis became widely used as its specific treatment. Although it was known that some cases of dropsy were refractory to digitalis, this drug continued to be used and recommended for general treatment of dropsy well into the middle of the 19th century when, with the discovery of the cardiac, renal, and other etiologies of edema, and the action of digitalis on the heart, the pathophysiology of edema was understood and digitalis therapy was more specifically applied. With the perfect vision of hindsight, one might imagine that if patients dramatically responsive and refractory to digitalis had been carefully compared with respect to both clinical presentation and pathological findings, the etiology, pathophysiology, and appropriate treatment of edema might have been discovered 50 years earlier.

Sufficient data are not yet available to accept or reject the hypothesis that neuroleptic-responsive and neuroleptic-refractory patients have different illnesses. However, medical history suggests that the burden of proof lies with the position that clear differences in neuroleptic responsiveness are not linked to differences in pathophysiology, and that clinical attention to the neuroleptic responsive–resistant distinction is long overdue. It is understandable in light of our limited treatment options—but paradoxical nonetheless—that neuroleptic-resistant patients are routinely treated indefinitely with high neuroleptic dosages. Identification of such patients should be followed by gradual neuroleptic dosage reduction and possible withdrawal. Faraone et al. (1989) showed that, with neuroleptic withdrawal or neuroleptic dosage reduction, close to half of neuroleptic-resistant patients either improve or show no clinical deterioration. In both cases, those patients are better off without neuroleptics. Neuroleptic-resistant patients deserve trials with other potentially useful agents, including β-adrenergic blockers, benzodiazepines, lithium, and anticonvulsants. (This issue is also addressed in Chapter 21 of this book.)

A methodological requirement of current schizophrenia research is that patients be diagnosed according to standard symptom-based criteria. I would suggest that studies examining the genetic, biological, and clinical correlates of schizophrenia also identify patients along the neuroleptic-response dimension. The distinction between neuroleptic-responsive and neuroleptic-refractory patients is often not easy to make, but this distinction exists, and on historical, theoretical, and clinical grounds it clamors for application.

References

Awad AG: Drug therapy in schizophrenia: variability of outcome and prediction of response. Can J Psychiatry 34:711–720, 1989

Ayers T, Liberman RP, Wallace CJ: Subjective response to antipsychotic drugs: failure to replicate predictions of outcome. J Clin Psychopharmacol 4:89–93, 1984

Bartko G, Frecska E, Zador G, et al: Neurological features, cognitive impairment and neuroleptic response in schizophrenic patients. Schizophr Res 2:311–313, 1989

Bartko G, Herczeg I, Zador G: Blink rate response to haloperidol as possible predictor of therapeutic outcome. Biol Psychiatry 27:113–115, 1990

Bersani G, Valeri M, Bersani I, et al: HLA antigens and neuroleptic response in clinical subtypes of schizophrenia. J Psychiatr Res 23:213–220, 1989

Bishop MP, Gallant DM, Sykes TF: Extrapyramidal side effects and therapeutic response. Arch Gen Psychiatry 13:155–162, 1965

Bowers MB Jr, Swigar ME, Jatlow PI, et al: Early neuroleptic response: clinical profiles and plasma catecholamine metabolites. J Clin Psychopharmacol 7:83–86, 1987

Brown W, Herz L: Neuroleptic response as a nosologic device, in Handbook of Schizophrenia, Vol 3. Edited by Tsuang MT, Simpson JC. Amsterdam, Netherlands, Elsevier, 1988, pp 139–149

Brown WA, Laughren TP, Chisholm E, et al: Low serum neuroleptic levels predict relapse in schizophrenic patients. Arch Gen Psychiatry 39:998–1000, 1982

Casey JF, Lasky JJ, Klett JC, et al: Treatment of schizophrenic reactions with phenothiazine derivatives. Am J Psychiatry 117:97–105, 1960

Crow TJ: Molecular pathology of schizophrenia: more than one disease process? BMJ 280:66–68, 1980

Csernansky JG, Yesavage JA, Maloney W, et al: The treatment response scale: a retrospective method of assessing response to neuroleptics. Am J Psychiatry 140:1210–1212, 1983

Czobor P, Volavka J: Pretreatment EEG predicts short-term response to haloperidol treatment. Biol Psychiatry 30:927–942, 1991

Czobor P, Volavka J: Level of haloperidol in plasma is related to electroencephalographic findings in patients who improve. Psychiatry Res 42:129–144, 1992

Davidson M, Kahn R, Powchik P: Changes in plasma homovanillic acid concentrations in schizophrenic patients following neuroleptic discontinuation. Arch Gen Psychiatry 48:73–76, 1991a

Davidson M, Kahn R, Knott P, et al: Effects of neuroleptic treatment on symptoms of schizophrenia and plasma homovanillic acid concentrations. Arch Gen Psychiatry 48:910–913, 1991b

Davila R, Manero E, Zumarraga M, et al: Plasma homovanillic acid as a predictor of response to neuroleptics. Arch Gen Psychiatry 45:564–567, 1988

Duncan E, Wolkin A, Angrist B, et al: Plasma HVA in neuroleptic responsive and nonresponsive schizophrenics. Poster presented at the 31st annual meeting of the American College of Neuropsychopharmacology, San Juan, Puerto Rico, December 1992

Faraone SV, Brown WA, Laughren TP: Serum neuroleptic levels, prolactin levels, and relapse: a two year study of schizophrenic outpatients. J Clin Psychiatry 48:151–154, 1987

Faraone SV, Green AI, Brown WA, et al: Clinical effects of an 80% neuroleptic dose reduction in neuroleptic refractory psychotic patients. Hosp Community Psychiatry 40:1193–1199, 1989

Friedman L, Lys C, Schultz C, et al: The relationship of structural brain imaging parameters to antipsychotic treatment response: a review. J Psychiatry Neurosci 17:42–54, 1992

Galbrecht CR, Klett CJ: Predicting response to phenothiazines: the right drug for the right patients. J Nerv Ment Dis 147:173–183, 1968

Garver DL, Sautter FJ, Magnusson M, et al: Heterogeneity of neuroleptic response in psychosis. Paper presented at the 140th annual meeting of the American Psychiatric Association, Chicago, IL, May 1987

Gelder M, Kolakowska T: Variability of response to neuroleptics in schizophrenia: clinical, pharmacologic, and neuroendocrine correlates. Compr Psychiatry 20:397–408, 1979

Goldberg SC: Negative and deficit symptoms in schizophrenia do respond to neuroleptics. Schizophr Bull 11:453–456, 1985

Goldberg SC, Frosch WA, Drossman AK, et al: Prediction of response to phenothiazines in schizophrenia: a cross-validation study. Arch Gen Psychiatry 26:367–373, 1972

Goldberg SC, Schooler NR, Hogarty GE, et al: Prediction of relapse in schizophrenic outpatients treated by drug and sociotherapy. Arch Gen Psychiatry 34:171–184, 1977

Goldstein MJ: Premorbid adjustment, paranoid status, and patterns of response to phenothiazine in acute schizophrenia. Schizophr Bull 3:24–37, 1970

Green AI, Faraone SV, Brown WA, et al: Neuroleptic dose reduction studies: clinical and neuroendocrine effects. Paper presented at the 31st annual meeting of the American College of Neuropsychopharmacology, San Juan, Puerto Rico, December 1992

Hogan TP, Awad AG: Subjective response to neuroleptics and outcome in schizophrenia: a re-examination comparing two measures. Psychol Med 22:347–352, 1992

Hogan TP, Awad AG, Eastwood MR: Early subjective response and prediction of outcome of drug therapy in schizophrenia. Can J Psychiatry 30:246–248, 1985

Hollister LE, Kim DY: Intensive treatment with haloperidol of treatment-resistant chronic schizophrenic patients. Am J Psychiatry 139:1466–1468, 1982

Hollister LE, Overall JE, Kimbell I, et al: Specific indications for different classes of phenothiazines. Arch Gen Psychiatry 30:94–99, 1974

Itil TM, Marasa J, Saletu B, et al: Computerized EEG: predictor of outcome in schizophrenia. J Nerv Ment Dis 160:188–203, 1975

Itil TM, Shapiro D, Schneider SJ, et al: Computerized EEG as a predictor of drug response in treatment resistant schizophrenics. J Nerv Ment Dis 169:629–637, 1981

Karson CN, Bigelow LB, Kleinman JE, et al: Haloperidol-induced changes in blink rates correlate with changes in BPRS score. Br J Psychiatry 140:503–507, 1982

Kay SR, Singh MM: The positive-negative distinction in drug-free schizophrenic patients. Arch Gen Psychiatry 46:711–718, 1989

Keefe RSE, Mohs RC, Losonczy MF, et al: Characteristics of very poor outcome schizophrenia. Am J Psychiatry 144:889–895, 1987

Kendell RE: The Role of Diagnosis in Psychiatry. Oxford, Scientific Publications, 1975

Klein DF: Importance of psychiatric diagnosis in prediction of clinical drug effects. Arch Gen Psychiatry 16:118–126, 1967

Knobler HY, Itzchaky S, Emanuel D, et al: A case of resistant schizophrenia. Br J Psychiatry 149:789–793, 1986

Kolakowska T, Gelder MG, Orr MW: Drug-related and illness-related factors in the outcome of chlorpromazine treatment: testing a model. Psychol Med 10:335–343, 1980

Kolakowska T, Williams AO, Ardern M, et al: Schizophrenia with good and poor outcome. Br J Psychiatry 146:229–246, 1985

Lindstrom EM, Ohlund LS, Lindstrom LH, et al: Symptomatology and electrodermal activity as predictors of neuroleptic response in young male schizophrenic inpatients. Psychiatry Res 42:145–158, 1992

Little KY, Gay TL, Vore M: Predictors of response to high dose antipsychotics in chronic schizophrenics. Psychiatry Res 30:1–9, 1989.

Losonczy MF, Song IS, Mohs RC: Correlation of lateral ventricle size in chronic schizophrenia, I: behavioral and treatment response measures. Am J Psychiatry 143:976–981, 1986

Marder SR, Asarnow RF, Van Putten T: Information processing and neuroleptic response in acute and stabilized schizophrenic patients. Psychiatry Res 13:41–49, 1984

May PRA, Van Putten T, Yale C: Predicting outcome of antipsychotic drug treatment from early response. Am J Psychiatry 137:1088–1089, 1980

Murray RM, Murphy DL: Drug response and psychiatric nosology. Psychol Med 8:667–681, 1978

Naber D, Wirz-Justice A, Kafka MS: Seasonal variations in the endogenous rhythms of dopamine receptor binding in rat striatum. Biol Psychiatry 16:831–839, 1981

Naber D, Wirz-Justice A, Kafka MS: Chronic fluphenazine treatment modifies circadian rhythms of neurotransmitter receptor binding in rat brain. J Neural Transm 55:277–288, 1982

National Institute of Mental Health Psychopharmacology Research Branch Collaborative Study Group: Differences in clinical effects of three phenothiazines in "acute" schizophrenia. Diseases of the Nervous System 28:369–383, 1967

Nedopil N, Ruther E: Initial improvement as predictor of outcome of neuroleptic treatment. Pharmacopsychiatria 14:205–207, 1981

Overall JE, Gorham DR: The Brief Psychiatric Rating Scale. Psychol Rep 17:799–812, 1962

Pandurangi AK, Goldberg SC, Brink DH, et al: Amphetamine challenge in schizophrenia. Paper presented at the annual meeting of the Society of Biological Psychiatry, Chicago, IL, May 1987

Peroutka SJ, Snyder SH: Relationship of neuroleptic drug effects at brain dopamine, serotonin, α-adrenergic, and histamine receptors to clinical potency. Am J Psychiatry 137:1518–1522, 1980

Pickar D, Labarca R, Doran AR, et al: Longitudinal measurement of plasma homovanillic acid levels in schizophrenic patients. Arch Gen Psychiatry 43:669–676, 1986.

Rimon R, Averbuch H, Rozick P, et al: Serum and CSF levels of haloperidol by radioimmunoassay and radioreceptor assay during high-dose therapy of resistant schizophrenic patients. Psychopharmacology (Berl) 73:197–199, 1981

Schulz SC, Conley RR, Kahn EM, et al: Nonresponders to neuroleptics: a distinct subtype, in Schizophrenia: Scientific Progress. Edited by Schultz SC, Tamminga CA, New York, Oxford University Press, 1989, pp 341–350

Severson J, Marcusson J, Winblad B, et al: Age-correlated loss of dopaminergic binding sites in human basal ganglia. J Neurochem 39:1623–1631, 1982

Smith RC, Largen J, Vroulis G, et al: Neuropsychological test scores and clinical response to neuroleptic drugs in schizophrenic patients. Compr Psychiatry 33:139–145, 1992

Van der Velde CD: Variability of schizophrenia: reflection of a regulatory disease. Arch Gen Psychiatry 33:489–496, 1976

Van Putten T, Marder SR: Low-dose treatment strategies. J Clin Psychiatry 41:12–16, 1986

Van Putten T, Marder SR, Aravagiri M, et al: Plasma homovanillic acid as a predictor of response to fluphenazine treatment. Psychopharmacol Bull 1:89–91, 1989

Van Tol HHM, Wu CM, Guan HC, et al: Multiple dopamine D_4 receptor variants in the human population. Nature 358:149–152, 1992

Whelton CL, Cleghorn JM, Atley S, et al: Developmental and neurologic correlates of treatment response in schizophrenia. J Psychiatry Neurosci 17:15–22, 1992

Wolkin A, Barouche F, Wolf AP, et al: Dopamine blockade and clinical response: evidence for two biological subgroups of schizophrenia. Am J Psychiatry 146:905–908, 1989

Zubin J: Negative symptoms: are they indigenous to schizophrenia? Schizophr Bull 11:461–469, 1985

CHAPTER 20

Recent Neuroleptic Maintenance Strategies in the Management of Schizophrenia

Steven R. Hirsch, M.D., F.R.C.Psych., and
Dora Kohen, M.D., M.R.C.Psych.

During the 1950s, when neuroleptic medication first began being used to treat acute episodes of schizophrenia, the usual practice was to discontinue medication before discharge or a few weeks later; medication was then reintroduced if the patient began to relapse. In current terminology, this practice is called *targeted therapy* or *brief intermittent therapy* (the former term will be used in this chapter).

After that first decade, psychiatrists began to treat patients with medication for longer periods of time than just during recovery, finding that this regimen could prevent relapse. Clinical trials in the United States and the United Kingdom in the late 1960s and early 1970s showed that maintenance medication significantly lowered relapse rates. The first double-blind, placebo-controlled trial of patients stabilized on maintenance therapy in the community was carried out by Hirsch et al. (1973), who randomly and blindly substituted placebo for active medication in about half of their cohort of 71 patients. They found that only 8% of the patients on active medication relapsed in the 9 months of follow-up, as opposed to 66% of the patients on placebo. Following that study, results from some 35 placebo-controlled trials have confirmed the increased risk of relapse in patients who lower or stop their neuroleptic treatment.

In this chapter, we review treatment strategies aimed at reducing patients' exposure to neuroleptic medication, either by lowering their dosage or by treating them only when early prodromal symptoms appear. The desired outcome of this review would be that lower exposure to medication is associated with a lower incidence of immediate and long-term side effects, better social functioning, and an improved sense of personal well-being, and that these benefits outweigh the increased risk of relapse that would be attenuated by low-dosage treatment or early intervention in the prodromal phases of relapse.

Limitations of Continuous Medication and the Need for a Reevaluation

The use of continuous oral and depot neuroleptic treatment for maintaining schizophrenic patients in a steady state and preventing relapse is probably one of the clinical practices in psychiatry best supported by scientific evidence. Since the initial study by Hirsch et al. (1973), there have been more than 35 double-blind, placebo-controlled maintenance medication trials in schizophrenia; these have involved more than 3,600 patients, follow-up periods of 4–24 months, and an average relapse rate across trials of 57% on placebo compared with 16% on active medication (Davis 1975). Although there is no doubt that patients avoided relapse longer when on continuous medication, in a 7-year follow-up of the 82 chronic schizophrenic patients originally identified for the trial by Hirsch et al. (1973), Curson et al. (1985) found that 83% of patients eventually relapsed during the 7-year follow-up and 63% relapsed while on maintenance medication.

Several investigators (Cheung 1981; Dencker et al. 1980; Hirsch et al. 1973; Hogarty et al. 1976; Johnson 1976; Johnson et al. 1987;

Wistedt 1981) have been able to show that discontinuation of neuro-leptic treatment following several years without relapse, even when the best-stabilized patients and patients with lower risks were studied, leads to a relapse rate between 80% and 100%, depending on patient selection (see summary of these studies in Table 20–1).

The serious disadvantages of standard neuroleptic drug therapy are widely known. Akathisia, acute dystonia, drug-induced parkinsonism, and, in the long term, tardive dyskinesia and tardive dystonia present a formidable challenge to treating chronic schizophrenia. These major side effects have led clinicians to reconsider the basis on which they evaluate the benefits of treatment. Might there be a greater advantage to patients if they can have their exposure to medication reduced, even if they run a higher risk of relapse? Furthermore, if patients benefit from a lower incidence of early and long-term side effects and experi-ence better social functioning and an improved sense of well-being with reduced exposure to neuroleptic treatment, would they be pre-pared for a higher risk of relapse?

Alternative Strategies

In reviewing the alternative strategies to continuous maintenance medication, we examine the arguments for low-dosage treatment, targeted (or early intervention) therapy, and a third approach, in

Table 20–1. Relapse rates following drug discontinuation and long-term remission

Study	Time patients in remission	Duration of study	Patient relapse rate (%)
Wistedt (1981)	< 6 months	1 year	100
Hirsch et al. (1973)	< 1 year	9 months	92
Johnson (1976)	1–2 years	6 months	53
Hirsch et al. (1973)	1–5 years	9 months	66
Hogarty et al. (1976)	2–3 years	1 year	65
Cheung (1981)	3–5 years	18 months	62
Johnson et al. (1987)	1–4 years	18 months	80
Dencker et al. (1980)	2 years	2 years	85

which low-dosage treatment is combined with dosage augmentation therapy at early signs of relapse.

Low-Dosage Treatment

Pioneering studies of low-dosage treatment were published by Caffey et al. (1964) and Prien et al. (1973). Both groups of investigators carried out 4-month investigations in which patients were randomly allocated either to continue their daily treatment regimen or to be in a low-dosage group in which patients received active medication on alternating days, 3 days of the week; in Caffey et al.'s study, a placebo group was also included. The outcomes of these initial studies demonstrated a significant disadvantage of the lower-dosage therapy. In Caffey et al.'s (1964) study, 16% of the patients in the low-dosage group relapsed in the first 4 months, compared with 5% of the patients in the daily treatment group and 45% of the patients in the placebo group. Prien et al. (1973) found that 8% in the low-dosage group relapsed with neuroleptic medication compared with 1% in the daily treatment group. These relapse rates were low compared with those of later studies, partly because the trials lasted only 4 months and the medication dosage that was given to the low-dosage group was still substantial.

In a study by Capstick (1980), patients were withdrawn from depot neuroleptic medication by gradually increasing the periods between injections by 1 week at each visit and slowly decreasing the dosage over a 6-month period. When the patients reached the level of 3 mg of fluphenazine decanoate every 8 weeks, medication was stopped. The relapse rate among the patients in the first 6 months as dosages were being lowered was 40%; a further 40% of patients relapsed in the next 18 months after they reached the point of receiving no neuroleptic treatment. Thus, there was an overall relapse rate of 80% over a 2-year period. In 1979, Kane et al. reported on an open study in which the neuroleptic medication of 57 patients was reduced to one-tenth of the usual dosage or to 1.25–5 mg of fluphenazine decanoate every 2–4 weeks. Twenty-six percent of the patients relapsed in the following 6 months. In both Capstick's and Kane et al.'s studies, symptoms quickly remitted when medication was reintroduced and patients often did not require admission to the hospital.

In a subsequent double-blind, controlled study, Kane et al. (1983) randomly allocated 126 patients to receive either 1.25–5 mg of fluphenazine decanoate or 12.5–50 mg of fluphenazine decanoate every 2 weeks. The results of this study revealed that the 90% dosage reduction (1.25–5 mg) brought about a 56% relapse rate in the first year compared with a 7% relapse rate in patients maintained on a standard neuroleptic dosage regimen. Still, only 7% of the low-dosage-treated patients required hospitalization, and the social sequelae of relapse were minimal. On the lower-dosage regimen, patients appeared to have a better adjustment with less social withdrawal and blunting of affect and less motor retardation. The results of this study suggested that a trade-off is associated with neuroleptic dosage reduction strategies—that is, low dosages of medication are associated with improved social functioning and a greater sense of well-being at the expense of a higher rate of symptom generation that nonetheless responds quickly to early treatment interventions.

In the United Kingdom, Johnson et al. (1987) reported on a double-blind trial comparing a 50% dosage reduction of flupenthixol decanoate with a standard dosage of 40 mg every 2 weeks. At the end of a 1-year period, a (statistically) significantly higher relapse rate was seen in the patients in the lower-dosage group (32%) than in the group receiving the standard-dosage regimen (10%). It is interesting to note, however, that the dosage of 40 mg every 2 weeks is about one-third higher than many United Kingdom clinicians would prescribe (40 mg every 3 weeks is the lowest recommended dosage).

To examine the long-term effects of neuroleptic dosage reduction, Johnson et al. (1987) maintained the 50% neuroleptic dosage reduction group for a total of 3 years. Patients who were on the standard dosage were switched to the 50% dosage reduction group, though these patients were then rated under nonblind conditions. For patients completing 2 years of the study, a 56% overall relapse rate was observed; for patients completing 3 years, a 70% relapse rate was observed. With respect to side effects, no differences were observed between the standard-dosage group and the 50%-dosage-reduction group during the first year of double-blind comparison (see Table 20–2). This finding indicates that a neuroleptic dosage reduction of 50%

Table 20–2.   Low-dosage neuroleptic maintenance studies

| | | | Relapse rates by treatment (%) | | |
	Study N	Follow-up period	Standard dosage	Reduced dosage	Placebo
Caffey et al. (1964)	43	4 months	5	16	45
Prien et al. (1973)	43	4 months	1	8	—
Kane et al. (1983)	90	1 year	7	56	—
Johnson et al. (1987)	50	1 year	10	32	—
Capstick (1980)	47	2 years	—	80	—
Johnson et al. (1987)	50	2 years	—	56	—
Marder et al. (1987)	80	2 years	36	69	—
Johnson et al. (1987)	50	3 years	—	20	—

or more by whatever means leads to a significantly higher rate of relapse, although the relapse can often be controlled at an early stage. Moreover, Johnson et al. (1987) found that a considerable proportion of patients did not relapse even at the end of 2 years, suggesting that this approach could be tried on a case-by-case basis.

Targeted (Early Intervention) Treatment

The second strategy to reduce exposure to medication had its origin in the retrospective study of K. Herz and Melville (1980), who questioned 145 schizophrenic patients and their relatives about symptoms that were present leading up to relapse. Depressed mood, agitation, anger, and social withdrawal were common in the 3-week prodromal period prior to the reemergence of florid schizophrenic symptoms. Prodromal symptoms were self-reported in 70% of patients, and were reported by both patients and their relatives in more than 90% of patients. Symptoms experienced in more than 50% of patients included tension and nervousness; loss of sleep, appetite, interest, and concentration; memory loss; thoughts of being laughed at or of being noticed; and a feeling of being excited, depressed, or worthless. Dencker et al. (1980), Wistedt (1981), and Capstick (1980) all reported similar findings.

Knights and Hirsch (1981) found that depressive and neurotic symptoms were prevalent in the acute phase of the illness; Knights et al. (1979) reported that those symptoms continued to come and go during the recovery phase. Both findings supported the view that these symptoms are an intrinsic part of schizophrenic pathology. Thus, the concept that one might be able to treat patients with neuroleptics for brief periods only when they are about to relapse, using early neurotic and nonspecific prodromal symptoms as warnings of impending relapse, suggested itself as a possible alternative strategy to continuous neuroleptic medication (K. Herz and Melville 1980).

K. Herz and Melville's concept has now been tested in four randomized, controlled clinical trials (Carpenter et al. 1990; M. I. Herz et al. 1991; Jolley et al. 1990; Pietzcker et al. 1986) in which targeted treatment (treatment triggered by patients who note an emergence of neurotic and nonspecific symptoms) was compared with standard, continuous, long-term prophylactic medication. Two of these studies were placebo controlled (M. I. Herz et al. 1991; Jolley et al. 1990), and 2-year follow-up results of both have been published. The patients in M. I. Herz et al.'s (1991) study took oral or depot medication, whereas the patients in Jolley et al.'s (1990) study received only depot neuroleptic medication. Carpenter et al. (1990) and Pietzcker and colleagues (Pietzcker et al. 1986, 1993) have carried out open studies. Patients in Carpenter et al.'s (1990) study were on oral medication, but patients in Pietzcker and colleagues' studies (Pietzcker et al. 1986, 1993) were on either oral or depot medication. In all four studies, patients were seen on a weekly, biweekly, or monthly basis for the research assessments. In all of the above-mentioned studies except one (Jolley et al. 1990), some sort of supportive psychotherapy was also provided.

Pietzcker et al.'s (1986) multicenter trial had a third cohort called a "crisis intervention group," in which patients were treated only when frank psychotic symptoms appeared or breakdown occurred. The purpose of this group was to test the hypothesis that early intervention (i.e., targeted treatment) decreases the rate of emergence of specific schizophrenic symptoms. Thus, patients receiving early intervention were expected to have lower relapse rates than patients treated at the time when psychosis was more readily identifiable using conventional criteria. The results from this study showed that early intervention at the prodromal stage did indeed have significant advantages over crisis intervention. The relapse rates were 23% for the continuous maintenance therapy group, 49% for the early intervention group, and 63% for the crisis intervention group (these differences were statistically significant). However, the patients who did not relapse while on targeted therapy but who completed the 2-year follow-up period did not benefit by having improved social adjustment or an improved sense of well-being despite having a significantly lower dosage of medication and spending less time on medication.

The 2-year clinical outcome of these four studies showed a large and significant disadvantage of the targeted intervention group as compared with the continuous maintenance therapy group. The dropout or readmission rate in patients receiving targeted neuroleptic therapy was 50% or more.

Prodromal symptoms were significantly greater or more frequently reported in the early intervention group than in the continuous treatment group by all investigators except in the Carpenter et al. (1990) study, in which prodromal symptoms were not assessed. Specific schizophrenic symptoms and readmission rates were significantly higher in the samples reported by Carpenter et al. (1990) and Pietzcker et al. (1993) at the first and second year of follow-up. Jolley et al. (1990) reported the readmission rate as not significantly different at the end of the first year but worse at the end of the second year.

M. I. Herz et al. (1991) reported higher rates of symptoms and readmissions that were not significantly different; they further observed a 46% dropout rate in their targeted therapy group, which consistently decreased the number of patients available in whom to study the differences between groups who completed the study.

Social functioning.   Social functioning was measured in all of these studies (Carpenter et al. 1990; M. I. Herz et al. 1991; Jolley et al.

1990; Pietzcker et al. 1986), but targeted therapy provided no advantage in this regard at any point for any of the studies. M. I. Herz et al. (1991) reported significantly higher rates of relapse and increased burden to relatives in the targeted therapy group. Carpenter et al. (1990) reported higher unemployment, and Pietzcker et al. (1986) reported poor social stability. Jolley et al. (1990) observed no differences in social functioning at any point during the 12 monthly assessments or in the frequency of neurotic symptoms. These findings clearly indicate that reducing exposure to neuroleptic dosage increased the rate of symptom emergence, relapse rates, and hospitalization over 2 years, but that this strategy offered no advantages to patients in terms of improved well-being or social functioning. A significant disadvantage in various elements of social functioning was also reported by these studies.

Other possible benefits of targeted therapy were considered. All targeted therapy groups had a significant neuroleptic dosage reduction ranging from 30% (Carpenter et al. 1990) to 63% (Jolley et al. 1990). Neurological side effects were assessed in three of the studies (M. I. Herz et al. 1991; Jolley et al. 1990; Pietzcker et al. 1986) at the start of the study and at various points throughout the first and second year. No significant differences between measurements of extrapyramidal side effects or tardive dyskinesia were observed. Nevertheless, it is worthwhile to indicate that some 40% or more of the patients survived 2 years on targeted treatment without relapse.

Combined Low-Dosage and Dosage Augmentation Treatment

Two studies (Hogarty et al. 1988; Marder et al. 1987) have compared a standard-dosage medication approach with a dosage augmentation strategy for patients on a low-dosage regimen as soon as prodromal or early schizophrenic symptoms appeared. Marder et al. (1987) compared a standard dosage of 25 mg of fluphenazine decanoate every 2 weeks with 5 mg every 2 weeks. They noted that approximately 30% of the patients in both groups showed an exacerbation of illness during the first year, whereas 69% of those in the low-dosage group showed a significantly higher rate of early signs of relapse at the end of the 2-year follow-up period. At the time of exacerbation, clinicians were given the flexibility to double the patients' dosage if early signs of relapse (excluding nonspecific prodromal symptoms) emerged. Symptoms were well controlled at this increased dosage, which was 50 mg of fluphenazine decanoate every 2 weeks in the standard-dosage group and 10 mg of the same medication every 2 weeks in the low-dosage group. Patients were considered survivors if their symptoms could be controlled within a few days; otherwise, they were considered to have relapsed. Symptom evaluation following dosage augmentation showed similar relapse rates in both groups—44% for the patients in the low-dosage group with augmentation and 31% for patients in the standard-dosage group with augmentation—with the difference between the two groups being found as nonsignificant.

Hogarty et al. (1988) carried out a similarly designed study in which the average low-dosage treatment of fluphenazine decanoate was 3.8 mg every 2 weeks and the average standard-dosage treatment of fluphenazine decanoate was 25.7 mg every 2 weeks. The results of their study did not show a significant difference in exacerbation rates between the two treatments prior to augmentation, but there was a significant reduction in relapse rates in both treatment groups following an increase in medication. They observed that 49% of the patients in the low-dosage treatment group showed an exacerbation of illness, but only 28% were regarded as having relapsed when compared with the 45% of patients who showed exacerbation while on the standard dosage, 22% of whom were considered to have relapsed, despite increased medication in both groups.

These findings suggested that one possible alternative to a full-dosage maintenance neuroleptic regimen could be a low-dosage regimen combined with a dosage augmentation strategy when prodromal or early symptoms of relapse appear. One potential strategy would be to implement a progressively lower-dosage neuroleptic treatment regimen (e.g., reducing the original dosage to one-half for 3–6 months and then perhaps to one-quarter but no more) in combination with a dosage augmentation program (which would involve giving at least double the dosage when prodromal or early symptoms of relapse appear) and to then return to the original low dosage when the symptoms had been controlled for 2 weeks.

Summary of Alternative Strategies

In summary, randomized controlled trials have conclusively shown that there is a significantly higher risk of relapse with targeted, early intervention therapy when patients were monitored for up to 2 years. However, 40%–64% of patients treated at the first sign of prodromal symptoms continued 2 years without relapse. Moreover, the risk of relapse did not increase after the first 18 months of treatment. One might conclude that there is a subgroup of patients for whom this treatment is advantageous. However, Pietzcker et al.'s (1993) study enables us to put targeted treatment in perspective. They screened 3,481 patients, of whom only 11% could enter their study. Of these, only 47% were able to complete the 2-year period on targeted neuroleptic treatment. This suggests that the treatment may be feasible for as small a group as 5% of schizophrenic patients, and—as has already been seen—there is no demonstrable benefit in measures of clinical or social functioning or personal well-being, even with respect to extrapyramidal side effects.

It could be concluded, therefore, that targeted treatment is indicated only as an alternative when patients otherwise refuse treatment or for patients who are highly motivated to reduce neuroleptic exposure despite a substantial risk of relapse. If these patients remain relapse free for 18 months, then there may not be any added risk by continuing targeted as opposed to continuous neuroleptic treatment. In addition, it is of paramount importance to note that the close observation and intense treatment offered in these trials is not likely to be achieved in ordinary community practice, where patients tend to be less closely supervised and followed up.

Neuroleptic Dosage and the Emergence of Movement Disorders

The risks of extrapyramidal side effects (EPS) associated with neuroleptic drug treatment—such as akathisia, drug-induced parkinsonism, acute dystonia, and tardive dyskinesia (TD) and tardive dystonia—

have had a powerful influence on the search to reduce exposure to neuroleptic medication by lowering the dosage and investigating the duration of treatment. In the absence of evidence to the contrary, the assumption has been that there ought to be an association among neuroleptic dosage, the duration of treatment, and the risk for EPS, including TD.

As is discussed in Chapter 25 of this book, the majority of patients do not develop TD; furthermore, investigators in case studies of dose-response relationships have mostly evaluated individuals manifesting signs of TD. It is likely that individual differences influence patients' vulnerability to developing TD, a vulnerability that might play an even greater role in the development of EPS than do dosage or duration of exposure to neuroleptics (Kane et al. 1992).

Hogarty et al. (1988) and Jolley et al. (1990) evaluated targeted versus continuous maintenance neuroleptic treatment in the emergence of EPS; both groups reported less EPS in the targeted treatment groups.

Kane et al. (1985) found less akathisia in the targeted treatment group in the first year of follow-up, and Marder et al. (1987) observed less akathisia in the first 6 months of targeted treatment but no difference thereafter. Hogarty et al. (1988) also reported less akathisia in their low-dosage–treated patients during the first year of the study, but no difference in the second year.

Investigators in the majority of cross-sectional studies (Jeste and Wyatt 1981; Morgenstern et al. 1987) and follow-up studies (Gardos et al. 1988; M. I. Herz et al. 1991; Jolley et al. 1990; Marder et al. 1987; Pietzcker et al. 1993) have not found an association between TD and drug variables, such as dosage and duration of neuroleptic treatment (Barnes et al. 1983a, 1983b; Kane and Smith 1982). Baldessarini et al. (1988) reported that the frequent use of relatively high dosages of neuroleptics may mask an association between the drug dosage and duration of treatment factors and the risk of TD, and suggested that the use of lower dosages of neuroleptics in patients could reveal dose-response effects during the course of long-term follow-up.

Hogarty et al. (1988), Johnson et al. (1987), and Kane et al. (1983) examined the efficacy of a low-dosage versus a standard-dosage neuroleptic treatment regimen, as well as the effects of these regimens on the emergence of TD. At the end of his 18-month follow-up period, Johnson et al. (1987) found significantly less TD in the low-dosage group only. Hogarty et al. (1988), who followed patients for 2 years, and Kane et al. (1983), who followed patients for 1 year, found no significant differences between the low-dosage versus the standard-dosage regimens and the emergence of TD (see summary of results in Table 20–3). However, in Kane et al.'s (1983) study, patients in the low-dosage group who were examined at the end of 24 weeks showed fewer signs of TD, but this effect was temporary, as there were no differences between that group and the standard-dosage group at 1-year follow-up.

Because increasing age is a known risk factor for TD, and older patients generally receive lower dosages of neuroleptics, the effect of dosage and age may be confounding factors in elderly patients and should probably be studied in younger patients.

Kane and Smith (1982) documented that studies reporting a significant relationship between TD and neuroleptic drug dosage or duration of neuroleptic treatment are based on samples of patients in early years of their drug treatment.

Marder et al. (1987) reported no differences in the incidence of TD at the end of a 1-year follow-up period between patients receiving targeted or continuous neuroleptic treatment. Jolley et al. (1990) also reported no significant differences between two groups of continuous treatment versus targeted treatment and the emergence of TD at the end of a 2-year follow-up period. Similar results, as summarized in Table 20–3, were reported in the studies by M. I. Herz et al. (1991) and Pietzcker et al. (1993).

Jeste et al. (1979) reviewed the information on drug treatment and TD and concluded that there was a lack of evidence supporting the commonly held belief that frequent lengthy interruptions of neuroleptic treatment decrease the incidence of TD. The effects of "drug holidays" were also examined by Levine et al. (1980) and Shenay et al. (1981). Although Levine et al. (1980) detected an increase of TD during the 3-month discontinuation period, Shenay et al. (1981) observed no change in TD status during their patients' 6-week fixed-length neuroleptic drug holiday.

Table 20–3.   Neuroleptic regimen and the emergence of tardive dyskinesia

Intermittent versus continuous maintenance neuroleptic treatment

Study	Instrument	Follow-up period	Intermittent versus continuous treatment
Pietzcker et al. (1993)	AIMS	2 years	No difference
M. I. Herz et al. (1991)	AIMS	1 year	No difference
M. I. Herz et al. (1991)	AIMS	2 years	No difference
Marder et al. (1987)	AIMS	1 year	No difference
Jolley et al. (1990)	Modified Simpson-Angus Scale	2 years	No difference

Low-dosage versus standard-dosage neuroleptic regimen

Study	Instrument	Follow-up period	Low-dosage versus standard-dosage regimen
Hogarty et al. (1988)	—	2 years	No difference
Johnson et al. (1987)	AIMS	8 months	No difference
Johnson et al. (1987)	AIMS	12 months	No difference
Johnson et al. (1987)	AIMS	18 months	↓ tardive dyskinesia in low-dosage group (sig)
Kane et al. (1983)	Simpson Dyskinesia Scale	24 weeks	Fewer signs of tardive dyskinesia with low dosages
Kane et al. (1983)	Simpson Dyskinesia Scale	1 year	No difference

Note. AIMS = Abnormal Involuntary Movement Scale: Guy 1976; Modified Simpson-Angus Scale: Knights et al. 1979; Simpson Dyskinesia Scale: Simpson et al. 1979.

Conclusion

Our review of controlled studies of low-dosage and brief, targeted neuroleptic treatment in long-term maintenance schizophrenic patients shows that a reduction of 50% or more below the standard recommended dosage carries a high risk of relapse over the ensuing 18-month period. In general, the results of the studies reported in this chapter indicate that low-dosage or targeted neuroleptic treatment strategies, which reduce a patient's exposure to neuroleptic medication, have failed to show consistent benefits for patients in terms of improved social functioning or improved sense of well-being. In addition, these studies and those looking at drug holidays have not demonstrated efficacy of these strategies in reducing the risk of TD.

Future controlled studies in large patient samples of different age groups treated with neuroleptics should examine possible relationships between neuroleptic treatment and demographic data, psychiatric history, and clinical variables. These studies should lead to a better understanding of treatment-related risk factors for TD in different patient groups. Nevertheless, the assumption that improved patient functioning and reduced risks of untoward side effects would be derived from these treatment studies has proven to be largely exaggerated. Progress is more likely to come from a new generation of psychotropic drugs acting on different pharmacological principles.

References

Baldessarini RJ, Cohen BM, Teicher MH: Significance of neuroleptic dose and plasma level in the pharmacological treatment of psychoses. Arch Gen Psychiatry 45:79–91, 1988

Barnes TRE, Kidger T, Gore SM: Tardive dyskinesia: a 3-year follow-up study. Psychol Med 13:71–81, 1983a

Barnes TRE, Rosser M, Trauer T: A comparison of purposeless movements in psychiatric patients treated with antipsychotic drugs and normal individuals. J Neurol Neurosurg Psychiatry 46:540–546, 1983b

Caffey EM, Diamond LS, Frank TV, et al: Discontinuation or reduction of chemotherapy in chronic schizophrenics. Journal of Chronic Diseases 17:347–359, 1964

Capstick N: Long-term fluphenazine decanoate maintenance dosage requirements of chronic schizophrenic patients. Acta Psychiatr Scand 61:256–262, 1980

Carpenter WT, Hanlon TE, Heinrichs DW, et al: Continuous versus targeted medication in schizophrenic out-patients: outcome results. Am J Psychiatry 147:1138–1148, 1990

Cheung HK: Schizophrenics fully remitted on neuroleptics for 3–5 years: to stop or continue medication? Br J Psychiatry 138:490–494, 1981

Curson DA, Barnes TRE, Bamber RW, et al: Long-term depot maintenance of chronic schizophrenic out-patients—the seven-year follow-up of the Medical Research Council fluphenazine/placebo trial, I: course of illness, stability of diagnosis and the role of the special maintenance clinic. Br J Psychiatry 146:464–480, 1985

Davis JM: Overview: maintenance therapy in psychiatry, I: schizophrenia. Am J Psychiatry 132:1237–1245, 1975

Dencker SJ, Lepp M, Malm U: Do schizophrenics well adapted in the community need neuroleptics? a depot withdrawal study. Acta Psychiatr Scand Suppl 279:64–66, 1980

Gardos G, Cole JO, Haskell D, et al: The natural history of tardive dyskinesia. J Clin Psychopharmacol 8 (4 suppl):31–37, 1988

Guy W (ed): Abnormal Involuntary Movement Scale, in ECDEU Assessment Manual for Psychopharmacology, Revised (DHEW Publ No ADM 76-338). Rockville, MD, U.S. Department of Health, Education, and Welfare: Alcohol, Drug Abuse, and Mental Health Administration, 1976, pp 534–537

Herz K, Melville C: Relapse in schizophrenia. Am J Psychiatry 137:801–805, 1980

Herz MI, Glazer WM, Mostert MA, et al: Intermittent versus maintenance medication in schizophrenia: two-year results. Arch Gen Psychiatry 48:333–339, 1991

Hirsch SR, Gaind R, Rohde PD, et al: Outpatient maintenance of chronic schizophrenic patients with long-acting fluphenazine: double-blind placebo trial. BMJ 1:633–637, 1973

Hogarty GE, Ulrich RF, Mussare F, et al: Drug discontinuation among long term, successfully maintained schizophrenic outpatients. Diseases of the Nervous System 37:494–500, 1976

Hogarty GE, McEvoy JP, Munetz M, et al: Dose of fluphenazine, familial expressed emotion, and outcome in schizophrenia. Results of a two-year controlled study. Arch Gen Psychiatry 45:797–805, 1988

Jeste DV, Wyatt RJ: Changing epidemiology of tardive dyskinesia: an overview. Am J Psychiatry 138:297–309, 1981

Jeste DV, Potkin SG, Sinha S, et al: Tardive dyskinesia—reversible and persistent. Arch Gen Psychiatry 36:585–590, 1979

Johnson DAW: The duration of maintenance therapy in chronic schizophrenia. Acta Psychiatr Scand 53:298–301, 1976

Johnson DAW, Ludlow JM, Street K, et al: Double-blind comparison of half-dose and standard-dose flupenthixol decanoate in the maintenance of stabilised outpatients with schizophrenia. Br J Psychiatry 151:634–638, 1987

Jolley AG, Hirsch SR, Morrison E, et al: Trial of brief intermittent neuroleptic prophylaxis for selected schizophrenic outpatients: clinical and social outcome at two years. BMJ 301:837–842, 1990

Kane JM, Smith JM: Tardive dyskinesia: prevalence and risk factors, 1959 to 1979. Arch Gen Psychiatry 39:473–481, 1982

Kane JM, Rifkin A, Quitkin F, et al: Low-dose fluphenazine decanoate in maintenance treatment of schizophrenia. Psychiatry Res 1:341–348, 1979

Kane JM, Rifkin A, Woerner M, et al: Low-dose neuroleptic treatment of outpatient schizophrenics. Arch Gen Psychiatry 40:839–896, 1983

Kane JM, Rifkin AM, Woerner M, et al: High dose versus low dose strategies in the treatment of schizophrenia. Psychopharmacol Bull 21:533–537, 1985

Kane JM, Jeste DV, Barnes TRE, et al: Tardive dyskinesia: a task force report of the American Psychiatric Association. American Psychiatric Association, Washington DC, 1992

Knights A, Hirsch SR: Revealed depression and drug treatment for schizophrenia. Arch Gen Psychiatry 38:806–811, 1981

Knights A, Okasha MS, Salih MA, et al: Depressive and extrapyramidal symptoms and clinical effects: a trial of fluphenazine versus flupenthixol in maintenance of schizophrenic outpatients. Br J Psychiatry 135:515–523, 1979

Levine J, Schooler NR, Severe J, et al: Discontinuation of oral and depot fluphenazine in schizophrenic patients after one year of continuous medication: a controlled study, in Long-Term Effects of Neuroleptics (Advances in Biochemical Psychopharmacology, Vol 24). Edited by Cattabeni F, Racagni G, Spano PF, et al. New York, Raven, 1980, pp 483–493

Marder SR, Van Putten T, Mintz J, et al: Low- and conventional-dose maintenance therapy with fluphenazine decanoate: two-year outcome. Arch Gen Psychiatry 44:518–521, 1987

Morgenstern H, Glaser WM, Gibowski LD, et al: Predictors of tardive dyskinesia: results of a cross-sectional study in an outpatient population. Journal of Chronic Diseases 40:319–327, 1987

Pietzcker A, Gaebel W, Kopcke W, et al: A German multi-centre study on the neuroleptic long-term therapy of schizophrenic patients: preliminary report. Pharmacopsychiatry 19:161–166, 1986

Pietzcker A, Gaebel W, Kopcke W, et al: Intermittent versus maintenance neuroleptic long-term treatment in schizophrenia: two-year results of a German multicenter study. J Psychiatr Res 27:321–339, 1993

Prien RF, Gillis RD, Caffey EM: Intermittent pharmacotherapy in chronic schizophrenia. Hosp Community Psychiatry 24:317–322, 1973

Shenay RS, Sadler AG, Solomon C, et al: Effects of six-week drug holiday on symptom status, relapse and tardive dyskinesia in chronic schizophrenics. J Clin Psychopharmacol 1:141–145, 1981

Simpson GM, Lee JH, Zoubok B, et al: A rating scale for tardive dyskinesia. Psychopharmacology 64:171–179, 1979

Wistedt B: A depot neuroleptic withdrawal study. Acta Psychiatr Scand 64:65–84, 1981

CHAPTER 21

Adjunctive Nonneuroleptic Agents in Treatment-Refractory Schizophrenia

Marc-Alain Wolf, M.D.; Pierre-Michel Llorca, M.D.; and
Christian L. Shriqui, M.D., M.Sc., F.R.C.P.C.

The treatment of schizophrenia was revolutionized with the introduction of chlorpromazine in the 1950s. Since then, results from several double-blind, placebo-controlled studies have confirmed the effectiveness of neuroleptics in the treatment and prevention of acute episodes of schizophrenia (Davis 1975, 1976; Davis et al. 1980; Gelder and Kolakowska 1979; Kane and Lieberman 1987; Kane et al. 1992). However, neuroleptic drug therapy does not constitute a cure for schizophrenia, and neuroleptics are of little or no therapeutic benefit to some 25%–30% of

This work was supported by a Scholarship Award from the Fonds de la Recherche en Santé du Québec (FRSQ) to C. Shriqui. The authors thank S. Champetier for assistance in the manuscript preparation.

schizophrenic patients. In addition, neuroleptics have limited efficacy in improving social and interpersonal functioning, and they produce a wide range of unpleasant adverse effects (Ayd 1961; Davis 1976; Kane et al. 1992; Losonczy et al. 1986; Meltzer 1992a; Rifkin and Siris 1987; Shriqui 1988; see also Chapters 22–26 in this book).

The management of treatment-refractory schizophrenic patients presents an enormous clinical challenge. The development of novel antipsychotic drugs and the use of nonneuroleptic adjunctive strategies in these patients is a rapidly evolving area. Novel antipsychotic agents (e.g., clozapine, risperidone; see discussion of these and other agents in Chapters 12 and 14 of this book) improve positive and negative symptoms of schizophrenia and induce fewer extrapyramidal side effects (EPS) compared with standard neuroleptics (Borison et al. 1992a, 1992b; Chouinard et al. 1993; Gerlach 1991; Kane et al. 1988; Meltzer 1992b).

Clozapine is effective in a significant proportion of treatment-refractory schizophrenic patients (Kane et al. 1988; Meltzer 1992b), yet the 1%–2% incidence rate of clozapine-induced agranulocytosis combined with clozapine's elevated dosage-dependent seizure risk and high cost are significant factors limiting the drug's use.

Results from multicenter clinical trials with novel antipsychotic agents, such as risperidone, lead to new therapeutic guidelines for treatment-refractory schizophrenic patients, depending on the agents' proven efficacy, side effect profile, cost-effectiveness, and benefit-to-risk ratio. Although the results of these trials are eagerly awaited, it can be realistically expected that some patients will continue to derive little or no benefit from these novel antipsychotics. In addition, the limited availability of these novel antipsychotic agents because of health care budget constraints is a major concern. In such cases, adjunctive nonneuroleptic treatment strategies represent a valuable treatment modality.

Factors that influence treatment response in schizophrenic patients include neuroleptic noncompliance, pharmacokinetic considerations (which can lead to inadequate plasma concentrations), interindividual differences in bioavailability and metabolism, psychosocial factors, and the heterogeneity of schizophrenia itself (Altamura 1992). Lack of therapeutic response to standard neuroleptics often leads to one of two possible treatment approaches: one is a trial with an atypical antipsychotic and the other is one or several trials with nonneuroleptic adjunctive agents, including bromocriptine, lithium, benzodiazepines, β-adrenergic antagonists, carbamazepine, valproic acid, L-deprenyl, reserpine, and fluoxetine. However, the usefulness of the data from many studies on the efficacy of nonneuroleptic agents has been questionable because some studies have had methodological difficulties and results between studies have been inconsistent (Lindenmayer 1992; Meltzer 1992a; Schulz et al. 1990). In this chapter, we review the literature on the use of adjunctive nonneuroleptic agents in treatment-refractory schizophrenia and present some of the methodological difficulties encountered in studies of these agents.

Methodological Considerations

Clinical studies addressing treatment refractoriness in schizophrenia have often been difficult to interpret for a variety of reasons. These are discussed below.

Reliability of the schizophrenic diagnosis. Wolkowitz et al. (1990a) reminded researchers of the importance of diagnostic reliability, recalling a 1977 study by Strauss and Gift in which between 4 and 68 patients out of the same sample of 272 patients were diagnosed as schizophrenic, depending on which diagnostic criteria were used. Commonly used diagnostic criteria for schizophrenia include DSM-III-R (American Psychiatric Association 1987), the Research Diagnostic Criteria (RDC; Spitzer et al. 1978), and the Feighner criteria (Feighner et al. 1972). Differences between these diagnostic criteria have limited the comparability of results across studies. Using DSM-III-R criteria, Smith et al. (1992) reported that 23 out of 50 treatment-refractory psychotic patients (46%) required a change in their psychiatric diagnosis. The DSM-IV (American Psychiatric Association 1994) has introduced several changes in the diagnostic criteria for schizophrenia (see Chapter 4). However, it is unclear how these newly established criteria will impact on the diagnostic reliability of the illness.

Clinical trials in treatment-refractory schizophrenic patients are increasingly using structured or semistructured diagnostic interviews to ensure diagnostic accuracy. In addition, the length and chronicity of illness and standardization of neuroleptic and other psychotropic medications are important to consider.

Definition of neuroleptic resistance.   The results from the pivotal double-blind, comparative study of clozapine versus chlorpromazine by Kane et al. (1988) suggested specific pharmacological criteria for neuroleptic treatment refractoriness: the patient must have had at least three periods of treatment in the preceding 5 years, with neuroleptic agents from at least two different chemical classes, at dosages equivalent to or greater than 1,000 mg/day of chlorpromazine, for a minimum period of 6 weeks each, without significant symptomatic relief and with no period of good functioning within the past 5 years.

Brenner et al. (1990) developed a rating scale to evaluate neuroleptic response and treatment refractoriness. This scale, which uses scores from a social adjustment index (Brenner et al. 1990), the Clinical Global Impression (CGI) scale (Guy 1976), and the Brief Psychiatric Rating Scale (BPRS; Overall and Gorham 1962), contains seven levels of neuroleptic response varying from 1 ("remission") to 7 ("severely treatment refractory").

Recognized pharmacological criteria for neuroleptic resistance have been considered by some investigators as potentially too restrictive. For example, Meltzer (1990) suggested that, at least in theory, a schizophrenic patient who has not fully recovered to his or her best premorbid level of functioning should be viewed as treatment refractory.

Definition of neuroleptic treatment response.   A statistically significant symptomatic improvement during a clinical trial may not correspond with a similar rate of improvement in the patient's quality of life. In the clozapine collaborative study by Kane et al. (1988), the improvement criteria were defined as a decrease in BPRS total score of at least 20% and either a CGI score greater than 4 or a BPRS score less than 36. Wolkowitz et al. (1990a) also suggested relying on the individual case study to determine treatment response.

Identification of schizophrenic patient subgroups responsive to nonneuroleptic adjunctive agents. The diagnostic, clinical, and demographic characteristics of patients responsive to nonneuroleptic adjunctive agents have been frequently neglected (Wolkowitz et al. 1990a). In clinical trials with adjunctive nonneuroleptic agents, treatment response should be systematically evaluated with regard to change in positive and negative symptoms.

Effect of nonneuroleptic adjunctive agents on neuroleptic side effects. Certain nonneuroleptic adjunctive agents such as beta-blockers can induce improvement in both psychopathology and neuroleptic side effects (e.g., akathisia). Possible correlations between changes in psychopathology and neuroleptic side effects should be examined whenever possible.

Major Classes of Nonneuroleptic Adjunctive Treatments in Schizophrenia

Benzodiazepines

Because of their gamma-aminobutyric acid (GABA) agonist properties, benzodiazepines can indirectly inhibit mesolimbic dopaminergic activity (Garbutt and van Kammen 1983). This effect has prompted the use of benzodiazepines in schizophrenic patients for the control of anxiety, insomnia, and agitation. Lingjaerde (1991) reported that benzodiazepines alone can reduce anxiety, stress, and insomnia in schizophrenic patients. At high dosages, however, benzodiazepines can exert an antipsychotic effect with consequent improvement in delusions and hallucinations. Nestoros (1980) reviewed 14 controlled studies; in only 1 of those studies (Kellner et al. 1979) was a beneficial effect of adding benzodiazepines to neuroleptics reported. However, the lack of positive findings in the remaining 13 studies is believed to have resulted from the use of inadequate dosages. Christison et al. (1991) reviewed 6 controlled studies subsequent to 1980 and reported a significant beneficial effect of benzodiazepines when compared with placebo in 4 (Jimerson et al. 1982; Nestoros et al. 1982; Wolkowitz et al. 1986, 1988) out of the 6 studies. The two remaining studies (Csernansky et al. 1988; Karson et al. 1982) showed no advantage of benzodiazepines over placebo.

Treatment-refractory schizophrenic patients who respond to the addition of a benzodiazepine generally improve after 2–3 weeks of benzodiazepine treatment. In schizophrenic patients, diazepam, clonazepam, estazolam, and alprazolam have been used in combination with neuroleptics. A summary of these controlled studies—reviewed elsewhere (Christison et al. 1991; Llorca et al. 1991; Wolkowitz and Pickar 1991)—is presented in Table 21–1.

In general, these studies suggest a beneficial effect of benzodiazepines in reducing psychotic anxiety. However, the effects of benzodiazepines on schizophrenic symptoms per se remain unclear. In some patients, their continued use can lead to a variety of complications, including substance abuse behavior, withdrawal symptoms, disinhibition, and psychotic exacerbation (Dixon et al. 1989; Little and Taghavi 1991; Meltzer 1992a).

As posed by Wolkowitz and Pickar (1991), unanswered questions concerning the use of benzodiazepines in patients with treatment-refractory schizophrenia include the following:

- What are potential predictors of benzodiazepine response?
- Which target symptoms are the most affected?
- How do benzodiazepines exert their pharmacological effects?
- What is the optimal treatment period with benzodiazepines in these patients?

Mood-Stabilizing Drugs

Lithium.   The use of lithium in schizophrenia is associated with the question of diagnostic boundaries between schizophrenia and schizoaffective disorders. In a review of the literature, Atre-Vaidya and Taylor (1989) observed that a number of chronic schizophrenic patients responding to lithium treatment had concomitant affective symptoms or a previous personal or family history of affective disorder. Despite several studies in which the efficacy of combining lithium and

Table 21–1. Studies of benzodiazepines added to neuroleptic medication in treatment-refractory schizophrenic patients

Study	N	Benzodiazepine	Neuroleptic associated	Patient description	Study design	Results
Ruskin et al. (1979)	8	Diazepam 40–80 mg/day	—	Chronic schizophrenic patients unresponsive to neuroleptics	Placebo crossover	Inefficacious (BPRS)
Lingjaerde et al. (1979)	23	Diazepam 15 mg/day	—	19 chronic schizophrenic patients unresponsive to neuroleptics	Placebo crossover	Improvement of suspiciousness and unusual thought content (BPRS)
Karson et al. (1982)	13	Clonazepam	Haloperidol Mesoridazine Fluphenazine	RDC diagnoses of chronic schizophrenia	Placebo crossover	Inefficacious; excitement in 4 patients (BPRS)
Lingjaerde (1982)	58	Estazolam	—	52 schizophrenic patients refractory to neuroleptics	Placebo crossover	Improvement: global ratings, auditory and visual hallucinations, compulsive thoughts (CGI, CPRS)
Altamura et al. (1987)	24	Clonazepam 3 mg/day	Haloperidol 3–19 mg/day	Schizophrenia, disorganized (DSM-III) in acute exacerbation	Double-blind versus placebo	Improvement in week one of anxiety, tension, and excitement; no difference in week 4 (BPRS)
Csernansky et al. (1988)	55	Alprazolam (mean dosage = 3.7 mg/day) Diazepam (mean dosage 39 mg/day)	—	Schizophrenic (RDC) outpatients with negative symptoms	Double-blind versus placebo Alprazolam ($n = 18$) Diazepam ($n = 20$) Placebo ($n = 17$)	Alprazolam superior to placebo during the first weeks; no persistent benefit (CGI, BPRS, SANS)

Table 21–1. Studies of benzodiazepines added to neuroleptic medication in treatment-refractory schizophrenic patients *(continued)*

Study	N	Benzodiazepine	Neuroleptic associated	Patient description	Study design	Results
Wollkowitz et al. (1988)	12	Alprazolam (mean dosage = 2.9 mg/day)	Fluphenazine (26 mg/day on average)	Schizophrenia (RDC and DSM-III)	Placebo crossover	Decrease of positive and negative symptoms (A-T RSEB, BHGRS, BPRS)
Pato et al. (1989)	17	Alprazolam (< 5 mg/day)	Fluphenazine	Chronic schizophrenic patients (RDC and DSM-III)	Placebo crossover	Mild decrease in psychosis (BHGRS, BHGPR)
Barbee et al. (1992)	28	Alprazolam	Haloperidol	Acutely psychotic patients with schizophrenia (DSM-III-R)	Double-blind versus placebo Duration: 72 hours	Efficacious on excitement and uncooperativeness (BPRS) in initial hours; dystonic reactions

Note. — = No details available; DSM-III (American Psychiatric Association 1980); DSM-III-R (American Psychiatric Association 1987); RDC = Research Diagnostic Criteria (Spitzer et al. 1978). **Psychometric tests:** A-T RSEB = Abrams-Taylor Rating Scale for Emotional Blunting (Abrams and Taylor 1978); BHGPR = Bunney-Hamburg Global Psychosis Rating Scale (Bunney and Hamburg 1963); BHGRS = Bunney-Hamburg Global Rating Scale (Bunney and Hamburg 1963); BPRS = Brief Psychiatric Rating Scale (Overall and Gorham 1962); CGI = Clinical Global Impression scale (Guy 1976); CPRS = Comprehensive Psychopathological Rating Scale (Asberg et al. 1978); SANS = Scale for the Assessment of Negative Symptoms (Andreasen 1983).

neuroleptics in schizophrenia has been evaluated, only a few investigators have examined this issue in treatment-refractory patients.

In four of the five controlled studies reviewed in Table 21–2 (Carman et al. 1981; Growe et al. 1979; Schulz et al. 1990; Small et al. 1975), all four of which included schizophrenic and schizoaffective disorder patients, a beneficial effect was reported with the addition of lithium to neuroleptics. In addition, lithium may also prevent relapses in schizoaffective patients. Until now, no clear predictors of lithium response have been identified in either schizophrenic or schizoaffective patients. Some reports have raised concerns about a potential neurotoxic effect of combining lithium with neuroleptics (Christison et al. 1991). Reported neurotoxic effects have usually consisted of reversible confusional episodes (Braden et al. 1982; F. Miller and Menninger 1987; Small et al. 1975), although some rare irreversible neurological effects (Cohen and Cohen 1974) have also occurred. The addition of lithium to neuroleptics has also been suggested as a potential risk factor for neuroleptic malignant syndrome (Addonizio and Susman 1991; Pope et al. 1986; Susman and Addonizio 1988).

Carbamazepine.   The use of carbamazepine in schizophrenia began in the 1980s. In Table 21–3, the results of five rigorously conducted studies in neuroleptic-resistant chronic schizophrenic or schizoaffective patients are presented. Investigators in four of these studies reported positive findings, although the alleviated symptoms were mostly nonspecific for schizophrenia (agitation, aggressivity, and mood disturbance). To our knowledge, there has been only one study in which the efficacy of carbamazepine added to neuroleptics in a homogeneous sample of chronic, neuroleptic-refractory schizophrenic patients was examined (Kidron et al. 1985); this study resulted in a negative finding. Overall, investigators have consistently found that carbamazepine treatment results in a decrease in aggressive and violent behaviors (Christison et al. 1991; Schulz et al. 1990). A decrease in positive or negative symptoms remains possible with carbamazepine, although this effect has not been clearly demonstrated. Similarly, the effectiveness of carbamazepine in patients with abnormal temporal electroencephalographic activity remains unclear (Christison et al. 1991; Schulz et al. 1990). The usual daily dosage requirements of

Table 21–2. Studies of lithium added to neuroleptic medication in treatment-refractory schizophrenic patients

Study	N	Patient description	Study design	Results
Small et al. (1975)	22	Neuroleptic-resistant patients; 14 chronic schizophrenic and 8 schizoaffective patients (Feighner)	2 possible sequences: A-B-A-B or B-A-B-A, with A = lithium and B = placebo (double-blind)	10 improved (4 schizoaffective) and 7 discharged for chronic care Improvement in global illness, social competence, and manifest psychosis (CGI, BPRS, NOSIE, MSRS)
Growe et al. (1979)	8	Neuroleptic-resistant patients; 6 schizophrenic and 2 schizoaffective patients (RDC)	16-week study with 2 possible sequences: A-B-A-B or B-A-B-A, with A = lithium and B = placebo (double-blind)	Only 1 of 8 syndromes, psychotic excitement, improved significantly (PIP)
Carman et al. (1981)	18	Patients with chronic or multiple hospitalizations or with poor social functioning; 11 schizophrenic and 7 schizoaffective patients (RDC)	2 possible sequences: A-B-A or B-A-B, with A = lithium and B = placebo (double-blind)	BPRS: decreased psychosis in 5 patients (3 schizoaffective); decreased arousal in 8 patients (4 schizoaffective)
Schulz et al. (1990)	14	Patients who were nonresponsive to acute haloperidol treatment; schizophrenic or schizoaffective patients (DSM-III)	2 groups randomly assigned to a 2-week trial with either lithium + haloperidol (n = 8) or carbamazepine + haloperidol (n = 6)	5 of 8 patients responded to lithium + haloperidol; 2 of 6 responded to carbamazepine + haloperidol Improvement of total BPRS score and BPRS thought disorder factor Briefer duration of illness, higher MMSE scores, and more family histories of schizophrenia in responsive patients

| Collins et al. (1991) | 44 | Neuroleptic-resistant schizophrenic patients detained in a maximum-security hospital (DSM-III-R) | Control group ($n = 23$) versus lithium group ($n = 21$); single-blind 4-week trial | No significant differences (MS, SANS) |

Note. DSM-III (American Psychiatric Association 1980); DSM-III-R (American Psychiatric Association 1987); Feighner = Feighner criteria (Feighner et al. 1972); RDC = Research Diagnostic Criteria (Spitzer et al. 1978). **Psychometric tests:** BPRS = Brief Psychiatric Rating Scale (Overall and Gorham 1962); CGI = Clinical Global Impression scale (Guy 1976); MMSE = Mini-Mental Status Exam (Folstein et al. 1975); MS = Manchester Scale (Krawiecka et al. 1977); MSRS = Manic State Rating Scale (Beigel et al. 1971); NOSIE = Nurses' Observation Scale for Inpatient Evaluation (Honigfeld et al. 1966); PIP = Psychotic Inpatient Profile (Lorr and Vestre 1968); SANS = Scale for the Assessment of Negative Symptoms (Andreasen 1983).

carbamazepine in treatment-resistant schizophrenic patients is 400–600 mg/day, although there is no evidence of a minimal effective dosage in these patients (Neppe 1983, 1988).

From a pharmacokinetic perspective, carbamazepine increases its own hepatic enzyme metabolism as well as that of haloperidol, whose plasma levels can be decreased by one-third (Kidron et al. 1985). Theoretically, this drug interaction could lead to a worsening of psychotic symptoms. However, in neuroleptic-resistant patients, the use of carbamazepine may decrease side effects such as akathisia.

Valproic acid.   McElroy et al. (1989) reviewed the use of valproic acid in schizophrenic disorders. Of a total of 107 schizophrenic patients in eight studies, approximately one-third responded favorably. However, inaccuracy of diagnostic criteria, frequent co-occurrence of manic symptoms, and a negative finding in two controlled studies (Fisk and York 1987; Ko et al. 1985) cast doubt on this agent's efficacy.

Wassef et al. (1989) observed a rapid improvement of hallucinations in three neuroleptic-treated schizophrenic patients who were administered 1 g/day of valproic acid. Van Valkenburg et al. (1990) reported a greater clinical efficacy of valproic acid at serum levels greater than 50 µg/ml, which is equivalent to the serum level required for an anticonvulsant effect.

Other antiepileptic agents.   Other antiepileptic agents may also be of benefit in the treatment of schizophrenia. Raptis et al. (1989) reported on the clinical effect of beclamide and found that it could potentiate the efficacy and tolerability of haloperidol in a sample of 12 acutely ill schizophrenic and schizoaffective patients. Chouinard and Sultan (1990) suggested that the efficacy of antiepileptic drugs—and particularly that of carbamazepine and valproic acid—in some schizophrenic patients may be linked to their antikindling effect, which could decrease supersensitivity psychosis (see Chapter 26).

Antidepressants

The use of antidepressant medication is not uncommon in schizophrenia. Depressive symptoms in schizophrenic patients were recognized

Table 21–3. Studies of carbamazepine added to neuroleptic medication in treatment-refractory schizophrenic patients

Study	N	Patient description	Study design	Results
Neppe (1983)	13	Chronic nonepileptic patients; patients with temporal lobe electroencephalographic abnormalities; 10 schizophrenic patients, 9 with neuroleptics	Crossover double-blind study	9 of 11 better on carbamazepine; 1 of 11 better on placebo; significant improvement of aggression; electroencephalogram recordings worse in 6 patients
Kidron et al. (1985)	11	Neuroleptic-resistant chronic schizophrenic patients (RDC)	Crossover double-blind study	No difference between carbamazepine and placebo (BPRS); lowered haloperidol levels during carbamazepine augmentation
Herrera et al. (1987)	6	Chronic schizophrenic patients (DSM-III) nonresponsive to high-dosage neuroleptics	Single-blind study	Depression, anxiety, and withdrawal significantly improved (BPRS)
Okuma et al (1989)	162	Neuroleptic-resistant schizophrenic ($n = 127$) patients or schizoaffective patients with acute psychosis ($n = 35$) (DSM-III)	Carbamazepine versus placebo added to neuroleptics for 4 weeks	Improvement of manic symptoms (CPRG mania scale), uncooperativeness, suspiciousness, and excitement (BPRS); aggressive patients more likely to respond
Schulz et al. (1990)	14	Schizophrenic or schizoaffective (DSM-III) patients nonresponsive to acute haloperidol treatment	2-week double-blind trial with either lithium + haloperidol or carbamazepine + haloperidol	2 responded to carbamazepine + haloperidol; improvement of total BPRS score and BPRS thought disorder factor

Note. DSM-III (American Psychiatric Association 1980); RDC = Research Diagnostic Criteria (Spitzer et al. 1978). **Psychometric tests:** BPRS = Brief Psychiatric Rating Scale (Overall and Gorham 1962); CPRG Mania Scale = Clinical Psychopharmacology Research Group of Japan Mania Scale (Takahashi et al. 1975).

by Kraepelin and Bleuler. Recently, attention has focused on a possible association between depressive symptoms and negative schizophrenic symptoms (Siris et al. 1988; see Chapter 7).

Very few investigators have examined the efficacy of antidepressant medication in nondepressed, neuroleptic-resistant, chronic schizophrenic patients. Tricyclic antidepressants and monoamine oxidase inhibitors can be of benefit to schizophrenic patients with depressive or negative symptoms. Clinical reports have also documented improvement in depressive and negative symptoms in schizophrenic patients treated with selective serotonin reuptake inhibitors. However, the evidence of their efficacy in schizophrenic patients is only preliminary. Fluoxetine, which has been reported to improve negative and depressive symptoms in schizophrenic patients, may also improve positive symptoms. It is clear that more studies are required to investigate fluoxetine's efficacy in these patients.

Because of their distinct mechanisms of action, tricyclic antidepressants (TCAs), monoamine oxidase inhibitors (MAOIs), and novel antidepressants (particularly selective serotonin reuptake inhibitors) are reviewed separately.

Tricyclic antidepressants.   Siris et al. (1978) reviewed 16 double-blind, controlled studies in which imipramine or amitriptyline was used in combination with chlorpromazine or perphenazine. Investigators in two studies reported positive findings with TCA use, particularly in patients with a concomitant depressive symptomatology. Siris and colleagues (Siris et al. 1987, 1988, 1989a, 1989b, 1990, 1991) conducted a series of studies, the results of which supported the efficacy of adding imipramine to neuroleptics in schizophrenic or schizoaffective patients with either predominantly negative symptoms or depressive features. However, Kramer et al. (1989) reported an increase in hallucinations and conceptual disorganization in a group of 58 depressed, haloperidol-treated, chronic schizophrenic patients when desipramine, amitriptyline, or placebo was added to haloperidol in a double-blind fashion.

Monoamine oxidase inhibitors.   Results from 3 of the 12 studies reviewed by Siris et al. (1978) supported a beneficial effect of combining an MAOI with neuroleptics. In an 8-month clinical trial with 30 depressed schizophrenic patients treated with either chlorpromazine monotherapy (300 mg/day) or chlorpromazine in combination with tranylcypromine (20 mg/day), Bucci (1987) reported improvement in both negative and depressive symptoms with the combination therapy.

Novel antidepressants. In an open study of 20 schizophrenic patients treated with neuroleptics, Mizuki et al. (1992) reported that mianserin improved negative schizophrenic symptoms. Selective serotonin reuptake inhibitors have recently been tried in the treatment of schizophrenia. Goff et al. (1990) and Chiaroni et al. (1991) conducted open-label trials of fluoxetine in small cohorts of schizophrenic patients treated with neuroleptics. In these trials, 4 out of 9 patients (Goff et al. 1990) and 5 out of 7 patients (Chiaroni et al. 1991) experienced improvement both in depressive symptoms and in positive and negative schizophrenic symptoms.

Silver and Nassar (1992) carried out a double-blind, placebo-controlled trial of fluvoxamine added to neuroleptics in a group of 30 treatment-resistant, chronic schizophrenic patients. They reported that negative symptoms improved with fluvoxamine, whereas positive and depressive symptoms improved with fluvoxamine and placebo.

Dopaminergic Strategies

Various agents affecting the presynaptic metabolism of dopamine have been tested clinically. Berlant (1990) reviewed the efficacy of α-methyl-p-tyrosine (metyrosine), a tyrosine hydroxylase inhibitor, and the use of λ-hydroxybutyrate (GHB), an inhibitor of dopamine release. Results from most open and controlled studies have suggested a positive effect of metyrosine combined with neuroleptics in comparison with neuroleptic monotherapy. However, no systematic clinical trials have examined this agent's efficacy in treatment-refractory schizophrenia. GHB, used alone or with neuroleptics, appears rather ineffective.

Other dopaminergic strategies tried in schizophrenic patients include the use of reserpine, tiospirone, dopamine agonists, partial dopamine agonists, and dopamine precursors.

Reserpine.   Reserpine induces a presynaptic depletion in dopamine not only in dopaminergic but also in noradrenergic and serotonergic pathways (Nasrallah et al. 1979). Its use in schizophrenia dates back to 1952, just prior to the introduction of chlorpromazine. Reserpine's antipsychotic effect has been demonstrated in more than 20 controlled studies, including two studies with entirely chronic schizophrenic samples (Berlant 1986, 1990; Christison et al. 1991). However, in the past 25 years, the demonstrated superiority and tolerability of neuroleptics has markedly reduced the use of reserpine in the treatment of schizophrenia. Investigators in a few open studies have observed a positive effect of combining neuroleptics and reserpine (Bacher and Lewis 1978, 1985; Barsa and Kline 1955, 1956; Berlant 1986), but the evidence from these trials is insufficient to predict treatment response. Although side effects to reserpine can be severe and potentially life-threatening (e.g., depression, hypotension, bradycardia), its use in treatment-refractory schizophrenia merits further study.

Tiospirone.   This nonneuroleptic dopamine receptor antagonist is believed not to induce dopamine receptor supersensitivity. Tiospirone has been clinically tested in two controlled trials (Borison et al. 1989; Moore et al. 1987) in which it was reported that its antipsychotic efficacy was comparable to that of standard neuroleptics.

Dopamine agonists and precursors; L-dopa.   In their review of the literature, Christison et al. (1991) cited three double-blind studies (Gerlach and Luhdorf 1975; Inanaga et al. 1975; Kay and Opler 1985) in which a beneficial effect of L-dopa in neuroleptic-treated schizophrenic patients with predominantly negative symptoms was reported. Despite these encouraging results, further replication studies are required to fully evaluate L-dopa's short- and long-term efficacy in treating negative symptoms and to determine which patients are most likely to respond and at what optimal dosage range.

Bromocriptine.   At a low dosage, bromocriptine is believed to act as a presynaptic dopamine receptor agonist and to exert an antipsychotic effect (Meltzer et al. 1983). When administered alone at dosages of 5 mg/day or less, bromocriptine demonstrated no significant clinical effects (Brambilla et al. 1983; Meltzer et al. 1983). When combined with neuroleptics, however, bromocriptine was more effective. Studying 11 schizophrenic patients on neuroleptics, Cutler et al. (1984) reported brief clinical improvement (over a 2-hour period) in hostility and formal thought disorder following a single 2-mg dose of bromocriptine. Gattaz and Kollisch (1986) noted the rapid onset and lasting beneficial effect of 2.5 mg/day of bromocriptine in a paranoid schizophrenic patient who was unresponsive to either fluperlapine or haloperidol. In a subsequent double-blind, controlled study with 30 acutely ill schizophrenic patients, Gattaz et al. (1989) reported that 2.5 mg/day of bromocriptine accelerated patients' clinical response to haloperidol, but that after a 10-day period, this difference was no longer significant when compared with haloperidol used alone.

Wolf et al. (1992a, 1992b) reported on the efficacy of bromocriptine in 9 patients and 11 patients, respectively. All patients were receiving neuroleptic medication and suffered from chronic, treatment-refractory schizophrenia. Clinical improvement was noted in both positive and negative symptoms with 1.25 mg/day and 2.5 mg/day of bromocriptine. At the 1.25-mg/day dosage, clinical improvement was short-lived, but at the 2.5-mg/day dosage, improvement was sustained throughout the 4-week follow-up period.

Partial dopamine D_2 receptor agonists. These compounds act as dopamine D_2 receptor agonists and antagonists and could, theoretically, compensate for either a hyperdopaminergic (linked to positive symptoms) or hypodopaminergic (associated with negative symptoms) state. The clinical efficacy of these agents (e.g., SDZ HDC 912, terguride, roxindole, B-HT 920) remains unclear (Gerlach 1991).

Noradrenergic Strategies

Propranolol and other beta-blockers. Propranolol is a nonselective beta-blocker. Berlant (1987) and Llorca and Wolf (1991) reviewed the effectiveness of propranolol alone (without concomitant neuroleptics) in treatment-refractory schizophrenic patients. Overall, investigators in open studies of propranolol alone, involving a total of

41 patients, have reported clinical improvement in up to 20% of subjects. Opposing findings have been reported in two double-blind, controlled trials with propranolol: Peet et al. (1981) observed no clinical efficacy, whereas Ecclestone et al. (1985) reported a significant beneficial effect in positive and negative symptoms.

In double-blind conditions, several studies have evaluated the efficacy of adding propranolol to neuroleptics in treatment-refractory patients; the results of these studies are summarized in Table 21–4.

Results of initial clinical trials with propranolol were more promising than those of recent studies. Overall, schizophrenic patients can benefit from the addition of propranolol to alleviate anxiety and impulsive or aggressive behavior, and possibly to improve positive symptoms as well. At high dosages, propranolol induces significant side effects, particularly hypotension. An increase in the plasma concentration of neuroleptics (e.g., thioridazine, chlorpromazine) has been associated with the use of propranolol. This pharmacological interaction may be responsible for propranolol's efficacy in schizophrenia (Lader 1988). Beta-blockers are also effective in the treatment of neuroleptic-induced akathisia (Dumon et al. 1992; Lader 1988). This extrapyramidal side effect often goes unrecognized and should always be considered in the agitated and anxious schizophrenic patient.

Another nonselective beta-blocker, oxprenolol, was clinically tested by Volk et al. (1972) in eight patients, four of whom were schizophrenic. Two of the schizophrenic patients demonstrated clinical improvement. Further research with more-selective beta-blockers is required before drawing any conclusions on the overall efficacy of these agents in the treatment of schizophrenia.

Clonidine.   This centrally acting antihypertensive drug stimulates presynaptic α_2-adrenergic receptors, which exert an inhibitory effect. Llorca and Wolf (1991) reviewed several clinical trials evaluating clonidine's efficacy in schizophrenia. In their double-blind studies, Freedman et al. (1982) and van Kammen et al. (1989) reported an antipsychotic effect when using clonidine alone; in their open studies, Angrist et al. (1988) and Lechin and Van Der Dijs (1981) reported positive results when clonidine was used in combination with neuro-

Table 21–4. Studies of propranolol added to neuroleptic medication in treatment-refractory schizophrenic patients

Authors	N	Patient description	Study design	Results
Yorkston et al. (1977)	14	Chronic schizophrenic patients with florid symptoms despite neuroleptics (PSE)	Chlorpromazine + propranolol (< 500 mg/day), $n = 7$, versus chlorpromazine + placebo, $n = 7$, for 12 weeks	Significant improvement of global symptomatology (BPRS)
Bigelow et al. (1978)	7	Schizophrenic patients with long-term hospitalizations despite neuroleptics (RDC)	Crossover study: propranolol (< 1,920 mg/day) versus placebo for 4 weeks each	No significant effect (BPRS)
King et al. (1980)	5	Chronic schizophrenic inpatients with florid symptoms despite neuroleptics (Feighner)	Crossover study: propranolol (1 g/day) versus placebo for 3 weeks each	No effect (modified BPRS, WWBS)
Lindström and Persson (1980)	12	Chronic schizophrenic inpatients	Crossover study: propranolol (1 g/day) versus placebo for 2 weeks each	Significant improvement of global symptomatology and thought disturbance index (CPRS)
Myers et al. (1981)	20	Neuroleptic-refractory schizophrenic inpatients (Schneider)	Neuroleptic + propranolol (< 1,920 mg/day), $n = 10$, versus neuroleptic + placebo, $n = 10$, for 12 weeks	No effect (BPRS)
Pugh et al. (1983)	41	Schizophrenic inpatients with florid symptoms despite neuroleptics (Feighner)	Neuroleptic + propranolol (< 640 mg/day), $n = 21$, versus neuroleptic + placebo, $n = 20$, for 12 weeks	Improvement of NOSIE scores but not of BPRS scores

Note. Feighner = Feighner criteria (Feighner et al. 1972); PSE = Present State Examination (Wing et al. 1974); RDC = Research Diagnostic Criteria (Spitzer et al. 1978). **Psychometric tests:** BPRS = Brief Psychiatric Rating Scale (Overall and Gorham 1962); Modified BPRS = Modified Brief Psychiatric Rating Scale (Yorkston et al. 1974); CPRS = Comprehensive Psychopathological Rating Scale (Asberg et al. 1978); NOSIE = Nurses' Observation Scale for Inpatient Evaluation (Honigfeld et al. 1966); WWBS = Wing Ward Behavior Scale (Wing 1961).
Source. Adapted from Christison et al. 1991; Llorca and Wolf 1991.

leptics. However, patients' response to clonidine has also been improved with neuroleptics alone (Donaldson et al. 1983). Nevertheless, low dosages of clonidine are of benefit to some treatment-refractory schizophrenic patients.

Serotonergic Strategies

Results from clinical studies with serotonergic agents in schizophrenia have generally been inconsistent (Bleich et al. 1988). When fenfluramine, a nonselective antiserotonergic agent, was used in combination with neuroleptics in schizophrenic patients, it was found to be ineffective in most studies (Alphs et al. 1989; Marshall et al. 1989; Shore et al. 1985). However, in an open study, cyproheptadine, a nonspecific serotonergic antagonist with anticholinergic and antihistaminic properties, significantly improved negative symptoms in 10 neuroleptic-treated schizophrenic patients (Silver et al. 1989). In a double-blind study, Llorca et al. (1992) administered cyproheptadine to 24 treatment-refractory schizophrenic patients, noting a significant improvement in 7 patients.

At least 14 separate serotonergic (5-HT) receptors have been identified in the central nervous system; these are divided into 7 main families (5-HT_1 through 5-HT_7; Roth 1994). Selective serotonergic agents are being developed for the treatment of schizophrenia, and agents considered to be potentially active as novel antipsychotics are frequently evaluated on the basis of their 5-HT_2–D_2 receptor antagonist properties. However, other potential antipsychotic agents with 5-HT_1 agonist and 5-HT_3 antagonist properties are under investigation (Gerlach 1991).

5-HT_1 agonists.   Clinical trials with buspirone (a 5-HT_{1A} partial agonist) in schizophrenic patients treated with neuroleptics have yielded inconclusive findings (Brody et al. 1990; D'Mello et al. 1989; Goff et al. 1991). However, the potential value of 5-HT_1 agonists in the treatment of schizophrenia remains to be established.

5-HT_2 antagonists.   Several neuroleptics, such as thioridazine and clozapine, are potent 5-HT_2 receptor antagonists. The novel antipsychotic compound risperidone combines dopamine D_2 receptor blockade with potent 5-HT$_2$ antagonist effects. Although risperidone has been shown to significantly improve positive and negative symptoms of schizophrenia and elicits significantly fewer EPS than haloperidol or placebo (Borison et al. 1992a, 1992b; Chouinard et al. 1993; Gelders et al. 1989; Janssen et al. 1988), its efficacy in treatment-refractory schizophrenic patients is presently the object of a large Canadian multicenter clinical trial.

Ritanserin (a potent and selective 5-HT$_2$ receptor antagonist) has been reported to improve negative schizophrenic symptoms and to decrease the frequency of EPS (particularly tremors and akathisia) when used concomitantly with neuroleptics (Bersani et al. 1986; Borison et al. 1992a; Gerlach 1991; C. H. Miller et al. 1990, 1992).

5-HT$_3$ antagonists. The antipsychotic potential of 5-HT$_3$ antagonists such as ondansetron and ICS 205-930 in the treatment of schizophrenia remains to be established (De Veaugh-Geiss et al. 1992; Gerlach 1991). However, the clinical development of ondansetron as a novel antipsychotic agent has been discontinued, and it has since been marketed as an antiemetic primarily for chemotherapy-treated patients.

Peptidergic Strategies

Opiate agonists and antagonists. Both an excess and a decreased availability of circulating endorphins have been hypothesized to play a role in schizophrenia, and these alternative hypotheses have been tested in various clinical trials (De Wied et al. 1978; Jacquet and Marks 1976; Terenius et al. 1976). Following an initial report by Gunne et al. (1977), several investigators evaluated the efficacy of naloxone, an opiate receptor antagonist, in neuroleptic-treated schizophrenic patients. The outcomes of these trials have been inconsistent. However, its parenteral administration and brief duration of action render naloxone of little clinical interest. Naltrexone, a similar compound, has also been shown to be ineffective (Gitlin et al. 1981). Wolkowitz et al. (1990b) have noted the relative efficacy of nalmefene.

Although β-endorphins generally appear ineffective in the treatment of schizophrenia (Berger et al. 1986), clinical results with γ-endorphins have been variable (Verhoeven et al. 1979, 1982, 1986, 1987). Early clinical findings with methadone, an opiate receptor agonist, supported a potential antipsychotic effect (Brizer et al. 1985; Feinberg and Hartman 1991).

Cholecystokinin-related peptides.   The behavioral, electrophysiological, and biochemical characteristics of cholecystokinin (CCK)-related peptides are similar to those of neuroleptics (Hommer and Skirboll 1983; Lindenmayer 1992). Although some open clinical trials of these compounds were initially promising, investigators in most double-blind, controlled studies have reported negative results. This outcome may be a consequence of their difficulty in crossing the blood-brain barrier (Peselow et al. 1987).

Other peptides.   Thyrotropin-releasing hormone (TRH) may have a beneficial effect in schizophrenia, although its role in improving positive (Mizuki et al. 1986) and negative symptoms (Brambilla et al. 1986) is unclear. Vasopressin was first used in the treatment of schizophrenia prior to the introduction of neuroleptics (Forizs 1952). A related compound, desmopressin, has been reported to improve negative symptoms (Brambilla et al. 1986; Iager et al. 1986).

Other Strategies

Electroconvulsive therapy.   Electroconvulsive therapy (ECT) has been suggested to enhance the passage of neuroleptics across the blood-brain barrier (Gujavarty et al. 1987). Schizophrenia-spectrum disorders that are most likely to respond to ECT include catatonic schizophrenia, schizoaffective disorder, and rapid-onset schizophrenia (Christison et al. 1991). Meltzer (1992a) reviewed the efficacy of ECT in treatment-refractory schizophrenic patients and noted four uncontrolled studies in which ECT was reported to be effective in more than 50% of cases (Friedel 1986; Gujavarty et al. 1987; Meltzer 1992a; Milstein et al. 1990).

Calcium channel inhibitors. Neuroleptics of the diphenylbutyl-piperidine class exert a calcium channel–blocking effect that has been linked to their clinical efficacy in improving negative schizophrenic symptoms (Gould et al. 1983). This suggestion has prompted the use of several calcium channel inhibitors in the treatment of schizophrenia (Bartko et al. 1991; Reiter et al. 1989; Stedman et al. 1991). In a review of the literature, Llorca and Wolf (1991) noted one study with nifedipine and four of six studies with verapamil in which the results were negative. The vast majority of studies in which the efficacy of calcium channel inhibitors have been examined in schizophrenia have had small sample sizes and were held under uncontrolled conditions. With nifedipine, Stedman et al. (1991) reported a statistically but not clinically significant effect in 10 chronic schizophrenic patients. Using verapamil, Bartko et al. (1991) observed a significant improvement in positive, negative, and anxiety-depressive symptoms in 22 partially responsive, neuroleptic-treated schizophrenic patients. However, the evidence supporting the use of calcium channel inhibitors in schizophrenia is inconclusive.

N-methyl-D-aspartate agonists. Modulation of glutamatergic synaptic transmission in schizophrenia might be involved in producing an antipsychotic effect. Because the action of L-glutamate at its N-methyl-D-aspartate (NMDA) receptor site is antagonized by phencyclidine (PCP), a drug known to induce psychotic symptoms, it is possible that stimulation of NMDA receptors could be antipsychotic in schizophrenia (Javitt 1987; Tamminga et al. 1992). Glycine and its agonist milacemide have been tested in schizophrenic patients, with negative results so far (Gerlach 1991; Tamminga et al. 1992). Nevertheless, the hypothesis that the NMDA-PCP receptor complex may be involved in schizophrenia warrants further study.

Miscellaneous agents. Other potential agents whose efficacy remains to be established in the treatment of schizophrenia have included prostaglandin E_1 (Kaiya 1987) and antioxidant agents such as vitamins C and E (Beauclair et al. 1987; Shriqui and Jones 1990; Suboticanec et al. 1990).

Conclusion

Despite numerous studies, no specific agent used alone or in combination with neuroleptics has been demonstrated to be consistently effective in treatment-refractory schizophrenic patients. Benzodiazepines, lithium, carbamazepine, and antidepressant medication are the most commonly used adjunctive agents in this population. The actual value of many of these targeted research strategies remains to be established. As stated at the beginning of this chapter, research in this area is fraught with methodological constraints.

Before we conclude, we wish to emphasize the importance of rendering psychosocial treatment interventions accessible to severely ill schizophrenic patients. Because of their illness severity or long-term inpatient status, these patients can be prematurely excluded from such therapeutic approaches.

References

Abrams R, Taylor MA: A rating scale for emotional blunting. Am J Psychiatry 135:226–229, 1978

Addonizio G, Susman VL: Neuroleptic Malignant Syndrome: A Clinical Approach. St. Louis, MO, Mosby-Year Book, 1991

Alphs LD, Lafferman JA, Ross L, et al: Fenfluramine treatment of negative symptoms in older schizophrenic inpatients. Psychopharmacol Bull 24:149–153, 1989

Altamura AC: A multidimensional (pharmacokinetic and clinical-biological) approach to neuroleptic response in schizophrenia, with particular reference to drug resistance. Schizophr Res 8:187–198, 1992

Altamura AC, Mauri MC, Mantero MM, et al: Clonazepam-haloperidol combination therapy in schizophrenia: a double-blind study. Acta Psychiatr Scand 76:702–706, 1987

American Psychiatric Association: Diagnostic and Statistical Manual of Mental Disorders, 3rd Edition. Washington, DC, American Psychiatric Association, 1980

American Psychiatric Association: Diagnostic and Statistical Manual of Mental Disorders, 3rd Edition, Revised. Washington, DC, American Psychiatric Association, 1987

American Psychiatric Association: Diagnostic and Statistical Manual of Mental Disorders, 4th Edition. Washington, DC, American Psychiatric Association, 1994

Andreasen NC: The Scale for the Assessment of Negative Symptoms (SANS). Iowa City, IA, University of Iowa, 1983

Angrist BM, Smith M, Adler L, et al: Preliminary studies of clonidine in psychotic patients. J Neural Transm 71:115–121, 1988

Asberg M, Montgomery SA, Perris C, et al: A comprehensive psychopathological rating scale. Acta Psychiatr Scand Suppl 271:1–62, 1978

Atre-Vaidya N, Taylor MA: Effectiveness of lithium in schizophrenia: do we really have an answer? J Clin Psychiatry 50:170–173, 1989

Ayd FJ: A survey of drug-induced extrapyramidal reactions. JAMA 175:1054, 1961

Bacher NM, Lewis HA: Addition of reserpine to antipsychotic medication in refractory chronic schizophrenic outpatients. Am J Psychiatry 135:488–489, 1978

Bacher NM, Lewis HA: Long-term reserpine use in selected refractory outpatients (letter). Am J Psychiatry 142:386–387, 1985

Barbee JG, Mancuso DM, Freed CR, et al: Alprazolam as a neuroleptic adjunct in the emergency treatment of schizophrenia. Am J Psychiatry 149:506–510, 1992

Barsa JA, Kline NS: Combined reserpine-chlorpromazine in treatment of disturbed psychotics. AMA Archives of Neurology and Psychiatry 74:280–286, 1955

Barsa JA, Kline NS: A comparative study of reserpine, chlorpromazine in treatment of disturbed psychotics. AMA Archives of Neurology and Psychiatry 76:90–97, 1956

Bartko G, Horvath S, Zador G, et al: Effects of adjunctive verapamil administration in chronic schizophrenic patients. Prog Neuropsychopharmacol Biol Psychiatry 15:343–349, 1991

Beauclair L, Vinogradov S, Riney SJ, et al: An adjunctive role for ascorbic acid in the treatment of schizophrenia? J Clin Psychopharmacol 7:282–283, 1987

Beigel A, Murphy DL, Bunney WE Jr: The Manic-State Rating Scale. Arch Gen Psychiatry 25:256–262, 1971

Berger PA, Watson SJ, Akil H, et al: Investigating opioid peptides in schizophrenia and depression, in Neuropeptides in Schizophrenia and Depression. Edited by Martin JB, Barchos JD. New York, Raven, 1986, pp 309–333

Berlant JL: Neuroleptics and reserpine in refractory psychoses. J Clin Psychopharmacol 6:180–184, 1986

Berlant JL: One more look at propranolol for the treatment of refractory schizophrenia. Schizophr Bull 13:705–714, 1987

Berlant JL: Presynaptic modulators of dopamine synthesis in the treatment of chronic schizophrenia, in The Neuroleptic Nonresponsive Patient: Characterization and Treatment. Edited by Angrist BM, Schulz SC. Washington, DC, American Psychiatric Press, 1990, pp 139–152

Bersani G, Grispini A, Marini S, et al: Neuroleptic-induced extrapyramidal side-effects: clinical perspectives with ritanserin (R 55667), a new selective 5-HT$_2$ receptor blocking agent. Current Therapeutic Research 40:492–499, 1986

Bigelow LB, Zalcman S, Kleinman J, et al: Propranolol treatment of chronic schizophrenia: clinical response, catecholamine metabolism and lymphocyte beta-receptors, in Catecholamines: Basic and Clinical Frontiers. Edited by Usdin E, Kapin I, Barchas J. New York, Pergamon, 1978, pp 1851–1853

Bleich A, Brown SL, Van Praag HM: The role of serotonin in schizophrenia. Schizophr Bull 14:297–315, 1988

Borison RL, Sinha D, Haverstock S, et al: Efficacy and safety of tiospirone vs haloperidol and thioridazine in a double-blind placebo-controlled trial. Psychopharmacol Bull 25:190–193, 1989

Borison RL, Diamond BI, Pathiraja AP, et al: Clinical overview of risperidone, in Novel Antipsychotic Drugs. Edited by Meltzer HY. New York, Raven, 1992a, pp 233–239

Borison RL, Pathiraja AP, Diamond BI, et al: Risperidone: clinical safety and efficacy in schizophrenia. Psychopharmacol Bull 28:213–218, 1992b

Braden W, Fink EB, Qualls CB, et al: Lithium and chlorpromazine in psychotic inpatients. Psychiatry Res 7:69–81, 1982

Brambilla F, Scarone S, Pugnetti L, et al: Bromocriptine therapy in chronic schizophrenia: effects on symptomatology, sleep patterns and prolactin response to stimulation. Psychiatry Res 8:159–169, 1983

Brambilla F, Aguglia E, Massironi R, et al: Neuropeptide therapies in chronic schizophrenia: TRH and vasopressin administration. Neuropsychobiology 15:114–121, 1986

Brenner HD, Dencker SJ, Goldstein MJ, et al: Defining treatment refractoriness in schizophrenia. Schizophr Bull 16:551–561, 1990

Brizer DA, Hartman N, Sweeny J, et al: Effect of methadone plus neuroleptics on treatment resistant chronic paranoid schizophrenia. Am J Psychiatry 142:1106–1107, 1985

Brody D, Adler LA, Kim T, et al: Effects of buspirone in seven schizophrenic subjects (letter). J Clin Psychopharmacol 10:68–69, 1990

Bucci L: The negative symptoms of schizophrenia and the monoamine oxidase inhibitors. Psychopharmacology (Berl) 91:104–108, 1987

Bunney WE Jr, Hamburg DS: Methods for reliable longitudinal observation of behavior. Arch Gen Psychiatry 9:280–294, 1963

Carman JS, Bigelow LB, Wyatt RJ: Lithium combined with neuroleptics in chronic schizophrenic and schizoaffective patients. J Clin Psychiatry 42:124–128, 1981

Chiaroni P, Azorin JM, Evrin C, et al: Intérêt de la fluoxétine dans le traitement des psychoses schizophréniques. L'information Psychiatrique 67:449–454, 1991

Chouinard G, Sultan S: Treatment of supersensitivity psychosis with antiepileptic drugs: report of a series of 43 cases. Psychopharmacol Bull 26:337–341, 1990

Chouinard G, Jones B, Remington G, et al: A Canadian multicenter placebo-controlled study of fixed doses of risperidone and haloperidol in the treatment of chronic schizophrenic patients. J Clin Psychopharmacology 13:25–40, 1993

Christison GW, Kirch DG, Wyatt RJ: When symptoms persist: choosing among alternative somatic treatments for schizophrenia. Schizophr Bull 17:217–245, 1991

Cohen WJ, Cohen NH: Lithium carbonate, haloperidol and irreversible brain damage. JAMA 230:1283–1287, 1974

Collins PJ, Larkin EP, Shubsachs APW: Lithium carbonate in chronic schizophrenia: a brief trial of lithium carbonate added to neuroleptics for treatment of resistant schizophrenic patients. Acta Psychiatr Scand 84:150–154, 1991

Csernansky JG, Riney SJ, Lombrozo L, et al: Double-blind comparison of alprazolam, diazepam and placebo for the treatment of negative schizophrenic symptoms. Arch Gen Psychiatry 45:655–659, 1988

Cutler NR, Jeste DV, Kaufmann CA, et al: Low dose bromocriptine: a study of acute effects in chronic medicated schizophrenics. Prog Neuropsychopharmacol Biol Psychiatry 8:277–283, 1984

Davis JM: Overview: maintenance therapy in psychiatry, I: schizophrenia. Am J Psychiatry 132:1237–1245, 1975

Davis JM: Recent developments in the drug treatment of schizophrenia. Am J Psychiatry 133:208–214, 1976

Davis JM, Schaffer CB, Killian GA, et al: Important issues in the drug treatment of schizophrenia. Schizophr Bull 6:70–87, 1980

De Veaugh-Geiss J, McBain S, Cooksey P, et al: The effects of a novel 5-HT$_3$ antagonist, ondansetron, in schizophrenia, in Novel Antipsychotic Drugs. Edited by Meltzer HY. New York, Raven, 1992, pp 225–232

De Wied D, Kovacs GL, Bohus B, et al: Neuroleptic activity of the neuropeptide beta-LPH 62-77. Eur J Pharmacol 49:427–436, 1978

Dixon L, Weiden PJ, Frances AJ, et al: Alprazolam intolerance in stable schizophrenic outpatients. Psychopharmacol Bull 25:213–214, 1989

D'Mello DA, McNeil JA, Harris W: Buspirone suppression of neuroleptic-induced akathisia: multiple case reports (letter). J Clin Psychopharmacol 9:151–152, 1989

Donaldson SR, Gelenberg AJ, Baldessarini RJ: The pharmacologic treatment of schizophrenia: a progress report. Schizophr Bull 9:504–527, 1983

Dumon JP, Catteau J, Lanvin F, et al: Randomized, double-blind, crossover, placebo-controlled comparison of propranolol and betaxolol in the treatment of neuroleptic-induced akathisia. Am J Psychiatry 149:647–650, 1992

Ecclestone D, Fairbairn AF, Hassanye HF, et al: The effect of propranolol and thioridazine on positive and negative symptoms of schizophrenia. Br J Psychiatry 147:623–630, 1985

Feighner JP, Robins E, Guze SB, et al: Diagnostic criteria for use in psychiatric research. Arch Gen Psychiatry 26:57–63, 1972

Feinberg DT, Hartman N: Methadone and schizophrenia (letter). Am J Psychiatry 148:1750–1751, 1991

Fisk GC, York SM: The effect of sodium valproate on tardive dyskinesia. Br J Psychiatry 150:542–546, 1987

Folstein MF, Folstein SE, McHugh PR: Mini-Mental State: a practical method for grading the cognitive state of patients for the clinician. J Psichiatr Res 12:189–198, 1975

Forizs L: The use of pitressin in the treatment of schizophrenia with deterioration. N C Med J 12:76–80, 1952

Freedman R, Kirch D, Bell J, et al: Clonidine treatment of schizophrenia. Acta Psychiatr Scand 65:35–45, 1982

Friedel RO: The combined use of neuroleptics and ECT in drug-resistant schizophrenic patients. Psychopharmacol Bull 22:928–930, 1986

Garbutt JC, van Kammen D: The interaction between GABA and dopamine: implications for schizophrenia. Schizophr Bull 9:336–353, 1983

Gattaz WF, Kollisch M: Bromocriptine in the treatment of neuroleptic-resistant schizophrenia. Biol Psychiatry 21:519–521, 1986

Gattaz WF, Rost W, VK Hübner C, et al: Acute and subchronic effects of low-dose bromocriptine in haloperidol treated schizophrenics. Biol Psychiatry 25:247–255, 1989

Gelder M, Kolakowska T: Variability of response to neuroleptics in schizophrenia: clinical, pharmacologic and neuroendocrine correlates. Compr Psychiatry 20:397–408, 1979

Gelders Y, Heylen S, Vanden Busche G, et al: Serotonin 5-HT$_2$ receptor antagonism in the treatment of schizophrenia. Abstracts, VIII World Congress of Psychiatry, International Congress Series 899. Amsterdam, Netherlands, Excerpta Medica, 1989

Gerlach J: New antipsychotics: classification, efficacy and adverse effects. Schizophr Bull 17:289–309, 1991

Gerlach J, Luhdorf K: The effect of L-dopa in young patients with simple schizophrenia, treated with neuroleptic drugs. Psychopharmacology (Berl) 44:105–110, 1975

Gitlin MJ, Gerner RH, Rosenblatt M: Assessment of naltrexone in the treatment of schizophrenia. Psychopharmacology (Berl) 74:51–53, 1981

Goff DC, Brotman AW, Waites M, et al: Trial of fluoxetine added to neuroleptics for treatment-resistant schizophrenic patients. Am J Psychiatry 147:492–494, 1990

Goff DC, Midha KK, Brotman AW, et al: An open trial of buspirone added to neuroleptics in schizophrenic patients. J Clin Psychopharmacol 11:193–197, 1991

Gould RJ, Murphy KMM, Reynolds IJ, et al: Antischizophrenic drugs of the diphenylbutylpiperidine type act as calcium channel antagonists. Proc Natl Acad Sci U S A 80:5122–5125, 1983

Growe GA, Crayton JW, Klass DB, et al: Lithium in chronic schizophrenia. Am J Psychiatry 136:454–455, 1979

Gujavarty K, Greenberg LB, Fink M: Electroconvulsive therapy and neuroleptic medication in therapy-resistant positive-symptom psychosis. Convulsive Therapy 3:185–195, 1987

Gunne LM, Lindström L, Terenius L: Naloxone-induced reversal of schizophrenic hallucinations. J Neural Transm 40:13–19, 1977

Guy W (ed): ECDEU Assessment Manual for Psychopharmacology, Revised (DHEW Publ No ADM 76-388). Rockville, MD, U.S. Department of Health, Education and Welfare, 1976

Herrera JM, Sramek JJ, Costa JF: Efficacy of adjunctive carbamazepine in the treatment of chronic schizophrenia. Drug Intelligence and Clinical Pharmacy 21:355–358, 1987

Hommer D, Skirboll L: Cholecystokinin-like peptides potentiate apomorphine-induced inhibition of dopamine neurons. Eur J Pharmacol 91:151–152, 1983

Honigfeld G, Roderic D, Klett JC: NOSIE-30: a treatment sensitive ward behavior scale. Psychol Rep 19:180–182, 1966

Iager AC, Kirch DG, Bigelow LB, et al: Treatment of schizophrenia with a vasopressin analogue. Am J Psychiatry 143:375–377, 1986

Inanaga K, Nakano T, Nagata T, et al: Double-blind controlled study of L-dopa therapy in schizophrenia. Folia Psychiatrica et Neurologica Japonica 29:123–143, 1975

Jacquet YF, Marks N: The C-fragment of beta-lipotropin: an endogenous neuroleptic or antipsychotogen. Science 194:632–636, 1976

Janssen PAJ, Niemegeers CJE, Awouters F, et al: Pharmacology of risperidone (R64-766): a new antipsychotic with serotonin-S_2 and dopamine D_2 antagonistic properties. J Pharmacol Exp Ther 244:685–693, 1988

Javitt DC: Negative symptomatology and the PCP (phencyclidine) model of schizophrenia. Hillside Journal of Clinical Psychiatry 9:12–35, 1987

Jimerson DC, van Kammen DP, Post RM, et al: Diazepam in schizophrenia: a preliminary double-blind trial. Am J Psychiatry 139:489–491, 1982

Kaiya H: Prostaglandin E₁ treatment of schizophrenia. J Clin Psychopharmacol 7:357–358, 1987.

Kane JM, Lieberman JA: Maintenance pharmacotherapy in schizophrenia, in Psychopharmacology: The Third Generation of Progress. Edited by Meltzer HY. New York, Raven, 1987, pp 1103–1109

Kane J, Honigfeld G, Singer J, et al: Clozapine for the treatment-resistant schizophrenic. Arch Gen Psychiatry 45:789–796, 1988

Kane JM, Jeste DV, Barnes TRE, et al: Tardive Dyskinesia: A Task Force Report of the American Psychiatric Association. Washington, DC, American Psychiatric Association, 1992

Karson CN, Weinberger DR, Bigelow L, et al: Clonazepam treatment of chronic schizophrenia: negative results in a double-blind, placebo controlled trial. Am J Psychiatry 139:1627–1628, 1982

Kay SR, Opler LA: L-dopa in the treatment of negative schizophrenic symptoms: a single-subject experimental study. Int J Psychiatry Med 15:293–298, 1985

Kellner R, Wilson RM, Muldawer MD: Anxiety in schizophrenia: the response to chlordiazepoxide in an intensive design study. Arch Gen Psychiatry 32:1246–1254, 1979

Kidron R, Averbuch I, Klein E, et al: Carbamazepine induced reduction of blood levels of haloperidol in chronic schizophrenia. Biol Psychiatry 20:219–222, 1985

King DJ, Turkson SNA, Liddle J, et al: Some clinical and metabolic aspects of propranolol in chronic schizophrenia. Br J Psychiatry 137:458–468, 1980

Ko G, Korpi E, Freed W, et al: Effect of valproic acid on behavior and plasma amino acid concentrations in chronic schizophrenic patients. Biol Psychiatry 20:199–228, 1985

Kramer MS, Vogel WH, DiJohnson C, et al: Antidepressants in "depressed" schizophrenic inpatients. Arch Gen Psychiatry 46:922–928, 1989

Krawiecka M, Goldberg D, Vaughan M: A standardized psychiatric assessment scale for rating chronic psychotic patients. Acta Psychiatr Scand 55:299–308, 1977

Lader MH: Beta-adrenoreceptor antagonists in neuropsychiatry: an update. J Clin Psychiatry 49:213–223, 1988

Lechin F, Van Der Dijs B: Clonidine therapy for psychosis and tardive dyskinesia. Am J Psychiatry 138:390, 1981

Lindenmayer JP: Pharmacological strategies for the neuroleptic nonresponder, in New Biological Vistas on Schizophrenia. Edited by Lindenmayer JP, Kay SR. New York, Brunner/Mazel, 1992, pp 241–258

Lindström LH, Persson E: Propranolol in chronic schizophrenia: a controlled study in neuroleptic treated patients. Br J Psychiatry 137:126–130, 1980

Lingjaerde O: Effect of the benzodiazepine derivative estazolam in patients with auditory hallucinations: a multi-centre double-blind, crossover study. Acta Psychiatr Scand 65:339–354, 1982

Lingjaerde O: Benzodiazepines in the treatment of schizophrenia: an updated survey. Acta Psychiatr Scand 84:453–459, 1991

Lingjaerde O, Engstrand E, Ellingsen P, et al: Antipsychotic effect of diazepam when given in addition to neuroleptics in chronic psychotic patients: a double-blind clinical trial. Current Therapeutic Research 26:505–514, 1979

Little JD, Taghavi EH: Disinhibition after lorazepam augmentation of antipsychotic medication (letter). Am J Psychiatry 148:109, 1991

Llorca PM, Wolf MA: Utilisation de certaines médications cardiologiques dans le traitement de la schizophrénie: revue de la littérature. J Psychiatry Neurosci 16:19–24, 1991

Llorca PM, Wolf MA, Estorges JP: The use of benzodiazepines in schizophrenia: a review. European Psychiatry 6:217–222, 1991

Llorca PM, Bougerol T, Wolf MA, et al: Bromocriptine, cyproheptadine and carbamazepine in combination to neuroleptics in chronic schizophrenia. Clin Neuropharmacol 15 (suppl 1, part B):227B, 1992

Lorr M, Vestre ND: The Psychotic Inpatient Profile Manual. Los Angeles, CA, Western Psychological Services, 1968

Losonczy M, Song IS, Mohs RC, et al: Correlates of lateral ventricular size in chronic schizophrenia, I: behavioral and treatment response measures. Am J Psychiatry 143:976–981, 1986

Marshall BD, Glynn SM, Midha KK, et al: Adverse effects of fenfluramine in treatment refractory schizophrenia. J Clin Psychopharmacol 9:110–115, 1989

McElroy SL, Keck PE, Pope HG, et al: Valproate in psychiatric disorders: literature review and clinical guidelines. J Clin Psychiatry 50:23–29, 1989

Meltzer HY: Commentary: defining treatment refractoriness in schizophrenia. Schizophr Bull 16:563–565, 1990

Meltzer HY: Treatment of the neuroleptic-nonresponsive schizophrenic patient. Schizophr Bull 18:515–542, 1992a

Meltzer HY: Clozapine: pattern of efficacy in treatment-resistant schizophrenia, in Novel Antipsychotic Drugs. Edited by Meltzer HY. New York, Raven, 1992b, pp 33–46

Meltzer HY, Kolokowska T, Robertson A, et al: Effect of low-dose bromocriptine in treatment of psychosis: the dopamine autoreceptor stimulation strategy. Psychopharmacology (Berl) 81:37–41, 1983

Miller CH, Fleischhacker WW, Ehrmann H, et al: Treatment of neuroleptic induced akathisia with the 5-HT₂ antagonist ritanserin. Psychopharmacol Bull 26:373–376, 1990

Miller CH, Hammer M, Pycha R, et al: The effect of ritanserin on treatment-resistant neuroleptic induced akathisia: case reports. Prog Neuropsychopharmacol Biol Psychiatry 16:247–251, 1992

Miller F, Menninger J: Lithium-neuroleptic neurotoxicity is dose dependent. J Clin Psychopharmacol 7:89–91, 1987

Milstein V, Small JG, Miller MJ, et al: Mechanisms of action of ECT: schizophrenia and schizoaffective disorder. Biol Psychiatry 27:1282–1292, 1990

Mizuki Y, Ushisima I, Yamada M, et al: A treatment trial with an analog of thyrotropin releasing hormone (DN-1417) and Des-tyrosine-gamma-endorphin in schizophrenia. Int Clin Psychopharmacol 1:303–313, 1986

Mizuki Y, Kajimura N, Kai S, et al: Effects of mianserin in chronic schizophrenia. Prog Neuropsychopharmacol Biol Psychiatry 16:517–528, 1992

Moore NC, Meyendorff E, Yeragani V, et al: Tiaspirone in schizophrenia. J Clin Psychopharmacol 7:98–101, 1987

Myers DH, Campbell PL, Cocks NM, et al: A trial of propranolol in chronic schizophrenia. Br J Psychiatry 139:118–121, 1981

Nasrallah HA, Risch SC, Fowler RC: Reserpine, serotonin and schizophrenia. Am J Psychiatry 136:856–857, 1979

Neppe VM: Carbamazepine as adjunctive treatment in nonepileptic chronic inpatients with EEG temporal lobe abnormalities. J Clin Psychiatry 44:326–331, 1983

Neppe VM: Carbamazepine in nonresponsive psychosis. J Clin Psychiatry 49 (suppl 4):22–28, 1988

Nestoros JN: Benzodiazepines in schizophrenia: a need for reassessment. International Pharmacopsychiatry 15:171–179, 1980

Nestoros J, Suranyi-Cadotte B, Spees RC, et al: Diazepam in high doses is effective in schizophrenia. Prog Neuropsychopharmacol Biol Psychiatry 6:513–516, 1982

Okuma T, Yamashita J, Takahashi R, et al: Clinical efficacy of carbamazepine in affective and schizophrenic disorders. Pharmacopsychiatry 22:47–53, 1989

Overall JE, Gorham DR: The brief psychiatric rating scale. Psychol Rep 10:799–812, 1962

Pato CN, Wolkowitz OM, Rapaport M, et al: Benzodiazepine augmentation of neuroleptic treatment in patients with schizophrenia. Psychopharmacol Bull 25:263–266, 1989

Peet M, Bethell MS, Coates A, et al: Propranolol in schizophrenia, I: comparison of propranolol, chlorpromazine and placebo. Br J Psychiatry 139:105–111, 1981

Peselow E, Angrist BM, Sudilovsky A, et al: Double-blind controlled trials of cholecystokinin octapeptide in neuroleptic-refractory schizophrenia. Psychopharmacology (Berl) 91:80–84, 1987

Pope HG Jr, Keck PE Jr, McElroy SL: Frequency and presentation of neuroleptic malignant syndrome in a large psychiatric hospital. Am J Psychiatry 143:1227–1233, 1986

Pugh CR, Steinert J, Priest RG: Propranolol in schizophrenia: a double-blind, placebo-controlled trial of propranolol as an adjunct to neuroleptic medication. Br J Psychiatry 143:151–155, 1983

Raptis C, Garcia-Borreguero D, Weber M, et al: Anticonvulsants as adjuncts for the neuroleptic treatment of schizophrenic psychoses: a clinical study with beclamide. Acta Psychiatr Scand 81:162–167, 1989

Reiter S, Adler L, Angrist BM, et al: Effects of verapamil on tardive dyskinesia and psychosis in schizophrenic patients. J Clin Psychiatry 50:26–27, 1989

Rifkin A, Siris S: Drug treatment of acute schizophrenia, in Psychopharmacology: The Third Generation of Progress. Edited by Meltzer HY. New York, Raven, 1987, pp 1095–1101

Roth BL: Multiple serotonin receptors: clinical and experimental aspects. Annals of Clinical Psychiatry 6:67–78, 1994

Ruskin P, Averbuch I, Belmaker RH: Benzodiazepines in chronic schizophrenia. Biol Psychiatry 14:557–558, 1979

Schulz SC, Kahn EM, Baker RW, et al: Lithium and carbamazepine augmentation in treatment-refractory schizophrenia, in The Neuroleptic Nonresponsive Patient: Characterization and Treatment. Edited by Angrist BM, Schulz SC. Washington, DC, American Psychiatric Press, 1990, pp 111–136

Shore D, Korpi ER, Bigelow LB, et al: Fenfluramine and chronic schizophrenia. Biol Psychiatry 20:329–352, 1985

Shriqui CL: Dyskinésie tardive: mise à jour. Can J Psychiatry 33:637–644, 1988

Shriqui C, Jones B: Free radical involvement in schizophrenia and tardive dyskinesia. Schizophr Res 3:81, 1990

Silver H, Nassar A: Fluvoxamine improves negative symptoms in chronic schizophrenia: an add-on double-blind, placebo-controlled study. Biol Psychiatry 31:698–704, 1992

Silver H, Blacker M, Weller MPJ, et al: Treatment of chronic schizophrenia with cyproheptadine. Biol Psychiatry 25:502–504, 1989

Siris SG, van Kammen DP, Docherty MD: Use of antidepressant drugs in schizophrenia. Arch Gen Psychiatry 35:1368–1377, 1978

Siris SG, Morgan V, Fagerstrom R, et al: Adjunctive imipramine in the treatment of post-psychotic depression. Arch Gen Psychiatry 42:533–539, 1987

Siris SG, Adan F, Cohen M, et al: Post-psychotic depression and negative symptoms: an investigation of syndromal overlap. Am J Psychiatry 145:1532–1537, 1988

Siris SG, Adan F, Strahan A, et al: A comparison of six- and nine-week trials of adjunctive imipramine in post-psychotic depression. Compr Psychiatry 30:483–489, 1989a

Siris SG, Cutler J, Owen K, et al: Adjunctive imipramine maintenance treatment in schizophrenic patients with remitted post-psychotic depression. Am J Psychiatry 146:1495–1497, 1989b

Siris SG, Mason SE, Bermanzohn PC, et al: Adjunctive imipramine maintenance in post-psychotic depression/negative symptoms. Psychopharmacol Bull 26:91–94, 1990

Siris SG, Bermanzohn PC, Gonzalez A, et al: The use of antidepressants for negative symptoms in a subset of schizophrenic patients. Psychopharmacol Bull 27:331–335, 1991

Small JG, Kellams JJ, Milstein V, et al: A placebo-controlled study of lithium combined with neuroleptics in chronic schizophrenic patients. Am J Psychiatry 132:1315–1317, 1975

Smith GN, MacEwan GW, Ancill RJ, et al: Diagnostic confusion in treatment-refractory psychotic patients. J Clin Psychiatry 53:197–200, 1992

Spitzer RL, Endicott J, Robins E: Research diagnostic criteria: rationale and reliability. Arch Gen Psychiatry 35:773–782, 1978

Stedman TJ, Whiteford HA, Eyles D, et al: Effects of nifedipine on psychosis and tardive dyskinesia in schizophrenic patients. J Clin Psychopharmacol 11:43–47, 1991

Strauss JS, Gift TE: Choosing an approach for diagnosing schizophrenia. Arch Gen Psychiatry 34:1248–1253, 1977

Suboticanec K, Folnegovic-Smalc V, Korbar M, et al: Vitamin C status in chronic schizophrenia. Biol Psychiatry 28:959–966, 1990

Susman VL, Addonizio G: Recurrence of neuroleptic malignant syndrome. J Nerv Ment Dis 186:234–240, 1988

Takahashi R, Itho K, Itho H, et al: Comparison of efficacy of lithium carbonate and chlorpromazine in mania by double-blind controlled study. Arch Gen Psychiatry 32:1310–1318, 1975

Tamminga CA, Cascella N, Fakouhi TD, et al: Enhancement of NMDA-mediated transmission in schizophrenia, in Novel Antipsychotic Drugs. Edited by Meltzer HY. New York, Raven, 1992, pp 171–177

Terenius L, Wahlstrom A, Lindström L, et al: Increased CSF levels of endorphins in chronic psychosis. Neurosci Lett 3:157–162, 1976 van Kammen DP, Peters JL, van Kammen WB, et al: Clonidine treatment of schizophrenia: can we predict treatment response? Psychiatry Res 27:297–311, 1989

Van Valkenburg C, Kluznik J, Merrill R, et al: Therapeutic levels of valproate for psychosis. Psychopharmacol Bull 26:254–255, 1990

Verhoeven WMA, Van Praag HM, Van Ree JM, et al: Improvement of schizophrenic patients treated with des-tyr-gamma-endorphin (DT-gamma-E). Arch Gen Psychiatry 36:294–298, 1979

Verhoeven WMA, Van Ree JM, Heezius-Van Bentum A, et al: Antipsychotic properties of des-enkephalin-gamma-endorphin in treatment of schizophrenic patients. Arch Gen Psychiatry 39:648–654, 1982

Verhoeven WMA, Westenberg HGM, Van Ree JM: A comparative study on the antipsychotic properties of desenkephalin-gamma-endorphins and ceruletide in schizophrenic patients. Acta Psychiatr Scand 37:372–382, 1986

Verhoeven WMA, Van Ree JM, De Wied D: Peptides de type neuroleptique dans la schizophrénie, in Manuel de Psychiatrie Biologique. Edited by Mendlewicz J. Paris, Masson, 1987, pp 210–228

Volk W, Bier W, Braun JP, et al: Behandlung von erregten psychosen mit einem beta-receptoren-blocker (oxprenolol) in hoher dosierung. Nervenarzt 43:491–492, 1972

Wassef A, Watson DJ, Morrisson P, et al: Neuroleptic-valproic acid combination in treatment of psychotic symptoms: a three cases report. J Clin Psychopharmacol 9:45–48, 1989

Wing JK: A simple and reliable subclassification of chronic schizophrenia. Journal of Mental Science 107:862–865, 1961

Wing JK, Cooper JE, Sartorius N: The Description and Classification of Psychiatric Symptoms: An Instruction Manual for the PSE and CATEGO System. Cambridge, UK, Cambridge University Press, 1974

Wolf MA, Diener JM, Lajeunesse C, et al: Low-dose bromocriptine in neuroleptic-resistant schizophrenia: a pilot study. Biol Psychiatry 31:1166–1168, 1992a

Wolf MA, Diener JM, Lajeunesse C, et al: Utilisation des faibles posologies de bromocriptine dans la schizophrénie chronique résistante aux neuroleptiques: une étude préliminaire. J Psychiatry Neurosci 17:68–71, 1992b

Wolkowitz OM, Pickar D: Benzodiazepines in the treatment of schizophrenia: a review and reappraisal. Am J Psychiatry 148:714–726, 1991

Wolkowitz OM, Pickar D, Doran AR, et al: Combination alprazolam-neuroleptic treatment of the positive and negative symptoms of schizophrenia. Am J Psychiatry 143:85–87, 1986

Wolkowitz OM, Breier A, Doran AR, et al: Alprazolam augmentation of the antipsychotic effects of fluphenazine in schizophrenic patients. Arch Gen Psychiatry 45:664–671, 1988

Wolkowitz OM, Bartko JJ, Pickar D: Drug trials and heterogeneity in schizophrenia: the mean is not the end. Biol Psychiatry 28:1021–1025, 1990a

Wolkowitz OM, Rapaport MH, Pickar D: Benzodiazepine augmentation of neuroleptics, in The Neuroleptic Nonresponsive Patient: Characterization and Treatment. Edited by Angrist BM, Schulz SC. Washington, DC, American Psychiatric Press, 1990b, pp 89–108

Yorkston NJ, Zaki SA, Malik MKU, et al: Propranolol in the control of schizophrenic symptoms. BMJ 4:633–635, 1974

Yorkston NJ, Zaki SA, Pitcher DR, et al: Propranolol as an adjunct to the treatment of schizophrenia. Lancet 2:575–578, 1977

SECTION IV

Neuroleptic-Induced Side Effects

CHAPTER 22

Acute Extrapyramidal Syndromes

Daniel E. Casey, M.D.

N euroleptic (antipsychotic) drugs are the mainstay of treatment for both acute and chronic psychoses. After being introduced in the 1950s, these agents were labeled *neuroleptics* to incorporate the concept of "taking control of the neuron." The underlying belief was that neuroleptic drugs produced both antipsychotic and motor side effects at approximately the same dosage (Delay et al. 1952; Deniker 1984), a level that was conceptualized as the *neuroleptic threshold*. Originally, it was believed that the effects on thinking and motor function were inextricably linked. However, subsequent research has shown that these drug actions are distinct and potentially separable. Unfortunately, the majority of patients (approximately 75%) (Casey and Keepers 1988; Keepers et al. 1983) experience acute extrapyramidal syndromes (EPS) at a neuroleptic dosage that also produces antipsychotic benefits.

In this chapter, I review current knowledge about acute EPS. It is

This work was supported by the DANICAS Foundation. The typescript was prepared by Crystal Berger.

important to consider each acute extrapyramidal syndrome as a separate entity because each has a different time course and treatment strategy, and each may be misdiagnosed as a psychiatric symptom. I also review the relative contributions of patient, drug, and temporal variables to the syndrome. Finally, I discuss an algorithm of strategies for clinically managing acute EPS.

Clinical Manifestations

Clinical manifestations of EPS are summarized in Table 22–1.

Akathisia.   Akathisia is a subjective feeling of restlessness. Although the original definition of akathisia was limited to the patient's subjective experience, many patients also demonstrate motor signs of this syndrome, such as shifting their weight from foot to foot while standing, or crossing and uncrossing their legs while sitting. Thus, there is some controversy over the issue of whether patients with typical motor signs of akathisia but no subjective complaints should be diagnosed as having akathisia or pseudoakathisia (Adler et al. 1989; Barnes and Braude 1985). Patients often described their subjective experience by using adjectives such as anxious, jittery, internally restless, antsy, and so on. Some psychotic patients are not able to describe accurately the feelings of akathisia and may use colorful or peculiar thought-disordered language to express their discomfort. It is important to distinguish neuroleptic-induced akathisia from the agitation that is intrinsically associated with psychoses. The treatment of the latter might lead the clinician to increase the neuroleptic dosage, which would only further aggravate the akathisia (Casey 1991a).

Neuroleptic-induced dystonia.   Neuroleptic-induced dystonia is characterized by briefly sustained or fixed abnormal postures that arise from involuntary muscular contractions. Symptoms of torticollis, trismus, oculogyric crises, laryngeal-pharyngeal constriction, tongue protrusion or thickness, and bizarre positions of the limbs and trunk can all be symptoms of neuroleptic-induced dystonia. These symptoms are sometimes diagnosed as malingering, hysterical conversion reactions,

Table 22–1. Acute extrapyramidal syndromes (EPS) and tardive dyskinesia (TD)

Syndrome	Symptoms	Distinguish from psychiatric symptoms	Period of symptom onset (days)	Treatment
Acute EPS				
Acute dystonia	Briefly sustained or fixed abnormal postures of the limbs, trunk, neck, face, eyes, or tongue	Manipulation, hysteria, seizures, catatonia	1–5	Benztropine (1–2 mg) or diphenhydramine (25–50 mg) im or iv are diagnostic and curative
Parkinsonism	Tremor, rigidity, bradykinesia (akinesia), mask face, decreased arm swing	Depression, negative symptoms of psychosis	5–30	Reduce neuroleptic dosage; administer anti-EPS agents
Akathisia	Subjective complaints of motor restlessness, pacing, rocking, shifting foot to foot	Severe agitation, psychotic decompensation	1–30	Reduce neuroleptic dosage; administer β-adrenergic blockers, propranolol, or anti-EPS agents
Rabbit syndrome	Perioral tremor (parkinsonian variant?)	—	Variable	Administer anti-EPS agents
TD				
Tardive dyskinesia	Orofacial-lingual dyskinesia, choreoathetosis in limbs and trunk	Stereotypy or mannerisms of psychosis	Months to years	No consistently effective treatment; lower neuroleptic dosage
Tardive dystonia	Persisting abnormal postures of the limbs, trunk, neck, face, eyes, or tongue	Acute dystonia, idiopathic dystonia	Months to years	No consistently effective treatment; high dosages of anticholinergics or clozapine may help
Tardive akathisia	Persisting subjective and objective restlessness	Acute akathisia, psychotic agitation	Months to years	No consistently effective treatment; propranolol or anti-EPS agents may help

Source. Reprinted from Casey DE: "Schizophrenia," in *Manual of Psychiatric Disorders.* Edited by Simpson G. New York, Impact Medical Communications (in press).

seizures, or catatonia (Casey 1991a). Failure to recognize an acute dystonic reaction will lead the patient to suffer unduly, resulting in treatment noncompliance (Casey 1991b).

Neuroleptic-induced parkinsonism.   Neuroleptic-induced parkinsonism, which is clinically similar to idiopathic parkinsonism, is characterized by tremor, rigidity, and bradykinesia (occasionally referred to as *akinesia*). The tremor is greater at rest, with a rhythmical to-and-fro motion. Cogwheel rigidity is detected as a ratchet-like sensation when testing for muscle tone. It is most easily evaluated in the upper limbs. Bradykinesia is characterized by a paucity of spontaneous activity. This can be as subtle as patients' changing position very little while sitting, exhibiting mild decreases in arm swing, or displaying decreased facial expression. More severe symptoms include stooped posture, substantially decreased arm swing, and a masklike facial expression. Bradykinesia is often misdiagnosed as depression, negative symptoms of psychosis, or withdrawal. As with the other acute EPS, it is important to properly make the differential diagnosis between neuroleptic drug–induced parkinsonism and psychoses, because the treatment strategies for each differ.

Rabbit syndrome.   The rabbit syndrome is an uncommon neuroleptic-induced side effect characterized by rhythmical tremors in the lips and perioral area (Casey 1992a; Villeneuve 1972). It is best thought of as a variant of drug-induced parkinsonism because the tremor is in the characteristic parkinsonian range of 3–6 Hz and improves with antiparkinsonian medicines. This disorder may occur at any time during neuroleptic treatment.

Paradoxical dyskinesia.   Paradoxical dyskinesia refers to a seldom-reported and poorly understood syndrome that clinically resembles tardive dyskinesia but pharmacologically responds like acute EPS. Phenomenologically, it appears as a cross between tardive dyskinesia and akathisia, as there are often repetitive, stereotyped, hyperkinetic dyskinesias of the mouth, face, limbs, and trunk (Casey 1992b). It improves with antiparkinsonian drugs or when neuroleptic drugs are discontinued (Casey and Denney 1977; Gerlach 1979).

Pathophysiology

Despite approximately 40 years of research on neuroleptics, little is known about the specific pathophysiologies of the underlying acute EPS. Although it is tempting to explain all of these side effects with a uniform and parsimonious theory, that may be unwise. The most common explanation of the underlying mechanism of acute EPS is dopamine D_2 receptor blockade, which is induced by all of the commercially available neuroleptics. However, one of the major problems with this hypothesis is that neuroleptic drugs block dopamine receptors within hours, whereas acute EPS may not develop for several days or weeks (Casey 1991a).

Akathisia.   Akathisia is the least well understood of the acute EPS. There is not a good neuroanatomical localization of this syndrome, and it responds less well to antiparkinsonian drugs (Adler et al. 1989; Casey 1991a; Keepers et al. 1983). The efficacy of propranolol, a nonselective β-adrenergic blocker, in akathisia (Adler et al. 1989; Lipinski et al. 1984) suggests that nondopaminergic mechanisms may be involved. Because neuroleptic drugs have very little direct action on β-adrenergic receptors, it is quite possible that the underlying pathophysiology of akathisia involves a secondary or tertiary effect of neuroleptics.

Dystonia.   Dystonia may be explained by either hyper- or hypodopaminergic influences in the basal ganglia (Casey 1991b; Rupniak et al. 1986). The hyperdopaminergic theory suggests that the increased release of dopamine induced by acute neuroleptic blockade overcomes this receptor blockade to produce dystonia. This hypothesis is supported by data that show that dystonia does not occur until the second day after a single dose, when neuroleptic blood levels are falling (Garver et al. 1976). The theory of hypodopaminergic function underlying dystonia proposes that neuroleptics effectively block dopamine at the postsynaptic site, and dystonia is the clinical consequence of that blockade. This hypothesis is supported by the observation that most dystonia occurs during the first few days of continuous neuroleptic treatment, when drug blood levels are rapidly increasing (Casey 1991b; Keepers et al. 1983).

Neuroleptic-induced parkinsonism.   Neuroleptic-induced parkinsonism usually takes several days or weeks to develop—an interval not consistent with the time course of rapidly occurring neuroleptic receptor blockade. Partial or complete tolerance to some or all of the drug-induced parkinsonian symptoms over several weeks and months also remains unexplained. The time course of tolerance is consistent with the evolution of dopamine receptor hypersensitivity, and may be a better fit of this model than its application to the pathophysiology of tardive dyskinesia (Casey 1987a, 1987b).

Epidemiology

The prevalence of acute EPS varies widely across studies, ranging from 2% to 100% of treated patients (Casey 1991a; Sovner and DiMascio 1978). This variability is influenced by patient, drug, and temporal factors. Over the past few decades, there has been a trend toward increasing prevalence of acute EPS, as it has become more common for clinicians to prescribe higher drug dosages with low-milligram, high-potency neuroleptics. Incidences of dystonia have steadily risen from 2.3% in 1960 (Ayd 1961) to 39% in 1980 (Keepers et al. 1983), and topped 90% in Boyer et al.'s (1989) review of high-risk young male patients. Akathisia occurs in approximately 25% of patients, with a range of 2%–75% (Adler et al. 1989). Drug-induced parkinsonism also occurs in approximately 25%–50% of patients, but its rate of incidence is highly influenced by age (Richardson et al. 1991).

Patient variables.   Age, gender, and history of previous EPS strongly influence whether a patient will develop these symptoms during current neuroleptic treatment. Akathisia is most often seen in middle-aged female patients (Adler et al. 1989; Ayd 1961; Keepers et al. 1983), although this disorder occurs at relatively similar prevalence rates for all the groups. Dystonia occurs most often in young male patients, and it is uncommonly seen in elderly patients receiving neuroleptics (Addonizio and Alexopoulos 1988; Keepers et al. 1983). Drug-induced parkinsonism occurs most often in adolescents, young adults, and elderly individuals (Moleman et al. 1982; Richardson et al. 1991).

A history of previous EPS is a very strong predictor of a patient's vulnerability to future EPS, if similar neuroleptic treatment is resumed. EPS rates can be predicted with approximately 75%–85% accuracy in these patients (Keepers and Casey 1991). Combining knowledge about prior EPS vulnerability with data from patient, drug, and temporal factors will give the most information about identifying EPS risk in the current course of treatment.

Drug factors. The intrinsic biochemical properties of neuroleptic drugs influence EPS rates. The relative balance of dopamine receptor and anticholinergic properties intrinsic to each neuroleptic drug correlates with the drug's propensity to produce acute EPS (Snyder et al. 1974), although other mechanisms of neuroleptic action may also account for EPS rates (Coward et al. 1989; Sayers et al. 1976). Low-milligram, high-potency drugs with minimal anticholinergic action (e.g., haloperidol, fluphenazine) produce more EPS than do high-milligram, low-potency compounds (e.g., thioridazine, chlorpromazine), which have more anticholinergic activity. Intermediate-potency compounds (e.g., perphenazine) produce intermediate rates of EPS. Clozapine is considered an atypical neuroleptic, at least in part, because it produces far fewer EPS (Casey 1989), although Cohen et al. (1991) raised questions about the possibility that akathisia occurred as frequently with clozapine as with other neuroleptics. However, EPS rates should not be the only consideration in neuroleptic drug choice because 1) EPS can usually be well managed with anti-EPS drugs, and 2) other undesirable drug effects (e.g., anticholinergic side effects, hypotension, leukopenia, agranulocytosis) should also be considered when selecting a neuroleptic.

The relationship between neuroleptic dosage and EPS is complex. Lower dosages produce fewer EPS than moderate or high dosages. However, megadosages produce the same or fewer EPS than moderate to high dosages (Keepers and Casey 1987). The correlation between neuroleptic dosage and EPS widely varies between no relationship (Tune and Coyle 1981) to a significant positive correlation (Baldessarini et al. 1988; Hansen et al. 1981). The seemingly intuitive and straightforward relationship between drug dosage and EPS may be absent because of several factors. If the EPS-dosage association is nonlinear, such as the inverted ∪-shaped curve function that is seen in dystonia, or if issues such as prophylactic use of antiparkinsonian drugs or specific factors of age or gender strongly influence EPS rates, it will be difficult to identify the role of specific drugs unless other factors are well controlled. Only by studying fixed dosages along the complete range of the dosage-response curve can the relationship between drug treatment and side effects be identified.

Several drugs that are dopamine receptor antagonists have the same potential to produce acute EPS, even though they are not marketed as neuroleptics. These include the antiemetic compounds (e.g., prochlorperazine, promethazine), the gastric motility–antiemetic agent metoclopramide, and the antidepressant amoxapine.

Temporal aspects.   Each acute EPS has a separate time course. Akathisia may occur within minutes, hours, or days of initiating neuroleptic drugs. Farde (1992) recently identified a correlation between acute dopamine D_2 receptor blockade and the onset of akathisia within 15 minutes of intravenous drug administration using positron-emission tomography scans. The large majority of dystonic reactions occur within the first 96 hours after starting or rapidly increasing neuroleptic drug dosages (Keepers et al. 1983; Sramek et al. 1986). Drug-induced parkinsonism most commonly develops by the end of the first or second week of treatment. This syndrome may gradually increase in severity for anywhere from a few to several more weeks (Ayd 1961). Eventually, many patients develop partial or full tolerance to this syndrome as they continue to take neuroleptics for several months.

Therapeutic Strategies

EPS can be managed with three separate strategies: 1) initial prophylaxis, 2) waiting for treatment-emergent EPS to develop, and 3) extended prophylaxis. *Initial prophylaxis* uses anti-EPS agents at the beginning of neuroleptic treatment to prevent EPS. There is considerable controversy about this approach. Proponents of prophylaxis argue that dystonic episodes and other EPS can be dangerous and often go unrecognized. Opponents argue that anti-EPS drugs have their own autonomic nervous system side effects and that routine use of these drugs exposes some patients to unnecessary side effects, as not all patients develop EPS. Both sides of the discussion contend that their approach seeks the maximum benefit with the fewest risks and will lead to the development of a therapeutic alliance and maintenance of treatment compliance with the patient.

Waiting for treatment-emergent EPS to develop is the standard approach to managing these disorders. It has the advantage of treating only those patients who need such treatment but has the risk that some patients will remain impaired from unrecognized EPS.

Extended prophylaxis is arbitrarily defined as continued anti-EPS drug therapy for 3 months or longer to suppress EPS. This can develop from continuing initial prophylaxis or from maintaining anti-EPS drug treatment that was initiated at the time of treatment-emergent EPS.

Managing Acute EPS

Managing acute EPS requires careful decision making at several points in therapy. The algorithm discussed in this section (and depicted in Figure 22–1) follows a logical course of clinical choices that parallel the time course of initiating neuroleptics, followed by maintaining long-term treatment of psychotic symptoms. Obtaining a thorough history and neuropsychiatric evaluation of the patient are essential elements for estimating the risk of EPS. Clearly documenting the psychiatric and neurological status of the patient prior to beginning drug therapy is important because it establishes a reference point for interpreting future clinical changes; furthermore, it will have medical-legal benefits if treatment decisions are later questioned.

Initial prophylaxis is indicated when there is 1) a high risk of EPS, 2) a predisposition to EPS based on prior history, or 3) detrimental sequelae of EPS (Casey 1991a; Casey and Keepers 1988). The risk assessment for EPS is made by evaluating patient factors (i.e., age, gender, and previous occurrence of EPS), drug properties (e.g., dosage, milligram potency, intrinsic anticholinergic properties), and temporal aspects of drug treatment (Keepers and Casey 1987, 1991; Keepers et al. 1983). If a patient previously had EPS with the drug dosage and type that is to be used in current treatment, it is highly likely that the patient will have EPS again. The concern for detrimental sequelae, such as in the paranoid patient who is unlikely to continue drug treatment if there is a dystonic reaction, is also an important consideration.

If the balance of factors suggests that initial prophylaxis is indicated, this approach should be utilized, since it is clearly effective (Boyer et al. 1989; Casey et al. 1980; Keepers et al. 1983; Sramek et al. 1986; Winslow et al. 1986). The most efficacious approach is to initiate prophylaxis for 1–2 weeks in the high-risk patient. Then, if EPS have not developed, the anti-EPS medicines should be gradually tapered to a level where EPS are present or should be discontinued if no EPS occur with tapering. This should give maximum protection in the initial period of vulnerability for those at greatest risk, yet reduce the risk of continuing anti-EPS drug side effects if patients do not need these drugs.

Initiating anti-EPS drug therapy for treatment-emergent EPS is standard practice. Dystonic reactions are best treated with parenteral anticholinergic (e.g., benztropine) or antihistaminic (e.g., diphenhydramine) agents. This approach is almost uniformly effective. If patients fail to improve after 1–3 repeated doses over a few hours, a search for other possible causes of dystonia should be initiated.

The primary strategy for managing drug-induced parkinsonism is to reduce the neuroleptic dosage. However, this is not possible in many patients in the early phases of a psychotic exacerbation. Therefore, adding anti-EPS drugs is the next alternative. The widely accepted anticholinergic and antihistaminic agents appear to be equally effective. Amantadine, a weak dopamine agonist, has fewer anticholinergic side effects. It is also an effective antiparkinsonian drug (Casey and Keepers 1988). Changing to another neuroleptic with a different side effect profile is also an option, but this is usually unnecessary.

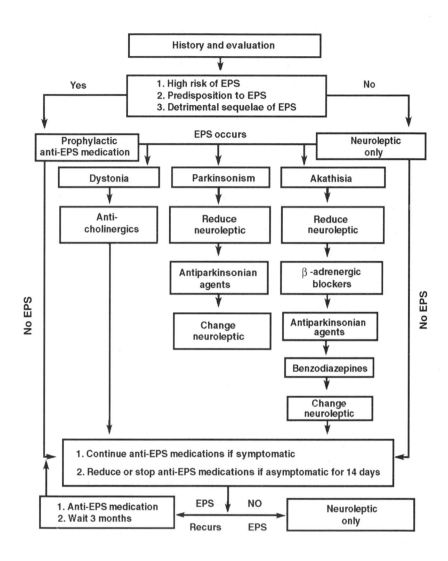

Figure 22–1. An algorithm for managing neuroleptic-induced acute extrapyramidal syndromes (EPS).

Source. Reprinted with permission from Casey DE, Keepers GA: "Neuroleptic Side Effects: Acute Extrapyramidal Syndromes and Tardive Dyskinesia," in *Psychopharmacology: Current Trends.* Edited by Casey DE, Christensen AV. Berlin, Springer, 1988, p. 2080.

Akathisia is the most difficult of the acute extrapyramidal syndromes to manage. The large number of treatment alternatives available attests to the limited efficacy of each of these treatments. Again, the best strategy is to reduce neuroleptic dosage, if possible. β-adrenergic blockers that penetrate the blood-brain barrier are effective antiakathisia drugs for many patients. Propranolol at 30–120 mg/day in divided doses is the recommended treatment range. If β-adrenergic blockers are not effective, then standard anti-EPS agents may be useful. If this approach fails, benzodiazepines can be considered. However, prescription of this class of drugs on an extended basis raises concerns about dependence and the potential for abuse. Another alternative is to change to another neuroleptic.

Extended prophylaxis or continued treatment with anti-EPS drugs will be necessary for many patients. In the ideal world, the anti-EPS drugs would be able to completely control acute EPS. Unfortunately, this is not always possible, because the anti-EPS dosage is limited by the troublesome side effects of these drugs. Many patients gain only partial control of their EPS and have to continue on anti-EPS agents indefinitely. The long-term strategy in managing extended prophylaxis or continuing anti-EPS treatment is to periodically attempt to gradually reduce the anti-EPS drugs. If EPS recur during this drug decrease, the previously effective anti-EPS dosage can be reinstituted. Casey and Keepers' (1988) review of extended prophylaxis studies published since 1980 indicated that 35%–90% of patients benefit from continued prophylaxis or treatment with anti-EPS drugs.

Much of the controversy regarding the use of anti-EPS drugs would not be relevant if lower neuroleptic dosages were used more often. Fortunately, there appears to be an emerging trend toward lower neuroleptic dosages for managing psychoses, as it becomes clear that high dosages of drug therapy do not produce the additional benefits that would outweigh the substantial risks (Baldessarini et al. 1988).

The algorithm illustrated in Figure 22–1 for therapeutic strategies to manage acute EPS offers a logical stepwise process for achieving the greatest benefit with the fewest risks. This multifactorial approach is preferred to using the inflexible "one strategy fits all" approach, since such a rigid approach cannot adequately address the complex interactions between patient, drug, and temporal factors. Failing to control acute EPS will produce additional impairments of the patient's functioning, lead to substantial medication noncompliance, and ultimately lead to drug discontinuation with probable psychotic exacerbations. On the other hand, unnecessarily exposing patients to the autonomic nervous system side effects of treatment from anti-EPS drugs will also eventually lead to poor compliance. Careful attention to EPS with flexible strategies that are periodically reevaluated will lead to the most effective use of antipsychotic drugs and minimize the effects of EPS, while research continues to seek the ideal neuroleptic that is efficacious yet free of acute EPS.

References

Addonizio G, Alexopoulos GS: Drug-induced dystonia in young and elderly patients. Am J Psychiatry 145:869–871, 1988

Adler LA, Angrist B, Reiter S, et al: Neuroleptic-induced akathisia: a review. Psychopharmacology (Berl) 97:1–11, 1989

Ayd FJ: A survey of drug-induced extrapyramidal reactions. JAMA 175:1054–1060, 1961

Baldessarini RJ, Cohen BM, Teicher MII: Significance of neuroleptic dose and plasma level in pharmacological treatment of psychosis. Arch Gen Psychiatry 45:79–91, 1988

Barnes TRE, Braude WM: Akathisia variants and tardive dyskinesia. Arch Gen Psychiatry 42:874–878, 1985

Boyer WF, Bakalar NH, Lake CR: Anticholinergic prophylaxis of acute haloperidol induced dystonic reactions. J Clin Psychopharmacol 7:164–166, 1989

Casey DE: Tardive dyskinesia, in Psychopharmacology: The Third Generation of Progress. Edited by Meltzer HY. New York, Raven, 1987a, pp 1411–1419

Casey DE: Neuroleptic-induced parkinsonism increases with repeated treatment in monkeys, in Clinical Pharmacology in Psychiatry IV: Selectivity in Psychotropic Drug Action—Promise or Problems. Edited by Dahl SG, Gram LF, Paul SM, et al. Berlin, Springer, 1987b, pp 243–247

Casey DE: Clozapine: neuroleptic-induced EPS and tardive dyskinesia. Psychopharmacology (Berl) 99:S47–S53, 1989

Casey DE: Neuroleptic drug-induced extrapyramidal syndromes and tardive dyskinesia. Schizophr Res 4:109–120, 1991a

Casey DE: Neuroleptic-induced acute dystonia, in Drug-Induced Movement Disorders. Edited by Lang AE, Weiner WJ. New York, Futura Press, 1991b, pp 21–40

Casey DE: The rabbit syndrome, in Disorders of Movement in Psychiatry and Neurology. Edited by Joseph AB, Young R. Cambridge, UK, Blackwell, 1992a, pp 139–142

Casey DE: Paradoxical tardive dyskinesia, in Disorders of Movement in Psychiatry and Neurology. Edited by Joseph AB, Young R. Cambridge, UK, Blackwell, 1992b, pp 67–69

Casey DE: Schizophrenia, in Manual of Psychiatric Disorders. Edited by Simpson G. New York, Impact Medical Communications (in press)

Casey DE, Denney D: Pharmacological characterization of tardive dyskinesia. Psychopharmacology (Berl) 54:1–8, 1977

Casey DE, Keepers GA: Neuroleptic side effects: acute extrapyramidal syndromes and tardive dyskinesia, in Psychopharmacology: Current Trends. Edited by Casey DE, Christensen AV. Berlin, Springer, 1988, pp 74–93

Casey DE, Gerlach J, Christensson E: Dopamine, acetylcholine, and GABA effects in acute dystonia in primates. Psychopharmacology (Berl) 70:83–87, 1980

Cohen BM, Keck PE, Satlin A, et al: Prevalence and severity of akathisia in patients on clozapine. Biol Psychiatry 29:1215–1219, 1991

Coward DM, Imperato A, Urwyler S, et al: Biochemical and behavioural properties of clozapine. Psychopharmacology (Berl) 99:S6–S12, 1989

Delay J, Deniker P, Hare JM: Utilisation en thérapeutique psychiatrique d'une phénothiazine d'action centrale élective (4560 RP). Ann Med Psychol (Paris) 110:112–117, 1952

Deniker P: Introduction of neuroleptic chemotherapy into psychiatry, in Discoveries in Biological Psychiatry. Edited by Ayd FJ, Blackwell B. Baltimore, Ayd Medical Communications, 1984, pp 155–164

Farde L: Selective D_1 or D_2 dopamine receptor blockade induces akathisia in humans—a PET study with [^{11}C] SCH 23390 and [^{11}C]-raclopride. Psychopharmacology (Berl) 107:23–29, 1992

Garver DL, Davis JM, Dekirmenjian H, et al: Dystonic reactions following neuroleptics: time course and proposed mechanisms. Psychopharmacology (Berl) 47:199–201, 1976

Gerlach J: Tardive dyskinesia. Dan Med Bull 26:209–245, 1979

Hansen LB, Larsen NE, Vestergard P: Plasma levels of perphenazine (Trilafon) related to development of extrapyramidal side effects. Psychopharmacology (Berl) 74:306–309, 1981

Keepers GA, Casey DE: Prediction of neuroleptic-induced dystonia. J Clin Psychopharmacology 7:342–344, 1987

Keepers GA, Casey DE: Use of neuroleptic-induced extrapyramidal symptoms to predict future vulnerability to side effects. Am J Psychiatry 148:85–89, 1991

Keepers GA, Clappison VJ, Casey DE: Initial anticholinergic prophylaxis for neuroleptic-induced extrapyramidal syndromes. Arch Gen Psychiatry 40:1113–1117, 1983

Lipinski JF, Zubenko GS, Cohen BM, et al: Propranolol in the treatment of neuroleptic-induced akathisia. Am J Psychiatry 141:412–415, 1984

Moleman P, Schmitz PJM, Ladee GA: Extrapyramidal side effects and oral haloperidol: an analysis of explanatory patient and treatment characteristics. J Clin Psychiatry 43:492–496, 1982

Richardson MA, Haugland G, Craig TJ: Neuroleptic use, Parkinson-like symptoms, tardive dyskinesia and associated factors in child and adolescent psychiatric patients. Am J Psychiatry 148:1322–1328, 1991

Rupniak NMJ, Jenner P, Marsden CD: Acute dystonia induced by neuroleptic drugs. Psychopharmacology (Berl) 88:403–419, 1986

Sayers AC, Burki HR, Ruch W, et al: Anticholinergic properties of antipsychotic drugs and their relation to extrapyramidal side effects. Psychopharmacology (Berl) 51:15–22, 1976

Snyder S, Greenberg D, Yamamura H: Antischizophrenic drugs and brain cholinergic receptors. Arch Gen Psychiatry 31:58–61, 1974

Sovner R, DiMascio A: Extrapyramidal syndromes and other neurological side effects of psychotropic drugs, in Psychopharmacology: A Generation of Progress. Edited by Lipton MA, DiMascio A, Killam DK. New York, Raven, 1978, pp 1021–1032

Sramek JJ, Simpson GM, Morrison RL, et al: Anticholinergic agents for prophylaxis of neuroleptic-induced dystonic reactions: a prospective study. J Clin Psychiatry 47:305–309, 1986

Tune L, Coyle JT: Acute extrapyramidal side effects: serum levels of neuroleptics. Psychopharmacology (Berl) 75:9–15, 1981

Villeneuve A: The rabbit syndrome: a peculiar extrapyramidal reaction. Canadian Psychiatric Association Journal 17:69–72, 1972

Winslow RS, Stillner V, Coons DJ, et al: Prevention of acute dystonic reactions in patients beginning with high-potency neuroleptics. Am J Psychiatry 143:706–710, 1986

CHAPTER 23

Neuroleptic Malignant Syndrome

Gerard Addonizio, M.D., and
Virginia L. Susman, M.D.

Neuroleptic malignant syndrome (NMS) is a rare but potentially fatal disorder that has been observed in psychiatric and nonpsychiatric patients who have been exposed to neuroleptics. First identified in the French literature in the 1960s (Delay et al. 1962), it has received significant recognition in the English-language literature only since Caroff's 1980 review. Since that review, a large number of anecdotal reports, additional reviews, and even prospective studies have followed. Although little controversy about the existence of the syndrome remains, there is still some debate about its diagnostic criteria and whether it exists in milder or partial forms (Addonizio et al. 1986; Adityanjee and Singh 1988).

Epidemiology

In the review by Caroff (1980), men with NMS outnumbered women 2:1 among the 60 patients studied. Subsequent reviews have also identified more male patients than female patients with NMS. In Pearlman's (1986) compilation of 302 patients with NMS, 58% were men, and in Addonizio et al.'s (1987) review of 115 NMS patients, 63% were men. The consistent pattern of more men than women having NMS is often attributed to clinicians' tendency to medicate men more aggressively than women because of the perception that psychotic men are potentially more violent than women.

Caroff (1980) found 80% of patients with NMS to be age 40 years or younger. Although the typical NMS patient is a young adult, it is also crucial for clinicians to be aware that NMS has developed in young children who accidentally ingested neuroleptics (Klein et al. 1985), in adolescents (Joshi et al. 1991), and in elderly patients (Addonizio 1991).

The incidence of NMS has varied considerably among the published reviews of the syndrome. The rate has been reported to be as low as .07% (Gelenberg et al. 1988) and as high as 2.2% (Hermesh et al. 1992). The reasons for this variability probably include differing thresholds for diagnosing the syndrome, diverse patient populations, and varying treatment practices. In addition, according to some investigators (Gelenberg et al. 1988; Keck et al. 1991), the incidence of NMS seems to be decreasing with early detection, active treatment, and more conservative dosing of neuroleptics.

Risk Factors

Many investigators have tried to identify risk factors for the development of NMS. Among those receiving the most attention are concomitant treatment with lithium and an underlying diagnosis of an affective disorder. To date, there have been inconsistent findings about both. In Pearlman's (1986) review, 40% of the patients with NMS had affective disorders, and in Addonizio et al.'s (1987) review, 44% had affective disorders. In Rosebush and Stewart's (1989) prospective analysis of 20 patients who developed NMS, it was observed that only 1 patient was schizophrenic, whereas 14 had affective disorders. In another prospective study of 223 patients treated with neuroleptic medication, Hermesh et al. (1992) found a heightened NMS risk for patients with bipolar affective disorder. On the other hand, in their prospective study of 9,792 neuroleptic-treated patients, Deng et al. (1990) reported 12 cases of NMS and no increased risk for those patients who had affective disorders. Deng et al. did acknowledge that their diagnostic criteria would overdiagnose schizophrenia.

Deng et al. (1990) found no association between lithium and NMS, nor did Keck et al. (1989a) in their case–control study of risk factors for NMS. However, many authors (Keck et al. 1987, 1989b; Pope et al. 1986; Rosebush and Stewart 1989) have reported what seems a disproportionately high number of cases of NMS developing in patients receiving lithium. In addition, Downey et al. (1984) and Gabuzda and Frankenberg (1987) each reported on a single patient who developed NMS-like signs on two separate occasions following exposure to lithium alone. Susman and Addonizio (1987) reported on two patients who developed recurrent NMS when exposed to lithium shortly after clinical recovery from NMS. Rosebush and Stewart (1989) reported a similar phenomenon in two NMS patients.

Electrolyte disturbances have also been considered a risk factor for the development of NMS. Both hyponatremia (Gibb et al. 1986; Tomson 1986; Wedzicha and Hoffbrand 1984) and hypernatremia (Addonizio et al. 1987; Rosebush and Stewart 1989) have been associated with the development of NMS. It should be recalled that electrolyte imbalances can also be a consequence of NMS.

The contribution of ambient temperature to the development of NMS is unclear. Shalev et al. (1988) concluded that high environmental temperatures could trigger NMS. Neuroleptics have α-adrenergic blocking and anticholinergic properties in addition to their anti-dopaminergic effects, and all of these can interfere with thermoregulation. Patients receiving neuroleptics are also at increased risk for heatstroke (Mann and Boger 1978). Therefore, it seems reasonable to consider high ambient temperature a potential risk factor for the development of NMS.

Patients with organic brain syndromes have been considered a population at greater risk for NMS since Delay and Deniker (1965) first observed this association. Other authors finding support for this include Addonizio et al. (1987), Caroff (1980), Rosebush and Stewart (1989), and Shalev and Munitz (1986).

Keck et al. (1989a) conducted a case–control study to assess risk factors for NMS. Age, gender, and diagnosis were matched in the patients and control subjects, so these variables were not assessable. Keck et al. did find increased risk for NMS associated with a greater amount of time in locked seclusion, larger overall neuroleptic dosage increase during the 5 days preceding the onset of NMS, higher mean and total neuroleptic dosages, and a greater number of intramuscular injections of neuroleptics. They interpreted these results as showing a correlation between psychomotor agitation and the risk for NMS. Hermesh et al. (1992) also found an association between intramuscular injections and the risk for NMS.

Role of Medication

Neuroleptic malignant syndrome can be caused by any type of neuroleptic medication (Addonizio et al. 1987). Although high-potency neuroleptics such as haloperidol and fluphenazine are most commonly implicated, there are numerous cases of NMS associated with low-potency neuroleptics. For example, several cases of NMS have been reported in patients on metoclopramide (L. S. Friedman et al. 1987; Robinson et al. 1985). Even clozapine-induced NMS has been reported in a handful of cases (Anderson and Powers 1991; DasGupta and Young 1991; Miller et al. 1991; Muller et al. 1988; Pope et al. 1986). In rare instances, antidepressants have also been implicated (Baca and Martinelli 1990; Halman and Goldbloom 1990; Langlow and Alarcon 1989; Lesaca 1987).

Although reviews of published cases seem to indicate that high-potency neuroleptics are more likely to cause NMS, these conclusions may only reflect prescribing practices for different neuroleptics. In fact, investigators in one large study (Deng et al. 1990) found that oral high-potency neuroleptics were not important risk factors for NMS, but that fluphenazine decanoate was a risk factor, especially if used without an antiparkinsonian agent. In addition, high-potency neuroleptics may be prescribed at higher average dosages than low-potency neuroleptics.

The dosage of the neuroleptic must also be accounted for in evaluating risk of developing NMS. NMS may occur with very small dosages of neuroleptics, but it is generally accepted that large dosages pose a greater risk. Keck et al. (1989a), in their case–control study, observed that patients with NMS received significantly higher dosages of neuroleptics and more parenteral medication than those who did not develop NMS. Further indirect evidence that NMS is related to higher neuroleptic dosages came from Gelenberg et al.'s (1988) study, in which a very low annual frequency of NMS was reported in a general hospital setting where physicians prescribed significantly modest dosages of neuroleptics.

In addition to potency and dosage, the rate of increase in dosage is an important risk factor for the development of NMS (Keck et al. 1989a; Shalev and Munitz 1986). Levinson and Simpson (1986) have argued that although neuroleptics regularly cause extrapyramidal side effects (EPS), a concurrent fever is often the result of a medical illness and not a direct neuroleptic effect. Contrary to this conclusion, Addonizio et al. (1987), in analyzing 115 published cases of NMS, found that medical workups usually did not reveal an underlying medical cause of the fever associated with EPS.

Several reports have indicated that lithium may potentiate the development of NMS (Keck et al. 1987), and in some cases lithium alone may trigger a recurrence of NMS in the immediate post-NMS period (Susman and Addonizio 1987). In a number of cases, an NMS-like syndrome has been reported in patients with Parkinson's disease who suddenly stopped taking L-dopa, bromocriptine, or amantadine (Addonizio and Susman 1991). The implication of these cases is that NMS can occur secondary to a sudden decrement in dopaminergic functioning. The observable syndrome may be the final common pathway of a sudden downregulation of the dopaminergic system in susceptible individuals.

Diagnostic Issues

Clinical Presentation

The core features of NMS include elevated temperature, rigidity, other EPS, and autonomic dysregulation. Elevated temperature is a central feature of NMS, and ranges in severity from mild elevations to severe hyperthermia. EPS are also central to NMS, particularly severe rigidity. Other EPS such as tremors and dystonias are also frequently seen. Hypertonic pharyngeal musculature may lead to dysphagia, dysarthria, and sialorrhea (Smego and Durack 1982). Blood pressure is often elevated or labile, and pulse rate is usually quite rapid. In one review of published cases of NMS, Addonizio et al. (1987) reported tachycardia in 97% of cases. Profuse diaphoresis, incontinence, and pallor are often seen. The patient is frequently confused and may become mute. Mental status changes range from stupor to coma (Caroff and Mann 1988).

Dramatic, fulminating cases that develop shortly after initiating treatment with neuroleptic medication begins are the most easily recognized. However, NMS has been reported in patients taking maintenance neuroleptics and may develop insidiously over several days. The syndrome is generally believed to be caused by impaired dopamine functioning secondary to neuroleptic administration. Support for this theory is derived from the overrepresentation of patients receiving high-potency neuroleptics (often administered at disproportionately high levels) among reported cases of NMS. Further support comes from the observation that NMS develops when adjunctive amantadine is discontinued (Lazarus 1985; Simpson and Davis 1984); in addition, patients with Parkinson's disease whose antiparkinsonian medications are discontinued will subsequently develop a syndrome identical to NMS (J. H. Friedman et al. 1985; Gibb and Griffith 1986; Toru et al. 1981). Nonetheless, it is essential that clinicians be aware that NMS may develop in patients receiving any neuroleptic—including the atypical neuroleptic clozapine—at any given dosage.

Diagnostic Criteria

Although a classic case of NMS includes hyperthermia, rigidity, autonomic instability, and altered consciousness, there is much debate about which of these features must be present to diagnose the syndrome and the degree of severity of each sign necessary to consider it present (Addonizio and Susman 1991). Some investigators feel that the syndrome must occur explosively with dramatic symptoms, whereas others feel that milder forms exist (Addonizio et al. 1986).

Various schema for diagnosing NMS have been proposed. One set of diagnostic criteria proposed by Levenson (1985) involves differentiating so-called major and minor manifestations and requiring a certain number of symptoms from each category to make the diagnosis. Fever, rigidity, and elevated levels of creatine phosphokinase (CPK) are the major manifestations, and several autonomic signs and altered consciousness are the minor manifestations. This schema has been criticized for designating elevated CPK as a major manifestation and for allowing NMS to be diagnosed in the absence of elevated temperature or rigidity. Keck et al. (1989b) proposed operational criteria that require a temperature of at least 38°C, at least two of several severe EPS, and at least two significant disturbances of autonomic function for definitively diagnosing NMS.

Laboratory Findings

Although laboratory data can help confirm the diagnosis of NMS, no laboratory finding is pathognomonic of this disorder. Laboratory tests often help in ruling out other disorders that may mimic NMS or in identifying one of the medical complications of NMS.

The muscle isoenzyme level of CPK is often elevated in NMS. Levels may be mild or extremely high (Addonizio and Susman 1991). Mild elevations in CPK are relatively nonspecific, since CPK rises with muscle trauma, exercise, cocaine intoxication, alcoholism, and intramuscular injections. Significant increases in CPK may be seen in acutely psychotic patients with no apparent reason for the elevation (Meltzer et al. 1980). With resolution of the NMS, CPK levels return to normal.

Reviews of NMS have consistently demonstrated leukocytosis as an associated feature of the syndrome (Shalev and Munitz 1986), with elevation in most cases ranging between 10,000 and 20,000/mm³. Both hyponatremia and hypernatremia are sometimes seen. In one study (Rosebush and Stewart 1989), 13 of 24 patients with NMS had serum calcium concentrations below the normal range. Ten of 16 patients had magnesium levels below the lower limit of normal in the same study. There have also been reports of low serum iron levels that returned to normal upon resolution of the syndrome (Rosebush and Stewart 1989).

Brain-imaging techniques, such as computed tomography scans, have not revealed any specific defect in NMS, and electroencephalograms are usually normal or demonstrate nonspecific slowing.

In most cases, analyses of cerebrospinal fluid (CSF) have been normal, with an occasional finding of elevated protein levels. Hepatic enzymes are occasionally mildly elevated. When rhabdomyolysis occurs, myoglobinuria may be seen (Smego and Durack 1982). This must be taken very seriously, since renal failure may soon follow.

To date, no characteristic autopsy findings have been revealed. In one case, necrosis of the anterior and lateral hypothalamic nuclei was demonstrated (Horn et al. 1988). As this represents the findings in only one case, the significance of necrosis in these areas remain to be determined. There is also evidence that patients with NMS have elevated levels of catecholamines (Gurrera and Romero 1992). In one study (Nisijima and Ishiguro 1990) in which CSF monoamine metabolites were measured in eight patients with NMS during the active phase of the disorder and after recovery, levels of homovanillic acid (HVA) were significantly lower in both instances. In addition, levels of 5-hydroxyindoleacetic acid were lower than those in the control patients both in the active phase of NMS and after recovery. These findings suggest a relationship between the development of NMS and disturbances of dopamine and serotonin metabolism.

Differential Diagnosis

Because NMS is a potentially fatal disorder, suspicion of NMS requires immediate attention and action on behalf of the clinician. On the other hand, it is also important that clinicians not be so conservative that they discontinue neuroleptics every time a patient develops rigidity and a mild febrile illness. Whereas the diagnosis of NMS may be absolutely clear in some cases, many times other causes of NMS symptoms must be ruled out.

Lethal catatonia may simulate NMS. Patients with this disorder develop motor excitement, clouding of consciousness, rigidity, fever, tachycardia, diaphoresis, and labile blood pressure (Mann et al. 1986).

If neuroleptic treatment has already commenced, it can be very difficult to distinguish NMS from lethal catatonia. Upon cessation of neuroleptics, symptoms may resolve and the diagnosis of NMS become clear. On the other hand, if symptoms of NMS continue, it is difficult to know if the cause of the problem is lethal catatonia or an NMS that has not resolved with cessation of neuroleptics.

Heatstroke is a potentially lethal disorder seen in patients on neuroleptics in a hot and often humid environment. Many of the symptoms of heatstroke are similar to NMS except that, unlike with NMS, the skin is usually hot and dry and in most cases sweating is absent (Petersdorf and Root 1987). Another important difference between the two disorders is that muscles are usually flaccid in heatstroke (Caroff 1980) whereas they are rigid in NMS.

Much has been written about the potential relationship between NMS and malignant hyperthermia (MH). *Malignant hyperthermia* is a potentially lethal syndrome in which a hypermetabolic state occurs in muscles after the administration of halogenated inhalational anesthetic agents or after receiving the depolarizing muscle relaxant succinylcholine (Nelson and Flewellen 1983). In MH, there is skeletal muscle rigidity and increase in body temperature as high as 43°C at a rate of 1°C every 5 minutes. Making the distinction between NMS and MH should be easy, given that MH—unlike NMS—occurs during administration of anesthetic agents. Concerns about potential pathophysiologic links between the two disorders, or concerns about one disorder predisposing an individual toward the other, have not been borne out. There are many differences between NMS and MH (Addonizio and Susman 1991):

- There is a clear muscle abnormality in MH.
- MH is a genetic disorder; there has been only one case reported of more than one family member developing NMS (Otani et al. 1991).
- MH is associated with anesthetic agents.
- MH has a higher mortality rate than NMS.
- MH develops over minutes.
- There are no reports of MH and NMS occurring in the same patient.
- Neuroleptics are used in patients with MH without inducing NMS.
- Curare and pancuronium cause flaccidity in NMS.

Other disorders can mimic NMS, but they usually can be recognized by physical and laboratory features that are not typical of NMS. Such disorders include central nervous system infection, akinetic mutism, "locked-in syndrome," tetany, thyrotoxicosis, pheochromocytoma, intermittent acute porphyria, and tetanus (Addonizio and Susman 1991). In addition, NMS-like syndromes may be caused by other pharmacological agents. The serotonin syndrome may resemble NMS (Sternbach 1991). This syndrome may occur when combining monoamine oxidase inhibitors (MAOIs) and fluoxetine or MAOIs and L-tryptophan. An NMS-like syndrome may also be seen with the MAOI-tricyclic combination (Lazarus et al. 1989). A florid NMS-like state can be precipitated when antiparkinsonian medication is suddenly stopped in a patient with Parkinson's disease (Figa-Talamanca et al. 1985). Lithium toxicity and anticholinergic delirium may resemble NMS. Other agents to be considered include amphetamines, fenfluramine, cocaine, phencyclidine, and strychnine (Addonizio and Susman 1991).

Pathophysiology

Hypotheses regarding the pathophysiology of NMS have largely revolved around known actions of neuroleptics on dopaminergic systems in the extrapyramidal system and the hypothalamus (Addonizio et al. 1987). Presumably, EPS and autonomic dysregulation are the end result of these pharmacological effects.

Another major model has revolved around similarities between the clinical presentation of NMS and MH. No model has adequately addressed why some people have the commonly observable neuroleptic-induced EPS whereas others develop a florid syndrome with multiple manifestations.

There is abundant evidence that impaired dopamine function is causally related to NMS. High-potency neuroleptics are most often implicated in cases of NMS (Addonizio et al. 1987), and high dosages as well as rapid increases in neuroleptic dosages (Shalev and Munitz 1986) increase risk. Also, dopaminergic agents such as bromocriptine and amantadine have been dramatically effective in treating individual cases of NMS (Addonizio and Susman 1991). In addition, patients with Parkinson's disease who suddenly discontinue dopaminergic medication can develop a syndrome that resembles NMS (Figa-Talamanca et al. 1985). In one study (Nisijima and Ishiguro 1990), CSF HVA was measured in eight patients with NMS. Compared with normal ("in good health") control subjects, levels of HVA were lower in patients with active NMS and were decreased after resolution of NMS. This same dopaminergic abnormality could lead to hypothalamic dysfunction, resulting in elevated temperature, tachycardia, labile blood pressure, and diaphoresis.

A different hypothesis suggests that much of the elevated temperature in NMS is secondary to the severe muscle contraction that occurs. In one review of NMS (Addonizio et al. 1987), the temporal correlation between development of EPS and elevated temperature was examined in 105 cases. Elevated temperature and EPS occurred simultaneously in 32% of the patients, EPS occurred before elevated temperature in 59%, and elevated temperature appeared before EPS in only 9%. Although this evidence is suggestive, the extent to which EPS contributes to the development of elevated temperature remains unclear.

Based on similarities between the clinical presentation of NMS and MH, there has been interest in attempting to identify common pathophysiologic links between the two disorders. Investigators have used a muscle contracture test developed for MH to research this issue. The results have been discrepant. Caroff et al. (1987) carried out a muscle contracture test after muscle biopsy exposure to halothane and incremental dosages of fluphenazine in seven NMS patients, six MH patients, and six nonpsychiatric control patients. There were no significant differences among the groups when comparing cumulative responses to fluphenazine. Yet the response to halothane in the NMS group was similar to that of the MH group, but was significantly greater than the response found in the control group. In a similar study, Araki et al. (1988) reported further evidence that muscle contracture in NMS was comparable to that in MH. On the other hand, results from other studies have conflicted with these reports (Bond 1984; Scarlett et al. 1983; Tollefson 1982). In a study by Krivosic-Horber et al. (1987), contracture tests were performed on six NMS patients. In five subjects the results were negative for MH and in one subject there were equivocal findings. Varying results may be a function of differing research techniques (Addonizio and Susman 1991). Further elucidation of this potential link will require larger controlled studies with standardized laboratory procedures. In their pilot study, Keck et al. (1990) investigated the porcine stress syndrome as a potential animal model for NMS. This syndrome is a genetic disorder of swine characterized by hyperthermia, rigidity, and autonomic dysfunction. The results of the study did not confirm the utility of the porcine stress syndrome as an animal model for NMS.

Other pathophysiologic models of NMS have emphasized the potential role of sympathoadrenomedullary activity (Gurrera and Romero 1992), λ-aminobutyric acid (Fricchione 1985), serotonin, and calcium metabolism (Addonizio and Susman 1991). Clearly, the field remains nascent in its exploration of pathophysiologic mechanisms of NMS.

Clinical Course

The majority of patients develop NMS within 2 weeks of beginning neuroleptic medication (Addonizio et al. 1987; Caroff and Mann 1988; Kurlan et al. 1984; Shalev and Munitz 1986). Rapid increments of neuroleptic dosages have also been associated with the development of NMS (Shalev and Munitz 1986). Most cases develop fulminantly, with major signs and symptoms manifest within hours to 2–3 days (Addonizio et al. 1987; Caroff 1980; Kurlan et al. 1984; Shalev and Munitz 1986). However, Addonizio et al. (1987) observed that the syndrome evolved more slowly—over the course of 4–30 days—in 21% of the cases they reviewed.

Some investigators have tried to identify patterns of symptom development in the hope of facilitating early detection and perhaps treatment. Careful review of reported cases by Addonizio and Susman (1991) clarified that no predictable sequence of symptom development has been established. Related to the study of symptom development is continuing consideration of the source of temperature elevation. The elevation of temperature appearing relatively late in the development of NMS has been construed as support for the theory that protracted muscle rigidity generates the temperature rise. Earlier development of temperature elevation has been taken as evidence that hypothalamic thermoregulation has been perturbed by the central dopaminergic blockade induced by neuroleptics.

The variability of data presented in case reports has made it somewhat difficult to identify the usual duration of an episode of NMS (Addonizio and Susman 1991). The time of onset is clearer in fulminant cases, but in slowly developing cases it has not been established whether onset is at the time of the first premonitory symptoms or when the full constellation of symptoms has developed. Likewise, the end of an episode could be the time of complete resolution or when temperature and other autonomic signs resolve, even though some residual stiffness continues. Allowing for these vagaries, it is generally accepted that NMS associated with oral neuroleptics lasts for approximately 2 weeks, and that NMS associated with depot neuroleptics lasts approximately 3–4 weeks (Addonizio et al. 1987; Shalev and Munitz 1986).

Medical Complications

The patient experiencing NMS is acutely and dangerously ill. Hyperthermia can be life threatening and should be managed with external cooling and hydration. Many of the pharmacological agents used to treat NMS have been selected because they have the potential to reverse the central or peripheral factors presumed to contribute to the elevated temperature. Because these patients are bedridden as the result of the severity of their illness, including its rigidity and altered levels of consciousness, they are at risk for pneumonia and thromboembolism. Dystonias and rigidity can compromise swallowing and respiration, rendering NMS patients vulnerable to aspiration pneumonia and tachypneic hypoventilation (Smego and Durak 1982). Muscle rigidity and perhaps even a primary neuroleptic-induced disorder of muscle metabolism (Martin and Swash 1987) contribute to heat production and muscle breakdown. Rhabdomyolysis, myoglobinuria, and consequent renal insufficiency or failure can result in considerable morbidity.

Rhabdomyolysis developed in 14 of 53 patients in one review (Levenson 1985), with 10 patients developing renal failure. In their reviews, Addonizio et al. (1987) and Shalev and Munitz (1986) reported that 16% and 8%, respectively, of their patients developed acute renal failure. In Rosebush and Stewart's (1989) prospective study, 7 of 24 patients (30%) experienced renal failure. In a later study, Shalev et al. (1989) found a significantly higher mortality rate in patients who had myoglobinuria and renal failure. They concluded that nearly 50% of patients with these complications died and that no other medical complication of NMS was predictably associated with mortality.

The use of varying diagnoses for respiratory problems in case reports has limited a quantitative review of the frequency of pulmonary disorders. Addonizio et al. (1987) found pneumonia to be the most frequently reported complication of NMS and the second most frequent cause of death. Twelve percent of the 120 patients whose cases were reviewed by Shalev and Munitz (1986) had so-called pulmonary insufficiency. Levenson (1985) reported that respiratory failure was the second most common complication among the 53 cases he reviewed. Shalev et al.'s (1989) study, in which renal failure and myoglobinuria were linked with increased risk for mortality, found no such association for respiratory distress. Other respiratory disorders identified in NMS patients include pulmonary edema, pulmonary emboli, pneumothorax, pneumomediastinum, and adult respiratory distress syndrome (Addonizio and Susman 1991).

A number of other complications have been linked to NMS, none of which have developed in a significant number of cases. Among the complications convincingly linked to NMS are disseminated intravascular coagulation (Eles et al. 1984; Kleinknecht et al. 1982), myocardial infarction (Becker et al. 1988; Bernstein 1979; Harsch 1987), cerebral infarction (Pullicino et al. 1991), and, as later sequelae, neuropsychological deficits (vanHarten and Kemperman 1991). Balzan and Cacciottolo (1992) and de Boer and Gaete (1992) described close temporal association between the development of NMS and diabetic ketoacidosis, prompting speculation that the metabolic derangement may have predisposed the patients to NMS.

In 1980, Caroff reported a death rate of 20% from NMS, a figure that was widely quoted at that time. Nonetheless, a comparison of the major reviews of NMS by Addonizio and Susman (1991) mirrored the observations of others (Pearlman 1986; Shalev et al. 1989) in documenting a decline in mortality rates to less than 10%. There are a number of plausible explanations for this decline. Wider recognition, earlier diagnosis with prompt cessation of neuroleptic medication, and active treatment have been suggested by a number of authors (Addonizio et al. 1987; Caroff and Mann 1988; Pearlman 1986; Shalev et al. 1989). An alternative possibility is that improved awareness and the notion that milder forms of NMS exist have increased the total number of reported cases but decreased the proportion of serious or fatal cases.

Treatment

Rapid and intensive supportive treatment is essential for the patient with NMS. Cooling by sponging or cooling blankets with vigorous efforts to maintain or reestablish good hydration are key. Because dysphagia and altered consciousness can interfere with oral intake, intravenous fluids may be necessary. In fact, the more precise measurement of intake and output afforded by intravenous fluids and catheterization may be desirable or even essential. Active nursing care, with emphasis on pulmonary therapy, positioning, and skin care, can help prevent pulmonary stasis and the development of decubitus or thrombosis. Some clinicians recommend the use of prophylactic heparin.

The potential lethality of the syndrome has driven many investigators to explore active treatments. The pharmacological agents used have included medications such as bromocriptine, amantadine, and L-dopa that counter the antidopaminergic properties of neuroleptics. Other agents, such as dantrolene, benzodiazepines, and antihypertensives, have been administered in hopes of targeting specific signs of NMS. The literature is replete with case reports of NMS treated with one or more of these agents. Unfortunately, the reports are highly variable in their quality. Deficiencies include failure to mention the dosages of medications, the duration of NMS prior to treatment, and the time from beginning treatment to symptom remission. In addition, there could be overreporting of successfully treated cases or of ones with unfavorable outcomes. Active treatment may be used only in the most serious cases.

Shalev et al. (1989) studied mortality rates in NMS. They observed that no protective effect was provided by bromocriptine, dantrolene, or amantadine, but presumed that active treatment might have been prescribed too late or in inadequate dosages. Addonizio and Susman (1991) analyzed treated NMS cases using fairly stringent criteria for treatment efficacy: either symptom reversal within 24 hours or improvement followed by relapse when treatment was withdrawn, then a second response upon reinstitution of treatment. Although there were convincing responses with each of the major agents used in the cases Addonizio and Susman reviewed, there was no single agent or combination that was always effective or clearly superior. In their review, Sakkas et al. (1991) studied 734 reports of NMS and used three measures of clinical efficacy: the authors' assessment, relapse of NMS upon discontinuation of active treatment, and the mortality rate. They identified consistently favorable ratings for bromocriptine, amantadine, and dantrolene on each of the measures. On the other hand, in the prospective study of 20 patients by Rosebush et al. (1991), 8 of whom received dantrolene, bromocriptine, or both, it was observed that active treatment was associated with both a longer course of illness and more sequelae, despite controlling for severity of NMS, neuroleptic exposure, and risk factors. However, Rosebush et al. did note that the group receiving active treatment had experienced a higher incidence of acute medical illness.

Although doubt has been cast on the effectiveness of pharmacological treatments, it seems reasonable to consider using them in severe cases when supportive care seems inadequate. Choosing bromocriptine or dantrolene as a first choice should be based on the side effect profile of each agent and the clinical profile of the patient. Adjunctive benzodiazepines may also be useful.

Finally, another treatment warranting careful consideration is electroconvulsive therapy (ECT). It has proven useful in the treatment of functional catatonia and, based on the similarities between catatonia and NMS, it has been used in a number of cases of NMS. In addition to treating the underlying psychiatric disorders of some patients, ECT has apparently helped to reverse some of signs of NMS in others (Abbott and Loizou 1986; Addonizio and Susman 1987; Hermesh et al. 1987). Concerns that succinylcholine might trigger malignant hyperthermia because of similarities between that syndrome and NMS have proven unfounded (Addonizio and Susman 1987). There have been several reports of cardiac complications developing in NMS patients treated with ECT (Hughes 1986; Lazarus 1986; Regestein et al. 1977; Ries and Schuckit 1980), which lead to the recommendation that cardiac status should be monitored very carefully when using ECT in patients with NMS.

Recurrence and Aftercare

Treating continuing or recurring psychosis in patients who have experienced NMS presents clinicians with difficult decisions. How susceptible any patient is to recurrent NMS is not known. There are numerous case reports of both safe resumption of neuroleptic treatment and recurrences of NMS with resumed treatment.

Results from several follow-up studies are now available. Most authors agree that the greatest risk for recurrence is posed by premature reintroduction of neuroleptics (i.e., giving neuroleptics before the original episode of NMS has completely resolved) (Rosebush et al. 1989; Susman and Addonizio 1988). The current recommendation is that neuroleptics should be withheld for 2 weeks following clinical resolution of an episode of NMS (Addonizio and Susman 1991; Gelenberg et al. 1989; Rosebush et al. 1989).

Although a number of investigators have made the commonsense recommendation that patients who have had NMS should be given low-dosage, low-potency neuroleptics and be observed closely for any signs of recurrence, the results of Rosebush et al.'s (1989) study of 15 patients who underwent 20 rechallenges indicated that neither the dosage nor the potency of the neuroleptic used for rechallenge was significant. Recalling Shalev and Munitz's (1986) observation about the risk of NMS being heightened by more rapid or dramatic dosing increments, it does seem most prudent to raise dosages slowly.

There is considerable interest in using clozapine to treat post-

NMS patients. Clozapine has been associated with NMS (Anderson and Powers 1991; Miller et al. 1991), but its safe use in a number of NMS patients (Burrell and Fewster 1991; Stoudemire and Clayton 1989; Weller and Kornhuber 1992) and its unique lack of EPS render it an inviting alternative. Another pharmacological approach to the post-NMS patient is pretreatment with an anti-NMS agent before reintroduction of neuroleptics. Total avoidance of neuroleptics by treating post-NMS patients with benzodiazepines, carbamazepine, lithium, or ECT are other approaches.

References

Abbott RJ, Loizou LA: Neuroleptic malignant syndrome. Br J Psychiatry 148:47–51, 1986

Addonizio G: The pharmacologic basis of neuroleptic malignant syndrome. Psychiatric Annals 21:152–156, 1991

Addonizio G, Susman VL: ECT as a treatment alternative for patients with symptoms of neuroleptic malignant syndrome. J Clin Psychiatry 48:102–105, 1987

Addonizio G, Susman VL: Neuroleptic Malignant Syndrome: A Clinical Guide. St. Louis, MO, Mosby-Year Book, 1991

Addonizio G, Susman VL, Roth SD: Symptoms of neuroleptic malignant syndrome in 82 consecutive inpatients. Am J Psychiatry 143:1587–1590, 1986

Addonizio G, Susman VL, Roth SD: Neuroleptic malignant syndrome: review and analysis of 115 cases. Biol Psychiatry 22:1004–1020, 1987

Adityanjee, Singh S: Spectrum concept of neuroleptic malignant syndrome. Br J Psychiatry 153:107–111, 1988

Anderson ES, Powers PS: Neuroleptic malignant syndrome associated with clozapine use. J Clin Psychiatry 52:102–104, 1991

Araki M, Takagi A, Higuchi I, et al: Neuroleptic malignant syndrome: caffeine contracture of single muscle fibers and muscle pathology. Neurology 38:297–301, 1988

Baca L, Martinelli L: Neuroleptic malignant syndrome: a unique association with a tricyclic antidepressant. Neurology 40:1797–1798, 1990

Balzan M, Cacciottolo JM: Neuroleptic malignant syndrome presenting as hyperosmolar non-ketotic diabetic coma. Br J Psychiatry 161:257–258, 1992

Becker D, Birger M, Samuel E, et al: Myocardial infarction: an unusual complication of neuroleptic malignant syndrome. J Nerv Ment Dis 176:377–378, 1988

Bernstein RA: Malignant neuroleptic syndrome: an atypical case. Psychosomatics 20:840–846, 1979

Bond WS: Detection and management of the neuroleptic malignant syndrome. Clin Pharm 3:302–307, 1984

Burrell MF, Fewster C, Szabadi E, et al: Clozapine-treated NMS (letter). Br J Psychiatry 158:577, 1991

Caroff SN: The neuroleptic malignant syndrome. J Clin Psychiatry 41:79–83, 1980

Caroff SN, Mann SC: Neuroleptic malignant syndrome. Psychopharmacol Bull 24:25–29, 1988

Caroff SN, Rosenberg H, Fletcher JE, et al: Malignant hyperthermia susceptibility in neuroleptic malignant syndrome. Anesthesiology 67:20–25, 1987

DasGupta K, Young A: Clozapine-induced neuroleptic malignant syndrome. J Clin Psychiatry 52:105–107, 1991

de Boer C, Gaete HP: Neuroleptic malignant syndrome and diabetic ketoacidosis. Br J Psychiatry 161:856–858, 1992

Delay J, Deniker P: Sur quelques erreurs de prescription des médicaments psychiatriques. Société Médicale des Hôpitaux de Paris 116:487–493, 1965

Delay J, Pichot P, Lemperiere T, et al: L'emploi des butyrophénones en psychiatrie: étude statistique et psychométrique. Symposium Internazionale Sull'Haloperidol E Triperidol, Milano, Italy, November 18, 1962, pp 305–319

Deng MZ, Chen GQ, Phillips MR: Neuroleptic malignant syndrome in 12 of 9,792 Chinese inpatients exposed to neuroleptics: a prospective study. Am J Psychiatry 147:1149–1155, 1990

Downey GP, Caroff S, Beck S, et al: Neuroleptic malignant syndrome: patient with unique clinical and psychologic features. Am J Med 77:338–340, 1984

Eles GR, Songer JE, DiPette DJ: Neuroleptic malignant syndrome complicated by disseminated intravascular coagulation. Arch Intern Med 144:1296–1297, 1984

Figa-Talamanca L, Gualandi C, DiMeo L, et al: Hyperthermia after discontinuance of levodopa and bromocriptine therapy: impaired dopamine receptors a possible cause. Neurology 35:258–261, 1985

Fricchione GL: Neuroleptic catatonia and its relationship to psychogenic catatonia. Biol Psychiatry 20:304–313, 1985

Friedman JH, Feinberg SS, Feldman RG: A neuroleptic malignantlike syndrome due to levodopa therapy withdrawal. JAMA 254:2792–2795, 1985

Friedman LS, Weinrauch LA, D'Elia JA: Metoclopramide-induced neuroleptic malignant syndrome. Arch Intern Med 147:1495–1497, 1987

Gabuzda DH, Frankenburg FR: Fever caused by lithium in a patient with neuroleptic malignant syndrome. J Clin Psychopharmacol 7:283–284, 1987

Gelenberg AJ, Bellinghausen B, Wojcik JD, et al: A prospective survey of neuroleptic malignant syndrome in a short-term psychiatric hospital. Am J Psychiatry 145:517–518, 1988

Gelenberg AJ, Bellinghausen B, Wojcik JD, et al: Patients with neuroleptic malignant syndrome histories: what happens when they are rehospitalized? J Clin Psychiatry 50:178–180, 1989

Gibb WRG, Griffith DNW: Levodopa withdrawal syndrome identical to neuroleptic malignant syndrome. Postgrad Med J 62:59–60, 1986

Gibb WRG, Wedzicha JA, Hoffbrand BI: Recurrent neuroleptic malignant syndrome and hyponatraemia. J Neurol Neurosurg Psychiatry 49:960–961, 1986

Gurrera RJ, Romero JA: Sympathoadrenomedullary activity in the neuroleptic malignant syndrome. Biol Psychiatry 32:334–343, 1992

Halman M, Goldbloom DS: Fluoxetine and neuroleptic malignant syndrome. Biol Psychiatry 28:518–521, 1990

Harsch HH: Neuroleptic malignant syndrome: physiological and laboratory findings in a series of nine cases. J Clin Psychiatry 48:328–333, 1987

Hermesh H, Aizenberg D, Weizman A: A successful electroconvulsive treatment of neuroleptic malignant syndrome. Acta Psychiatr Scand 75:237–239, 1987

Hermesh H, Aizenberg D, Weizman A, et al: Risk for definite neuroleptic malignant syndrome: a prospective study in 223 consecutive inpatients. Br J Psychiatry 161:254–257, 1992

Horn E, Lach B, Lapierre Y, et al: Hypothalamic pathology in the neuroleptic malignant syndrome. Am J Psychiatry 145:617–620, 1988

Hughes JR: ECT during and after the neuroleptic malignant syndrome: case report. J Clin Psychiatry 47:42–43, 1986

Joshi PT, Capozzoli JA, Coyle JT: Neuroleptic malignant syndrome: life-threatening complication of neuroleptic treatment in adolescents with affective disorder. Pediatrics 87:235–239, 1991

Keck PE, Pope HG, McElroy SL: Frequency and presentation of neuroleptic malignant syndrome: a prospective study. Am J Psychiatry 114:1344–1346, 1987

Keck PE, Pope HG, Cohen BM, et al: Risk factors for neuroleptic malignant syndrome: a case control study. Arch Gen Psychiatry 46:914–918, 1989a

Keck PE, Sebastianelli J, Pope HG, et al: Frequency and presentation of neuroleptic malignant syndrome in a state psychiatric hospital. J Clin Psychiatry 50:352–355, 1989b

Keck PE Jr, Seeler DC, Pope HG Jr, et al: Porcine stress syndrome: an animal model for the neuroleptic malignant syndrome? Biol Psychiatry 28:58–62, 1990

Keck PE, Pope HG, McElroy SL: Declining frequency of neuroleptic malignant syndrome in a hospital population. Am J Psychiatry 148:880–882, 1991

Klein SK, Levinsohn MW, Blumer JL: Accidental chlorpromazine ingestion as a cause of neuroleptic malignant syndrome in children. J Pediatr 107:970–973, 1985

Kleinknecht D, Parent A, Blot P, et al: Rhabdomyolyses avec insuffisance rénale aiguë et syndrome malin des neuroleptiques. Ann Med Interne 133:549–552, 1982

Krivosic-Horber R, Adnet P, Guevart E, et al: Neuroleptic malignant syndrome and malignant hyperthermia. Br J Anaesth 59:1554–1556, 1987

Kurlan R, Hamill R, Shoulson I: Neuroleptic malignant syndrome. Clin Neuropharmacol 7:109–120, 1984

Langlow JR, Alarcon RD: Trimipramine-induced neuroleptic malignant syndrome after transient psychogenic polydipsia in one patient. J Clin Psychiatry 50:144–145, 1989

Lazarus A: Neuroleptic malignant syndrome and amantadine withdrawal. Am J Psychiatry 142:142, 1985

Lazarus A: Treatment of neuroleptic malignant syndrome with electroconvulsive therapy. J Nerv Ment Dis 174:47–49, 1986

Lazarus A, Mann SC, Caroff SN: The Neuroleptic Malignant Syndrome and Related Conditions. Washington, DC, American Psychiatric Press, 1989

Lesaca T: Amoxapine and neuroleptic malignant syndrome. Am J Psychiatry 144:1514, 1987

Levenson JL: Neuroleptic malignant syndrome. Am J Psychiatry 142:1137–1145, 1985

Levinson DF, Simpson GM: Neuroleptic-induced extrapyramidal symptoms with fever. Arch Gen Psychiatry 43:839–848, 1986

Mann SC, Boger WP: Psychotropic drugs, summer heat and humidity, and hyperpyrexia: a danger restated. Am J Psychiatry 135:1097–1100, 1978

Mann SC, Caroff SN, Bleier HR, et al: Lethal catatonia. Am J Psychiatry 143:1374–1381, 1986

Martin DT, Swash M: Muscle pathology in the neuroleptic malignant syndrome. J Neurol 235:120–121, 1987

Meltzer HY, Ross-Stanton J, Schlessinger S: Mean serum creatine kinase activity in patients with functional psychoses. Arch Gen Psychiatry 37:650–655, 1980

Miller DD, Sharafuddin MJA, Kathol RG: A case of clozapine-induced neuroleptic malignant syndrome. J Clin Psychiatry 52:99–101, 1991

Muller T, Becker T, Fritze J: Neuroleptic malignant syndrome after clozapine plus carbamazepine. Lancet 2:1500, 1988

Nelson TE, Flewellen EH: Current concepts: the malignant hyperthermia syndrome. N Engl J Med 309:416–418, 1983

Nisijima K, Ishiguro T: Neuroleptic malignant syndrome: a study of CSF monoamine metabolism. Biol Psychiatry 27:280–288, 1990

Otani K, Horiuchi M, Kondo T, et al: Is the predisposition to neuroleptic malignant syndrome genetically transmitted? Br J Psychiatry 158:850–853, 1991

Pearlman CA: Neuroleptic malignant syndrome: a review of the literature. J Clin Psychopharmacol 6:257–273, 1986

Petersdorf RG, Root RG: Alterations in body temperature, in Harrison's Principles of Internal Medicine. Edited by Braunwald E, Isselbacher KJ, Petersdorf RG. New York, McGraw-Hill, 1987

Pope HG, Jr, Cole JO, Choras PT, et al: Single case study: apparent neuroleptic malignant syndrome with clozapine and lithium. J Nerv Ment Dis 174:493–495, 1986

Pullicino P, Galizia AC, Azzopardi C: Cerebral infarction in neuroleptic malignant syndrome. J Neuropsychiatry Clin Neurosci 3:75–77, 1991

Regestein QR, Alpert JS, Reich P: Sudden catatonic stupor with disastrous outcome. JAMA 238:618–620, 1977

Ries RK, Schuckit MA: Catatonia and autonomic hyperactivity. Psychosomatics 21:349–350, 1980

Robinson MB, Kennett RP, Harding AE: Neuroleptic malignant syndrome associated with metoclopramide. J Neurol Neurosurg Psychiatry 40:1304, 1985

Rosebush P, Stewart T: A prospective analysis of 24 episodes of neuroleptic malignant syndrome. Am J Psychiatry 146:717–725, 1989

Rosebush P, Stewart T, Gelenberg A: Twenty neuroleptic rechallenges after neuroleptic malignant syndrome in 15 patients. J Clin Psychiatry 50:295–298, 1989

Rosebush PI, Stewart T, Mazurek MF: The treatment of neuroleptic malignant syndrome: are dantrolene and bromocriptine useful adjuncts to supportive care? Br J Psychiatry 159:709–712, 1991

Sakkas P, Davis JM, Hua J, et al: Pharmacotherapy of neuroleptic malignant syndrome. Psychiatric Annals 21:157–164, 1991

Scarlett JD, Zimmerman R, Berkovic SF: Neuroleptic malignant syndrome. Aust N Z J Med 13:70–73, 1983

Shalev A, Munitz H: The neuroleptic malignant syndrome: agent and host interaction. Acta Psychiatr Scand 73:337–347, 1986

Shalev A, Hermesh H, Munitz H: The role of external heat load in triggering the neuroleptic malignant syndrome. Am J Psychiatry 145:110–111, 1988

Shalev A, Hermesh H, Munitz H: Mortality from neuroleptic malignant syndrome. J Clin Psychiatry 50:18–25, 1989

Simpson SM, Davis GC: Case report of neuroleptic malignant syndrome associated with withdrawal from amantadine. Am J Psychiatry 141:796–797, 1984

Smego RA, Durack DT: The neuroleptic malignant syndrome. Arch Intern Med 142:1183–1185, 1982

Sternbach H: The serotonin syndrome. Am J Psychiatry 148:705–713, 1991

Stoudemire A, Clayton L: Successful use of clozapine in a patient with a history of neuroleptic malignant syndrome. Journal of Neuropsychiatry 1:303–305, 1989

Susman VL, Addonizio G: Reinduction of neuroleptic malignant syndrome by lithium. J Clin Psychopharmacol 7:339–341, 1987

Susman VL, Addonizio G: Recurrence of neuroleptic malignant syndrome. J Nerv Ment Dis 176:234–241, 1988

Tollefson G: A case of neuroleptic malignant syndrome: in vitro muscle comparison with malignant hyperthermia. J Clin Psychopharmacol 2:266–270, 1982

Tomson CRV: Neuroleptic malignant syndrome associated with inappropriate antidiuresis and psychogenic polydipsia. BMJ 292:171, 1986

Toru M, Matsuda O, Makiguchi K, et al: Neuroleptic malignant syndrome-like state following a withdrawal of antiparkinsonian drugs. J Nerv Ment Dis 169:324–327, 1981

vanHarten PN, Kemperman CJF: Organic amnestic disorder: a long-term sequel after neuroleptic malignant syndrome. Biol Psychiatry 29:407–410, 1991

Wedzicha JA, Hoffbrand BI: Neuroleptic malignant syndrome and hyponatraemia. Lancet 1:963, 1984

Weller M, Kornhuber J: Clozapine rechallenge after an episode of 'neuroleptic malignant syndrome'. Br J Psychiatry 161:855–856, 1992

Nonextrapyramidal Side Effects of Typical Antipsychotic Drugs

Scott A. West, M.D., and
S. Craig Risch, M.D.

The management of schizophrenia dramatically changed with the introduction of chlorpromazine in the 1950s. Since that time, advances in psychopharmacology have led to the development of numerous classes of antipsychotic medications. The antipsychotic efficacy of typical antipsychotic medications appears to be equal, and all classes share a common side-effect profile. However, antipsychotic medications vary markedly in the degree to which they produce both beneficial and adverse side effects. The majority of side effects are manageable and attributable to expected pharmacological actions, but there remains the potential for toxic and even lethal reactions. Although there is considerable overlap between the side effects of typical and atypical antipsychotic drugs, atypical antipsychotics such as clozapine have unique pharmacological properties and side effects. In this chapter, we focus on the side effects of typical antipsychotic drugs. (See Chapters 12, 14, and 25 in this volume for discussions of side effects of atypical antipsychotic medications.)

Introduction

Antipsychotic medications act on a variety of receptor systems and affect the physiologic function of virtually every organ system in the body. There is a peripheral blockade of cholinergic, α-adrenergic, histaminergic, and tryptaminergic activity (Risch et al. 1981). These medications also affect numerous pathways within the central nervous system (CNS), including the serotonergic, noradrenergic, and cholinergic systems, in addition to the central dopaminergic blockade that is thought to produce the antipsychotic activity (Risch et al. 1981; Snyder 1976).

The selection of a particular antipsychotic medication is typically based on the expected side effects. For example, acutely agitated patients are commonly treated with low-potency, relatively sedating medications such as chlorpromazine or thioridazine. Conversely, these medications are generally avoided in elderly patients because of their strong anticholinergic and anti–α-adrenergic activity, which may result in urinary retention, constipation, blurred vision, and orthostatic changes in blood pressure and pulse rate. High-potency medications are also generally preferred for use in elderly patients with concurrent dementia or delirium to minimize the anticholinergic effects that may cause further confusion.

The nonextrapyramidal side effects of typical antipsychotic medications can be divided into two groups for the purpose of clinical selection of a particular medication. The first group consists of three primary side effects: sedation, anticholinergic effects, and cardiovascular effects. These side effects commonly occur in patients and should be carefully considered when selecting a particular medication, as they may lead to further complications in certain patients and may also contribute to noncompliance (especially the anticholinergic effects). The second group consists of numerous side effects that are relatively uncommon in patients and that generally do not influence the selection of a particular medication; two examples include agranulocytosis and cholestatic jaundice. Although uncommon, these side effects may cause considerable morbidity and even mortality, so close monitoring is warranted.

Common Side Effects

Sedation

Sedation is unfortunately common, and there is no real antidote for this side effect. It is likely the result of central antihistaminergic activity, and is much more common with lower potency than with higher potency drugs (Rifkin and Siris 1987). Tolerance generally develops to the medication, which at least partially alleviates this effect. If sedation is intolerable, it may be helpful to reduce the dosage or to use a single dose at bedtime. This strategy may be especially desirable and beneficial in patients who are acutely agitated or anxious and in patients who have insomnia.

Anticholinergic Effects

The anticholinergic properties of these medications produce by far the most undesirable side effects and play a major role in noncompliance. The most common complaints include dry mouth, blurred vision, impaired micturition, and constipation (Rifkin and Siris 1987). These may not only be bothersome but may lead to more serious conditions such as fecal impaction, paralytic ileus, or urinary retention, with the subsequent development of a urinary tract infection (Rifkin and Siris 1987; Schatzberg and Cole 1991). In addition, cholinergic blockade may exacerbate symptoms of delirium and dementia, resulting in further confusion and cognitive impairment. Some degree of tolerance generally develops, and starting with low dosages and increasing dosages gradually often helps to minimize these adverse effects. The use of higher potency medications often completely avoids the development of these side effects; medications such as haloperidol and fluphenazine are often preferred in sensitive or elderly patients for this reason.

Cardiovascular Effects

Antipsychotic medications affect the cardiovascular system at numerous levels, creating a complex picture because of both the direct and the indirect effects (Risch et al. 1981). Orthostatic hypotension secondary to α-adrenergic blockade may result in serious head injuries and fractures (e.g., hip), especially in elderly patients, who are much more sensitive to these effects (Schatzberg and Cole 1991). It is more typical for systolic blood pressure to be affected than diastolic blood pressure, and low-potency medications are implicated much more frequently than high-potency medications. Numerous electrocardiographic (ECG) changes also occur, and both atrial and ventricular conduction time may be prolonged (Risch et al. 1981). These changes are thought to reflect a direct myocardial depressant action rather than a disruption of the autonomic nervous system or the CNS. Common ECG changes include abnormal T waves (blunting or notching), a prolonged QT interval, the appearance of U waves, and ST segment depression. These occur most frequently with the phenothiazines, but may also occur with other classes. It is fortunate that these effects seldom progress to heart blockages and typically resolve once the medication is discontinued. The use of high-potency medications is generally preferable in elderly patients and patients with a history of cardiovascular disease; in addition, these patients should be carefully monitored during the course of treatment.

Uncommon Side Effects

The following side effects occur relatively infrequently and therefore do not typically influence medication selection, although there are occasional exceptions. For example, grand mal seizures may occur with the use of any typical antipsychotic medication, but they have been most frequently reported with the use of chlorpromazine and seem least likely to occur with fluphenazine or thiothixene (Baldessarini 1990). Therefore, in patients with a known seizure disorder, it may be prudent to use either of the latter.

Central Nervous System Effects

Behavioral changes, affective flattening, and psychomotor slowing have all been associated with antipsychotic medications (American Medical Association 1992; Hollister 1983). These may be particularly bothersome in schizophrenic patients, who have a large degree of morbidity because of negative symptomatology. Hypothalamic dysregulation may also occur, with signs of hypo- and hyperthermia and weight gain. As previously mentioned, all phenothiazines have been implicated in lowering the seizure threshold; therefore, it is best to avoid these medications if possible in patients with a history of epilepsy. In patients withdrawing from CNS depressants (e.g., alcohol, barbiturates, benzodiazepines), a seizure may be more readily induced by the addition of antipsychotic medications.

Neuroendocrine Effects

Alterations in the regulation of the hypothalamic-pituitary axis may also occur. Typical antipsychotic medications cause an increase in circulating levels of prolactin, probably because of suppression of the hypothalamic inhibitory factor. Galactorrhea, lactation, and amenorrhea have all been reported in female patients on long-term maintenance with antipsychotic medication. Hyperprolactinemia in male patients is associated with decreased libido, impotence, and sterility (Hollister 1983). The syndrome of inappropriate secretion of antidiuretic hormone has been associated with antipsychotic medications, although it is unclear whether this is because of a direct effect on the hypothalamic-pituitary axis or a local effect on the renal tubules (Baldessarini 1990). This condition may lead to electrolyte abnormalities, most notably hyponatremia. Chlorpromazine is associated with increased plasma cholesterol, impairment in glucose tolerance, and inhibition of the release of corticotropin releasing factor and growth hormone (Baldessarini 1990); however, there have not been any clinical correlations (e.g., depression, growth retardation) with these alterations to date.

Ocular Effects

The most serious ocular complication is the pigmentary retinopathy associated with the use of thioridazine, typically with dosages exceeding 800 mg/day (American Medical Association 1992). This characteristically begins with deposits surrounding the macula lutea (bull's-eye lesion) and progresses to involve the entire retina. Loss of visual acuity may progress to total blindness if this condition is not detected early and the medication immediately discontinued.

Chlorpromazine may cause granular deposits in the cornea and lens; patients who are maintained on this medication should have periodic eye examinations for early detection of the deposits, because they resolve with discontinuation of the medication (Schatzberg and Cole 1991).

Hepatic Effects

Liver function abnormalities have been reported with the use of phenothiazines and the butyrophenone haloperidol (Levenson and Simpson 1987). Chlorpromazine has been by far the most commonly implicated antipsychotic medication, but this may be because chlorpromazine has been prescribed since the 1950s, when it became a model for drug-induced cholestatic hepatitis. Results from a Danish survey by Dossing and Andreasen (1982) indicated that the hepatitis was primarily cholestatic in 80% of cases and primarily cytotoxic in the remaining 20% of cases. In the same survey, it was also reported that the hepatitis progressed to chronic biliary cirrhosis in approximately 10% of patients. The mechanism behind this progression is still unclear, although it is most likely a hypersensitivity reaction that occurs in susceptible individuals. Because of the potential seriousness of hepatitis, it is recommended that liver function be monitored during the first 2–4 weeks of therapy; for patients with preexisting liver disease, monitoring should be extended to include at least the first 2 months of treatment.

Renal Effects

The effects of typical antipsychotic medications on renal function vary, possibly because of interactions at multiple levels of regulation. Chlorpromazine appears to have weak diuretic properties because of either suppression of antidiuretic hormone or direct action on the renal tubules (Baldessarini 1990). Conversely, haloperidol, thiothixene, fluphenazine, and thioridazine have all been associated with the syndrome of inappropriate secretion of antidiuretic hormone (SIADH) (Hollister 1983). These effects may lead to electrolyte abnormalities (i.e., hypernatremia and hyponatremia, respectively). Although such abnormalities are very uncommon, it may be prudent to initially monitor electrolytes in patients, especially in patients with impaired renal function or those on diuretic therapy.

Blood Dyscrasias

Numerous blood dyscrasias have been reported, including leukopenia, leukocytosis, and eosinophilia (Baldessarini 1990). However, the most serious and potentially fatal side effect is agranulocytosis, first reported in 1954, which occurs at a rate of less than 1:10,000 patients (Levenson and Simpson 1987). Agranulocytosis most frequently occurs with the use of high dosages of low-potency phenothiazines, such as chlorpromazine and thioridazine, during the first 2–3 months of treatment. It is hypothesized that this is because of the inhibition of mitosis (which arrests cell division), resulting in a progressive and sometimes rapid decline in the white blood cell count (Levenson and Simpson 1987). Periodic complete blood counts may lead to early detection, but because of the low incidence with typical antipsychotic medications, it is generally sufficient to monitor patients clinically for early signs of infection. If this side effect does occur, patients typically recover over the course of 1–3 weeks by discontinuing the medication and receiving supportive medical treatment. A nonphenothiazine may be initiated after recovery to manage persistent psychotic symptoms, provided blood counts are closely monitored.

Dermatologic Effects

Dermatologic reactions are relatively common with the phenothiazines, occurring in approximately 5% of patients (Baldessarini 1990). The two adverse effects include a hypersensitivity reaction and photosensitivity. The hypersensitivity reaction may be urticarial, maculopapular, petechial, or edematous. These reactions typically occur during the first few weeks of treatment and resolve with discontinuation of the medication. Photosensitivity may also occur, making patients susceptible to severe sunburn if not protected from the ultraviolet rays by a sunscreen containing p-aminobenzoic acid (Schatzberg and Cole 1991). In addition, chronic administration of high dosages of antipsychotic medication has been implicated (although rarely) in the development of abnormal pigmentation, typically a gray-blue pigmentation of the dermis in sun-exposed areas. This may gradually fade once the medication is discontinued.

Sexual Dysfunction

The α-adrenergic blockade that is typically produced by the lower potency medications may result in ejaculatory dysfunction (i.e., retrograde ejaculation) in male patients (Baldessarini 1990). Erectile dysfunction and priapism have also been reported, and, although these adverse effects are extremely unpleasant and often intolerable, they are rare. Female patients may experience anorgasmia, but this is also a relatively uncommon side effect. Because patients are often reluctant to mention adverse sexual effects, it is worthwhile to periodically inquire about any alterations in sexual performance.

Sudden Death

At this time, there is no clear relationship between the use of antipsychotic medications and sudden death (Levenson and Simpson 1987). The rates of death for patients taking antipsychotic medication do not differ from those of the general psychiatric population when controlling for concurrent medical illnesses. Results from numerous epidemiological studies have failed to demonstrate any clear association, and it is thought that if antipsychotic medications do contribute in some way to sudden death, it is so infrequent that it does not affect patient outcomes statistically. There are some authors who believe that antipsychotic medications are related to sudden death; they propose two possible mechanisms: aspiration with subsequent asphyxia and cardiovascular collapse attributable to a dysrhythmia or severe hypotension (Levenson and Simpson 1987). This clearly needs further investigation, but at this time antipsychotic medications do not appear to be a causative factor in the very rare cases of sudden death.

Conclusion

The introduction of typical antipsychotic drugs revolutionized the treatment of schizophrenia, and advances in psychopharmacology have led to the development of numerous classes of typical antipsychotic medications. However, these drugs have the potential to cause numerous bothersome and occasionally serious side effects. Because the efficacy of typical antipsychotic drugs is similar across classes, selection of a particular drug is based largely on the expected side effects. Although all classes share a common side effect profile, they vary markedly in the degree to which they produce adverse effects. The most common side effects include sedation and anticholinergic effects, which can often lead to noncompliance in sensitive patients. Cardiovascular effects, including hypotension and conduction delays, are also a primary consideration when selecting a particular medication. There are numerous other side effects, including CNS, neuroendocrine, ocular, hepatic, renal, and dermatological effects; blood dyscrasia; sexual dysfunction; and possibly sudden death. However, these are relatively uncommon and do not typically influence medication selection, although there are occasional exceptions. These potential side effects emphasize the need for close monitoring of all patients on typical antipsychotic medications; with close scrutiny of bothersome adverse effects, the use of antipsychotic medications is quite safe in the vast majority of patients.

References

American Medical Association: Antipsychotic drugs, in Drug Evaluations. Chicago, IL, American Medical Association, 1992, pp 245–267

Baldessarini RJ: Drugs and the treatment of psychiatric disorders, in The Pharmacological Basis of Therapeutics, 8th Edition. Edited by Gilman AG, Rall TW, Neis AS, et al. New York, Pergamon, 1990, pp 383–414

Dossing M, Andreasen PB: Drug-induced liver disease in Denmark: an analysis of 572 cases of hepatotoxicity reported to the Danish Board of adverse reaction to drugs. Scand J Gastroenterol 17:205–211, 1982

Hollister LE: Clinical Pharmacology of Psychotherapeutic Drugs, 2nd Edition, New York, Churchill Livingstone, 1983, pp 151–171

Levenson DF, Simpson GM: Serious nonextrapyramidal adverse effects of neuroleptics: sudden death, agranulocytosis, and hepatotoxicity, in Psychopharmacology: The Third Generation of Progress. Edited by Meltzer HY. New York, Raven, 1987, pp 1431–1436

Rifkin A, Siris S: Drug treatment of acute schizophrenia, in Psychopharmacology: The Third Generation of Progress. Edited by Meltzer HY, New York, Raven, 1987, pp 1095–1101

Risch SC, Groom GP, Janowski DS: Interfaces of psychopharmacology and cardiology—part 2. J Clin Psychiatry 42:47–59, 1981

Schatzberg AS, Cole JO: Manual of Clinical Psychopharmacology, 2nd Edition. Washington, DC, American Psychiatric Press, 1991, pp 85–143

Snyder SH: The dopamine hypothesis of schizophrenia. Am J Psychiatry 133:197–202, 1976

CHAPTER 25

Tardive Dyskinesia

Christian L. Shriqui, M.D., M.Sc., F.R.C.P.C., and
Lawrence Annable, B.Sc., Dip. Stat.

Tardive dyskinesia (TD) is a hyperkinetic syndrome of heterogeneous and involuntary abnormal movements continually present for at least 4 weeks, which occurs in predisposed individuals during or shortly following the cessation of long-term neuroleptic drug therapy (generally defined as a minimum of 3 months of total cumulative neuroleptic exposure), and which is not attributable to other causes (American Psychiatric Association 1992; Casey 1987; Shriqui 1988). Its prevalence, persistence, lack of effective treatment, and medicolegal implications are of major concern to clinicians prescribing maintenance neuroleptic drug therapy (American Psychiatric Association 1992; Baldessarini 1985; Casey 1985a, 1987; Feltner and Hertzman 1993; Kane and Smith 1982; Shriqui et al. 1990). The reversibility of the syndrome has been recognized since its earliest description (Schönecker 1957), but nevertheless, in many cases, TD is persistent and at times irreversible. In the great majority

This research was supported by a Scholarship Award and Research Grant 920852 from the Fonds de la Recherche en Santé du Québec (FRSQ) to Dr. Shriqui. **This chapter is dedicated to the memory of the late Dr. Ramzy Yassa.** The authors thank Serge Champetier for assistance in the manuscript preparation.

of cases, TD is of mild intensity, and patients are frequently unaware of its presence (Haag et al. 1992; Macpherson and Collis 1992). However, the involuntary movements of the face, lips, jaw, and tongue, with frequent protrusion or twisting of the tongue, constitute a further social handicap for patients with TD. In more severe cases, which are estimated to occur in fewer than 10% of patients (Haag et al. 1992), dyskinesias may interfere with speech and eating; cause irregular breathing; impair manual dexterity, mobility, and sexual intercourse; and pose a life-threatening danger (Casey and Rabins 1978; Chiang et al. 1985; Yassa and Jones 1985; Yassa and Lal 1985). Severe forms of TD may be associated with an increased risk of mortality, although the results of studies addressing this issue have been inconsistent (Kucharski et al. 1978; McClelland et al. 1986; Mehta et al. 1978; Yassa et al. 1984; Youssef and Waddington 1987).

Clinical Manifestations and Outcome

Clinical Description

Clinically, TD is characterized by involuntary, repetitive, purposeless hyperkinetic movements of a choreoathetoid and dystonic nature, varying in location and intensity (American Psychiatric Association 1992; Casey 1987). The word *dyskinesia* is a broad and nonspecific term that means "difficulty or abnormality in performing voluntary muscular movements" (Random House 1987, p. 611). The definitions of *chorea, athetosis,* and *dystonia,* as stated in the 1992 American Psychiatric Association (APA) Task Force Report on Tardive Dyskinesia (p. 9), are the following:

- *Chorea:* Rapid, jerky, quasi-purposive, nonrhythmic movements, especially of proximal body parts
- *Athetosis:* Slow, sinuous, writhing movements of distal parts of extremities
- *Dystonia:* Slow, sustained muscular contractions or spasms that may produce involuntary movements

The initial descriptions of TD emphasized orofacial movements, which are particularly frequent in elderly patients (Baldessarini 1985; Casey

1985a; Schönecker 1957; Sigwald et al. 1959). These movements include tongue protrusion, puckering and smacking of the lips, pouting, chewing, lateral jaw movements, and puffing of the cheeks. Other facial movements can include grimacing, blinking, and frowning. However, TD frequently involves other body areas, such as the upper and lower limbs, neck, and trunk. At times, the fingers and toes move in a repetitive pattern that resembles piano-playing movements (Casey 1987). The abnormal movements tend to increase with emotional stress, decrease or disappear during relaxation, and disappear during sleep (American Psychiatric Association 1992). Respiratory dyskinesia, once believed to be a rare complication of TD, was recently observed in 45% of a cohort of 76 patients with typical orofacial TD (Youssef and Waddington 1989). As mentioned earlier, severe forms of TD can be crippling and potentially life threatening (Casey and Rabins 1978; Gardos et al. 1987).

Types of Dyskinesias

Three types of dyskinesia have been described with respect to their time of onset (Casey 1987; Gardos et al. 1978; Schooler and Kane 1982):

- *Covert dyskinesia* is unmasked when neuroleptic drugs are reduced or discontinued.
- *Withdrawal dyskinesia* appears under similar circumstances but, by definition, resolves spontaneously within 3 months.
- *Overt dyskinesia* is present during the course of neuroleptic treatment.

The Schooler and Kane research diagnostic criteria for TD were proposed in 1982 to introduce some uniformity into the diagnosis of TD (Schooler and Kane 1982). These research diagnostic criteria are composed of three prerequisites: the patient must 1) have received at least 3 months of cumulative neuroleptic drug exposure; 2) display at least moderate abnormal involuntary movements in one or more body areas, or mild involuntary movements in two or more body areas; and 3) not have other conditions that produce involuntary hyperkinetic dyskinesias.

Related Movement Disorders

Two other late-developing movement disorders that have recently been described, and that are generally considered to be distinct from TD, are *tardive dystonia* and *tardive akathisia*. However, the extent to which these atypical tardive syndromes—particularly tardive dystonia—have their own distinct pathophysiology or represent symptom clusters of a general TD syndrome remains highly controversial (American Psychiatric Association 1992; Casey 1991).

Tardive dystonia is characterized by a sustained and often torsional abnormal posture involving the face, neck, trunk, or limbs, and is commonly associated with pain and disability (American Psychiatric Association 1992; Burke and Kang 1988; Burke et al. 1982; Wojcik et al. 1991). Tardive dystonia clinically resembles acute dystonia, but can persist for months and years following the withdrawal of neuroleptics (Burke et al. 1982; Gardos et al. 1987). The reported prevalence of tardive dystonia in schizophrenic outpatients and chronic hospitalized psychiatric patients is estimated at 1%–2% (Friedman et al. 1987; Sachdev 1991). Sachdev (1993) reported on the clinical characteristics of 15 patients with tardive dystonia, observing that the syndrome occurred in all age groups and in both genders. Consistent with previous findings by other investigators, there was a slight preponderance of tardive dystonia in male patients; furthermore, a frequent overlap of tardive dystonia with TD and tardive akathisia was reported.

Tardive akathisia is characterized by a compulsive and persistent restlessness (Barnes and Braude 1985), with repetitive actions primarily involving the limbs, face, and trunk. The acute form of akathisia is a well-known side effect of neuroleptic drug therapy, but the tardive form has only recently been recognized as a late-occurring or persistent side effect (American Psychiatric Association 1992; Burke et al. 1989).

The appearance of TD is often preceded by other neuroleptic-induced extrapyramidal side effects (EPS), such as parkinsonism, dystonia, and akathisia. At a later stage, TD frequently coexists with neuroleptic-induced parkinsonism and tardive forms of akathisia and dystonia (Chouinard et al. 1988; Hoffman et al. 1987; Richardson and Craig 1982; Sandyk et al. 1991).

Long-Term Course

The long-term outcome of TD has varied widely across studies, probably as a result of the different patient populations and different treatment regimens studied (Casey 1987; Casey and Gerlach 1986; Chouinard et al. 1988; Gardos et al. 1994; Nair and Yassa 1994; Yassa and Nair 1989, 1992). Generally speaking, investigators have found that, in most patients, the severity of the disorder tends to plateau at a mild level or shows a fluctuating course with periods of spontaneous remission (American Psychiatric Association 1992; Chouinard et al. 1988; Gardos et al. 1994). However, in certain patients, notably those over age 55 years, the disorder may progress to more severe forms that constitute a major physical impairment (Altamura et al. 1990; American Psychiatric Association 1992; Gardos et al. 1987; Giménez-Roldàn et al. 1985; Johnson et al. 1982; Yassa et al. 1990).

Although the course of TD can improve with or without cessation of neuroleptic treatment, results from several naturalistic and controlled studies have suggested that dosage reduction or discontinuation of neuroleptics leads to a better outcome for many patients with TD (American Psychiatric Association 1992; Casey 1985a; Chouinard et al. 1988; Fornazzari et al. 1989; Gardos et al. 1988; Glazer et al. 1990, 1991; Kane et al. 1983; Morns et al. 1993; Nair and Yassa 1994). (For example, see the review of studies using low-dosage as opposed to standard-dosage neuroleptic drug therapy and brief intermittent or targeted neuroleptic treatment and their influence on the course of TD in Chapter 20 of this book).

There have been very few systematic studies of TD in children and adolescents; in these populations, the treatment-emergent type of TD is the most frequent. Richardson et al. (1991), in their study of 104 neuroleptic-treated children and adolescents, reported a 12% prevalence of treatment-emergent TD. In this age group, none of the patients manifested signs of tardive dystonia.

Patient variables (e.g., age, gender, psychiatric diagnosis), treatment parameters (e.g., drug dosage, cumulative exposure, duration of treatment [continuous versus intermittent]), and temporal aspects (e.g., TD duration, length of follow-up) are factors that can influence the outcome of TD (Baldessarini 1985; Casey 1985a, 1987, 1991;

Casey and Gerlach 1986; Chouinard et al. 1988; Jeste and Caligiuri 1992; Kane and Smith 1982; Kane et al. 1984, 1988; Nair and Yassa 1994; Shriqui and Annable 1994). These factors are discussed in the section on risk factors for TD.

Diagnostic Issues

Diagnosing Tardive Dyskinesia

The diagnosis of TD is based on clinical observations and patient report rather than on objective laboratory test results, and should be considered in any patient with abnormal involuntary movements and a neuroleptic medication history of at least 3 months (Kane et al. 1984). Extensive laboratory tests are unnecessary for most patients who potentially have TD (American Psychiatric Association 1992). However, when a patient has a clinical history or physical signs that reveal a rapidly progressive dyskinesia, a positive family history of movement disorder, a history suggestive of a brain lesion, a dementia or significant cognitive impairment of unknown origin, or signs of neurologic, metabolic, or endocrine dysfunction, the clinician should order a laboratory workup for that patient, including a complete blood count, serum electrolytes, liver function tests, serum copper, ceruloplasmin, connective tissue screen, and, in suspected cases of Wilson's disease, urinary copper and amino acids (American Psychiatric Association 1992). Furthermore, in the presence of a rapidly progressive dyskinesia, a computed tomography (CT) or, preferably, a magnetic resonance imaging (MRI) brain scan is strongly recommended. Nonetheless, in addition to conducting a full patient history and physical and neurological examinations, some authors recommend that a skull X ray, electroencephalogram, and detailed blood chemistry be done in all patients presumed to have TD (Haag et al. 1992).

In recent years, clinical psychiatrists appear to be increasingly using clinical rating scales for TD, such as the Abnormal Involuntary Movement Scale (Guy 1976), the Abbreviated Rockland Simpson Scale for TD (Simpson et al. 1979), or the Extrapyramidal Symptom Rating

Scale (Chouinard et al. 1980b). Most likely, this increased usage is a direct consequence of greater physician awareness and training in the recognition, diagnosis, and management of acute and tardive EPS. Focused physician training in neuroleptic-induced movement disorders, including TD, takes only a few hours and has been shown to increase diagnostic skills (Dixon et al. 1989). Such training seminars are increasingly becoming an integral part of the psychiatric residency curricula of many medical faculties. Specific nursing training in the recognition of EPS and TD is often less systematic.

Differential Diagnosis

Because the diagnosis of TD is made largely by exclusion, clinicians should be careful not to overdiagnose the syndrome (Khot and Wyatt 1991). The differential diagnosis of TD is extensive (American Psychiatric Association 1992; Casey 1987; Cummings and Wirshing 1989; Kane et al. 1984; Lohr et al. 1986; Shriqui 1988) and is summarized in Table 25–1.

Spontaneous dyskinesias occur primarily in elderly patients and are usually orofacial in their distribution. The prevalence rate of this type of dyskinesia has been estimated at 4%–7% (Casey 1985b). However, recent reports indicate significantly higher rates for spontaneous oral dyskinesias, and edentulousness has been suggested to contribute to

Table 25–1. Differential diagnosis of tardive dyskinesia

Stereotyped movements and mannerisms associated with schizophrenia

Spontaneous oral dyskinesias of advanced age or senility

Huntington's disease, Wilson's disease, Tourette syndrome

Rheumatic (Sydenham's) chorea; postanoxic and postencephalitic extrapyramidal syndromes

Drug intoxications (L-dopa, amphetamines, anticholinergics, antidepressants, lithium, phenytoin)

Central nervous system complications of systemic metabolic disorders (e.g., hepatic or renal failure, hyperthyroidism, hypoparathyroidism, hypoglycemia)

Brain neoplasm (thalamic, basal ganglia)

Fahr's syndrome (familial calcification of the basal ganglia)

Focal dystonias (Meige syndrome, spasmodic torticollis)

the high rate of orofacial dyskinetic movements in elderly patients (Woerner et al. 1991).

The rabbit syndrome (Villeneuve 1972), a rare condition characterized by a rapid tremor of the lips, was once thought to be a manifestation of TD. It is now considered to be a parkinsonian side effect of neuroleptics and is responsive to antiparkinsonian agents (American Psychiatric Association 1992; Jus et al. 1974; Simpson et al. 1986; Wada and Yamaguchi 1992).

TD also needs to be distinguished from acute EPS (see Chapter 22 of this book) and from involuntary choreoathetoid movements induced by a wide variety of nonneuroleptic drugs (Lohr et al. 1986). However, it is only with neuroleptic agents that cases of persistent TD have been reported. Among the nonneuroleptics, the long-term use of metoclopramide (a drug commonly used for the treatment of gastrointestinal disorders) is associated with the occurrence of dyskinetic movements (Grimes et al. 1982; Mahler and Brown 1987).

Epidemiology

Prevalence and Incidence

Prevalence estimates for TD have varied greatly across studies, depending on the patient population studied and the method of diagnosis followed. Authors of the 1992 APA Task Force Report on Tardive Dyskinesia concluded that probably 15%–20% of patients receiving chronic neuroleptic treatment have some evidence of dyskinesia, ranging from a transient form of the condition to moderate or extreme forms. In a review of 76 studies of the prevalence of TD, Yassa and Jeste (1992) found an overall prevalence of 24.2% among a total of 39,187 patients. Likewise, Kane and Smith (1982) estimated the mean prevalence rate of TD to be about 20%, based on a retrospective analysis of 34,555 patients enrolled in 56 studies published from 1959 to 1979. In a sample of 1,745 patients, the overall prevalence of TD was 19.1% (Muscettola et al. 1993). Altamura et al. (1990) examined a population of 148 chronic schizophrenic patients and observed a

32% prevalence of TD. Other studies have reported even higher prevalence estimates of TD (Annable et al. 1989; Chouinard et al. 1988; Fleischauer et al. 1985; Hoffman et al. 1987; Saltz et al. 1989; Toenniessen et al. 1985; Yassa et al. 1983a, 1983b, 1988a), particularly in elderly patients (Crane and Smeets 1974; Lieberman et al. 1985; Yassa et al. 1988b).

Differences in the patient populations studied are probably a major factor in the wide variations among studies in the prevalence of TD. Studies of risk factors for TD have suggested that vulnerability to TD may depend on age, gender, psychiatric diagnosis, neuroleptic drug history (including dosage, mode of delivery, and duration and continuity of treatment), concomitant medications, and organic brain dysfunction, (American Psychiatric Association 1992), among other factors. (See the review of risk factors in following section.) In addition, differences in diagnostic methods and in the timing of evaluations for patients on injectable neuroleptics may also contribute to differences in prevalence estimates.

The extent to which some of these dyskinetic movements may be forms of abnormal involuntary movements that occur spontaneously in schizophrenic patients has been widely debated (American Psychiatric Association 1992). In 1991, Khot and Wyatt estimated that the true prevalence rate of TD, corrected for spontaneous dyskinesia, was below 20% for all age groups except the age range of 70–79 years. Those authors concluded that, after age 40 years, the prevalence of spontaneous dyskinesia is sufficiently high to warrant the consideration that many patients with a diagnosis of TD may in fact have abnormal movements attributable to causes other than neuroleptic medication. Because the likelihood of developing abnormal involuntary movements during neuroleptic treatment increases with age, Khot and Wyatt (1991) suggested that TD movements could be physiologically identical to spontaneous movements, but that neuroleptics facilitate the onset of the former. Nevertheless, the prevailing view is that neuroleptic drugs do play a major role in producing or precipitating dyskinetic movements in schizophrenic patients (American Psychiatric Association 1992).

In a follow-up study of 169 largely middle-aged schizophrenic outpatients, Chouinard et al. (1988) found that the prevalence of TD increased from 22% at baseline to 44% after 5 years. Of 131 patients who did not manifest TD at the start of the study, 35% developed it at an annual incidence rate of 8.4%. On the other hand, TD apparently remitted in 9 of the 38 patients in whom it had been present at the beginning of the study. Ninety-eight patients were followed for an additional 5 years, at the end of which (i.e., at 10 years) the prevalence of TD had increased to 56% (Annable et al. 1989). For the majority of these patients, the TD was of mild intensity.

In another 10-year outcome study of TD, Gardos et al. (1994) followed 63 of 122 neuroleptic-treated patients over 5- and 10-year periods. In this group of patients, the overall prevalence of TD remained stable at around 30%. Not only was there no overall increase in TD, but no subgroup showed a significant increase in severity of TD over the 10-year follow-up period. The results of this study are encouraging, as they suggest that TD can have a benign long-term course, even in the face of continued use of neuroleptics. However, these study results contrast with those reported by Chouinard et al. (1988) and Annable et al. (1989), who observed a high and increasing prevalence of TD during the course of a 10-year follow-up. A possible reason for this difference may relate to the much higher dosages of neuroleptics used in the patient cohort studied by Chouinard et al. (1988) and Annable et al. (1989).

In a cohort of 101 patients followed for 4 years, Bergen et al. (1989) reported that 24% of the patients had fluctuating TD status. These authors also reported that the proportion of TD-negative or TD-positive patients was relatively stable during the follow-up period.

In a 10-year follow-up study of 44 patients with TD, Yassa and Nair (1992) reported that a majority of the patients had no change in TD severity. However, patients whose TD improved had received a lower dosage of neuroleptics than those whose TD worsened. Yassa and Nair further reported that female patients showed a higher rate of improvement in their TD than did male patients.

In a 16-year follow-up study of facial dyskinesia in 99 female patients from a mental hospital population, McClelland et al. (1991) reported an increase in the prevalence of dyskinesia from 18.4% to 46.5%, which was significantly associated with the total dosage and duration of neuroleptics.

Several follow-up studies have examined the incidence of new cases of TD in cohorts of patients over varying periods of time. Results from an ongoing prospective study by Kane and colleagues (1988, 1994) in a large, diagnostically heterogeneous cohort of patients have suggested a cumulative TD incidence rate of approximately 5% per year in adult populations during the first 5 years of antipsychotic drug exposure. However, the incidence rate of TD in elderly patients treated for the first time with antipsychotic medication is considerably higher. In an ongoing cohort study of 215 newly treated, neuroleptic-naive elderly patients with a mean age of 77 years, Saltz et al. (1991) reported a 31% cumulative incidence rate after 43 weeks of cumulative neuroleptic exposure. Jeste et al. (1994), in their ongoing study, examined 275 psychiatric outpatients over age 45 years suffering from Alzheimer's disease, schizophrenia, and mood disorder. The patients included in the study had a median duration of total lifetime neuroleptic exposure at baseline of 26 days, and a current average neuroleptic dosage of less than 150 mg chlorpromazine equivalents. Although TD was diagnosed using slightly modified Schooler and Kane (1982) research diagnostic criteria, the results to date indicate that 26% of the patients developed TD by the end of 12 months of treatment, 52% by the end of 24 months, and 60% by the end of 36 months.

Risk Factors

Age. Numerous studies have identified age as the principal risk factor for the development of TD in schizophrenic patients on long-term neuroleptic therapy, a finding that cannot be attributed to an increased duration of neuroleptic treatment alone (American Psychiatric Association 1992). The risk of developing TD in elderly patients receiving neuroleptics for the first time is much higher than in younger patients (Jeste et al. 1994; Kane et al. 1994; Saltz et al. 1991). It also appears that elderly patients are vulnerable to more severe and persistent forms of the disorder (Kane and Smith 1982). The cause of this increased risk of TD with aging is unknown, but it seems likely that age-related changes in neuroreceptors and neuronal degeneration may play a role (American Psychiatric Association 1992).

Gender. A second consistent finding is that neuroleptic-treated women seem to be at a slightly greater overall risk for TD, and also tend to develop more severe forms of TD than men (American Psychiatric Association 1992; Muscettola et al. 1993; Yassa and Jeste 1992). In a review of 76 selected studies, Yassa and Jeste (1992) observed that the prevalence of TD in 39,187 patients was significantly higher in women (26.6%) than in men (21.6%).

Results from several studies have suggested that the risk of TD increases appreciably after menopause (Yassa and Jeste 1992). It has been proposed that estrogen might have a protective antidopaminergic effect in premenopausal women (Raymond et al. 1978), and that the decline in estrogen levels at menopause would account for the increased prevalence of TD in older women (Chouinard et al. 1980a).

Psychiatric diagnosis. The issue of whether the abnormal movements seen in untreated schizophrenic patients are of the dyskinetic type, and of whether schizophrenia constitutes a risk factor for TD, has been widely debated (Awouters et al. 1990; Barnes and Liddle 1985; Chorfi and Moussaoui 1989; Marsden 1985; Marsden et al. 1975; Owens 1985; Rogers 1992; Waddington and Youssef 1990). Owens (1985), for example, considered that antipsychotic drugs act to promote or exacerbate the inherent tendency for schizophrenic patients to develop spontaneous movement disorders.

A related finding has been that schizophrenic patients with negative symptoms (e.g., emotional withdrawal, flattening of affect, motor retardation, reduced social interest) or a poor prognosis have been found to have a higher prevalence of TD than those without these features (Barnes and Liddle 1985; Barnes et al. 1989; Chouinard et al. 1988; Jeste et al. 1984; Johnstone et al. 1991; Waddington 1987). In an age-matched group of schizophrenic patients, those with negative symptoms were found to have developed TD at an earlier age (Barnes et al. 1989). However, opposite findings, associating TD with positive schizophrenic symptoms, have also been reported (Gureje 1988; Sandyk and Kay 1991, 1992; Sandyk et al. 1991). At the present time, a majority of studies favor an association between TD and negative schizophrenic symptoms; however, most studies reporting this association generally included older patients.

Several but not all investigators (Inada and Yagi 1992) have indicated that schizoaffective and affective disorder patients treated with antipsychotic drugs have a higher TD prevalence than schizophrenic patients (Kane and Smith 1982; Kane et al. 1988; Parepally et al. 1989; Waddington 1989; Waddington and Youssef 1988; Yassa et al. 1983a, 1983b, 1992). A positive family history of affective illness in schizophrenic patients has also been associated with an increased risk of neuroleptic-induced parkinsonism (Galdi et al. 1981) and TD (Richardson et al. 1985).

Specific neuroleptic prescribed. No differences have been demonstrated among the standard neuroleptics with respect to their propensity to induce TD (Morgenstern and Glazer 1993). However, studies of this issue are limited by the practice of polypharmacy and the fact that most patients have been treated at different times with different neuroleptics. Certain novel antipsychotics, such as clozapine and possibly risperidone, may carry a lower risk of TD. Differences in the relative binding affinities between central dopamine D_2 and serotonin $5\text{-}HT_2$ receptors at the mesolimbic and nigrostriatal regions of the brain are thought to be involved in the reduced EPS and TD liability of novel antipsychotic drugs (American Psychiatric Association 1992; Casey 1992; Meltzer et al. 1989). It has been suggested that typical and atypical antipsychotics can be differentiated based on the lower dopamine D_2 and higher serotonin $5\text{-}HT_2$ pKi values of the atypical agents. Meltzer et al. (1989) proposed that a $5\text{-}HT_2\text{-}D_2$ ratio greater than or equivalent to 1.12 defines an atypical antipsychotic.

Depot neuroleptics, particularly depot fluphenazine (Gardos et al. 1977; Smith et al. 1978), have been associated with a higher prevalence of TD, but there is no consistent evidence supporting this association (Glazer and Kane 1992; Yassa et al. 1988a). Rather, TD may be more easily uncovered during treatment with depot neuroleptics as the result of a decline in neuroleptic plasma levels that may occur toward the end of the injection interval (Chouinard et al. 1982).

Neuroleptic dosage. Recent studies have reported a greater prevalence and incidence of TD in elderly patients receiving low dosages of neuroleptics (Chiu et al. 1992, 1993; Harris et al. 1992). However, this finding could be a consequence of the masking effect of higher dosages of neuroleptics and may also be related to age, as older patients are at greater risk for TD but are commonly prescribed lower dosages of neuroleptics. Nevertheless, results from some studies (Kane et al. 1994; Morgenstern and Glazer 1993) have suggested that the TD rate is greatest during the first 5 years of neuroleptic treatment, and that the rate increases with treatment duration and higher cumulative dosages of neuroleptics (American Psychiatric Association 1992; Annable et al. 1989; Chouinard et al. 1988; Kane et al. 1989). There is also evidence that, in the subgroup of patients who can be successfully maintained on lower dosages of neuroleptic medications, the short-term risk of TD is lower (Kane et al. 1983; Morgenstern and Glazer 1993). Findings as to the relationship between neuroleptic plasma levels and TD have been inconsistent, with some studies reporting a positive correlation and others not (American Psychiatric Association 1992).

Interrupted medication regimen.   "Drug holidays" for patients on long-term neuroleptic drug therapy were first advocated as a possible means of reducing the risk of TD in the American College of Neuropsychopharmacology's Food and Drug Administration Task Force 1973 report. However, results from the few clinical trials that have investigated this possibility have indicated that interrupted treatment with neuroleptics may actually increase the likelihood of persistent TD as well as of schizophrenic relapse (Goldman and Luchins 1984; Jeste et al. 1979).

Presence of other extrapyramidal side effects.   Several investigators (Annable et al. 1989; Casey 1991; Chouinard et al. 1988; Crane 1972; Kane et al. 1988; Saltz et al. 1991) have suggested that susceptibility to neuroleptic-induced parkinsonism is a risk factor for subsequent development of TD, and that drug-induced parkinsonism frequently coexists with TD. It has also been reported that patients with acute akathisia may be more likely to manifest TD (Barnes and Braude 1985; Chouinard et al. 1979a). On the basis of case reports, Nasrallah et al. (1980) and Munetz (1980) suggested that acute dystonic reactions might also predict a future disposition to TD.

Concomitant use of other drugs. Use of anticholinergic drugs, dopamine-blocking antiemetics, metoclopramide, and amoxapine are potential treatment-related risk factors for TD. Although anticholinergic agents can uncover or worsen existing TD, and their withdrawal can improve the condition (Chouinard et al. 1979b; Yassa 1988), there is no evidence indicating that the long-term use of these agents clearly increases the development of TD (American Psychiatric Association 1992; Yassa 1988). Because patients with EPS are more likely to receive antiparkinsonian anticholinergic medication, and EPS frequently precede the development of or coexist with TD, any association between anticholinergic medication and TD may in fact be an epiphenomenon (American Psychiatric Association 1992; Barnes 1990). However, in a population of 1,745 patients, Muscettola et al. (1993) reported that the use of high dosages of neuroleptics, increased duration of treatment, and regular combined use of neuroleptic and antiparkinsonian drugs were significantly associated with TD.

Other risk factors. Some studies have suggested an association between various types of organic brain dysfunction—resulting from toxic insult, epilepsy, alcoholism, or other neuropathology—and the development or intensity of TD (Chouinard et al. 1979a; Edwards 1970; Perris et al. 1979). In support of this association, Youssef and Waddington (1988) observed an overrepresentation of primitive (developmental) reflexes in schizophrenic and bipolar affective disorder patients with TD.

Cognitive impairment is frequently reported in patients with TD (Brown and White 1991a, 1991b, 1992; Brown et al. 1992b; Cooper et al. 1991; Davis et al. 1992; Famuyiwa et al. 1979; Karson et al. 1993; Sorokin et al. 1988; Waddington 1987; Waddington and Youssef 1986, 1988; Waddington et al. 1987), although a robust correlation has not been found in all studies (Gold et al. 1991).

In recent years, diabetes mellitus (specifically, type II, noninsulin-dependent diabetes mellitus) has been identified as a significant risk factor for TD. Cross-sectional prevalence studies have shown that diabetes mellitus increases the risk of TD by 50%–100% (Casey and Ganzini 1994; Ganzini et al. 1992; Mukherjee et al. 1991).

Other risk factors that have been reported for TD include alcohol abuse (Dixon et al. 1992; Olivera et al. 1990), ethnic origin (in particular, having an African American heritage; Morgenstern and Glazer 1993), and displaying a standard cerebral dominance pattern (right-handedness) (Barr et al. 1989; Brown et al. 1992a; Kern et al. 1991). Attempts to correlate TD with specific human leukocyte antigens have yielded equivocal results (Brown and White 1991c; Metzer et al. 1990).

With regard to nicotine exposure, results from two studies have shown a positive correlation with TD (Binder et al. 1987; Yassa et al. 1987). Menza et al. (1991) observed a positive association between smoking and the use of higher dosages of neuroleptics, although patients who smoked did not have increased TD. Zaretsky et al. (1993) examined the relationship between psychoactive substance use (as opposed to abuse) and TD in a sample of 51 neuroleptic-treated, chronic schizophrenic outpatients. Current weekly cannabis use was positively correlated with the presence and severity of TD. However, because patients in this sample used cannabis as the sole nonalcoholic substance, further studies are required to evaluate the relative risk specificity of cannabis.

Pathophysiology

Despite considerable research efforts, a clear understanding of the pathophysiological mechanisms involved in TD is still lacking (American Psychiatric Association 1992; Casey 1991; Egan 1994; Jeste and Wyatt 1982a; Lieberman et al. 1988). The current view is that TD is not a unitary syndrome (American Psychiatric Association 1992). Two subsyndromes of TD—orofacial and limb-truncal—with potentially distinct pathophysiologies are often distinguished clinically (Brown and White 1992; Gureje 1988, 1989; Kidger et al. 1980). In elderly patients, orofacial dyskinesia has been associated with aging and schizophrenia, whereas limb-truncal dyskinesia has been linked with treatment variables (Gureje 1988).

Investigators have begun using positron-emission tomography (PET) to study the dopaminergic system of patients with TD. Blin et al. (1989) examined eight neuroleptic-free patients with persistent TD and found that the striatal D_2 receptor density was not elevated in those patients when compared with that of age-matched normal (non-psychiatric) control subjects, but was positively correlated with the severity of orofacial dyskinesia. In another PET study, Andersson et al. (1990) compared 11 patients, 8 of whom had TD, with 5 healthy control subjects. All subjects had been off neuroleptics for at least 4 weeks. No differences could be found in D_2 receptor density between the control subjects and the patients with and without TD. Although investigators in some postmortem studies have reported upregulation of D_2 receptors following neuroleptic treatment, these studies have not shown differences in D_2 receptor numbers between patients with and without TD (Crow et al. 1982; Kornhuber et al. 1989).

There is considerable evidence supporting biochemical and pharmacological heterogeneity in TD and its various subtypes (Jeste and Wyatt 1982a, 1982b; Jeste et al. 1988; Lieberman et al. 1988; Nasrallah et al. 1986). For example, the dopamine-blocking agent papaverine has been reported to improve orofacial dyskinesia but to worsen limb dyskinesia (Gardos et al. 1976).

Dopaminergic receptor hypothesis.   Among the many biochemical hypotheses suggested for TD, the one that has received the most attention, despite numerous limitations, is that of dopamine receptor supersensitivity in the nigrostriatal dopamine pathway (American Psychiatric Association 1980; Casey 1987; Jenner and Marsden 1986; Jeste and Wyatt 1981, 1982a; Jeste et al. 1986; Lieberman 1989; Waddington 1985). By chronically blocking postsynaptic dopamine receptors, neuroleptics would create a chemical state analogous to surgical denervation, with prolonged receptor blockade sensitizing the receptors (by increasing the affinity of postsynaptic dopamine receptors), increasing the number of these receptors, or both. Limitations of this hypothesis include the fact that neuroleptic-treated rats and monkeys develop dopamine receptor supersensitivity within a few hours or days, whereas TD in humans is a late-occurring side effect in only some patients (Casey 1987; Jenner and Marsden 1986; Jeste and Wyatt 1981, 1982a; Jeste et al. 1986; Lieberman 1989; Waddington 1985). Although dyskinesias that emerge during neuroleptic withdrawal might result from a supersensitivity mechanism, it is unlikely that this hypothesis can explain persistent forms of TD, as the receptor supersensitivity in animals is frequently short-lived and can often be elicited after only a single injection of a neuroleptic (Jeste and Wyatt 1981, 1982a; Jeste et al. 1986).

Another objection to the dopaminergic supersensitivity hypothesis is that TD and neuroleptic-induced parkinsonism are frequently observed simultaneously in the same patient, despite the fact that, according to this theory, they result from increased and decreased amounts, respectively, of dopamine activity in the basal ganglia.

The heterogeneity of TD, both in its clinical manifestations and in its response to various agents, makes it likely that, apart from dopamine, other neurotransmitters (particularly norepinephrine, gamma-aminobutyric acid [GABA], acetylcholine, and serotonin) may be involved in its pathophysiology (Casey 1987; Glazer 1989; Jenner and Marsden 1986; Jeste and Wyatt 1981, 1982a; Jeste et al. 1986; Lieberman et al. 1988; Nasrallah et al. 1986; Sandyk and Fisher 1988; Seibyl et al. 1989; Shriqui 1988; Waddington 1985).

Catecholaminergic hyperactivity.   Evidence in favor of catecholaminergic hyperactivity in TD patients is suggested by elevated plasma dopamine-β-hydroxylase activity (Jeste and Wyatt 1982a; Jeste et al. 1986; Kaufmann et al. 1986).

GABAergic dysfunction.   GABA is frequently implicated in the pathophysiology of TD (Casey 1987; Jeste and Wyatt 1982a; Jeste et al. 1986; Thaker et al. 1987, 1989). The inhibitory effect of GABA on dopaminergic neurons is the rationale for increasing GABA activity as a treatment for TD (Casey 1987). Now, however, clinical use of GABAmimetic drugs is based on the critical role that GABAergic neurons play in the substantia nigra pars reticulata in mediating dyskinetic movements (Scheel-Kruger 1986). These substantia nigra pars reticulata GABA-containing neurons form an important inhibitory efferent pathway from the basal ganglia (Thaker et al. 1990). In animals, disruption of these GABAergic efferents can produce hyperkinetic involuntary movements (Arnt and Scheel-Kruger 1980). Chronic neuroleptic treatment in animals has resulted in a loss of striatal neurons (which could be GABAergic) and in a reduction of glutamic acid decarboxylase—the enzyme that catalyzes the synthesis of GABA activity in the substantia nigra (Gunne and Häggström 1985; Jeste and Wyatt 1982a; Jeste et al. 1986). In an experimental model, Gunne and Häggström (1985) found that monkeys chronically treated with neuroleptics that developed a dyskinetic syndrome demonstrated a reduction in glutamic acid decarboxylase activity, whereas similarly treated animals without dyskinesia did not. Treatment with GABAergic drugs (e.g., clonazepam, muscimol, gamma-acetylenic GABA) has reduced symptom severity in patients with TD (Jeste and Wyatt 1982a; Jeste et al. 1986; Tamminga et al. 1979; Thaker et al. 1990). These observations have led to the proposal that a GABAergic dysfunction may be an important underlying mechanism in TD (Fibiger and Lloyd 1984; Gunne et al. 1984; Jeste et al. 1986; Tamminga et al. 1979; Thaker et al. 1990).

Free-radical mechanisms. Whereas dopamine receptor supersensitivity is a frequent or essential component of TD, it is most likely insufficient to explain the heterogeneous and complex nature of the syndrome (Lieberman 1989). Biochemical mechanisms contributing to neuronal damage in patients with persistent TD are unknown, but may involve the action of cytotoxic free radicals (Cadet 1988; Cadet and Lohr 1989; Cadet et al. 1986, 1987; Cohen 1984; Fridovich 1983; Lohr 1991; Lohr et al. 1988; Shriqui and Jones 1990a, 1990b; Szymanski et al. 1992). This hypothesis suggests that neuronal damage in TD, particularly in the nigrostriatal region, would result from the cytotoxic effects of free radicals through membrane lipid peroxidation. The basal ganglia, by virtue of their high lipid and oxygen consumption, elevated concentration of transition metals (Riederer et al. 1989), and high metabolic activity derived from hydrogen peroxide formation, are particularly vulnerable to the cytotoxic effects of free radicals. By increasing catecholamine turnover, neuroleptics would stimulate an increased production of oxidative free radicals (Korpi and Wyatt 1984). Some investigators (Lohr 1991; Lohr et al. 1989, 1990; Pall et al. 1987; Peet et al. 1993a) have reported increased levels of lipid peroxidation products in the plasma and cerebrospinal fluid of dyskinetic compared with nondyskinetic patients treated with neuroleptics. This neurodegenerative process could in turn contribute to a disruption of inhibitory, potentially GABAergic, efferent pathways from the basal ganglia.

Other hypotheses. Altered serotonin neurotransmission has also been suggested to play a role in the development of TD (Sandyk and Fisher 1988; Seibyl et al. 1989). According to this hypothesis, 5-HT neurons projecting from the raphe nuclei to the striatum would exert an inhibitory effect on dopamine function, which has resulted in the testing of serotonergic agents such as the serotonin precursor 5-hydroxytryptophan (5-HTP) in the treatment of TD (Nasrallah et al. 1982, 1986).

Other neurochemical abnormalities, such as cholinergic hypoactivity, may also play a role in the occurrence of specific subtypes of persistent TD (Casey 1987; Jeste and Wyatt 1982a; Jeste et al. 1986; Shriqui 1988). Finally, another neurodegenerative hypothesis of TD involves the toxic effects to cell membranes of long-term accumulation of neuroleptics in neuromelanin granules and neuroleptic myelin (Seeman 1988).

Current evidence indicates that a combination of neurochemical and neuroanatomical abnormalities (discussed in the following section) occur in patients with TD (Jeste and Wyatt 1981, 1982a; Jeste et al. 1986).

Evidence for Structural Abnormalities in Tardive Dyskinesia

Some neuropathological studies have reported increased nigral degeneration and gliosis in TD patients (Arai et al. 1987; Christensen et al. 1970). In schizophrenic and bipolar patients, pineal gland calcification has been suggested as a potential neuroradiological marker of persistent TD (Sandyk 1988, 1990a, 1990b).

Increased iron deposits in the basal ganglia of TD patients (Campbell et al. 1985; Hunter et al. 1968) have been associated with MRI findings of abnormal (shortened) T2 relaxation times in the basal ganglia of patients with TD (Bartzokis et al. 1990, 1991; Drayer 1987; Drayer et al. 1986; Lohr 1991; Rutledge et al. 1987). Cytotoxic free radicals would be actively involved in this process by way of an iron–neuroleptic drug interaction (Bartzokis et al. 1990; Lohr 1991).

X rays, CT scans, and, more recently, MRI scans have been used to investigate neuroanatomical abnormalities in patients with TD. Because of its widespread availability and lower cost compared with MRI (Andreasen et al. 1989), CT is the most frequently used brain-imaging technique for investigating patients with possible TD. Nevertheless, because of its superior spatial and anatomical resolution, MRI allows for more adequate visualization and measurement of basal ganglia structures than CT (Coffman and Nasrallah 1986), and is preferable for the neuroradiological investigation of patients with TD.

Since 1976, 9 out of 24 English-language CT studies and 6 out of 9 English-language MRI studies have reported significant—albeit heterogeneous—abnormal findings in patients with TD. A thorough analysis of these findings is presented elsewhere (Hoffman and Casey 1991; Krishnan et al. 1988; Shriqui, in press). In addition, results from two recent MRI studies (Elkashef et al. 1994; Shriqui et al. 1994a) revealed no significant differences in basal ganglia signal intensity ratios or T2 relaxation times between schizophrenic patients with and without TD.

Overall, current evidence from CT and MRI studies has indicated that structural brain abnormalities occur in a significant proportion of patients with TD. However, because of several confounding factors, and increasing MRI findings that basal ganglia abnormalities occur in schizophrenic and affective disorder patients (Jernigan et al. 1991; Krishnan et al. 1992; Nasrallah et al. 1993; Young et al. 1991), no characteristic neuroanatomical picture of TD can be derived from available studies.

Prevention

Because of a lack of effective treatment, prevention of TD is essential. Primary prevention consists of limiting the long-term use of neuroleptics as much as possible to treating schizophrenia. Chronic use of neuroleptics for other psychiatric conditions rests mainly on clinical judgment, and alternative treatment strategies should be considered whenever possible (American Psychiatric Association 1992). Patients should be examined for the presence of any preexisting movement disorder before neuroleptic treatment is initiated, as well as be reevaluated periodically. Secondary prevention consists of limiting the duration of neuroleptic exposure, particularly in first-break-episode patients, and using minimal effective dosages of neuroleptics (American Psychiatric Association 1992; Kane et al. 1984; Shriqui 1988; M. A. Wolf and Wertenschlag 1989). Clinical rating scales, such as the Abnormal Involuntary Movement Scale (Guy 1976), the Abbreviated Dyskinesia Rating Scale (Simpson et al. 1979), or the Extrapyramidal Symptom Rating Scale (Chouinard et al. 1980b), when used every 6 months, may detect early signs of TD so that steps may be taken to try to slow or reverse its progression.

Informed Consent

Numerous articles on informed consent and medicolegal issues related to TD are widely available (Amabile and Cavanaugh 1988; American Psychiatric Association 1992; Gualtieri et al. 1986; Kennedy and Sanborn 1992; Kleinman et al. 1989; Munetz and Roth 1985; Shriqui et al. 1990; Tancredi 1988; Wettstein 1988; M. A. Wolf et al. 1988). Nevertheless, general guidelines with regard to the prescription of neuroleptics include the following:

1. Regular assessment of indication, duration, and dosage of neuroleptics
2. Use of minimal effective dosages of neuroleptics
3. Periodic renewal of informed consent
4. Examination of patients at regular intervals to detect early signs of TD
5. Documentation of these steps in the medical chart

Treatment

Despite numerous therapeutic trials with many different agents, no consistently effective treatment for TD has been found (American

Psychiatric Association 1992; Casey 1987, 1991; Feltner and Hertzman 1993; Jeste and Wyatt 1982a, 1982b; Jeste et al. 1988; Kane et al. 1984; Simpson et al. 1986). Since the 1980s, there has been a noticeable improvement in the quality of published treatment studies of TD, with more double-blind trials being done and an increased usage of standardized rating scales (Jeste et al. 1988). However, most treatment studies of TD have been of short duration only, with no established long-term efficacy noted.

The best currently available management strategy is gradual neuroleptic dosage reduction whenever possible (American Psychiatric Association 1992; Casey 1991). Discontinuing drug treatment can stabilize or improve TD, but this is not a realistic option for the majority of chronic schizophrenic patients (Casey and Gerlach 1986). Decreasing maintenance neuroleptic drug therapy to low to moderate dosages (i.e., 300–600 mg/day of chlorpromazine equivalents or less), where possible, will often lead to improvement of TD (Casey 1985c; Casey and Gerlach 1986). Nonpharmacological treatments for TD, based on anecdotal case reports, have included the use of electroconvulsive therapy in depressed patients with concomitant TD (American Psychiatric Association 1992; Chacko and Root 1983).

An abundant number of pharmacological agents have been used in the treatment of TD (American Psychiatric Association 1992; Casey 1987, 1991; Feltner and Hertzman 1993; Jeste and Wyatt 1982a, 1982b; Jeste et al. 1988; Simpson et al. 1986). These are summarized in the following section.

Pharmacological Strategies

Dopamine and catecholaminergic drugs. Increasing the dosage of a standard neuroleptic will consistently mask TD (Casey 1987; Jeste and Wyatt 1982a, 1982b; Jeste et al. 1988). This antidyskinetic (or rather, dyskinesia-suppressant) effect of neuroleptics appears to be separate from their sedative and antipsychotic effects (Jeste et al. 1988). This strategy is primarily indicated in patients who present with a moderate to severe form of TD that is unresponsive to other agents, and who require continuation of neuroleptic treatment.

The novel antipsychotic clozapine rarely, if at all, induces TD (de Leon et al. 1991; Kane et al. 1993). Its use has led to varying degrees of improvement in patients with TD (Leppig et al. 1989; Lieberman et al. 1989; Naber et al. 1989; Owen et al. 1989), particularly in those with tardive dystonia (Lamberti and Bellnier 1993; Lieberman et al. 1991). The low propensity of clozapine to induce TD (and other EPS) may be related to its lower dopamine D_2 receptor affinity in the nigrostriatal region compared with that of standard neuroleptic agents (Farde et al. 1992). In addition, it has been suggested that clozapine's effect on multiple neurotransmitters and its preferential $5\text{-}HT_2\text{--}D_2$ receptor ratio could be responsible for its atypical side effect profile (Casey 1992; Meltzer et al. 1989). In addition to its clinical use in treatment-refractory schizophrenia, clozapine is a potentially valuable treatment alternative for patients with moderate to severe forms of TD who require continued neuroleptic drug therapy.

Another atypical antipsychotic, risperidone, recently marketed in North America and the United Kingdom, may also be a promising treatment alternative for patients with TD who require continued neuroleptic drug therapy, on the basis of reports suggesting that it may have an antidyskinetic or, at the least, a dyskinesia-suppressant effect (Borison et al. 1992; Chouinard and Arnott 1992; Chouinard et al. 1993; Kopala and Honer 1994; Shriqui et al. 1994b). However, in their single-blind placebo-controlled crossover study of 10 schizophrenic patients with TD, Meco et al. (1989a) were unable to demonstrate a dyskinesia-suppressant effect of risperidone at a maximum daily dosage of 6 mg. At the present time, judgments on the potential value of risperidone in the treatment of TD, as well as on its potential to induce TD, await results from ongoing clinical trials and long-term clinical use.

Agents that decrease presynaptic catecholamine (and serotonin) activity via depletion or false neurotransmission (e.g., reserpine, tetrabenazine, α-methyl-p-tyrosine) have produced variable changes in the severity of TD (American Psychiatric Association 1992; Casey 1987; Jeste and Wyatt 1982a, 1982b; Jeste et al. 1986, 1988) in addition to side effects (e.g., drowsiness, akathisia, depression.) Bromocriptine, a dopamine agonist that at low dosages decreases synaptic release via dopamine autoreceptor stimulation, has been tried with little success

(Lenox et al. 1985; Tamminga and Chase 1980); in addition, it can induce hypertension, psychotic exacerbation, and even a worsening of TD. Desensitizing hypersensitive DA receptors by temporarily increasing DA levels is another potential treatment strategy (Yadalam and Simpson 1990).

Acetylcholine. Anticholinergic drugs are frequently reported to be of benefit in tardive dystonia (Jeste et al. 1988; M. E. Wolf and Koller 1985). However, these agents will usually have no effect and frequently worsen other forms of TD (Casey 1987; Chouinard et al. 1979b; Jeste et al. 1988; Yassa 1988). Although anticholinergic withdrawal can improve TD and is advisable in most cases (Yassa 1988), the common co-occurrence of drug-induced parkinsonism and TD is a frequent obstacle to reducing antiparkinsonian medication.

Attempts to increase cholinergic function with physostigmine, an acetylcholine esterase inhibitor, have produced inconsistent results (Kane et al. 1988). Clinical trials with cholinergic agents such as deanol, choline, and lecithin have been largely unsuccessful (American Psychiatric Association 1992; Casey 1987; de Montigny et al. 1979; Gelenberg et al. 1990; Nasrallah et al. 1984; Tanner 1983). In addition, these cholinergic agonists produce a wide range of side effects that include depression, diarrhea, and bronchospasm.

GABAergic drugs. GABA is closely linked to nigrostriatal dopaminergic function, and a reduction of nigrostriatal GABA activity in TD is the rationale for using GABA agonists. In general, the evidence supporting the use of GABAergic treatments in TD is encouraging, although considerable heterogeneity exists as to the individual efficacy of various GABAmimetic agents. Results from studies with baclofen and valproic acid either have been inconsistent or have shown these drugs to be frankly ineffective (Casey 1987; Jeste et al. 1988; Nair et al. 1978; Thaker et al. 1990). However, promising results with the potent GABA agonist muscimol, and with direct (e.g., progabide) and indirect (e.g., gamma-vinyl GABA) GABA agonist drugs, have been reported (Tamminga et al. 1979; Thaker et al. 1987). Results from Thaker et al.'s (1990) 12-week, double-blind placebo-controlled randomized crossover trial of clonazepam in 19 patients with TD have been of particular interest; in that study, clonazepam treatment produced a 35% decrease in dyskinesia ratings. The authors reported that tolerance to the antidyskinetic effect of clonazepam developed after long-term use, but that a 2-week clonazepam-free period was sufficient to recapture its antidyskinetic effect. Apart from drug tolerance, sedation is an additional side effect of GABAergic agents that has limited their clinical use.

Vitamin E. The hypothesis that free radicals are involved in the pathophysiology of TD (Cadet 1988; Cadet and Lohr 1989; Cadet et al. 1986, 1987; Lohr 1991; Lohr et al. 1988, 1990; Shriqui and Jones 1990a, 1990b) is central to the use of antioxidants, such as vitamin E (α-tocopherol; Burton et al. 1983), in the treatment of TD.

Since 1987, investigators in 14 clinical trials, 12 of which were double-blind placebo-controlled studies, have examined the therapeutic effect of vitamin E on TD (Adler et al. 1993a, 1993b; Akhtar et al. 1993; Dabiri et al. 1994; Egan et al. 1992; Elkashef et al. 1990; Junker et al. 1992; Lam et al. 1994; Lohr 1993; J. B. Lohr and M. P. Caligiuri, unpublished data, December 1994; Lohr et al. 1987; Peet et al. 1993b; Schmidt et al. 1991; Shriqui et al. 1992; Spivak et al. 1992). Positive effects have been shown in 10 of these 14 trials. However, several of these clinical trials included a small sample size (generally less than 20 patients) (Adler et al. 1993a; Dabiri et al. 1994; Egan et al. 1992; Elkashef et al. 1990; Junker et al. 1992; Lam et al. 1994; Lohr et al. 1987; Peet et al. 1993b; Schmidt et al. 1991; Spivak et al. 1992), brief treatment periods (6 weeks or less) (Akhtar et al. 1993; Egan et al. 1992; Elkashef et al. 1990; Junker et al. 1992; Lam et al. 1994; Lohr et al. 1987; Peet et al. 1993b; Schmidt et al. 1991; Shriqui et al. 1992; Spivak et al. 1992), and varying dosage regimens of vitamin E. So far, the results from these studies suggest that duration of TD, duration of vitamin E treatment, and dosage of vitamin E may influence treatment response. Although the optimal dose level of vitamin E remains to be confirmed, a dosage regimen of 1,600 IU/day of vitamin E is generally well tolerated and may be of greater therapeutic benefit than are lower dosage regimens (Shriqui 1993).

Although vitamin E is considered one of the most promising strategies to have emerged in the treatment and possible prevention of

TD, large-scale and long-term treatment studies to establish the general clinical value of vitamin E are required (American Psychiatric Association 1992). A large-scale collaborative study of vitamin E in the treatment of TD is presently ongoing. The efficacy of other antioxidants such as idebenone, coenzyme Q_{10} (ubiquinone$_{10}$; Greenberg and Frishman 1988), and Trolox-C (an analogue of vitamin E; Britt et al. 1992) in the treatment of TD still remains to be studied.

Finally, the synergistic potential of combining β-carotene (vitamin A; Palozza and Krinsky 1992), ascorbic acid (vitamin C is a potent antioxidant that also recycles the tocpheroxyl radical of vitamin E), or both with α-tocopherol (vitamin E) in the treatment of TD is currently being investigated.

Other agents. Various agents used to treat TD, such as L-tryptophan and 5-HTP (both serotonin precursors), cyproheptadine (a serotonin antagonist), prednisolone (a corticosteroid), estrogen, the ergoloid mesylate Hydergine, lithium, propranolol, and others have generally been unsuccessful (American Psychiatric Association 1992; Benecke et al. 1988; Casey 1987; Jeste and Wyatt 1982a, 1982b; Jeste et al. 1988; Seibyl et al. 1989; Yassa and Ananth 1980).

A double-blind placebo-controlled crossover trial in 10 chronic schizophrenic patients found ritanserin, a selective serotonin 5-HT$_2$ antagonist, to be ineffective in the treatment of TD (Meco et al. 1989b). However, further studies evaluating the efficacy of ritanserin are anticipated.

L-Deprenyl, a selective monoamine oxidase-B inhibitor that may decrease the production of free radicals, may have potential value in the treatment of TD (Szymanski et al. 1992). Essential fatty acids have been tried alone or in combination with vitamin E in the treatment of TD, but judgments of their efficacy await further study (Vaddadi 1991, 1992; Vaddadi et al. 1989).

Clonidine, an α-adrenergic receptor agonist, has shown some efficacy in patients with TD, but side effects, notably hypotension, limit the use of this drug (Jeste and Wyatt 1982b; Jeste et al. 1986).

Preliminary results with low dosages of insulin indirectly support the hypothesis that decreased glucose availability can influence receptor hypersensitivity (Mouret et al. 1991). The rationale behind the use of insulin is that hypersensitivity following DA receptor blockade results from an increased synthesis of receptors that, in the brain, is primarily dependent on the availability of glucose.

Calcium channel blockers such as diltiazem (Adler et al. 1988; Falk et al. 1988; Leys et al. 1988; Loonen et al. 1992; Ross et al. 1987), nifedipine (Duncan et al. 1990; Stedman et al. 1991; Suddath et al. 1991), and verapamil (Abad and Ovsiew 1993; Adler et al. 1988; Barrow and Childs 1986; Bartko et al. 1991; Dinan and Capstick 1989; Reiter et al. 1989) have been used in the treatment of classical manifestations of TD and tardive dystonia with varying success.

Conclusion

In recent years there has been significant progress in the understanding of the epidemiology of TD, particularly regarding its risk factors. Much of the pathophysiology of TD still remains a mystery, and current etiologic theories rely mainly on indirect evidence. Current hypotheses involve multiple neurotransmitter systems and free-radical mechanisms. The recent cloning of five human dopamine receptor subtypes (D_1–D_5; Schwartz et al. 1992; Seeman 1992; Sokoloff et al. 1990; Sunahara et al. 1991; Van Tol et al. 1991) and their role as target sites in the mechanism of action of antipsychotic drugs will likely further the understanding of the pathophysiology of TD.

Despite considerable research efforts, there has been little progress in the treatment of TD (Feltner and Hertzman 1993). The strategy of the treating clinician must therefore center on prevention and minimization of TD, with the risk-benefit ratio of neuroleptic treatment being carefully weighed on an ongoing basis. Future research will continue to investigate the many heterogeneous aspects of TD, which may in fact represent several conditions with distinct clinical manifestations, pathophysiology, neuroanatomical substrates, and treatment response.

With the introduction of novel antipsychotic agents with demonstrated clinical efficacy and a lower propensity to cause EPS, it is to be hoped that future generations of patients will be exposed to a substantially lower risk of TD.

References

Abad V, Ovsiew F: Treatment of persistent myoclonic tardive dystonia with verapamil. Br J Psychiatry 162:554–556, 1993

Adler LA, Duncan E, Reiter S, et al: Effects of calcium-channel antagonists on tardive dyskinesia and psychosis. Psychopharmacol Bull 24:421–425, 1988

Adler LA, Peselow E, Duncan E, et al: Vitamin E in tardive dyskinesia: time course of effect after placebo substitution. Psychopharmacol Bull 29:371–374, 1993a

Adler LA, Peselow E, Rotrosen J, et al: Vitamin E treatment of tardive dyskinesia. Am J Psychiatry 150:1405–1407, 1993b

Akhtar S, Jajor TR, Kumar S: Vitamin E in the treatment of tardive dyskinesia. J Postgrad Med 39:124–126, 1993

Altamura AC, Cavallaro R, Regazzetti MG: Prevalence and risk factors for tardive dyskinesia: a study in an Italian population of chronic schizophrenics. Eur Arch Psychiatry Clin Neurosci 240:9–12, 1990

Amabile PE, Cavanaugh JL: Legal liability for tardive dyskinesia: guidelines for practice, in Tardive Dyskinesia: Biological Mechanisms and Clinical Aspects. Edited by Wolf ME, Mosnaim AD. Washington, DC, American Psychiatric Press, 1988, pp 260–279

American College of Neuropsychopharmacology, Food and Drug Administration Task Force: Neurological syndromes associated with antipsychotic drug use. N Engl J Med 289:20 23, 1973

American Psychiatric Association: Tardive Dyskinesia: A Task Force Report of the American Psychiatric Association on Late Neurological Effects of Antipsychotic Drugs. Edited by Baldessarini RJ, Cole JO, Davis JM, et al. Washington, DC, American Psychiatric Association, 1980

American Psychiatric Association: Tardive Dyskinesia: A Task Force Report of the American Psychiatric Association. Edited by Kane JM, Jeste DV, Barnes TRE, et al. Washington, DC, American Psychiatric Association, 1992

Andersson U, Eckrnas SA, Hartvig P, et al: Striatal binding of C-NMSP studied with positron emission tomography in patients with persistent tardive dyskinesia: no evidence for altered dopamine D_2 receptor binding. J Neural Transm 79:215–226, 1990

Andreasen NC, Ehrhardt J, Yuh W, et al: Magnetic resonance imaging in schizophrenia: an update, in Schizophrenia: Scientific Progress. Edited by Schulz SC, Tamminga CA. London, Oxford University Press, 1989, pp 207–215

Annable L, Chouinard G, Ross-Chouinard A, et al: A ten-year follow-up study of tardive dyskinesia (abstract #533). Excerpta Medica International Conference Series 899:144, 1989

Arai N, Amano N, Iseki E, et al: Tardive dyskinesia with inflated neurons of the cerebellar dentate nucleus. Acta Neuropathol 73:38–42, 1987

Arnt T, Scheel-Kruger J: Intranigral GABA antagonists produce dopamine-independent biting in rats. Eur J Pharmacol 62:51–61, 1980

Awouters F, Niemegeers CJE, Janssen PAJ: "Tardive" dyskinesia: etiological and therapeutic aspects. Pharmacopsychiatry 23:33–37, 1990

Baldessarini RJ: Clinical and epidemiologic aspects of tardive dyskinesia. J Clin Psychiatry 46:8–13, 1985

Barnes TRE: Comment on the WHO Consensus Statement. Br J Psychiatry 156:413–414, 1990

Barnes TRE, Braude WM: Akathisia variants and tardive dyskinesia. Arch Gen Psychiatry 42:874–878, 1985

Barnes TRE, Liddle PF: Tardive dyskinesia: implications for schizophrenia? in Schizophrenia: New Pharmacological Clinical Development. Edited by Schiff AA, Roth M, Freeman HL. London, Royal Society of Medicine Services, 1985, pp 81–87

Barnes TRE, Liddle PF, Curson DA, et al: Negative symptoms, tardive dyskinesia, and depression in chronic schizophrenia. Br J Psychiatry 155:99–103, 1989

Barr WB, Mukherjee S, Degreef G, et al: Anomalous dominance and persistent tardive dyskinesia. Biol Psychiatry 25:826–834, 1989

Barrow N, Childs A: An anti-tardive dyskinesia effect of verapamil. Am J Psychiatry 143:1485, 1986

Bartko G, Horvath S, Zador G, et al: Effects of adjunctive verapamil administration in chronic schizophrenic patients. Prog Neuropsychopharmacol Biol Psychiatry 15:343–349, 1991

Bartzokis G, Garber HJ, Marder SR, et al: MRI in tardive dyskinesia: shortened left caudate T2. Biol Psychiatry 28:1027–1036, 1990

Bartzokis G, Marder SR, Oldendorf WH, et al: Tardive dyskinesia: MRI implicates brain iron in hypothesized damage from oxydative processes, in Proceedings of the Third International Congress on Schizophrenia Research. Tucson, AZ, April 1991

Benecke R, Conrad B, Klingelhofer J: Successful treatment of tardive dyskinesias with corticosteroids. Eur Neurol 28:146–149, 1988

Bergen JA, Eyland EA, Campbell JA, et al: The course of tardive dyskinesia in patients on long-term neuroleptics. Br J Psychiatry 154:523–528, 1989

Binder RL, Kazamatsuri H, Nishimura T, et al: Smoking and tardive dyskinesia. Biol Psychiatry 22:1280–1282, 1987

Blin J, Baron JC, Cambon H, et al: Striatal dopamine D_2 receptors in tardive dyskinesia: PET study. J Neurol Neurosurg Psychiatry 52:1248–1252, 1989

Borison RL, Pathiraja AP, Diamond BI, et al: Risperidone: clinical safety and efficacy in schizophrenia. Psychopharmacol Bull 28:213–218, 1992

Britt SG, Chiu VWS, Redpath GT, et al: Elimination of ascorbic acid-induced membrane lipid peroxidation and serotonin receptor loss by Trolox-C, a water-soluble analogue of Vitamin E. J Recept Res 12:181–200, 1992

Brown KW, White T: The psychological consequences of tardive dyskinesia: the effect of drug-induced parkinsonism and the topography of the dyskinetic movements. Br J Psychiatry 159:399–403, 1991a

Brown KW, White T: The association among negative symptoms, movement disorders, and frontal lobe psychological deficits in schizophrenic patients. Biol Psychiatry 30:1182–1190, 1991b

Brown KW, White T: Human leukocyte antigens and tardive dyskinesia. Br J Psychiatry 158:270–272, 1991c

Brown KW, White T: The influence of topography on the cognitive and psychopathological effects of tardive dyskinesia. Am J Psychiatry 149:1385–1389, 1992

Brown KW, White T, Anderson F, et al: Handedness as a risk factor for neuroleptic-induced movement disorders. Biol Psychiatry 31:746–748, 1992a

Brown KW, White T, Palmer D: Movement disorders and psychological tests of frontal lobe function in schizophrenic patients. Psychol Med 22:69–77, 1992b

Burke RE, Kang UJ: Tardive dystonia: clinical aspects and treatment. Adv Neurol 49:199–210, 1988

Burke RE, Fahn S, Jankovic J, et al: Tardive dystonia: late-onset and persistent dystonia caused by antipsychotic drugs. Neurology 32:1335–1346, 1982

Burke RE, Kang UJ, Jankovic J, et al: Tardive akathisia: an analysis of clinical features and response to open therapeutic trials. Mov Disord 4:157–175, 1989

Burton GW, Cheeseman KH, Doba T, et al: Vitamin E as an antioxidant in vitro and in vivo, in Ciba Foundation Symposium 101: Biology of Vitamin E. London, Pitman, 1983, pp 5–18

Cadet JL: Free radical mechanisms in the central nervous system: an overview. Int J Neurosci 40:13–18, 1988

Cadet JL, Lohr JB: Possible involvement of free radicals in neuroleptic-induced movement disorders: evidence from treatment of tardive dyskinesia with vitamin E. Ann N Y Acad Sci 570:176–185, 1989

Cadet JL, Lohr JB, Jeste DV: Free radicals and tardive dyskinesia. Trends Neurosci 9:107–108, 1986

Cadet JL, Lohr JB, Jeste DV: Tardive dyskinesia and schizophrenic burnout: the possible involvement of cytotoxic free radicals, in Handbook of Schizophrenia, Vol 2: Neurochemistry and Neuropharmacology of Schizophrenia. Series edited by Nasrallah HA; volume edited by Henn FA, DeLisi LE. Amsterdam, Netherlands, Elsevier, 1987, pp 425–438

Campbell WG, Raskind MA, Gordon T, et al: Iron pigment in the brain of a man with tardive dyskinesia. Am J Psychiatry 142:364–365, 1985

Casey DE: Tardive dyskinesia: epidemiologic factors as a guide for prevention and management. Adv Biochem Psychopharmacol 40:15–24, 1985a

Casey DE: Spontaneous and tardive dyskinesias: clinical and laboratory studies. J Clin Psychiatry 46:42–47, 1985b

Casey DE: Tardive dyskinesia: reversible and irreversible, in Dyskinesia Research and Treatment (Psychopharmacology Supplementum 2). Edited by Casey DE, Chase TN, Christensen AV, et al. Berlin, Springer-Verlag, 1985c, pp 88–97

Casey DE: Tardive dyskinesia, in Psychopharmacology: The Third Generation of Progress. Edited by Meltzer HY. New York, Raven, 1987, pp 1411–1419

Casey DE: Neuroleptic drug-induced extrapyramidal syndromes and tardive dyskinesia. Schizophr Res 4:109–120, 1991

Casey DE: What makes a neuroleptic atypical? in Novel Antipsychotic Drugs. Edited by Meltzer HY. New York, Raven, 1992, pp 241–251

Casey DE, Ganzini LK: Diabetes mellitus and tardive dyskinesia. Paper presented at the annual meeting of the American Psychiatric Association, Philadelphia, PA, May 25, 1994

Casey DE, Gerlach J: Tardive dyskinesia: what is the long-term outcome? in Tardive Dyskinesia and Neuroleptics: From Dogma to Reason (Clinical Insights Series). Edited by Casey DE, Gardos G. Washington, DC, American Psychiatric Press, 1986, pp 75–97

Casey DE, Rabins P: Tardive dyskinesia as a life-threatening illness. Am J Psychiatry 135:486–488, 1978

Chacko RC, Root L: ECT and tardive dyskinesia: two cases and a review. J Clin Psychiatry 44:265–266, 1983

Chiang E, Pitts WM, Rodriguez-Garcia M: Respiratory dyskinesia: review and case reports. J Clin Psychiatry 46:232–234, 1985

Chiu H, Shum P, Lau J, et al: Prevalence of tardive dyskinesia, tardive dystonia, and respiratory dyskinesia among Chinese psychiatric patients in Hong Kong. Am J Psychiatry 149:1081–1085, 1992

Chiu HFK, Wing YK, Kwong PK, et al: Prevalence of tardive dyskinesia in samples of elderly people in Hong Kong. Acta Psychiatr Scand 86:266–268, 1993

Chorfi M, Moussaoui D: Lack of dyskinesia in unmedicated schizophrenics. Pharmacology 97:423, 1989

Chouinard G, Arnott W: The effect of risperidone on extrapyramidal symptoms in chronic schizophrenic patients (abstract). Biol Psychiatry 31:158A, 1992

Chouinard G, Annable L, Ross-Chouinard A, et al: Factors related to tardive dyskinesia. Am J Psychiatry 136:79–83, 1979a

Chouinard G, de Montigny C, Annable L: Tardive dyskinesia and antiparkinsonian medication. Am J Psychiatry 136:228–229, 1979b

Chouinard G, Jones BD, Annable L, et al: Sex differences and tardive dyskinesia. Am J Psychiatry 137:507, 1980a

Chouinard G, Ross-Chouinard A, Annable L, et al: Extrapyramidal symptom rating scale. Can J Neurol Sci 7:233, 1980b

Chouinard G, Creese I, Boisvert D, et al: High neuroleptic plasma levels in patients manifesting supersensitivity psychosis. Biol Psychiatry 17:849–852, 1982

Chouinard G, Annable L, Ross-Chouinard A, et al: A 5-year prospective longitudinal study of tardive dyskinesia: factors predicting appearance of new cases. J Clin Psychopharmacol 8:21S–26S, 1988

Chouinard G, Jones B, Remington G, et al: A Canadian multicenter placebo-controlled study of fixed doses of risperidone and haloperidol in the treatment of chronic schizophrenic patients. J Clin Psychopharmacol 13:25–40, 1993

Christensen E, Moller J, Faurbye A: Neuropathological investigation of 28 brains from patients with dyskinesia. Acta Psychiatr Scand 46:14–23, 1970

Coffman JA, Nasrallah HA: Magnetic resonance brain imaging in schizophrenia, in Handbook of Schizophrenia, Vol 1: The Neurology of Schizophrenia. Edited by Nasrallah HA, Weinberger DR. Amsterdam, Elsevier, 1986, pp 251–266

Cohen G: Oxy-radical toxicity in catecholamine neurons. Neurotoxicology 5:77–82, 1984

Cooper SJ, Doherty MM, Foster J, et al: The relationship of involuntary movements to treatment variables, symptomatology and CT scan variables in chronic schizophrenia. Biol Psychiatry 29:408S, 1991

Crane GE: Pseudoparkinsonism and tardive dyskinesia. Arch Neurol 27:426–430, 1972

Crane GE, Smeets RA: Tardive dyskinesia and drug therapy in geriatric patients. Arch Gen Psychiatry 30:341–343, 1974

Crow TJ, Cross AJ, Johnstone EC, et al: Abnormal involuntary movements in schizophrenia: are they related to the disease process or its treatment? are they associated with changes in D_2 receptors? J Clin Psychopharmacol 5:336–340, 1982

Cummings JL, Wirshing WC: Recognition and differential diagnosis of tardive dyskinesia. International Journal of Psychiatry 19:133–144, 1989

Dabiri LM, Pasta D, Darby JK, et al: Effectiveness of vitamin E for treatment of long-term tardive dyskinesia. Am J Psychiatry 151:925–926, 1994

Davis EJB, Borde M, Sharma LN: Tardive dyskinesia and type II schizophrenia. Br J Psychiatry 160:253–256, 1992

de Leon J, Moral L, Camunas C: Clozapine and jaw dyskinesia: a case report. J Clin Psychiatry 52:494–495, 1991

de Montigny C, Chouinard G, Annable L: Ineffectiveness of deanol in tardive dyskinesia: a placebo controlled study. Psychopharmacology 65:219–223, 1979

Dinan TG, Capstick C: A pilot study of verapamil in the treatment of tardive dyskinesia. Human Psychopharmacology 4:55–58, 1989

Dixon L, Weiden PJ, Frances AJ, et al: Management of neuroleptic-induced movement disorders: effects of physician training. Am J Psychiatry 146:104–106, 1989

Dixon L, Weiden PJ, Haas G, et al: Increased tardive dyskinesia in alcohol-abusing schizophrenic patients. Compr Psychiatry 33:121–122, 1992

Drayer BP: Magnetic resonance imaging and brain iron: implications in the diagnosis and pathochemistry of movement disorders and dementia. British Neuroimaging Quarterly 3:15–30, 1987

Drayer BP, Burger P, Darwin R, et al: MRI of brain iron. American Journal of Roentgenology 147:103–110, 1986

Duncan E, Adler LA, Angrist B, et al: Nifedipine in the treatment of tardive dyskinesia. J Clin Psychopharmacol 10:414–416, 1990

Edwards H: The significance of brain damage in oral dyskinesia. Br J Psychiatry 116:271–275, 1970

Egan MF: The pathophysiology of tardive dyskinesia. Paper presented at the annual meeting of the American Psychiatric Association, Philadelphia, PA, May 25, 1994

Egan MF, Hyde TM, Albers GW, et al: Treatment of tardive dyskinesia with vitamin E. Am J Psychiatry 149:773–777, 1992

Elkashef AM, Ruskin PE, Bacher N, et al: Vitamin E in the treatment of tardive dyskinesia. Am J Psychiatry 147:505–506, 1990

Elkashef AM, Egan MF, Frank JA, et al: Basal ganglia iron in tardive dyskinesia: an MRI study. Biol Psychiatry 35:16–21, 1994

Falk WE, Wojick JD, Gelenberg AJ: Diltiazem for tardive dyskinesia and tardive dystonia. Lancet 1:824–825, 1988

Famuyiwa OO, Eccleston D, Donaldson AA, et al: Tardive dyskinesia and dementia. Br J Psychiatry 135:500–504, 1979

Farde L, Nordström AL, Wiesel FA, et al: Positron-emission tomographic analysis of central D_1 and D_2 dopamine receptor occupancy in patients treated with classical neuroleptics and clozapine. Arch Gen Psychiatry 49:538–544, 1992

Feltner DE, Hertzman M: Progress in the treatment of tardive dyskinesia: theory and practice. Hosp Community Psychiatry 44:25–34, 1993

Fibiger HC, Lloyd KG: Neurobiological substrates of tardive dyskinesia: the GABA hypothesis. Trends Neurosci 7:462–464, 1984

Fleischauer J, Kocher R, Hobi V, et al: Prevalence of tardive dyskinesia in a clinic population, in Dyskinesia Research and Treatment (Psychopharmacology Supplementum 2). Edited by Casey DE, Chase TN, Christensen AV, et al. Berlin, Springer-Verlag, 1985, pp 162–172

Fornazzari X, Grossman H, Thornton J, et al: Tardive dyskinesia: a five year follow-up. Can J Psychiatry 34:700–703, 1989

Fridovich I: Superoxide radical: an endogenous toxicant. Annu Rev Pharmacol Toxicol 23:239–257, 1983

Friedman JH, Kuraski LT, Wagner RI: Tardive dystonia in a psychiatric hospital. J Neurol Neurosurg Psychiatry 50:801–803, 1987

Galdi J, Rieder RO, Silber D, et al: Genetic factors in response to neuroleptics: a psychopharmacogenetic study. Psychol Med 11:713–728, 1981

Ganzini L, Casey DE, Hoffman WF, et al: Tardive dyskinesia and diabetes mellitus. Psychopharmacol Bull 28:281–286, 1992

Gardos G, Cole JO, Sniffin C: An evaluation of papaverine in tardive dyskinesia. J Clin Psychopharmacol 16:304–310, 1976

Gardos G, Cole JO, La Brie RA: Drug variables in the etiology of tardive dyskinesia: application of discriminant analysis. Progress in Neuropsychopharmacology 1:147–154, 1977

Gardos G, Cole JO, Tarsy D: Withdrawal syndromes associated with antipsychotic drugs. Am J Psychiatry 135:1321–1324, 1978

Gardos G, Cole JO, Salomon M, et al: Clinical forms of severe tardive dyskinesia. Am J Psychiatry 144:895–902, 1987

Gardos G, Cole JO, Haskell D, et al: The natural history of tardive dyskinesia. J Clin Psychopharmacol 8:S31–S37, 1988

Gardos G, Casey DE, Cole JO, et al: Ten-year outcome of tardive dyskinesia. Am J Psychiatry 151:836–841, 1994

Gelenberg AJ, Dorer DJ, Wojcik RN, et al: A crossover study of lecithin treatment of tardive dyskinesia. J Clin Psychiatry 51:149–153, 1990

Giménez-Roldán S, Mateo D, Bartolomé P: Tardive dystonia and severe tardive dyskinesia: a comparison of risk factors and prognosis. Acta Psychiatr Scand 71:488–494, 1985

Glazer WM: Noradrenergic function and tardive dyskinesia. Psychiatric Annals 19:297–301, 1989

Glazer WM, Kane JM: Depot neuroleptic therapy: an underutilized treatment option. J Clin Psychiatry 53:426–433, 1992

Glazer WM, Morgenstern H, Schooler N, et al: Predictors of improvement in tardive dyskinesia following discontinuation of neuroleptic medication. Br J Psychiatry 157:585–592, 1990

Glazer WM, Morgenstern H, Doucette JT: The prediction of chronic persistent versus intermittent tardive dyskinesia: a retrospective follow-up study. Br J Psychiatry 158:822–828, 1991

Gold JM, Egan MF, Kirch DG, et al: Tardive dyskinesia: neuropsychological, computerized tomographic, and psychiatric symptom findings. Biol Psychiatry 30:587–599, 1991

Goldman MB, Luchins DJ: Intermittent neuroleptic therapy and tardive dyskinesia: a literature review. Hosp Community Psychiatry 35:1215–1219, 1984

Greenberg SM, Frishman WH: Coenzyme Q_{10}: a new drug for myocardial ischemia? Med Clin North Am 72:243–258, 1988

Grimes JD, Hassan MN, Preston DN: Adverse neurologic effects of metoclopramide. Can Med Assoc J 126:23–25, 1982

Gualtieri CT, Sprague RL, Cole JO: Tardive dyskinesia: litigation and the dilemmas of neuroleptic treatment. Journal of Psychiatry and Law 14:187–216, 1986

Gunne LM, Häggström JE: Experimental tardive dyskinesia. J Clin Psychiatry 46 (sect 2):48–50, 1985

Gunne LM, Häggström JE, Sjokvist B: Association with persistent neuroleptic-induced dyskinesia of regional changes in the brain GABA synthesis. Nature 309:347–349, 1984

Gureje OYE: Topographic subtypes of tardive dyskinesia in schizophrenic patients aged less than 60 years: relationship to demographic, clinical, treatment, and neuropsychological variables. J Neurol Neurosurg Psychiatry 51:1525–1530, 1988

Gureje OYE: The significance of subtyping tardive dyskinesia: a study of prevalence and associated factors. Psychol Med 19:121–128, 1989

Guy W (ed): ECDEU assessment manual for psychopharmacology (DHHS Publ No ADM-76-338). Washington, DC, US Government Printing Office, 1976

Haag H, Ruther E, Hippius H: Tardive Dyskinesia: WHO Expert Series on Biological Psychiatry, Vol 1. Göttingen, Germany, Hogrefe & Huber, 1992

Harris MJ, Panton D, Caligiuri MP, et al: High incidence of tardive dyskinesia in older outpatients on low doses of neuroleptics. Psychopharmacol Bull 28:87–92, 1992

Hoffman WF, Casey DE: Computed tomographic evaluation of patients with tardive dyskinesia. Schizophr Res 5:1–12, 1991

Hoffman WF, Labs SM, Casey DE: Neuroleptic-induced parkinsonism in older schizophrenics. Biol Psychiatry 22:427–439, 1987

Hunter R, Blackwood W, Smith MC, et al: Neuropathological findings in three cases of persistent dyskinesia following phenothiazine medication. J Neurol Sci 7:263–273, 1968

Inada T, Yagi G: Incidence of tardive dyskinesia in affective disorder patients. J Clin Psychopharmacol 12:299–300, 1992

Jenner P, Marsden CD: Is the dopamine hypothesis of tardive dyskinesia completely wrong? Trends Neurosci 9:259–261, 1986

Jernigan TL, Zisook S, Heaton RK, et al: Magnetic resonance imaging abnormalities in lenticular nuclei and cerebral cortex in schizophrenia. Arch Gen Psychiatry 48:881–890, 1991

Jeste DV, Caligiuri MP: Tardive dyskinesia. Schizophr Bull 19:303–315, 1993

Jeste DV, Wyatt RJ: Dogma disputed: is tardive dyskinesia due to postsynaptic dopamine receptor supersensitivity? J Clin Psychiatry 42:455–457, 1981

Jeste DV, Wyatt RJ: Understanding and Treating Tardive Dyskinesia. New York, Guilford, 1982a

Jeste DV, Wyatt RJ: Therapeutic strategies against tardive dyskinesia: two decades of experience. Arch Gen Psychiatry 39:803–816, 1982b

Jeste DV, Potkin SG, Sinha S, et al: Tardive dyskinesia, reversible and persistent. Arch Gen Psychiatry 36:585–590, 1979

Jeste DV, Karson CM, Iager AC, et al: Association of abnormal involuntary movements and negative symptoms. Psychopharmacol Bull 20:380–381, 1984

Jeste DV, Lohr JB, Kaufmann CA, et al: Pathophysiology of tardive dyskinesia: evaluation of supersensitivity theory and alternative hypotheses, in Tardive Dyskinesia and Neuroleptics: From Dogma to Reason (Clinical Insights Series). Edited by Casey DE, Gardos G. Washington, DC, American Psychiatric Press, 1986, pp 15–32

Jeste DV, Lohr JB, Clark K, et al: Pharmacological treatments of tardive dyskinesia in the 1980s. J Clin Psychopharmacol 8:38S–48S, 1988

Jeste DV, Paulsen J, Caligiuri MP, et al: Late-life tardive dyskinesia. Paper presented at the annual meeting of the American Psychiatric Association, Philadelphia, PA, May 25, 1994

Johnson GFS, Hunt GE, Rey JM: Incidence and severity of tardive dyskinesia increase with age. Arch Gen Psychiatry 39:486, 1982

Johnstone EC, Owens DGC, Frith CD, et al: Disabilities and circumstances of schizophrenic patients—a follow-up study, III: clinical findings: abnormalities of the mental state and movement disorder and their correlates. Br J Psychiatry 159 (suppl 13):21–25, 1991

Junker D, Steigleider P, Gattaz WF: α-tocopherol in the treatment of tardive dyskinesia. Clin Neuropharmacol 15 (suppl 1):639B, 1992

Jus K, Jus A, Gautier J, et al: Studies of the actions of certain pharmacological agents on tardive dyskinesia and on the rabbit syndrome. International Journal of Clinical Pharmacology 9:138–145, 1974

Kane JM, Smith JM: Tardive dyskinesia prevalence and risk factors: 1959 to 1979. Arch Gen Psychiatry 39:473–481, 1982

Kane JM, Rifkin A, Woerner M, et al: Low-dose neuroleptic treatment of outpatient schizophrenics. Arch Gen Psychiatry 40:893–896, 1983

Kane JM, Woerner M, Lieberman J, et al: Tardive dyskinesia, in Neuropsychiatric Movement Disorders (Clinical Insights Series). Edited by Jeste DV, Wyatt RJ. Washington, DC, American Psychiatric Press, 1984, pp 85–118

Kane JM, Woerner MG, Lieberman J: Tardive dyskinesia: prevalence, incidence, and risk factors. J Clin Psychopharmacol 8:52S–56S, 1988

Kane J, Lieberman J, Woerner MG, et al: Tardive dyskinesia: new research, in Schizophrenia: Scientific Progress. Edited by Schulz SC, Tamminga CA. London, Oxford University Press, 1989, pp 381–386

Kane JM, Woerner MG, Pollack S, et al: Does clozapine cause tardive dyskinesia? J Clin Psychiatry 54:327–330, 1993

Kane JM, Woerner MG, Borenstein M, et al: Incidence and prevalence of tardive dyskinesia. Paper presented at the annual meeting of the American Psychiatric Association, Philadelphia, PA, May 25, 1994

Karson CN, Lyon N, Amick R, et al: The profile of cognitive impairment in elderly dyskinetic subjects. Journal of Neuropsychiatry 5:61–65, 1993

Kaufmann CA, Jeste DV, Shelton RC, et al: Noradrenergic and neuroradiological abnormalities in tardive dyskinesia. Biol Psychiatry 21:799–812, 1986

Kennedy NJ, Sanborn JS: Disclosure of tardive dyskinesia: effect of written policy on risk disclosure. Psychopharmacol Bull 28:93–100, 1992

Kern RS, Green MF, Satz P, et al: Patterns of manual dominance in patients with neuroleptic-induced movement disorders. Biol Psychiatry 30:483–492, 1991

Khot V, Wyatt RJ: Not all that moves is tardive dyskinesia. Am J Psychiatry 148:661–666, 1991

Kidger T, Barnes TRE, Trauer T, et al: Subsyndromes of tardive dyskinesia. Psychol Med 10:513–520, 1980

Kleinman I, Schachter D, Koritar E: Informed consent and tardive dyskinesia. Am J Psychiatry 146:902–904, 1989

Kopala LC, Honer WG: Schizophrenia and severe tardive dyskinesia responsive to risperidone. J Clin Psychopharmacol 14:430–431, 1994

Kornhuber J, Riederer P, Reynolds GP, et al: [3H]spiperone binding sites in post-mortem brains from schizophrenia patients: relationship to neuroleptic drug treatment, abnormal movements and positive symptoms. J Neural Transm 75:1–10, 1989

Korpi ER, Wyatt RJ: Reduced haloperidol: effects on striatal dopamine metabolism and conversion to haloperidol in the rat. Psychopharmacology 83:34, 1984

Krishnan KRR, Ellinwood EH, Rayasam K: Tardive dyskinesia: structural changes in the brain, in Tardive Dyskinesia: Biological Mechanisms and Clinical Aspects. Edited by Wolf ME, Mosnaim AD. Washington, DC, American Psychiatric Press, 1988, pp 167–177

Krishnan KRR, McDonald WM, Escalona PR, et al: Magnetic resonance imaging of the caudate nuclei in depression. Preliminary observations. Arch Gen Psychiatry 49:553–557, 1992

Kucharski LT, Smith JW, Dunn DD: Mortality and tardive dyskinesia. Am J Psychiatry 136:1228, 1978

Lam LCW, Chiu HFK, Hung SF: Vitamin E in the treatment of tardive dyskinesia: a replication study. J Nerv Ment Dis 182:113–114, 1994

Lamberti JS, Bellnier T: Clozapine and tardive dystonia. J Nerv Ment Dis 181:137–138, 1993

Lenox RH, Weaver LA, Saran BM: Tardive dyskinesia: clinical and neuroendocrine response to low dose bromocriptine. J Clin Psychopharmacol 5:286–292, 1985

Leppig M, Bosch B, Naber D, et al: Clozapine in the treatment of 121 outpatients. Psychopharmacology 99:S77–S79, 1989

Leys D, Vermersch P, Danel T, et al: Diltiazem for tardive dyskinesia. Lancet 1:250–251, 1988

Lieberman J: Dopamine pathophysiology in tardive dyskinesia. Psychiatric Annals 19:289–296, 1989

Lieberman J, Kane JM, Woerner M, et al: Prevalence of tardive dyskinesia in elderly patients. Psychopharmacol Bull 20:22–26, 1985

Lieberman J, Pollack S, Lesser M, et al: Pharmacologic characterization of tardive dyskinesia. J Clin Psychopharmacol 8:254–260, 1988

Lieberman J, Johns C, Cooper T, et al: Clozapine pharmacology and tardive dyskinesia. Psychopharmacology 99:S54–S59, 1989

Lieberman JA, Saltz BL, Johns CA, et al: The effects of clozapine on tardive dyskinesia. Br J Psychiatry 158:503–510, 1991

Lohr JB: Oxygen radicals and neuropsychiatric illness: some speculations. Arch Gen Psychiatry 48:1097–1106, 1991

Lohr JB: Vitamin E treatment of tardive dyskinesia. Paper presented at the annual meeting of the American Psychiatric Association, San Francisco, CA, May 1993

Lohr JB, Wisniewski A, Jeste DV: Neurological aspects of tardive dyskinesia, in Handbook of Schizophrenia, Vol 1: The Neurology of Schizophrenia. Edited by Nasrallah HA, Weinberger DR. Amsterdam, Netherlands, Elsevier, 1986, pp 97–119

Lohr JB, Cadet JL, Lohr MA, et al: α-tocopherol in tardive dyskinesia. Lancet 1:913–914, 1987

Lohr JB, Cadet JL, Lohr MA, et al: Vitamin E in the treatment of tardive dyskinesia: the possible involvement of free radical mechanisms. Schizophr Bull 14:291–296, 1988

Lohr JB, Underhill S, Moir M, et al: Lipid peroxidation in CSF: relationship to catecholamines and tardive dyskinesia. Biol Psychiatry 25:71A, 1989

Lohr JB, Kuczenski R, Bracha HS, et al: Increased indices of free radical activity in the cerebrospinal fluid of patients with tardive dyskinesia. Biol Psychiatry 28:535–539, 1990

Loonen AJM, Verwey HA, Roels PR, et al: Is diltiazem effective in treating the symptoms of (tardive) dyskinesia in chronic psychiatric inpatients? a negative, double-blind, placebo-controlled trial. J Clin Psychopharmacol 12:39–42, 1992

Macpherson R, Collis R: Tardive dyskinesia: patients' lack of awareness of movement disorder. Br J Psychiatry 160:110–112, 1992

Mahler JC, Brown RP: More on metoclopramide and tardive dyskinesia. N Engl J Med 316:412–413, 1987

Marsden CD: Is tardive dyskinesia a unique disorder? in Dyskinesia Research and Treatment (Psychopharmacology Supplementum 2). Edited by Casey DE, Chase TN, Christensen AV, et al. Berlin, Springer-Verlag, 1985, pp 64–71

Marsden CD, Tarsy D, Baldessarini RJ: Spontaneous and drug-induced movement disorders in psychotic patients, in Psychiatric Aspects of Neurological Disease. Edited by Benson DF, Blumer D. New York, Grune & Stratton, 1975, pp 219–266

McClelland HA, Dutta D, Metcalfe A, et al: Mortality and facial dyskinesia. Br J Psychiatry 148:310–316, 1986

McClelland HA, Metcalfe TA, Kerr TA, et al: Facial dyskinesia: a 16-year follow-up study. Br J Psychiatry 158:691–696, 1991

Meco G, Bedini L, Bonifati V, et al: Risperidone in the treatment of chronic schizophrenia with tardive dyskinesia. Current Therapeutic Research 46:876–883, 1989a

Meco G, Bedini L, Bonifati V, et al: Ritanserin in tardive dyskinesia: a double-blind crossover study versus placebo. Current Therapeutic Research 46:884–894, 1989b

Mehta D, Mallya A, Volavka J, et al: Mortality of patients with tardive dyskinesia. Am J Psychiatry 135:371–372, 1978

Meltzer HY, Matsubara S, Lee J-C: The ratios of serotonin$_2$ and dopamine$_2$ affinities differentiate atypical and typical antipsychotic drugs. Psychopharmacol Bull 25:390–392, 1989

Menza MA, Grossman N, Van Horn M, et al: Smoking and movement disorders in psychiatric patients. Biol Psychiatry 30:109–115, 1991

Metzer WS, Newton JEO, Steele RW, et al: HLA antigens in tardive dyskinesia. J Neuroimmunol 26:179–181, 1990

Morgenstern H, Glazer WM: Identifying risk factors for tardive dyskinesia among long-term outpatients maintained with neuroleptic medications: results of the Yale tardive dyskinesia study. Arch Gen Psychiatry 50:723–733, 1993

Morns P, Thaker G, Moran M, et al: Course of tardive dyskinesia in schizophrenic patients attending a motor disorder clinic for two years. Schizophr Res 9:278, 1993

Mouret J, Khomais M, Lemoine P, et al: Low doses of insulin as a treatment of tardive dyskinesia: conjuncture or conjecture? European Neurology 31:199–203, 1991

Mukherjee S, Reddy R, Schnur DB: Diabetes mellitus and tardive dyskinesia, in Biological Psychiatry, Vol 1. Edited by Racagni G, Brunello N, Fukada T. Amsterdam, Netherlands, Elsevier, 1991, pp 624–627

Munetz MR: Oculogyric crisis and tardive dyskinesia. Am J Psychiatry 137:1628, 1980

Munetz MR, Roth LH: Informing patients about tardive dyskinesia. Arch Gen Psychiatry 42:866–871, 1985

Muscettola G, Pampallona S, Barbato G, et al: Persistent tardive dyskinesia: demographic and pharmacological risk factors. Acta Psychiatr Scand 87:29–36, 1993

Naber D, Leppig M, Grohmann R, et al: Efficacy and adverse effects of clozapine in the treatment of schizophrenia and tardive dyskinesia: a retrospective study of 387 patients. Psychopharmacology 99:S73–S76, 1989

Nair NPV, Yassa R: Course and prognosis of tardive dyskinesia: a meta-analysis. Paper presented at the annual meeting of the American Psychiatric Association, Philadelphia, PA, May 25, 1994

Nair NPV, Yassa R, Ruizz-Navarro J, et al: Baclofen in the treatment of tardive dyskinesia. Am J Psychiatry 135:1562–1563, 1978

Nasrallah HA, Pappas NJ, Crowe BR: Oculogyric dystonia in tardive dyskinesia. Am J Psychiatry 137:850–851, 1980

Nasrallah HA, Smith RE, Dunner FJ, et al: Serotonin precursor effects in tardive dyskinesia. Psychopharmacology 77:234–235, 1982

Nasrallah HA, Dunner FJ, Smith RE, et al: Variable clinical response to choline in tardive dyskinesia. Psychol Med 14:697–700, 1984

Nasrallah HA, Dunner FJ, McCalley-Whitters M, et al: Pharmacologic probes of neurotransmitter systems in tardive dyskinesia: implications for clinical management. J Clin Psychiatry 47:56–59, 1986

Nasrallah HA, Chu O, Olson SC, et al: Increased caudate volume in schizophrenia: a controlled MRI study. Schizophr Res 9:204, 1993

Olivera AA, Kiefer MW, Manley NK: Tardive dyskinesia in psychiatric patients with substance use disorders. Am J Drug Alcohol Abuse 16:57–66, 1990

Owen RR, Beake BJ, Marby D, et al: Response to clozapine in chronic psychotic patients. Psychopharmacology 25:253–256, 1989

Owens DG: Involuntary disorders of movement in chronic schizophrenia: the role of the illness and its treatment, in Dyskinesia Research and Treatment (Psychopharmacology Supplementum 2). Edited by Casey DE, Chase TN, Christensen AV, et al. Berlin, Springer-Verlag, 1985, pp 79–87

Pall HS, Williams AC, Blake DR, et al: Evidence of enhanced lipid peroxidation in the cerebrospinal fluid of patients taking phenothiazines. Lancet 2:596–599, 1987

Palozza P, Krinsky NI: β-carotene and α-tocopherol are synergistic antioxidants. Arch Biochem Biophys 297:184–187, 1992

Parepally H, Mukherjee S, Schnur DB, et al: Tardive dyskinesia in bipolar patients. Biol Psychiatry 25:163A, 1989

Peet M, Laugharne J, Rangarajan N, et al: Tardive dyskinesia, lipid peroxidation and vitamin E. Schizophr Res 9:279, 1993a

Peet M, Laugharne J, Rangarajan N, et al: Tardive dyskinesia, lipid peroxidation, and sustained amelioration with vitamin E treatment. Int Clin Psychopharmacol 8:151–153, 1993b

Perris C, Dimitrijevic P, Jacobsson L, et al: Tardive dyskinesia in psychiatric patients treated with neuroleptics. Br J Psychiatry 135:509–514, 1979

Random House Dictionary of the English Language, 2nd Edition, Unabridged. New York, Random House, 1987

Raymond V, Beaulieu M, Labrie F: Potent antidopaminergic activity of estradiol at the pituitary level on prolactin release. Science 200:1173–1175, 1978

Reiter S, Adler LA, Angrist B, et al: Effects of verapamil on tardive dyskinesia and psychosis in schizophrenic patients. J Clin Psychiatry 50:26–27, 1989

Richardson MA, Craig TJ: The coexistence of parkinsonism-like symptoms and tardive dyskinesia. Am J Psychiatry 139:341–343, 1982

Richardson MA, Pass R, Bregman Z, et al: Tardive dyskinesia and depressive symptoms in schizophrenics. Psychopharmacol Bull 21:130–135, 1985

Richardson MA, Haugland G, Craig TJ: Neuroleptic use, parkinsonian symptoms, tardive dyskinesia, and associated factors in child and adolescent psychiatric patients. Am J Psychiatry 148:1322–1328, 1991

Riederer P, Sofic E, Rausch WD, et al: Transition metals, ferritin, glutathione, and ascorbic acid in parkinsonian brains. J Neurochem 52:515–520, 1989

Rogers D: Motor Disorder in Psychiatry: Towards a Neurological Psychiatry. New York, Wiley, 1992, pp 65–77

Ross JL, Mackenzie TB, Hanson DR, et al: Diltiazem for tardive dyskinesia. Lancet 1:268, 1987

Rutledge JN, Hilal SK, Silver AJ, et al: Study of movement disorders and brain iron by MR. American Journal of Neuroradiology 8:397–411, 1987

Sachdev P: The prevalence of tardive dystonia in patients with chronic schizophrenia (letter). Aust N Z J Psychiatry 25:446–448, 1991

Sachdev P: Clinical characteristics of 15 patients with tardive dystonia. Am J Psychiatry 150:498–500, 1993

Saltz BL, Kane JM, Woerner MG, et al: Prospective study of tardive dyskinesia in the elderly. Psychopharmacol Bull 25:52–56, 1989

Saltz BL, Woerner MG, Kane JM, et al: Prospective study of tardive dyskinesia: incidence in the elderly, preliminary findings. JAMA 266:2402–2406, 1991

Sandyk R: Tardive dyskinesia and the pineal gland. Int J Neurosci 43:111–114, 1988

Sandyk R: Pineal calcification and subtypes of tardive dyskinesia. Int J Neurosci 53:223–229, 1990a

Sandyk R: The relationship of pineal calcification to subtypes of tardive dyskinesia in bipolar patients. Int J Neurosci 54:307–313, 1990b

Sandyk R, Fisher H: Serotonin in involuntary movement disorders. Int J Neurosci 42:185–205, 1988

Sandyk R, Kay SR: The relationship of tardive dyskinesia to positive schizophrenia. Int J Neurosci 56:107–139, 1991

Sandyk R, Kay SR: "Positive" and "negative" movement disorders in schizophrenia. Int J Neurosci 66:143–151, 1992

Sandyk R, Awerbuch GI, Kay SR: Pineal gland classification and tardive dyskinesia. Lancet 23:1528, 1990

Sandyk R, Kay SR, Awerbuch GI, et al: Risk factors for neuroleptic-induced movement disorders. Int J Neurosci 61:148–188, 1991

Scheel-Kruger J: Dopamine-GABA interactions: evidence that GABA transmits, modulates, and mediates dopaminergic functions in the basal ganglia and the limbic system. Acta Neurol Scand Suppl 107:1–54, 1986

Schmidt M, Meister P, Baumann P: Treatment of tardive dyskinesias with vitamin E. European Psychiatry 6:201–207, 1991

Schönecker M: Ein eigentumliches Syndrom im oralen Bereich bei Megaphenapplikation. Nervenarzt 28:35, 1957

Schooler NR, Kane JM: Research diagnoses for tardive dyskinesia. Arch Gen Psychiatry 39:486–487, 1982

Schwartz J-C, Sokoloff P, Giros B, et al: The dopamine D_3 receptor as a target for antipsychotics, in Novel Antipsychotic Drugs. Edited by Meltzer HY. New York, Raven, 1992, pp 135–144

Seeman P: Tardive dyskinesia, dopamine receptors, and neuroleptic damage to cell membranes. J Clin Psychopharmacol 8 (suppl 4):3–9, 1988

Seeman P: Receptor selectivities of atypical neuroleptics, in Novel Antipsychotic Drugs. Edited by Meltzer HY. New York, Raven, 1992, pp 145–154

Seibyl JP, Glazer WM, Innis RB: Serotonin function in tardive dyskinesia. Psychiatric Annals 19:310–313, 1989

Shriqui CL: Dyskinésie tardive: mise à jour. Can J Psychiatry 33:637–644, 1988

Shriqui CL: Vitamin E in the treatment of tardive dyskinesia: does it really work? Schizophr Res 9:280, 1993

Shriqui CL: CT and MRI studies in tardive dyskinesia, in Neuroleptic-Induced Movement Disorders: A Comprehensive Survey. Edited by Yassa R, Jeste DV, Nair NPV. London, Cambridge University Press (in press)

Shriqui C, Annable L: Risk factors for tardive dyskinesia. Paper presented at the annual meeting of the American Psychiatric Association, Philadelphia, PA, May 25, 1994

Shriqui C, Jones B: Free radicals and tardive dyskinesia. Can J Psychiatry 35:282–284, 1990a

Shriqui C, Jones B: Free radical involvement in schizophrenia and tardive dyskinesia. Schizophr Res 3:81, 1990b

Shriqui CL, Bradwejn J, Jones BD: Tardive dyskinesia: legal and preventive aspects. Can J Psychiatry 35:576–580, 1990

Shriqui CL, Bradwejn J, Annable L, et al: Vitamin E in the treatment of tardive dyskinesia: a double-blind placebo-controlled study. Am J Psychiatry 149:391–393, 1992

Shriqui CL, Annable L, Bouchard G, et al: Tardive dyskinesia in schizophrenic subjects: a controlled magnetic resonance imaging (MRI) study. Paper presented at the annual meeting of the Canadian College of Neuropsychopharmacology, Quebec City, Canada, May 1994a

Shriqui CL, Nobecourt P, Rousseau F, et al: Clinical efficacy of risperidone in a patient with severe tardive dyskinesia. Schizophr Res 11:194, 1994b

Sigwald J, Bouttier D, Raymondeau C, et al: Quatre cas de dyskinésie facio-bucco-linguo-masticatrice à évolution prolongée secondaire à un traitement par les neuroleptiques. Rev Neurol (Paris) 100:751–755, 1959

Simpson GM, Lee JH, Zoubok B, et al: A rating scale for tardive dyskinesia. Psychopharmacology 64:171–179, 1979

Simpson GM, Pi EH, Sramek JJ: An update on tardive dyskinesia. Hosp Community Psychiatry 37:362–369, 1986

Smith RC, Strizick M, Klass D: Drug history and tardive dyskinesia. Am J Psychiatry 135:1402–1403, 1978

Sokoloff P, Giros B, Martres M, et al: Molecular cloning and characterization of a novel dopamine receptor (D_3) as a target for neuroleptics. Nature 347:146–151, 1990

Sorokin JE, Giordani B, Mohs RC, et al: Memory impairment in schizophrenic patients with tardive dyskinesia. Biol Psychiatry 23:129–135, 1988

Spivak B, Schwartz B, Radwan M, et al: α-tocopherol treatment for tardive dyskinesia. J Nerv Ment Dis 180:400–401, 1992

Stedman TJ, Whiteford HA, Eyles D, et al: Effects of nifedipine on psychosis and tardive dyskinesia in schizophrenic patients. J Clin Psychopharmacol 11:43–47, 1991

Suddath RL, Straw GM, Freed WJ, et al: A clinical trial of nifedipine in schizophrenia and tardive dyskinesia. Pharmacol Biochem Behav 39:743–745, 1991

Sunahara RK, Guan H-C, O'Dowd BF, et al: Cloning of the gene for a human dopamine D_5 receptor with higher affinity for dopamine than D_1. Nature 350:614–619, 1991

Szymanski SR, Lieberman JA, Saltz B, et al: Free radicals: do they cause tardive dyskinesia? Paper presented at the annual meeting of the American Psychiatric Association, Washington, DC, May 1992

Tamminga CA, Chase TN: Bromocriptine and CF 25-397 in the treatment of tardive dyskinesia. Arch Neurol 37:204-205, 1980

Tamminga CA, Crayton JW, Chase TN: Improvement in tardive dyskinesia after muscimol therapy. Arch Gen Psychiatry 36:595–598, 1979

Tancredi LR: Malpractice and tardive dyskinesia: a conceptual dilemma. J Clin Psychopharmacol 8 (suppl 4):71–76, 1988

Tanner CM: Treatment of tardive dyskinesia: other therapies. Clin Neuropharmacol 6:159–167, 1983

Thaker GK, Tamminga CA, Alphs LD, et al: Brain gamma-aminobutyric acid abnormality in tardive dyskinesia. Arch Gen Psychiatry 44:522–529, 1987

Thaker GK, Nguyen JA, Tamminga CA: Increased saccadic distractibility in tardive dyskinesia: functional evidence for subcortical GABA dysfunction. Biol Psychiatry 25:49–59, 1989

Thaker GK, Nguyen JA, Strauss ME, et al: Clonazepam treatment of tardive dyskinesia: a practical GABAmimetic strategy. Am J Psychiatry 147:445–451, 1990

Toenniessen LM, Casey DE, McFarland BH: Tardive dyskinesia in the aged: duration of treatment relationships. Arch Gen Psychiatry 42:278–284, 1985

Vaddadi KS: Essential fatty acids and α-tocopherol supplementation in tardive dyskinesia. Biol Psychiatry 1:618–620, 1991

Vaddadi KS: Use of gamma-linolenic acid in the treatment of schizophrenia and tardive dyskinesia. Prostaglandins Leukot Essent Fatty Acids 46:67–70, 1992

Vaddadi KS, Courtney P, Gilleard CJ, et al: A double-blind trial of essential fatty acid supplementation in patients with tardive dyskinesia. Psychiatry Res 27:313–323, 1989

Van Tol HHM, Bunzow JR, Guan H-C, et al: Cloning of the gene for a human dopamine D_4 receptor with high affinity for the antipsychotic clozapine. Nature 350:610–614, 1991

Villeneuve A: The rabbit syndrome: a peculiar extrapyramidal reaction. Can J Psychiatry 17:69–72, 1972

Wada Y, Yamaguchi N: The rabbit syndrome and antiparkinsonian medication in schizophrenic patients. Neuropsychobiology 25:149–152, 1992

Waddington JL: Further anomalies in the dopamine receptor supersensitivity hypothesis of tardive dyskinesia. Trends Neurosci 8:200, 1985

Waddington JL: Tardive dyskinesia in schizophrenia and other disorders: associations with aging, cognitive dysfunction and structural brain pathology in relation to neuroleptic exposure. Human Psychopharmacology 2:11–22, 1987

Waddington JL: Schizophrenia, affective psychoses, and other disorders treated with neuroleptic drugs: the enigma of tardive dyskinesia, its neurobiological determinants, and the conflict of paradigms. Int Rev Neurobiol 31:297–353, 1989

Waddington JL, Youssef HA: An unusual cluster of tardive dyskinesia in schizophrenia: association with cognitive dysfunction and negative symptoms. Am J Psychiatry 143:1162–1165, 1986

Waddington JL, Youssef HA: Tardive dyskinesia in bipolar affective disorder: aging, cognitive dysfunction, course of illness, and exposure to neuroleptics and lithium. Am J Psychiatry 145:613–616, 1988

Waddington JL, Youssef HA: The lifetime outcome and involuntary movements of schizophrenia never treated with neuroleptic drugs: four rare cases in Ireland. Br J Psychiatry 156:106–108, 1990

Waddington JL, Youssef HA, Dolphin C, et al: Cognitive dysfunction, negative symptoms, and tardive dyskinesia in schizophrenia. Arch Gen Psychiatry 44:907–912, 1987

Wettstein RM: Informed consent and tardive dyskinesia. J Clin Psychopharmacol 8 (suppl 4):65–70, 1988

Woerner MG, Kane JM, Lieberman JA, et al: The prevalence of tardive dyskinesia. J Clin Psychopharmacol 11:34–42, 1991

Wojcik JD, Falk WE, Fink JS, et al: A review of 32 cases of tardive dystonia. Am J Psychiatry 148:1055–1059, 1991

Wolf MA, Wertenschlag N: Facteurs de risque et prévention des dyskinésies tardives. Can J Psychiatry 34:177–181, 1989

Wolf MA, Grunberg F, Garneau Y: Aspects médico-légaux des dyskinésies tardives aux Etats–Unis. Encephale 14:133–138, 1988

Wolf ME, Koller WC: Tardive dystonia: treatment with trihexyphenidyl. J Clin Psychopharmacol 5:247–248, 1985

Yadalam KG, Simpson GM: Dopamine receptor sensitivity and tardive dyskinesia. Schizophr Res 3:80, 1990

Yassa R: Tardive dyskinesia and anticholinergic drugs: a critical review of the literature. Encephale 14:233–239, 1988

Yassa R, Ananth J: Lithium carbonate in the treatment of movement disorders. International Pharmacopsychiatry 15:301–308, 1980

Yassa R, Jeste DV: Gender differences in tardive dyskinesia: a critical review of the literature. Schizophr Bull 18:701–715, 1992

Yassa R, Jones BD: Complications of tardive dyskinesia: a review. Psychosomatics 26:305–313, 1985

Yassa R, Lal S: Impaired sexual intercourse as a complication of tardive dyskinesia. Am J Psychiatry 142:1514–1515, 1985

Yassa R, Nair NPV: Mild tardive dyskinesia: an 8-year follow-up study. Acta Psychiatr Scand 81:139–140, 1989

Yassa R, Nair NPV: A 10-year follow-up study of tardive dyskinesia. Acta Psychiatr Scand 86:262–266, 1992

Yassa R, Ghadirian AM, Schwartz G: Prevalence of tardive dyskinesia in affective disorder patients. J Clin Psychiatry 44:410–412, 1983a

Yassa R, Ananth J, Cordozo S, et al: Tardive dyskinesia in an outpatient population: prevalence and predisposing factors. Can J Psychiatry 28:391–394, 1983b

Yassa R, Mohelsky H, Dimitri R: Mortality rate in tardive dyskinesia. Am J Psychiatry 141:1018–1019, 1984

Yassa R, Lal S, Korpassy A, et al: Nicotine exposure and tardive dyskinesia. Biol Psychiatry 22:67–72, 1987

Yassa R, Iskandar H, Ally J: The prevalence of tardive dyskinesia in fluphenazine-treated patients. J Clin Psychopharmacol 8 (suppl 4):17–20, 1988a

Yassa R, Nastase C, Camille Y, et al: Tardive dyskinesia in a psychogeriatric population, in Tardive Dyskinesia: Biological Mechanisms and Clinical Aspects. Edited by Wolf ME, Mosnaim AD. Washington, DC, American Psychiatric Press, 1988b, pp 125–133

Yassa R, Nair NPV, Iskandar II, et al: Factors in the development of severe forms of tardive dyskinesia. Am J Psychiatry 147:1156–1163, 1990

Yassa R, Nastase C, Dupont D, et al: Tardive dyskinesia in the elderly psychiatric patients: a 5-year study. Am J Psychiatry 149:1206–1211, 1992

Young AH, Blackwood DHR, Roxborough H, et al: A magnetic resonance imaging study of schizophrenia: brain structure and clinical symptoms. Br J Psychiatry 158:158–164, 1991

Youssef HA, Waddington JL: Morbidity and mortality in tardive dyskinesia: associations in chronic schizophrenia. Acta Psychiatr Scand 75:74–77, 1987

Youssef HA, Waddington JL: Primitive (developmental) reflexes and diffuse cerebral dysfunction in schizophrenia and bipolar affective disorder: over-representation in patients with tardive dyskinesia. Biol Psychiatry 23:791–796, 1988

Youssef HA, Waddington JL: Characterization of abnormal respiratory movements in schizophrenic, bipolar and mentally handicapped patients with typical tardive dyskinesia. Int Clin Psychopharmacol 4:55–59, 1989

Zaretsky A, Rector NA, Seeman MV, et al: Current cannabis use and tardive dyskinesia. Schizophr Res 11:3–8, 1993

CHAPTER 26

Tardive Psychosis

Barry D. Jones, M.D., F.R.C.P.C.

It has been shown that dopamine (DA) receptor-binding sites increase in the neostriatum after chronic treatment with neuroleptics; based on this correlation, DA supersensitivity has been implicated in the etiology of tardive dyskinesia (Burt et al. 1977). Similar changes in DA receptor-binding sites could occur in other areas of the brain thought to be more directly linked to the production of psychotic symptoms. One such area may be the mesolimbic area; results from both animal and human studies support the development of increased DA receptor-binding sites in this region after chronic exposure to neuroleptics (Muller and Seeman 1977; Owen et al. 1979).

Because increases in DA activity in humans tend to be related to exacerbation or production of psychotic symptoms, an increase in DA activity in the mesolimbic area, analogous to the mechanism in tardive dyskinesia, should result in the appearance of psychotic symptoms at times when neuroleptic medication is decreased or held at constant dosage for a certain period of time (just as tardive dyskinesia can emerge or worsen under similar conditions). This would result in a neuroleptic-induced tardive psychosis that is separate from the illness-related psychosis (Chouinard et al. 1978a).

In this chapter, I examine the clinical literature for evidence supportive of four predictions that follow from this hypothesis of neuroleptic-induced tardive psychosis:

1. Psychosis may occur in patients with nonpsychotic disorders who are being treated with or have been withdrawn from neuroleptics, even though they have never been psychotic prior to receiving neuroleptics.
2. Psychosis is worse in neuroleptic-treated patients (i.e., there is a greater rate of relapse subsequent to drug withdrawal and more severe psychotic episodes with new symptoms) than in non–neuroleptic-treated patients.
3. Tolerance to the antipsychotic effect of neuroleptics should be seen.
4. Tendency to relapse because of tardive psychosis may be correlated with the presence and severity of tardive dyskinesia.

Onset of Psychosis in Nonpsychotic Patients When Neuroleptics Are Withdrawn

In 1978, Sale et al. described the case of a previously nonpsychotic patient who had received neuroleptic therapy for many years as treatment for anxiety and obsessional symptoms. When the medication was withdrawn, the patient experienced a psychotic episode. Caine et al. (1978) described the case of a 15-year-old patient with Tourette syndrome treated with haloperidol for 3 years at 20–30 mg/day. The patient had never previously manifested any psychotic symptoms, nor was there a family history of psychiatric illness. Upon withdrawal of haloperidol, the patient presented with severe dyskinetic movements and corresponding psychotic symptoms of feeling that his mind could be read, he was hearing voices, and his thoughts were disorganized. Both syndromes remitted upon reinstitution of the neuroleptic.

Hollister (1961) reported on 36 patients treated with chlorpromazine, 300 mg/day, for 3–12 months for the purpose of examining the effect of this drug on tuberculosis. None of the patients had previously manifested psychotic symptoms. However, during treatment, 4 patients became psychotic, with 2 requiring transfer to the psychiatry service. Upon termination of treatment, 4 other patients became restless and anxious and experienced insomnia. A major limitation of Hollister's findings was that some of the patients were treated concomitantly with isoniazid, which has been reported to induce psychotic symptoms.

Witschy et al. (1984) reported on the case of a patient with manic depressive illness who, after neuroleptics were withdrawn, developed psychotic symptoms. The authors speculated that this was an example of neuroleptic-induced tardive psychosis, as the patient had not suffered from the same psychotic symptoms in the past and the symptoms had rapidly appeared.

Psychosis Worse in Neuroleptic-Treated Patients Than in Non–Neuroleptic-Treated Patients

Results from a number of studies have suggested that patients treated with neuroleptics subsequently experience a worse form of illness, in some respects, than they had prior to treatment. Bockoven and Solomon (1975) compared the course of patients in two 5-year follow-up studies of newly admitted patients hospitalized in community-oriented hospitals. The first group was followed from 1947 to 1952, before the introduction of neuroleptics. Patients in the second group, followed from 1967 to 1972, were treated with drugs both during hospitalization and after discharge as clinically indicated. At the end of 5 years, 85% of the non–drug-treated patients and 83% of the drug-treated patients remained in the community. Although there were many complicating factors in this study, these results would suggest that, despite the use of neuroleptics with their proven antipsychotic effect in short-term application, no difference in terms of remaining out of hospital 5 years after discharge occurred between these groups, as if the drug effect had "worn off." Alternatively, these results could be explained by assuming that some patients retain beneficial effects from the drugs, whereas others may actually develop a more malignant form of the illness after discontinuing drug treatment.

Mosher and Menn (1978) compared the 2-year outcome data for young schizophrenic patients (ages 15–31 years) admitted to either a nonmedical psychological treatment program or a short-stay, crisis-oriented service in a community mental health center, where all patients received neuroleptics. Readmissions rates over the 2 years were 53% for the nondrug group versus 67% for the drug group.

Carpenter et al. (1977) compared the course of acute schizophrenic patients who received psychosocial treatment either with or without drug treatment; both groups of patients had had similar symptomatology and prognosis prior to treatment. They found the outcome at the end of 1 year to be similar for both groups. The non–drug-treated patients tended to have a shorter length of hospitalization (108 versus 126 days) and were less likely to be rehospitalized (35% versus 45%). These differences, however, did not reach statistical significance.

May and Goldberg (1978) found that schizophrenic patients who had been treated with neuroleptics showed a greater decrease of psychotic symptoms when compared with a group receiving only electroconvulsive therapy (ECT). However, at 5-year follow-up, the ECT-treated group showed fewer readmissions than the drug-treated group.

A major limitation of these studies was that the patients receiving no medication were receiving active treatment of another kind. Also, there remains the question of whether patients selected for nondrug treatment could have been healthier than those selected for drug treatment. In their study, Rappaport et al. (1978) controlled for these variables by examining young first- or second-break schizophrenic patients withdrawn from medication at follow-up, who had been randomly assigned to receive either placebo or neuroleptic medication during hospitalization. Patients in the no-medication group had fewer rehospitalizations and less functional disturbance than did those who had received medication over the subsequent year. However, the results of this study were contaminated by a greater loss to follow-up of non–drug-treated patients, which may have reflected psychotic relapse.

Schooler et al. (1967) found that within a 1-year follow-up of mainly first- or second-admission schizophrenic patients, those who had been randomly treated with neuroleptics had a greater risk of relapse—as manifested by number of readmissions—than did patients maintained on placebo. However, placebo-treated patients had been hospitalized for longer periods of time, raising the possibility that their increased hospitalization, rather than a lack of deleterious effect from drug treatment, accounted for their decreased rate of relapse. Thus, because of problems in study design, all of these results can only be described as suggestive, and not supportive or definitive.

A second approach to the question of patients' psychosis being worsened when they are treated with neuroleptics is to use the patients as their own controls. Upon cessation of neuroleptic treatment, the psychosis should be more severe than that previously seen in the same patient when his or her illness began, and maintenance of remission should be more closely dependent on continuation of neuroleptics than was the case earlier in the illness. Chouinard and Jones (1980) noted this finding anecdotally in their patient population. Patients reported that, when they first became ill, they could remain out of the hospital for a year or more despite a lack of compliance with medication. After a number of years of treatment, however, they would relapse within weeks of missing only one injection of their long-acting maintenance intramuscular neuroleptic. Whitaker and Hoy (1963) described the unexpected finding of four patients in their perphenazine withdrawal study who "relapsed to a state markedly worse than their condition before the original introduction of perphenazine" (p. 425). They were careful to rule out accompanying nonspecific withdrawal symptoms, such as nausea, sweating, and insomnia, as being contributory to the marked relapse. Blackburn and Allen (1961) reported that the illness of 12 of 15 patients relapsing from abrupt withdrawal of medication was severe enough to require emergency reinstitution of medication and transfer to a closed ward. Finally, Capstick (1980) found a significant tendency for 25 patients relapsing during withdrawal from fluphenazine decanoate to show symptoms other than those usually associated with their illness, in comparison with a group of 22 patients who relapsed during a 2-year follow-up period while off medication and who demonstrated their normal illness-related symptoms.

Of course, all of the above findings cannot control for the course of the original illness in the patient, which might have worsened or changed with or without neuroleptic treatment.

At this point, it becomes important to draw a distinction between two types of neuroleptic-induced psychosis that may exist as analogues of withdrawal dyskinesia (a disorder seen in younger patient populations that is generally reversible and closely related to cessation or abrupt decrease of neuroleptic medication) and tardive dyskinesia (a disorder seen in older patient populations that is generally irreversible and manifested as a breakthrough of abnormal movements at relatively constant dosages of neuroleptic medication). *Withdrawal psychosis,* therefore, may be seen as a psychotic relapse that occurs soon after medication dosage is abruptly decreased and that is seen most frequently in younger populations. *Tardive psychosis* would be more often seen as a breakthrough of psychotic symptoms in older patients chronically maintained on neuroleptics. Both entities would still require a minimum period of neuroleptic exposure and presumably some type of constitutional predisposition to developing the syndrome.

If such a distinction is valid, a group that would be expected to be at great risk to manifest withdrawal psychosis compared with chronic older patients would be children. Polizos et al. (1973) examined 34 schizophrenic children who had been treated with neuroleptics for an average of 1 year. Upon discontinuation of medication, 32 of the 34 children suffered "massive relapse" within 1–2 weeks after drug withdrawal, a remarkably high relapse rate and one that occurred relatively early. Also, 14 of these patients manifested dyskinetic movements concomitant with psychotic relapse.

Of course, this different relapse profile in children may be related to severity of illness or to altered drug kinetics in children. However, if one examines young adult patients who have also been exposed to medication for a period adequate to develop this putatively drug-induced syndrome (Levine et al. 1980), a similar pattern can be found in that relapse tends to occur early after abrupt withdrawal of medication and parallels the time course of withdrawal dyskinesia exacerbation. In fact, relapse rates in this younger patient population favor the medication group only during the withdrawal period, since, after 3 weeks, no difference in rate of relapse was found between those receiving drug and those receiving placebo.

Another group of patients that would possibly be more prone to show withdrawal psychosis would be those treated with the antipsychotic drug clozapine. Given that clozapine has a relatively short half-life and a greater affinity for mesolimbic than for striatal DA receptors, discontinuation of this drug could lead to greater rebound DA activity in the mesolimbic area, and subsequently to a higher frequency of withdrawal psychosis. Cases of withdrawal or supersensitivity psychosis have been reported after discontinuation of clozapine (Ekblom et al. 1984). In addition to case reports, Diamond and Borison (1986, 1988) showed that only patients treated with clozapine, in comparison with patients on haloperidol and chlorpromazine, showed rebound in psychopathology during a placebo wash-out period. They also reported that a subgroup of clozapine-withdrawal patients experienced a 17%–126% worsening of psychopathology in the withdrawal period compared with the period prior to clozapine treatment.

These clozapine withdrawal findings raise interesting questions about the underlying mechanisms governing tardive and withdrawal psychoses. Given clozapine's unusual efficacy in blocking the D_4 receptor (Van Tol et al. 1991), the clozapine withdrawal psychosis may represent a D_4 supersensitivity. My colleagues and I recently observed a patient who, after being treated with clozapine for over 1 year, had his clozapine therapy discontinued in preparation for starting the atypical antipsychotic drug risperidone (a potent dopamine D_2 and serotonin antagonist; Janssen et al. 1988). The patient showed a severe increase in psychotic symptoms upon discontinuation of the clozapine that could not be managed with risperidone. Only the reintroduction of clozapine brought these psychotic symptoms under relative control. Although other explanations may be entertained, the withdrawal psychosis appearing after clozapine discontinuation in this patient may have been attributable to a D_4 supersensitivity that risperidone and other typical neuroleptics were unable to treat at usual therapeutic doses. The possibility that clozapine-induced withdrawal psychosis is related to D_4 supersensitivity raises concerns about using this drug in patients other than those who are truly refractory to typical neuroleptic treatment.

Tolerance to Antipsychotic Effect of Neuroleptics

The phenomenon of tolerance has been demonstrated for extrapyramidal side effects but has not been demonstrated for antipsychotic effects from neuroleptic medications. However, in examining patients receiving injectable fluphenazine, Chouinard et al. (1978b) reported on the need to increase dosages of medication over the course of a 7-month follow-up of chronic, remitted schizophrenic outpatients.

The question arises as to why antipsychotic tolerance has not otherwise been reported in the literature. One possibility is that such tolerance is difficult to observe in patients on oral medication when compliance is not ensured. However, a more likely explanation could be that tolerance does occur in a certain number of patients but is not recognized as such. Tolerance to extrapyramidal side effects is reflected in a decrease of severity of these symptoms over time on constant dosage. Tolerance to antipsychotic effect might only be expressed with increase or breakthrough of psychotic symptoms over time at a constant dosage, as may occur in the tardive psychosis type of neuroleptic-induced psychosis previously described. It is, in fact, interesting that some 16% of chronic schizophrenic patients followed over months to a few years relapse despite evidence indicating adequate medication compliance (Baldessarini and Davis 1980).

Examining this question from a different perspective, one would expect, as outlined earlier, that patients who develop tolerance will present clinically with a higher dosage of drug while in remission than those who do not. This would be manifested as higher dosages for patients who have been treated long enough to develop neuroleptic-induced tardive psychosis compared with those who have not, and higher dosages for those patients who relapse when medication is decreased or discontinued compared with patients who do not.

Young and Meltzer (1980) retrospectively examined two groups of schizophrenic patients: those who had been treated successfully on low-dosage medication (200 chlorpromazine units) and those who had required higher dosages (800 chlorpromazine units). The low-dosage group tended to be experiencing their first psychotic episode, whereas the high-dosage group had had a significantly greater number of psychotic episodes.

One consistent finding in studies of patients on chronic neuroleptic maintenance is that the patients receiving higher dosages of medication are those most likely to relapse when medication is withdrawn.

Prien et al. (1969) found this to be one of the few predictive factors of relapse among the many patients examined in the context of a large, multicenter collaborative study. Andrews et al. (1976) observed a direct positive correlation between relapse following medication withdrawal and prestudy dosage levels of neuroleptics. This finding could be related to the fact that patients with a history of more severe illness and a higher number of previous psychotic episodes required higher dosages of neuroleptics, thus exposing them to a greater risk of relapse.

Case reports of patients requiring progressively higher dosages of neuroleptics to control psychosis would support the theory of tolerance to antipsychotic effect. Degwitz et al. (1970) reported on one patient who received progressive increases of oral haloperidol to control psychotic symptoms until the patient was finally receiving 600 mg/day of haloperidol. Csernansky and Hollister (1982) presented a case in which neuroleptic dosages were greatly increased over 20 years from an initial 800 mg/day of chlorpromazine to 280 mg/day of trifluoperazine and 160 mg/day of thiothixene. Chouinard and Jones (1980) reported on 10 patients receiving injectable, long-acting fluphenazine who required increasing dosages in order to maintain remission of psychosis. Also, Sramek et al.'s (1990) retrospective review of neuroleptic dosages over a 5-year period in 19 chronic schizophrenic patients revealed that 9 patients showed consistent yearly increases in their dosages, although their clinical status remained unchanged.

Of course, tolerance to a drug may be a peripheral metabolic tolerance rather than a central neurophysiological adaptation. However, when blood levels of neuroleptics were examined in two patients showing obvious evidence for tardive psychosis by Chouinard et al. (1982), and in 77 patients rated for the presence or absence of tardive psychosis by Cohen et al. (1980), patients with features of tardive psychosis were found to have 2½ times the blood levels of patients without those features. Oral or intramuscular doses of neuroleptics were similarly 2½ times higher in the tardive psychosis patients. Thus, metabolic tolerance would seem to be unimportant in accounting for increased dosages in such patients.

Despite this indirect evidence supporting a central tolerance to the antipsychotic effect of neuroleptics, most clinicians continue to feel that such an effect, if present, is rare. Palmstierna and Wistedt (1987) followed 38 schizophrenic outpatients for up to 8 years and found that the majority (93%) did not develop tolerance as evidenced by changes in neuroleptic dosage or clinical status. Accordingly, it must be concluded that the phenomenon of tolerance to antipsychotic effect, although supported by some indirect evidence, is relatively rare.

Tendency to Relapse Correlated With Tardive Dyskinesia

Tardive dyskinesia has been hypothesized to be caused by the induction of dopaminergic supersensitivity in the neostriatum by neuroleptics (Baldessarini 1985). Thus, the tendency to experience increased relapse of psychosis because of a similar phenomenon occurring in areas of the brain responsible for psychotic symptoms would be expected to be associated with tardive dyskinesia, assuming that both regions show similar response and adaptation to neuroleptic action, and that the neuroleptics themselves are reasonably equal in their potential to act in the two regions. Of course, dopaminergic supersensitivity need not be the specific phenomenon involved.

Jones et al. (1979) found the severity of tardive dyskinesia prior to drug discontinuation to be related to the degree of relapse in chronic schizophrenic patients after withdrawal from their maintenance neuroleptic dosage. However, the sample size in this study was small. Degwitz et al. (1970) reported on 53 chronic schizophrenic patients treated with neuroleptics for a minimum of 2 years. Twenty-five patients showed either an exacerbation or an emergence of tardive dyskinesia when their neuroleptics were discontinued. All of these patients concomitantly showed an increase of psychotic symptoms. In contrast, the patients who did not show signs of tardive dyskinesia did not relapse. Also, psychotic relapse showed a time course similar to that of the increase of dyskinetic symptoms.

Using a slightly different approach, Kurcharski et al. (1980) reported on 291 schizophrenic inpatients, observing that the severity of tardive dyskinesia positively correlated with inpatient status at the end of a 2-year follow-up. The authors hypothesized that tardive psychosis could have played a role in this association.

Levine et al. (1980) examined tardive dyskinetic changes in patients undergoing discontinuation of their neuroleptics and found a tendency—not statistically significant—for patients showing increased severity of dyskinesia over a 3-week period to also manifest early psychotic relapse.

Despite these positive findings of a relationship between tardive dyskinesia and a tendency to relapse when neuroleptic drugs are withdrawn, there have been many negative findings also reported in the literature. Hunt et al. (1988) found that one-third of patients who meet criteria for supersensitivity psychosis present with concomitant tardive dyskinesia. Chouinard et al. (1986) suggested that the discrepancy between Hunt et al.'s and others' findings could be related to the fact that supersensitivity psychosis is more likely to occur in patients with a good schizophrenic prognosis, whereas tardive dyskinesia is more likely to occur in patients with a poor schizophrenic prognosis. Alternatively, the data supporting the theory that a withdrawal psychosis appears after clozapine discontinuation (i.e., that patients who are sensitive to drugs that act preferentially on mesolimbic DA systems may be more prone to demonstrate supersensitivity or tardive psychosis) may offer a more suitable explanation for the lack of association between the clinical presentation of supersensitivity psychosis and the clinical manifestation of tardive dyskinesia.

Discussion

From this review, it can be seen that there is suggestive evidence for the hypothesis of neuroleptic-induced psychosis in the clinical psychiatric literature. However, the evidence is weak, and alternative explanations can be advanced to explain all findings. The importance of further investigations in this area cannot be underestimated. If neuroleptic withdrawal—or chronic maintenance neuroleptic therapy—can induce psychotic symptoms that mimic functional psychosis, that is a matter of theoretical and practical significance. For example, it can be speculated that lifetime neuroleptic treatment required after two or more psychotic episodes may in fact be needed not because of a chronic illness but because of drug-induced tardive psychosis. This would be the case, however, only in rare circumstances.

The inability to use factors such as premorbid personality or severity of illness to predict which patients will relapse off medication may be attributable to the confounding of these variables by neuroleptic induction of psychosis in a proportion of patients.

Confusion surrounding the diagnosis of schizophrenic patients when compared with patients with a bipolar disorder may be attributable to the neuroleptic induction of psychosis in the latter patient group, resulting in neuroleptic-dependent bipolar patients. Such confusion can contaminate research examining these different entities if a proportion of patients with bipolar disorders are incorrectly included within the schizophrenic population.

Studies examining the effectiveness of new antipsychotics in patients previously treated with neuroleptics may negatively influence results in patients suffering from neuroleptic-induced psychosis. Just as tardive dyskinesia can be suppressed in the short term by neuroleptics, so, too, could neuroleptic-induced psychotic symptoms resulting from neuroleptic withdrawal.

What type of studies clarify whether neuroleptic-induced psychoses could exist from the perspective of the four subheadings outlined previously?

Psychosis occurring in patients not previously psychotic. Studies placing patients without psychosis on neuroleptics are not ethical. However, patients who have previously been placed on neuroleptics for control of abnormal behavior, such as children suffering from mental retardation without psychosis, could be examined for psychotic symptoms if the medication is lowered or discontinued. Given their age, patients in this group should be especially prone to developing withdrawal psychosis.

Psychosis made worse after chronic neuroleptic exposure. Studies examining this prediction would also be unethical unless some form of active treatment is offered to patients who are acutely psychotic. One study design allowing for this but still testing the hypothesis would place acute, first-episode patients on neuroleptic treatment for variable lengths of time (e.g., 1 month, 3 months, 6 months, and 1 year). Patients would subsequently be withdrawn from medication—some gradually, others abruptly—and the incidence of relapse in each group would be recorded. Those patients receiving drugs for longer intervals should show greater rates of relapse. Similarly, patients with abrupt withdrawal should show greater rates of relapse than those with gradual withdrawal.

Tolerance to the antipsychotic effect of neuroleptics. The availability of assay techniques to measure neuroleptic plasma levels enables investigators to properly examine the question of tolerance to antipsychotic effect. However, the feasibility of such studies is restricted by a lack of knowledge concerning the natural course of psychotic illnesses, which presumably could become worse with time, thus requiring more medication to maintain remission. To control for this would require a group of randomly assigned patients who received medication only during psychotic episodes but were withdrawn from medication between episodes to be compared with a group of patients maintained constantly on neuroleptic therapy. Compared with patients receiving only episode-related medication, those receiving long-term treatment should, over time, require increased neuroleptic levels to maintain a similar clinical state. Also, after a sufficient length of follow-up, the two groups should show a differential relapse rate when neuroleptics were withdrawn in the maintenance group.

A related study design would involve placing two randomly assigned groups of patients on high- and low-dosage maintenance therapy and then discontinuing medication. Again, the high-dosage group should show a greater rate of relapse after medication was stopped and should require higher neuroleptic levels to reestablish remission. Positive findings in both of these study designs would require that tardive psychosis, withdrawal psychosis, or both occur in a sufficient number of patients.

Tendency to relapse related to incidence and severity of tardive dyskinesia. This association may not be causally related but linked instead to the severity of illness, requiring more medication and consequently placing the patient at greater risk for tardive dyskinesia. However, if two groups of patients, one with tardive dyskinesia and the other without, were matched according to history of drug exposure and other relevant variables, then one could predict an increased risk of relapse in the tardive dyskinesia patient group on the basis of neuroleptic-induced psychosis.

Finally, the growing understanding of the mechanism by which clozapine and other novel antipsychotics act, as well as recent clinical evidence supporting the occurrence of withdrawal psychosis in clozapine-treated patients, opens the door to potential new methods by which to understand tardive or withdrawal psychosis. Unlike clozapine, typical neuroleptic drugs do not possess a high affinity for the dopamine D_4 receptor at usual therapeutic dosages. It is possible, however, that patients who are exposed to very high dosages of typical neuroleptics or who have slowed peripheral metabolism leading to high plasma levels at usual dosages may sufficiently antagonize D_4 receptors to induce D_4 receptor supersensitivity over time. These patients in turn would relapse dramatically when drugs were discontinued and might only respond to reinstitution either of relatively high dosages of a typical neuroleptic or of atypical agents such as clozapine. According to this scheme, patients on clozapine would then develop increased D_4 receptor supersensitivity and would demonstrate similar extreme withdrawal psychosis when the drug was either decreased or discontinued.

The relative rarity of an association between tardive dyskinesia and supersensitivity psychosis, as well as evidence for tolerance to antipsychotic drug effect, might in fact be attributable to low D_4 receptor blockade with typical neuroleptics. A key question that arises is the ability of novel antipsychotics—such as clozapine—to induce tolerance to the antipsychotic drug effect. My colleagues and I are unaware of any studies reporting such a phenomenon, although we have observed patients who demonstrated a gradual loss of effectiveness with clozapine over time.

Finally, the long-term use of clozapine or clozapine-like agents and their subsequent withdrawal in animals may ultimately serve as an animal model for the study of either neuroleptic-induced tardive psychosis or schizophrenia itself.

References

Andrews P, Hall JN, Snaith RP: A controlled trial of phenothiazine withdrawal in chronic schizophrenic patients. Br J Psychiatry 128:451–455, 1976

Baldessarini RJ: Chemotherapy in Psychiatry: Principles and Practice. Cambridge, MA, Harvard University Press, 1985, p 78

Baldessarini RJ, Davis JM: What is the best maintenance dose of neuroleptics in schizophrenia? Psychiatry Res 3:115–122, 1980

Blackburn NH, Allen J: Behavioral effects of interrupting and resuming tranquilizing medication among schizophrenics. J Nerv Ment Dis 133:303–308, 1961

Bockoven JS, Solomon HC: Comparison of two five-year follow-up studies, 1947 to 1957 and 1967 to 1972. Am J Psychiatry 132:796–801, 1975

Burt DR, Creese I, Snyder SH: Antischizophrenic drugs: chronic treatment elevates dopamine receptor binding in brain. Science 196:326–328, 1977

Caine ED, Margolin DI, Brown GL, et al: Gilles de la Tourette's syndrome, tardive dyskinesia and psychosis in an adolescent. Am J Psychiatry 135:241–243, 1978

Capstick N: Long-term fluphenazine decanoate maintenance dosage requirements of chronic schizophrenic patients. Acta Psychiatr Scand 61:256–262, 1980

Carpenter WT, McGlashan TH, Strauss JS: The treatment of acute schizophrenia without drugs: an investigation of some current assumptions. Am J Psychiatry 134:14–20, 1977

Chouinard G, Jones BD: Neuroleptic-induced supersensitivity psychosis: clinical and pharmacological characteristics. Am J Psychiatry 137:16–21, 1980

Chouinard G, Jones BD, Annable L: Neuroleptic-induced supersensitivity psychosis. Am J Psychiatry 135:1409–1410, 1978a

Chouinard C, Annable L, Ross-Chouinard A: A double-blind controlled study of fluphenazine decanoate and enanthate in the maintenance treatment of schizophrenic outpatients, in Depot Fluphenazines: Twelve Years of Experience. Edited by Ayd JF Jr. Baltimore, MD, Ayd Medical Communications, 1978b

Chouinard G, Creese I, Boisvert D, et al: High neuroleptic plasma levels in patients manifesting supersensitivity psychosis. Biol Psychiatry 17:849–851, 1982

Chouinard G, Annable L, Ross-Chouinard A: Neuroleptic-induced psychological supersensitivity syndromes: are these syndromes myth or reality? supersensitivity psychosis and tardive dyskinesia: a survey in schizophrenic outpatients. Psychopharmacol Bull 22:891–896, 1986

Cohen BM, Lipinski JF, Pope HG Jr: Radioreceptor assays for neuroleptic drugs and clinical research in psychiatry. Psychopharmacol Bull 6:82–84, 1980

Csernsansky J, Hollister LE: Probable case of supersensitivity psychosis. Hospital Formulary 3:395–399, 1982

Degwitz VR, Bauer MP, Gruber M, et al: Der zeitliche zusammenhang zwischen dem auftreten persistierender extrapyramidaler hyperkinesen und psychoserecidiven nach abrupter unterbrechung langfristiger neuroleptischer behandlung chronisch schizophrener kranken. Arzneimittelforschung 20:890, 1970

Diamond BI, Borison RL: Basic and clinical studies of neuroleptic-induced supersensitivity psychosis and dyskinesia. Psychopharmacol Bull 22:900–905, 1986

Diamond BI, Borison RL: Rebound psychosis and dyskinesias after clozapine treatment. Psychopharmacology Ser 96:187, 1988

Ekblom B, Eriksson K, Lindstrom LH: Supersensitivity psychosis in schizophrenic patients after sudden clozapine withdrawal. Psychopharmacology 83:293–294, 1984

Hollister L: Chlorpromazine in the treatment of tuberculosis. Am Rev Respir Dis 81:562, 1961

Hunt JI, Singh H, Simpson GM: Neuroleptic-induced supersensitivity psychosis: retrospective study of schizophrenic inpatients. J Clin Psychiatry 49:258–261, 1988

Janssen PAJ, Niemegeers CJE, Awouters F, et al: Pharmacology of risperidone (R64766), a new antipsychotic with serotonin-S_2 and dopamine-D_2 antagonistic properties. J Pharmacol Exp Ther 244:685–693, 1988

Jones BD, Chouinard G, Annable L: Neuroleptics and pituitary dopaminergic receptors. Paper presented at the annual meeting of the American Psychiatric Association, Chicago, IL, May 1979

Kucharski LT, Smith JM, Dunn DD: Tardive dyskinesia and hospital discharge. J Nerv Ment Dis 168:215, 1980

Levine J, Schooler NR, Severe J, et al: Discontinuation of oral and depot fluphenazine in schizophrenia patients after one year of continuous medication: a controlled study. Adv Biochem Psychopharmacol 24:483–493, 1980

May PRA, Goldberg SC: Prediction of schizophrenic patients' response to pharmacotherapy, in Psychopharmacology: A Generation of Progress. Edited by Lipton MA, DiMascio A, Killam KF. New York, Raven, 1978, pp 1139–1153

Mosher LR, Menn AZ: Community residential treatment for schizophrenia: two year follow-up. Hosp Community Psychiatry 29:715–723, 1978

Muller P, Seeman P: Brain neurotransmitter receptors after long-term haloperidol: dopamine, acetylcholine, serotonin, α-noradrenergic, and naloxone receptors. Life Sci 21:1751, 1977

Owen F, Cross AJ, Crow TJ, et al: Increased dopamine-receptor sensitivity in schizophrenia. Lancet 2:223, 1979

Palmstierna T, Wistedt B: Absence of acquired tolerance to neuroleptics in schizophrenic patients. Am J Psychiatry 144:1084–1085, 1987

Polizos P, Englehardt DM, Hoffman SP, et al: Neurological consequences of psychotropic drug withdrawal in schizophrenic children. Journal of Autism and Developmental Disorders 3:247, 1973

Prien RF, Cole JO, Belkin NF: Relapse in chronic schizophrenics following abrupt withdrawal of tranquilizing drugs. Br J Psychiatry 115:679–686, 1969

Rappaport M, Hopkins HK, Hall K, et al: Are there schizophrenics for whom drugs may be unnecessary or contraindicated? International Pharmacopsychiatry 13:100, 1978

Sale I, Kristall H: Schizophrenia following withdrawal from chronic phenothiazine administration: a case report. Aust N Z J Psychiatry 12:73, 1978

Schooler NR, Goldberg SC, Boothe H, et al: One year after discharge: community adjustment of schizophrenic patients. Am J Psychiatry 123:986–995, 1967

Sramek JJ, Gaurano V, Herrera JM, et al: Patterns of neuroleptic usage in continuously hospitalized chronic schizophrenic patients: evidence for development of drug tolerance. Ann Pharmacother 24:7–9, 1990

Van Tol HHM, Bunzow JR, Guan HC, et al: Cloning of the gene for a human dopamine D_4 receptor with high affinity for the antipsychotic clozapine. Nature 350:610–614, 1991

Whitaker CB, Hoy RM: Withdrawal of perphenazine in chronic schizophrenia. Br J Psychiatry 109:422–427, 1963

Witschy JK, Malone GL, Holden LD: Psychosis after neuroleptic withdrawal in a manic-depressive patient. Am J Psychiatry 141:105–106, 1984

Young MA, Meltzer HY: The relationship of demographic, clinical, and outcome variables to neuroleptic treatment requirements. Schizophr Bull 6:88–101, 1980

SECTION V

Psychosocial Treatments

CHAPTER 27

The Interaction of Biopsychosocial Factors, Time, and Course of Schizophrenia

Courtenay M. Harding, Ph.D.

A good rule to follow before beginning to create a chapter is to investigate the derivations of key words commonly assumed and often reconstructed by a field to serve a specific purpose. Such jargon serves as convenient shorthand for unchallenged constructs permeated with assumptions (some generalizable and some very idiosyncratic). These constructs, therefore, tend to constrict thinking, restrict problem solving, and create the illusion that there is a common ground on which the field is built.

Psychosocial is just such a jargon word. The Greek derivation *psyche,* meaning "breath, spirit, and soul," is now converted to a combining form meaning "the mind; mental processes or activities" (Merriam-

The author is most grateful to have this manuscript supported by Grant 000193 from the Robert Wood Johnson Foundation.

Webster 1993, p. 942). *Social* is derived from the Latin *socialis,* based on *socius,* meaning "companion," but ends up meaning the following:

1. Involving allies or confederates
2. Marked by or passed in pleasant companionship with one's friends or associates; of, relating to, or designed for sociability
3. Of or relating to human society, the interaction of the individual and the group, or the welfare of human beings as members of society;
4. Tending to form cooperative and interdependent relationships with others of one's kind; living and breeding in more or less organized communities
5. Of, relating to, or based on rank or status in a particular society; of, relating to, or characteristic of the upper classes (Merriam-Webster 1993, p. 1114)

Therefore, *psychosocial factors,* at least under this definition, appear to cover the provision of 1) residential options, 2) social skills building, 3) vocational training, 4) consumer advocacy, 5) recreational opportunities, and 6) understanding of family interaction, all of which have been appropriately subsumed under the current meaning of *psychosocial rehabilitation.*

However, when the prefix *psych-* or *psycho-* is added to other words, the definition applies to effects that take place in only one direction; thus, according to *Merriam-Webster's Collegiate Dictionary* (1993), *psychotherapy* means "the treatment of mental or emotional disorder or of related bodily ills by psychological means" (p. 943); *psychogenic,* "originating in the mind or in mental or emotional conflict" (p. 942); *psychomotor,* "of or relating to motor action directly proceeding from mental activity" (p. 943); and *psychotropic,* "acting on the mind" (p. 943).

Therefore, by *psychosocial,* do we mean 1) society acting on mental processes of individuals, 2) mental processes affecting social functioning and thus society, or 3) the interaction of mental processes and society? Further, because our understanding of mental processes in serious mental illnesses now includes a plastic biological substrate (e.g., Greenough and Schwark 1984; Harding 1991; Kandel and Schwartz 1981; Sheflen 1981), we have shed the Cartesian dualism of the past in exchange for the person-illness-environment interaction (Strauss et al. 1985; also see Restak 1984 for overview) and the continuities and discontinuities of development (Emde and Harmon 1984).

I have been significantly influenced by nonlinear, interactionist, and dynamic modern thinkers such as M. Bleuler (1978), Ciompi (1989), Engel (1980), Gleick (1988), Kandel and Schwartz (1981), Selye (1956), Strauss and Carpenter (1981), and Tritton (1986), as well as by data from my longitudinal studies of schizophrenic patients and those with other prolonged psychiatric disorders (e.g., Harding et al. 1987a, 1987b). Therefore, it is my belief that interactions within and across the biopsychosocial contexts of the person, the family, the treatment, and the community (as well as just plain luck) (Bandura 1982; Rutter 1984) all play significant roles in the overall course of schizophrenia and the life of the person. Thus, having declared these acquired biases, and because excellent traditional reviews of psychosocial factors are already available (e.g., American Psychiatric Association 1989; M. J. Goldstein 1991; Liberman and Mueser 1989; McGlashan 1986a; Mosher and Keith 1979; Wyatt et al. 1988), in this chapter I now focus on the influence of biopsychosocial factors on the course of schizophrenia. I endeavor to chart the state of our understanding—as derived from longitudinal studies—of the impact of time on these biopsychosocial interactions and to present treatment strategies that appear to be helpful to the illness.

A Myopic View of Illness Course

Despite disclaimers to the contrary, there is a tendency in American psychiatry to persist in looking at schizophrenia as a single disorder whose course is based on what is seen during the clinician's short contact with the patient or during a cross-sectional research study (Cohen and Cohen 1984). The patient's outcome is often presumed either to remain stable or to deteriorate from whatever point the clinician-investigator last saw the patient (American Psychiatric Association 1980, 1987). This notion, taken to its zenith, was the Kraepelinian idea that "prognosis confirmed the diagnosis" (Kraepelin 1902). Thus, a good outcome in dementia praecox demanded a complete rediagnosis to manic depression. This perception was largely derived from retrospective studies of hospitalized samples (Kraepelin 1902; E. Bleuler 1911/1950; see also Harding et al. 1992 for a discussion of other significant methodological problems with this view).

Short-term longitudinal studies (i.e., lasting 15 years or less) have created lists of critical physiological, psychological, and social variables that appear to influence and predict the course and outcome of illness (Andreasen and Black 1991; Carone et al. 1991). These include diagnosis, type and age of onset, duration of illness, psychiatric history, degree of affectivity, other symptom dimensions, sensorium status, obsessive compulsions, assaultiveness, premorbid functioning, marital status, psychosexual behavior, neurological functioning, structural brain anomalies, gender, social class, and family history (Andreasen and Black 1991). Once identified, the prognostic power of such factors has often been presumed to remain the same thereafter (with the exception of McGlashan [1986b], who determined different predictors for what he defined as short-, medium-, and long-term outcomes, although his long-term outcome period matched the shortest outcome epoch of the very long-term studies in the world literature).

The Long-Term View of Illness Course

Yet patients and clinical reports persist in muddying the waters for Occam's razor[1] by their consistent feedback that challenges conceptions of the long-term course of schizophrenia (Beers 1908/1960; M. Bleuler 1978; Breier and Strauss 1983; Chamberlin 1979; Ciompi 1989; Leete 1987; Lovejoy 1982, 1984; Strauss et al. 1989).

Several investigators have followed intact cohorts over decades, regardless of whether the group members remained patients

---

[1] *Occam's razor* was named after an English philosopher, William of Occam. The name was applied to "a philosophical or scientific principle according to which the best explanation of an event is the one that is the simplest, using the fewest assumptions or hypotheses" (Merriam-Webster 1993, p. 810). It is otherwise known as the *principle of parsimony* or *Lloyd Morgan's canon* in comparative psychology (Marx and Hillix 1973).

(M. Bleuler 1978; Ciompi and Müller 1976; Harding et al. 1987a, 1987b; Hinterhuber 1973; Huber et al. 1975; Ogawa et al. 1987; Tsuang et al. 1979). Results from long-term studies have consistently indicated that time is a critical covariate that changes most factors that were thought to remain stable. Such studies have rebalanced psychiatry's viewpoint with findings of wide heterogeneity of functioning across a patient's life course. Levels of functioning—measured by symptom presentation, work, sociability, and basic self-care—can significantly improve or reconstitute over time, even for some chronic patients. Adult development continues despite delays by serious illness or impediments presented by the service delivery system (McCrory et al. 1980; Strauss and Harding 1990). The brain appears to be able to recompensate or even recalibrate itself over time (Greenough and Schwark 1984; Harding 1991; Kandel and Schwartz 1981; Restak 1984). For many more patients than is usually assumed, but unfortunately not for all, symptoms can ameliorate and disappear entirely. Age at onset and even gender effects lose much of their predictive power.

Therefore, in this chapter I endeavor to examine many widely held assumptions about variables thought to significantly and negatively impact on the course of schizophrenia, and to correct the misperception that such factors (e.g., diagnosis, symptom expression, gender, early work incapacity, poor social functioning, age at onset, delays in adult development) propel a person toward a uniformly poor long-term trajectory. Time can radically alter early expectations by producing a very different picture of course of illness and life than is expected for at least half of all members of a cohort, even the chronic ones. The key questions yet to be answered are, What kind of treatment for which kind of person and when in his or her trajectory? Who are those who are nonresponsive? What are the factors that impede rehabilitation?

Diagnosis as a Cross-Sectional Working Hypothesis

Mental health professionals used to think that a diagnosis came with a lifetime warranty. If patients appeared to improve, they were only in remission. For some patients, the diagnostic label became loaded with extra meaning (e.g., a deteriorating course for schizophrenia) (Harding et al. 1987c). To paraphrase Kraepelin (1902), once dementia praecox, always dementia praecox.

The results of the Vermont Longitudinal Study (Harding et al. 1987a, 1987b), however, challenged this notion. The patient cohort in that study has since been demonstrated to have been the most chronically ill cohort ever studied in the world literature (Harding 1988; Harding et al. 1987a, 1987b). The project presented the most conservative findings from the poorest prognostic groups, yet more than two-thirds of these subjects, all of whom met DSM-III criteria for schizophrenia, went on to demonstrate significant improvement and even recovery. It should be noted that their average age at onset (men = 24.2 years; women = 27.1 years) was 5–6 years younger than the estimate of 30 years made by McGlashan (1988) in his review of North American follow-up studies and corrected in a later version (McGlashan 1991; see also Childers and Harding 1990). Furthermore, the instrumental capacity of these patients was also at issue, with McGlashan assuming that they were among the best workers in the hospital. Additional retrospective review revealed that this representation may have been partially true of the larger sample but not of the schizophrenic subsample in question.

The finding of wide heterogeneity of outcome in schizophrenic patients was supported by the findings of 10 other recent world studies in which patients have been followed for two and three decades (see entire issue of *Schizophrenia Bulletin*, Volume 14, Number 4, 1988, for a review of these studies). Results from all of these studies indicated significant improvement and a wide heterogeneity of outcome for patients with schizophrenia. The only exception has been the findings of diagnostic stability reported by Tsuang et al. (1981), but because of artifacts introduced by significant methodological problems, the Tsuang et al. data represent only a weak challenge to this hypothesis—or perhaps the Feighner criteria (Feighner et al. 1972), which this team used, actually delineated one legitimate subgroup of the poor end of the continuum.

In addition, during the mid-20th century—years of some optimism in American psychiatry—subgroups of patients were identified who appeared to have a better prognosis. To test the notion that a certain cluster of variables would predict a better outcome for schizophrenia, Vaillant (1978) conducted a 10-year follow-up study of schizophrenic patients who demonstrated the following profile: acute onset, precipitating events, family history of affective disorders, affectivity in symptom presentation, confusion, and resolution of episode within 2 years. These "good prognostic" patients also demonstrated wide heterogeneity at follow-up, with 40% of the patients showing a chronic course at that point in their trajectory. Vaillant concluded that "prognosis and diagnosis are two different dimensions of psychosis" (Vaillant 1975).

After conducting both long and short follow-up studies of schizophrenia and other serious illnesses, Harding and Strauss (1984) concluded that the course of schizophrenia is a much

> more complex, dynamic, and heterogeneous process than has heretofore been appreciated or predicted by diagnostic specificity. The longitudinal picture of course . . . reveals nonlinear patterns and trends. . . . The individual has been documented as an active, developing person in interaction with his or her environment. These important modifiers reshape the course of illness and the person's life in which schizophrenia is but a part." (p. 339)

This more optimistic view is in direct opposition to the current neo-Kraepelinian stance of DSM-III (American Psychiatric Association 1980) and DSM-III-R (American Psychiatric Association 1987). According to the results of the Vermont Longitudinal Study (Harding et al. 1987a, 1987b), diagnosis (even using the narrower strategies of DSM-III) failed to predict outcome status an average of 32 years later (Harding et al. 1987b). Thus, we (Harding 1986; Harding et al. 1987b) agreed with Vaillant in concluding that a diagnosis represents a cross-sectional profile of the patient and could not be expected to withstand the impact of the wide variety of biopsychosocial factors that influence the course of illness and life across decades. Common sense and data have prevailed.

Because the findings of heterogeneity in onset, symptom presentation, course, and outcome persist, E. Bleuler (1911/1950) appears to have been on the right track when he proposed that there was a group of schizophrenias, a position now held by most clinicians and investigators (Stephens 1970). Perhaps the study of other dimensional or biological subtypes might prove to be more profitable than the study of a single disorder, such as the deficit syndrome versus the nondeficit categorization described below; however, so far, prognostic studies have been able to predict only 8%–27% of the variance in even short-term outcomes of less than 15 years (Bland et al. 1978; Shapiro and Shader 1979).

Change, Disappearance, or Stabilization of Symptoms Over Time

Docherty et al. (1978) and Ciompi (1989) outlined time-related series of symptomatic changes through which patients travel to descend into a psychosis. Once in a psychosis, male patients have often been found to display asociality, withdrawal, anhedonia, and apathy, whereas female patients have been described as flamboyantly psychotic, aggressive, and agitated (J. M. Goldstein and Link 1988; Haas et al. 1989; Lewine 1981). The notion that there may be at least two different types of illnesses with different biological correlates and outcomes has been put forward by Crow et al. (1982), Andreasen and Olsen (1982), and others. Negative symptoms of schizophrenia (Strauss et al. 1974) have been heralded as predisposing the patient to a poorer outcome (Andreasen and Olsen 1982; Andreasen et al. 1990). One problem that has persisted with this dichotomous categorization is the difficulty of identifying pure types of schizophrenia, because most patients display mixed symptoms. To complicate matters, symptoms can change over time, begin later, disappear, and reappear.

Carpenter et al. (1988) and others have described negative symptoms as states (instead of traits) that change over time in their configuration and strength. To bring some clarity to the situation, Carpenter et al. (1988) have proposed the *deficit syndrome,* which appears to operate independently of psychosis and which requires the addition of 12 months of temporal stability to at least two of the following symptoms: restricted affect, diminished emotional range, poverty of speech, curbing of interests, and diminished social drive. These symptoms must not be secondary to other factors such as anxiety, drug effects, suspiciousness, depression, or mental retardation (Carpenter et al. 1988). Thus, these investigators have contributed a system of criteria whereby more stable trait types can be distinguished. The lifelong stability of this syndrome has yet to be clearly established, but hints of its stability have come from a retrospective application of the Carpenter et al. criteria to the data from the Chestnut Lodge Study (Fenton and McGlashan 1992).

To increase reliability and validity of the deficit syndrome construct, Kirkpatrick et al. (1989) devised a structured rating scale—the Schedule for the Deficit Syndrome. Biological correlates of the deficit syndrome have also been found, such as neuropsychological measures (Thaker et al. 1988), eye-tracking impairments (Wagman et al. 1987), and anomalies on magnetic resonance imaging scans (Buchanan et al. 1990). This research represents a major methodological advance in the field.

Strauss et al. (1989) also suggested that negative symptoms have probable social and psychological aspects as well as biological correlates (Andreasen 1982; Crow et al. 1982; Flaum et al. 1990). Such aspects include responses to

1. Stave off the pain of positive symptoms
2. Apathy based in loss of hope
3. Reduce the possibility of bizarre behavior
4. Resist giving up patienthood
5. Deal with guilt over past dysfunction
6. Resist stress
7. Giving up in the face of overwhelming social "stigma, discouraging 'therapeutic' messages, and social dysfunction" (Strauss et al. 1989, p. 131)

These factors and cognitive impairment all play a role in the process, with the suggestion that such ingredients should be appreciated and incorporated into the study and treatment of negative symptoms.

Age at Onset Is Not Predictive of Illness Course

Age at onset has been a traditional and consistent factor in the studies of schizophrenia (American Psychiatric Association 1987). Early onset has been persistently associated with male gender (Lewine 1980), poor premorbid functioning (Childers and Harding 1990; Farina et al. 1962; Gittleman-Klein and Klein 1969; Zigler and Levine 1981), severity of illness (Crow et al. 1982), brain anomalies (Flor-Henry 1990; Nasrallah et al. 1990), and poorer short-term outcomes. Part of the explanation may be the 10% early suicide rate of severely ill, young male patients (Grebb and Cancro 1989) and the decline in good outcomes among moderately physically healthy, menopausal female patients who have lost their protective estrogen and succumbed to more neuroleptic side effects, such as tardive dyskinesia (Gardos and Cole 1980; Seeman 1983; Seeman and Lang 1990).

However, results from long-term studies, especially the Vermont Longitudinal Study (Harding et al. 1987a, 1987b), the Bonn Study (Huber et al. 1975), and two Swiss projects—the Lausanne Investigations (Ciompi 1980) and the Burghölzli Hospital Study (M. Bleuler 1978), have indicated that the impact of age at onset as a predictor of outcome is reduced to only a trend level after two to three decades.

Other possible explanations for differences in age at onset have targeted differential family reports of role expectations and symptom display of sons versus daughters, societal differences in help-seeking behaviors (Test and Berlin 1981), the neurodevelopmental theories of Taylor (1969) and Weinberger (1987), and studies of hormonal differences, such as the estrogen-protection theories of Seeman (1988).

Several problems have existed in determining patients' ages at onset of illness. Onset is notoriously difficult to define and thus to demarcate: Does onset mean a clear decline from the usual level of functioning, the appearance of first symptoms, or both? Thus, there is a fuzzy boundary between wellness and illness. In addition, the data regarding onset are often generated by family recollections, with patients' recollections frequently differing. Both retrospective and prospective studies suffer from inaccurate assessment. Investigators in high-risk studies are still struggling to find "markers" (e.g., Cornblatt et al. 1989), and studies of school-age children show that a wide range of early pathology displayed by children often gets resolved by adulthood (Watt and Saiz 1991).

Thus, although researchers continue to define the criteria and search for evidence, clinicians need to resist prognostication. The implications for treatment are considerable. Clinicians and investigators need to understand the extreme difficulty of making a diagnosis of schizophrenia during adolescence, given the emotional lability of that period (Conger 1991; Weiner 1982), the tendency for historical revisionism by parents and patients in the search for reasons for the illness, and the possibility that a particular patient may be fortunate enough to be in the group that experiences only one episode in a lifetime.

Gender Issues

Most of the gender issues in schizophrenia are described in Chapter 11 of this book. Until recently, there were few biological gender difference studies in schizophrenia (J. M. Goldstein and Tsuang 1990). The early focus was on age at onset and premorbid functioning. But now a significant number of other contrasts have been uncovered. Female schizophrenic patients have been found to present with the following characteristics: higher family risk for morbidity (Flor-Henry 1990; J. M. Goldstein et al. 1990), less obstetric and birth complications (Mednick 1970; Mirdal et al. 1974), and differential structural (Lewine et al. 1990; Nasrallah et al. 1990) and functional brain anomalies (Goldberg et al. 1991; Green 1993). However, because the technology and understanding of the importance of gender research have been developed only within the last decade, the impact of such factors has yet to be examined in long-term biological investigations.

In addition, the Colorado Longitudinal Research Consortium (Harding 1993) has suggested that two groups have remained clinically known but hidden by lack of research. The first group is composed of the female patients with early onset, who may have the same profiles as their male counterparts. Conversely, the second group is made up of male patients with late onset. It is proposed that each of these subgroups has been masked by gender mean comparisons. It is time to target such groups for study.

However, what work has been accomplished from the very long-term studies may add further to psychiatry's understanding. As mentioned above, female patients, in general, have the advantage over male patients across the life course from prenatal neurodevelopment to menopause (J. M. Goldstein and Tsuang 1990; Seeman 1983; Seeman and Lang 1990). If obstetrical complications add to brain vulnerability, then the female brain, which develops earlier prenatally than the male brain, is less at risk than the male brain (McMillen 1979). Age at onset for female patients is generally well into the 20s, after they have completed their education and often have married or established a work history (Seeman and Lang 1990). With their premorbid level of functioning better developed, female patients, therefore, have a broader baseline from which to draw strength for improvement, recovery, and reintegration back into the community (Childers and Harding 1990; Farina et al. 1962; Gittleman-Klein and Klein 1969; Zigler and Levine 1981).

Long-term studies have consistently found that the advantage that female patients appear to have for many years seems to taper off to only a trend level at follow-up in their later years (M. Bleuler 1978; Childers and Harding 1990; Ciompi 1980; Huber et al. 1980). Based on their work on the effects of estrogen, Seeman and Lang (1990) suggested that young female patients should receive less neuroleptics early on and be treated very carefully postmenopausally.

Furthermore, gender affects social and cultural expectations as well. Female patients face day-to-day risks of traumatic sexual events and motherhood, as well as dealing with pregnancy and medication complications. The desire for a normal dating process with patients and nonpatients is felt by both genders. Such desires and behaviors are often ignored or contravened by counselors and living situations. Moreover, little in the way of education occurs on these issues (Test and Berlin 1981). (See Bachrach and Nadelson [1988], in which the special considerations needed to treat chronically mentally ill women are targeted.)

The Role of Personality and Psychological Coping Over Time

One of Zubin et al.'s (1985) many contributions was a reminder that patients return to the premorbid personality with which they entered the illness. Therefore, clinicians and researchers need to know if any

Axis II disorder is present, and to separate Axis I behavior from Axis II behavior, although there may be underlying or overlapping substrate problems for which treatment of one axis may help with treatment of the other (R. Cloninger, presidential address at American Psychopathological Association meeting, New York, NY, March 1993). Agreeing with both Cloninger and Zubin, the Vermont Longitudinal Study team (Harding et al. 1987a, 1987b) was convinced that Axis II behavior played a much greater clinical role in the lack of recovery shown in many patients who once qualified for DSM-III schizophrenia. Huber et al. (1975; the Bonn Study), M. Bleuler (1978; the Burghölzli Hospital Study), and Ciompi (1980; the Lausanne Investigations) also found that good premorbid personality functioning led to better outcome. Huber et al. (1980) reported that marked abnormality in premorbid personality uniformly led to poor outcome.

In the Yale 2-year follow-up study, Breier and Strauss (1983) reported on the acquisition of self-control mechanisms for psychotic symptoms. Their patients learned over time to stop feeling hopeless and helpless by becoming frustrated enough to search for their own individual prodromal sequence, identify their earliest red flag, and then implement simple commonsense strategies to avoid a downward spiral. Patients often taught one another. These strategies shifted the power of control back to the patients and appeared to affect their course trajectories.

Patients in the Yale study also described finding a time, in trying to cope with their illness, that for them was "the last straw." They called it their "low turning point"—the point at which they decided to reorganize their lives toward recovery. Many subjects were able to pinpoint the precise episode in which this occurred (Rakfeldt and Strauss 1989).

Catching Up on Adult Developmental Tasks

The interplay between adult development and the recovery process is the bedrock stratum on which the fields of psychiatry and psychology were built (Colarusso and Nemiroff 1987; Sullivan 1956; Vaillant 1977). Yet the active role of the person in this process is often forgotten in the treatment process (Strauss and Harding 1990; Strauss et al. 1985, 1987).

Crucial adult developmental tasks are often delayed by having such a serious illness. Often, the first thing a patient wishes to try, once having reached a new (but fragile) stabilization of psychosis and psychopharmacology, is to go back to school, ask someone for a date, leave the parental home, or get a job. McCrory et al. (1980) suggested that these events constitute "rehabilitation crises." Instead of discouraging the patient in a fragile state from attempting such stressful tasks, at the expense of adult development, McCrory et al. suggested a series of strategies for working with patients to face the tasks, such as acknowledging with them the upcoming stress, role-playing, closely titrating their medication, and scheduling more frequent visits to support them while they undertake these ventures. Such strategies enable clinicians who are concerned about their patients' vulnerability to stress and relapse to promote the patients' continuing adult human development in a "rehabilitation alliance" (McCrory 1988).

Reconstitution of Social Functioning Over Time

One of the most significant elements in the description of schizophrenia is the decline in or absence of interpersonal functioning (American Psychiatric Association 1987). As patients succumb to the illness, they often withdraw into an autistic-like world (E. Bleuler 1911/1950), much to the consternation of family and friends. Some patients were asocial as children and simply slowly withdraw further. Others functioned well until overcome by an episode (Watt and Saiz 1991). Social network researchers have found that individuals with schizophrenia always tended to have smaller, narrower, more loosely connected social networks (Beels 1979; Hammer 1981). Harding et al. (1984) found that the recovered patients in the Vermont Longitudinal Study had significantly more normalized networks. One of the strategies used in the Vermont study was placing patients into natural community social situations (e.g., church choirs, bowling leagues). Perhaps this programmatic decision aided in the more complete reintegration of these patients (Chittick et al. 1961; Harding et al. 1987a, 1987b).

In their short-term longitudinal study, Strauss and Carpenter (1974) found that future social functioning was predicted by past social functioning and not by symptoms or duration of hospitalization. Social functioning also helped to predict work functioning as the one domain that crossed over to partially predict another domain. Strauss and Carpenter (1974) initiated the idea of "open-linked systems."

Longer-term studies have systematically discovered that social functioning is often restored and developed further over decades. Ciompi (1980) found that 33% of the patients they studied were restored to social functioning after an average of 37 catamnestic years. Huber et al. (1980) found 56% of their patients to have restored social functioning after an average 23-year duration of illness, with a 99% concordance of symptom recovery as well. In a multitrait, multimethod protocol, Harding et al. (1987b) rated 68% of the DSM-III schizophrenic patients in their study as having restored social functioning after a 32-year duration of illness (Harding et al. 1987b); for a matched cohort in Maine, they found 48% to have restored social functioning after an illness duration of 36 years (DeSisto et al., in press). Ogawa et al. (1987), in their 21- to 27-year follow-up study in Japan, found that 47% of their patients were self-supportive and functioning well socially and independently, with a normal family life. In fact, it is predicted that 10–20 years after acute hospitalization, 60% of patients will be socially recovered as well as part-time employed (American Psychiatric Association 1989). Therefore, once again, time appears to play a critical role in this type of functioning.

Given these findings, attention has been paid to psychosocial rehabilitation strategies (Chittick et al. 1961; Liberman et al. 1986) to augment and increase the natural restoration process. In the 2-year iterative, intensive follow-up of patients after admission for psychosis in the Yale Longitudinal Study (Strauss et al. 1985), Breier and Strauss (1984) found that there were changes in how patients used social relationships during the different stages of illness. In the convalescent stage, patients in the Yale study needed social relationships for ventilation, reality testing, social approval and integration, material supports, problem solving, and constancy. Later, during the rebuilding phase, patients shifted away from their identity of patienthood. Their use of social relationships changed to needs for motivation, reciprocal relating, symptom monitoring, empathetic understanding, modeling, and insight. Time again played a major role in this pattern.

To increase the level of social functioning for chronic patients, several strategies have proven successful for many. The Vermont cohort received a comprehensive model program that targeted both social integration and vocational rehabilitation (Chittick et al. 1961; Harding et al. 1987a). In the 1960s, Paul and colleagues found that a social learning–token economy program could significantly improve levels of functioning of chronic patients. Those patients were eventually improved enough to be released to the community (Paul and Lentz 1977). Other well-known social rehabilitation programs have included the Fountain House model in New York (Beard et al. 1982), which has been widely copied across the world. That model stresses interdependence, self-help, and self-reliance.

Eventually, transitional employment programs have augmented the social aspects of programs (Beard et al. 1978). Assertive outreach programs, such as Training in Community Living and the Program for Assertive Community Treatment (PACT) in Madison, Wisconsin (Test and Stein 1978), have demonstrated considerable effectiveness. The Soteria House in San Francisco (Mosher and Menn 1979) and in Bern, Switzerland (Ciompi and Bernasconi 1986) has provided yet another model for quiet space, titrated social interaction, acceptance, and little or no medication to help young patients recompensate from a severe psychotic experience and stay within the community. Liberman et al. (1986) provided a set of manuals and videotapes, along with a highly structured program—Social Skills Training—to teach a wide variety of specific social skills. This program uses role-playing, modeling, vicarious learning, focused instructions, social reinforcements, and feedback to assess and target social deficits.

Family psychoeducational programs (Anderson et al. 1980; M. J. Goldstein et al. 1986) have also made a dramatic contribution to the reduction of relapse rates, especially for young male schizophrenic patients (Hogarty 1984). These types of programs and supports for families have consistently produced the same advantageous results across cultures and countries (e.g., Leff and Vaughn 1985). Families have begun to play major roles in the care and treatment of their loved ones (Hatfield and Lefley 1987). Thus, time and social engineering contribute to the reduction of symptoms and the increased reconnection of patients with their families and their communities.

Some environmental factors that have been identified as impeding progress toward improvement (Harding et al. 1992) include the following: institutionalization, socialization into the patient role, lack of rehabilitation programs, reduced social status, reduced economic opportunities, side effects of medication, lack of staff expectations, self-fulfilling prophecies, and loss of hope. Many of these factors are never included in the study of course of illness; they reflect imposed stigma and societal, public policy, and treatment ignorance rather than the nature of the patient or his or her illness process.

Work Functioning as Treatment

Freud (1930/1953) declared that "work has greater effect than any other technique of living in the direction of binding the individual closely to reality . . . in his work at least, he is securely attached to a part of reality . . . the human community" (p. 80). Work was one of the cornerstones of treatment in the era of "moral treatment" (Bockoven 1963). Dr. Kirkbride (quoted in Bond 1947), a superintendent of one of the then-new hospitals, said,

> The value of employment . . . is now so universally conceded that no arguments are required in its favor. Its value cannot be estimated in dollars and cents. The object is to restore mental health and tranquillize [sic] the restlessness and mitigate the sorrows of disease. (Bond 1947, p. 60)

But once minimum wage was instituted, hospitals closed their large farm operations, and vocational rehabilitation became a sporadic experience for patients. In fact, with medicalization of care, vocational rehabilitation has often been given a secondary role after treatment has occurred instead of being considered part of treatment (Harding et al. 1987d).

Reports from long-term studies on work functioning have shown a wide range of results. In Ciompi's (1980) cohort of patients, who averaged 75 years of age at follow-up, 15% were doing full-time work and 37% were performing part-time work (1980). Ogawa et al. (1987) found 47% of their patient cohort to be self-supportive at the 2-decade mark, and Huber et al. (1980) found 56% of their patient cohort to be employed full-time at the 2-decade mark as well. In the Vermont study (Harding et al. 1987a, 1987b), vocational rehabilitation was used as a principal ingredient in the treatment of severely ill patients. These patients responded positively to the program, and 45% of the patients were employed over the years, with 40% employed at an average of 32 years later (the average age of the patients was 61, with a range up to 86 years). In comparison with the matched cohort from Maine (followed up for an average of 36 years), who did not receive rehabilitation, the Vermont patients achieved a (statistically) significantly better vocational outcome, despite the fact that both cohorts were equivalent in work histories (Harding et al. 1990).

Anthony and Jansen (1984), of the Boston University Center for Rehabilitation, have suggested the following:

- Previous psychiatric symptomatology, diagnostic category, intelligence, aptitude, and personality tests are poor predictors of future work performance or response to vocational rehabilitation.
- A person's ability to function in one environment does not predict his or her ability to function in another setting.
- Prior work performance and social functioning do predict future work performance.
- The best pencil-and-paper tests are those of a person's concept of being a worker.

These findings echo those from Strauss and Carpenter's (1974) "open-linked systems," in which work history predicted future work behavior. Systems of mental health and vocational rehabilitation tend to be fragmented, disconnected, and rigid, and to use ad hoc compensatory operations (Harding et al. 1987d). Furthermore, Strauss et al. (1985) found that a strategy that works for a patient at one point in time may cause problems later. One such strategy would be the provision of a highly structured environment for a disorganized patient; at an early stage of recovery, such an environment might enable that patient to become organized in his or her thought processes; later in the course of recovery, however, that environment could become highly stressful and psychotogenic by being too organized. Drake and Sederer (1986) wrote about the need to titrate treatment carefully around the current status of each patient, including performing periodic reassessments to make certain of the best fit.

Conclusion

In this chapter, I have switched the focus from psychosocial to biopsychosocial factors affecting the course of schizophrenia to illustrate the nature of the person-illness-environment interaction. Across the long-term worldwide studies, the passage of time has been found to affect all of the factors that challenge our list of so-called stable predictors for good or poor outcome. Such changeable factors that impinge on the course and outcome of schizophrenia include the following:

- Diagnosis as only a cross-sectional working hypothesis
- Symptom fluidity
- Age at onset, which not only is difficult to determine but also weakens with time as a predictor
- Gender effects, which are influenced by both biology and the environment
- The continuities and discontinuities of personality and the role of ongoing adult developmental tasks
- The reconstitution of social and vocational functioning whether or not symptoms disappear
- The impact of environmental engineering

The picture of schizophrenia is one of halts and advances, continuities and discontinuities, innate and acquired abilities and disabilities, acquisition of skills and buffers, biological and environmental recalibrations and compensations, and just plain luck. Hawking (1988) defined three "arrows" of time; the psychological arrow of time permits knowledge only of the past and not of the future, which is entirely in flux and unpredictable because of the two other arrows of time: the thermodynamic and the cosmic.

Brooks (G. W. Brooks, personal communication, February 1982), who followed his patients in Vermont for nearly four decades, once remarked to me that "the more one got to know a patient, the more normal he or she became. Conversely, the more one got to know a colleague, the more abnormal they became." In fact, to paraphrase a well-known aphorism, "Do patients have to try twice as hard to be considered half as well?" (Harding 1986). In an article entitled "The Clouded Crystal Ball" (1986), Aldrich assessed the likelihood that floundering medical students would fail and leave school. Thirty-five years later, when these predictions were cross-checked, the findings indicated that few of the predicted students suffered such dire consequences and, in fact, most achieved success. Patients in the Vermont Longitudinal Study admitted that the most important ingredient in their improvement—and, in some cases, their complete recovery—was hope: "Someone believed in me, someone who told me I might have a chance to recover, and my own persistence" (Harding et al. 1992). Working with hope connects to the natural self-healing capacities within each patient and encourages the process by instilling a sense of self-efficacy (Bandura 1977; Cousins 1979; Lovejoy 1982). Instead of using the old pessimistic statements of the past when asked by a patient about the course of schizophrenia,

> You have a severe and chronic illness and you will have to be on medication all the rest of your life.

clinicians should say,

> Yes, you have a serious illness, but results from 10 worldwide studies show that you have a 50-50 or better chance of significant improvement and perhaps recovery. It may take quite a long time, but we will be here to help maximize the return to functioning.

The last statement bespeaks no false hope, relies on worldwide data, and may help reduce the disastrous 10% suicide rate of young male schizophrenic patients and the 40% rate of suicide attempts by all schizophrenic patients (Grebb and Cancro 1989).

As Huber et al. (1980) declared after completing the Bonn Studies, "Schizophrenia does not seem to be a disease of slow, progressive deterioration. Even in the second and third decades of illness, there is still potential for full or partial recovery" (p. 595). Other investigators in long-term follow-up studies, such as Ciompi (1980), M. Bleuler (1978), and Brooks and Deane (1965), all argued that the best treatment for schizophrenic patients is "therapists relating constantly and actively to the healthy aspects of the psychotic patient" (M. Bleuler 1978, p. 297).

References

Aldrich CK: The clouded crystal ball: a 35-year follow-up of psychiatrists' predictions. Am J Psychiatry 143:45–49, 1986

American Psychiatric Association: Diagnostic and Statistical Manual of Mental Disorders, 3rd Edition. Washington, DC, American Psychiatric Association, 1980

American Psychiatric Association: Diagnostic and Statistical Manual of Mental Disorders, 3rd Edition, Revised. Washington, DC, American Psychiatric Association, 1987

American Psychiatric Association: Schizophrenia, in Treatments of Psychiatric Disorders: A Task Force Report of the American Psychiatric Association. Washington, DC, American Psychiatric Association, 1989, pp 1483–1606

Anderson CM, Hogarty GE, Reiss DJ: Family treatment of adult schizophrenic patients: a psycho-educational approach. Schizophr Bull 6:490–505, 1980

Andreasen NC: Negative symptoms in schizophrenia: definition and reliability. Arch Gen Psychiatry 39:789–794, 1982

Andreasen NC, Black DW: Schizophrenia, in Introductory Textbook of Psychiatry. Washington, DC, American Psychiatric Press, 1991, pp 225–254

Andreasen NC, Olsen S: Negative versus positive schizophrenia definition and validation. Arch Gen Psychiatry 39:789–794, 1982

Andreasen NC, Flaum M, Swayze VW II, et al: Positive and negative symptoms in schizophrenia: a critical reappraisal. Arch Gen Psychiatry 47:615–621, 1990

Anthony WA, Jansen MA: Predicting the vocational capacity of the chronically mentally ill: research and policy implications. Am Psychol 39:537–544, 1984

Bachrach LL, Nadelson CC (eds): Treating chronically mentally ill women. Washington DC, American Psychiatric Press, 1988

Bandura A: Self-efficacy: toward a unifying theory of behavioral change. Psychol Rev 84:191–215, 1977

Bandura A: The psychology of chance encounters and life paths. Am Psychol 37:747–755, 1982

Beard JH, Malamud TJ, Rossman E: Psychiatric rehabilitation and long-term rehospitalization rates: the findings of two research studies. Schizophr Bull 4:622–635, 1978

Beard JH, Propst R, Malamud TJ: The Fountain House model of psychiatric rehabilitation. Psychosocial Rehabilitation Journal 5:47–53, 1982

Beels CC: Social networks and schizophrenia. Psychiatr Q 51:209–215, 1979

Beers CW: A Mind That Found Itself (1908), 5th Edition. Garden City, NY, Doubleday, 1960

Bland RC, Parker JH, Orn H: Prognosis in schizophrenia. Arch Gen Psychiatry 35:72–77, 1978

Bleuler E: Dementia Praecox or The Group of Schizophrenias (1911). Translated by Zinkin J. New York, International Universities Press, 1950

Bleuler M: The Schizophrenic Disorders: Long-Term Patient and Family Studies. Translated by Clemens SM. New Haven, CT, Yale University Press, 1978

Bockoven JS: Moral Treatment in American Society. New York, Springer, 1963

Bond ED: Dr. Kirkbride and His Mental Hospital. Philadelphia, PA, JB Lippincott, 1947

Breier A, Strauss JS: Self-control in psychotic disorders. Arch Gen Psychiatry 40:1114–1145, 1983

Breier A, Strauss JS: Social relationships in the recovery from psychotic disorder. Am J Psychiatry 141:949–955, 1984

Brooks GW, Deane WN: The chronic mental patient in the community. Diseases of the Nervous System 26:85–90, 1965

Buchanan RW, Kirkpatrick B, Heinrichs DW, et al: Clinical correlates of the deficit syndrome of schizophrenia. Am J Psychiatry 147:290–294, 1990

Carone BJ, Harrow M, Westermeyer JF: Posthospital course and outcome in schizophrenia. Arch Gen Psychiatry 48:247–253, 1991

Carpenter WT Jr, Heinrich DW, Wagman AMI: Deficit and non-deficit forms of schizophrenia: the concept. Am J Psychiatry 145:578–583, 1988

Chamberlin J: On Our Own—Patient Controlled Alternative to the Mental Health System. New York, McGraw-Hill, 1979

Childers SE, Harding CM: Gender, premorbid social functioning, and long-term outcome in DSM-III schizophrenia. Schizophr Bull 16:309–318, 1990

Chittick RA, Brooks GW, Irons FS, et al: The Vermont Story. Burlington, VT, Queen City Printers, 1961

Ciompi L: Catamnestic long-term study on the course of life and aging schizophrenics. Schizophr Bull 6:606–618, 1980

Ciompi L: The Psyche and Schizophrenia: The Bond Between Affect and Logic. Cambridge, MA, Harvard University Press, 1989

Ciompi L, Bernasconi R: "Soteria Bern:" Erste Erfarungen mit einer neu-artigen Milieutherapie für akute Schizophrene. Psychiatrie Prax 13:172–176, 1986

Ciompi L, Müller C: Lebensweg und alter der Schizophrenen: Eine katamnestische Langzeitstudie bis ins Senium. Berlin, Springer Verlag, 1976

Cohen P, Cohen J: The clinician's illusion. Arch Gen Psychiatry 41:1178–1182, 1984

Colarusso CA, Nemiroff RA: Clinical implications of adult developmental theory. Am J Psychiatry 144:1263–1270, 1987

Conger JJ: Adolescence and Youth: Psychological Development in a Changing World. New York, Harper Collins, 1991

Cornblatt B, Winters L, Erlenmeyer-Kimling L: Attentional markers of schizophrenia: evidence from the New York High Risk Study, in Schizophrenia: Scientific Progress. Edited by Schulz SC, Tamminga CA. New York, Oxford University Press, 1989

Crow TJ, Cross AJ, Johnstone EC, et al: Two syndromes in schizophrenia and their pathogenesis, in Schizophrenia as a Brain Disease. Edited by Henn FA, Nasrallah HA. New York, Oxford University Press, 1982, pp 196–234

Cousins N: Anatomy of an Illness as Perceived by the Patient: Reflections on Healing and Regeneration. New York, Norton, 1979

DeSisto MJ, Harding CM, McCormick RJ, et al: The Maine-Vermont three-decade series of serious mental illness: a matched comparison of cross-sectional outcome. Br J Psychiatry (in press)

Docherty JP, VanKammen DP, Siris SG, et al: Stages of onset of schizophrenic psychosis. Am J Psychiatry 135:420–426, 1978

Drake RE, Sederer LI: The adverse effects of intensive treatment of chronic schizophrenia. Compr Psychiatry 27:313–326, 1986

Emde RN, Harmon RJ (eds): Continuities and Discontinuities in Development. New York, Plenum, 1984

Engel GL: The clinical application of the biopsychosocial model. Am J Psychiatry 137:535–544, 1980

Farina A, Garmezy N, Zalusky M, et al: Premorbid behavior and prognosis in female schizophrenic patients. Journal of Consulting Psychology 26:56–60, 1962

Feighner JP, Robbins E, Guze SB, et al: Diagnostic criteria for use in psychiatric research. Arch Gen Psychiatry 26:57–63, 1972

Fenton WS, McGlashan TH: Natural history of the deficit syndrome. Paper presented at the annual meeting of the American Psychiatric Association, Washington, DC, May 1992

Flaum M, Arndt S, Andreasen NC: The role of gender in studies of ventricle enlargement in schizophrenia: a predominantly male effect. Am J Psychiatry 147:1327–1332, 1990

Flor-Henry P: Influence of gender in schizophrenia as related to other psychopathological syndromes. Schizophr Bull 16:211–227, 1990

Freud S: Civilization and its discontents (1930), in The Standard Edition of the Complete Psychological Works of Sigmund Freud, Vol 21. Translated and edited by Strachey J. London, Hogarth Press, 1953, pp 54–145

Gardos G, Cole JO: Overview: public health issues of tardive dyskinesia. Am J Psychiatry 137:776–781, 1980

Gittleman-Klein R, Klein DF: Premorbid social adjustment and prognosis in schizophrenia. J Psychiatr Res 7:35–53, 1969

Gleick J: Chaos: Making a New Science. New York, Viking, 1988

Goldberg TE, Gold JM, Braff DL: Neuropsychological functioning and time-linked information processing in schizophrenia, in American Psychiatric Press Review of Psychiatry, Vol 10. Edited by Tasman A, Goldfinger SM. Washington, DC, American Psychiatric Press, 1991, pp 60–78

Goldstein JM, Link BG: Gender differences in the clinical expression of schizophrenia. J Psychiatr Res 22:141–155, 1988

Goldstein J, Tsuang MT: Gender and schizophrenia: an introduction and synthesis of findings. Schizophr Bull 16:179–183, 1990

Goldstein JM, Santangelo SL, Simpson JC, et al: The role of gender in identifying subtypes of schizophrenia: a latent class analytic approach. Schizophr Bull 16:263–275, 1990

Goldstein MJ: Psychosocial (nonpharmacologic) treatments for schizophrenia, in American Psychiatric Press Review of Psychiatry, Vol. 10. Edited by Tasman A, Goldfinger SM. Washington, DC, American Psychiatric Press, 1991, pp 116–135

Goldstein MJ, Hand I, Hahlweg K: Treatment of Schizophrenia: Family Assessment and Intervention. Berlin, Springer-Verlag, 1986

Grebb JA, Cancro R: Schizophrenia: clinical features, in Comprehensive Textbook of Psychiatry, 5th Edition. Edited by Kaplan HI, Sadock BJ. Baltimore, MD, Williams & Wilkins, 1989, pp 757–777

Green MF: Cognitive remediation in schizophrenia: is it time yet? Am J Psychiatry 150:178–187, 1993

Greenough WT, Schwark HD: Age-related aspects of experience effects upon brain structure, in Continuities and Discontinuities in Development. Edited by Emde RN, Harmon RJ. New York, Plenum, 1984, pp 69–91

Haas GL, Sweeney JA, Keilp J, et al: Sex differences in neurocognition. Paper presented at the annual meeting of the American Psychiatric Association, San Francisco, CA, May 1989

Hammer M: Social support, social networks and schizophrenia. Schizophr Bull 7:45–57, 1981

Harding CM: Speculations on the measurement of recovery from severe psychiatric disorder and the human condition. J Psychiatry Neurosci 11:199–294, 1986

Harding CM: Course types in schizophrenia: an analysis of European and American studies. Schizophr Bull 14:633–643, 1988

Harding CM: Aging and schizophrenia: a possible beneficial interaction, in Schizophrenia: A Life Span Developmental Perspective. Edited by Walker EF. New York, Academic Press, 257–273, 1991

Harding CM: The Colorado Longitudinal Research Consortium: A Large Scale PAL Model (Models of Public-Academic Linkages). Boulder, CO, Western Commission on Higher Education Press, 1993

Harding CM, Strauss JS: The course of schizophrenia: an evolving concept, in Controversies in Schizophrenia: Changes and Constancies. Edited by Alpert M. New York, Guilford, 1984, pp 333–347

Harding CM, Brooks GW, Ashikaga T, et al: Social competence and life course after psychosis. Symposium presentation at the annual meeting of the American Psychiatric Association, Los Angeles, May 1984

Harding CM, Brooks GW, Ashikaga T, et al: The Vermont longitudinal study of persons with severe mental illness, I: methodology, study sample, and overall status 32 years later. Am J Psychiatry 144:718–726, 1987a

Harding CM, Brooks GW, Ashikaga T, et al: The Vermont longitudinal study, II: long-term outcome of subjects who retrospectively met DSM-III criteria for schizophrenia. Am J Psychiatry 144:727–735, 1987b

Harding CM, Zubin J, Strauss JS: Chronicity in schizophrenia: fact, partial fact, or artifact? Hosp Community Psychiatry 38:477–486, 1987c

Harding CM, Strauss JS, Hafez H, et al: Work and mental illness, I: toward an integration of the rehabilitation process. J Nerv Ment Dis 175:317–326, 1987d

Harding CM, DeSisto MJ, McCormick RV, et al: Maine's replication of Vermont's 32-year outcome study: recent findings and surprising implications (abstract). Schizophr Res (special issue) 3:9–10, 1990

Harding CM, Zubin J, Strauss JS: Chronicity in schizophrenia revisited. Br J Psychiatry 161 (suppl 18):27–37, 1992

Hatfield AB, Lefley HP (eds): Families of the Mentally Ill. New York, Guilford, 1987

Hawking SW: A Brief History of Time. New York, Bantam Books, 1988

Hinterhuber H: Zur Katamnese der Schizophrenien. Fortschr Neurol Psychiatr 41:527–558, 1973

Hogarty GE: Expressed emotion and schizophrenia relapse: implication from the Pittsburgh study, in Controversies in Schizophrenia. Edited by Alpert M. New York, Guilford, 1984, pp 354–365

Huber G, Gross G, Schüttler R: A long-term follow-up study of schizophrenia: psychiatric course of illness and prognosis. Acta Psychiatr Scand 52:49–57, 1975

Huber G, Gross G, Schüttler R, et al: Longitudinal studies of schizophrenic patients. Schizophr Bull 6:592–605, 1980

Kandel ER, Schwartz JH: Principles of Neural Science. Amsterdam, Netherlands, Elsevier/North-Holland, 1981

Kirkpatrick B, Buchanan RW, McKenney PD, et al: The schedule for the deficit syndrome: an instrument for research in schizophrenia. Psychiatry Res 30:119–123, 1989

Kraepelin E: Clinical Psychiatry—A Textbook for Students and Physicians, 6th Edition. Translated by Diefendorf AR. New York, Macmillan, 1902

Leete E: The treatment of schizophrenia: a patient's perspective. Hosp Community Psychiatry 38:486–491, 1987

Leff J, Vaughn C: Expressed Emotion in Families: Its Significance for Mental Illness. New York, Guilford, 1985

Lewine RRJ: Sex differences in age of symptom onset and first hospitalization in schizophrenia. Am J Orthopsychiatry 50:316–322, 1980

Lewine RRJ: Sex differences in schizophrenia: timing or subtypes? Psychol Bull 90:432–434, 1981

Lewine RRJ, Gulley LR, Risch SC, et al: Sexual dimorphism, brain morphology, and schizophrenia. Schizophr Bull 16:195–204, 1990

Liberman RP, Mueser KT: Schizophrenia: psychosocial treatment, in Comprehensive Textbook of Psychiatry, 5th Edition. Edited by Kaplan HI, Sadock BJ. Baltimore, MD, Williams & Wilkins, 1989, pp 792–806

Liberman RP, Mueser KT, Wallace CJ: Social skills training for schizophrenics at risk for relapse. Am J Psychiatry 143:523–526, 1986

Lovejoy M: Expectations and the recovery process. Schizophr Bull 8:605–609, 1982

Lovejoy M: Recovery from schizophrenia: a personal odyssey. Hosp Community Psychiatry 35:809–812, 1984

Marx MH, Hillix WA: Systems and Theories in Psychology, 2nd Edition. New York, McGraw-Hill, 1973

McCrory DJ: The human dimension of vocational rehabilitation: some reflections, in Vocational Rehabilitation of Persons With Prolonged Psychiatric Disorders. Edited by Ciardiello JA, Bell MD. Baltimore, MD, Johns Hopkins University Press, 1988, pp 208–218

McCrory DJ, Connolly PS, Hanson-Mayer TP, et al: The rehabilitation crisis: the impact of growth. Journal of Applied Rehabilitation Counseling 11:136–139, 1980

McGlashan TH: Schizophrenia: psychosocial treatments and the role of psychosocial factors in its etiology and pathogenesis, in American Psychiatric Association Annual Review, Vol 5. Edited by Francis AJ, Hales RE. Washington, DC, American Psychiatric Press, 1986a, pp 96–111

McGlashan TH: Predictors of shorter-, medium-, and longer-term outcome in schizophrenia. Am J Psychiatry 143:50–55, 1986b

McGlashan TH: A selective review of recent North American long-term follow-up studies of schizophrenia. Schizophr Bull 14:515–542, 1988

McGlashan TH: A selective review of recent North American long-term follow-up studies of schizophrenia, in Psychiatric Treatment: Advances in Outcome Research. Edited by Marin S, Gosset J, Grob M. Washington, DC, American Psychiatric Press, 1991, pp 61–105

McMillen MM: Differential mortality by sex in fetal and neonatal deaths. Science 204:89–91, 1979

Mednick SA: Breakdown in individuals at high risk for schizophrenia: possible predispositional perinatal factors. Mental Hygiene 5:50–63, 1970

Merriam-Webster's Collegiate Dictionary, 10th Edition. Springfield, MA, Merriam-Webster, 1993

Mirdal GKM, Mednick SA, Schulsinger F, et al: Perinatal complications in children of schizophrenic mothers. Acta Psychiatr Scand 50:552–568, 1974

Mosher LR, Keith SJ: Research on the psychosocial treatment of schizophrenia: a summary report. Am J Psychiatry 136:623–631, 1979

Mosher LR, Menn AZ: Soteria: an alternative to hospitalization for schizophrenia, in New Directions for Mental Health Services: Alternatives to Acute Hospitalization. Edited by Lamb HR. San Francisco, CA, Jossey-Bass, 1979, pp 73–84

Nasrallah HA, Schwarzkopf SB, Olson SC, et al: Gender differences in schizophrenia on MRI brain scans. Schizophr Bull 16:205–210, 1990

Ogawa K, Miya M, Watarai A, et al: A long-term follow-up study of schizophrenia in Japan, with special reference to the course of social adjustment. Br J Psychiatry 151:758–765, 1987

Paul GL, Lentz RJ: Psychosocial Treatment of Chronic Mental Patients: Milieu Versus Social Learning Programs. Cambridge, MA, Harvard University Press, 1977

Rakfeldt J, Strauss JS: The low turning point: a control mechanism in the course of psychiatric disorder. J Nerv Ment Dis 177:32–37, 1989

Restak RM: The Brain. New York, Bantam Books, 1984

Rutter M: Continuities and discontinuities in socioemotional development, in Continuities and Discontinuities in Development. Edited by Emde RN, Harmon RJ. New York, Plenum, 1984, pp 41–68

Seeman MV: Interaction of sex, age and neuroleptic dose. Compr Psychiatry 24:125–128, 1983

Seeman M: Schizophrenia in women and men, in Treating Chronically Mentally Ill Women. Edited by Bachrach L, Nadelson C. Washington, DC, American Psychiatric Press, 1988, pp 19–28

Seeman MV, Lang M: The role of estrogens in schizophrenia gender differences. Schizophr Bull 16:185–194, 1990

Selye H: The Stress of Life. New York, McGraw-Hill, 1956

Shapiro R, Shader R: Selective review of results of previous follow-up studies of schizophrenia and other psychoses, in Schizophrenia: An International Follow-Up Study. Geneva, World Health Organization, 1979, pp 11–44

Sheflen A: Levels of Schizophrenia. New York, Brunner/Mazel, 1981

Stephens JH: Long-term course and prognosis in schizophrenia. Seminars in Psychiatry 2:464–485, 1970

Strauss JS, Carpenter WT Jr: The prediction of outcome in schizophrenia, II: relationships between predictor and outcome variables. Arch Gen Psychiatry 31:37–42, 1974

Strauss JS, Carpenter WT Jr: Schizophrenia. New York, Plenum, 1981

Strauss JS, Harding CM: Relationships between adult development and the course of mental disorder, in Risk and Protective Factors in the Development of Psychopathology. Edited by Rolf J, Master A, Cicchetti D, et al. New York, Cambridge University Press, 1990, pp 514–535

Strauss JS, Carpenter WT Jr, Bartko JJ: An approach to the diagnosis and understanding of schizophrenia, III: speculations on the processes that underlie schizophrenic symptoms and signs. Schizophr Bull 11:61–70, 1974

Strauss JS, Hafez H, Lieberman P, et al: The course of psychiatric disorder, III: longitudinal principles. Am J Psychiatry 142:289–296, 1985

Strauss JS, Harding CM, Hafez H, et al: The role of the patient in recovery from psychosis, in Psychosocial Management of Schizophrenia. Edited by Strauss JS, Böker W, Brenner H. Toronto, Hans Huber Publications, pp 160–166, 1987

Strauss JS, Rakfeldt J, Harding CM, et al: Psychological and social aspects of negative symptoms. Br J Psychol 155 (suppl 7):128–132, 1989

Sullivan HS: The interpersonal theory of mental disorder, in Clinical Studies in Psychiatry. Edited by Perry HS, Gawel ML, Gibbon M. New York, WW Norton, 1956, pp 3–11

Taylor DC: Differential rates of cerebral maturation between sexes and between hemispheres. Lancet 2:140–142, 1969

Test MA, Berlin SB: Issues of special concern to chronically mentally ill women. Professional Psychology 12:136–145, 1981

Test MA, Stein LI: Training in community living: research designs and results, in Alternatives to Mental Hospital Treatment. Edited by Stein LI, Test MA. New York, Plenum, 1978, pp 57–74

Thaker G, Buchanan R, Kirkpatrick B, et al: Eye movements in schizophrenia: clinical and neurobiological correlates. Society for Neuroscience Abstracts 14:339, 1988

Tritton D: Chaos in the swing of a pendulum. New Scientist, July 24, 1986, p 37

Tsuang M, Woolson R, Fleming J: Long-term outcome of major psychoses, I: schizophrenia and affective disorders compared with psychiatrically symptom-free surgical conditions. Arch Gen Psychiatry 36:1295–1301, 1979

Tsuang MT, Woolson RF, Winokur G, et al: Stability of psychiatric diagnosis. Arch Gen Psychiatry 38:535–539, 1981

Vaillant GE: Ten- to 15-year follow-up of remitting schizophrenics. Paper presented at the 128th annual meeting of the American Psychiatric Association, Anaheim, CA, May 1975

Vaillant GE: Adaptation to Life. Boston, Little, Brown, 1977

Vaillant GE: A ten-year follow-up of remitting schizophrenics. Schizophr Bull 4:78–85, 1978

Wagman AMI, Heinrichs DW, Carpenter WT Jr: Deficit and nondeficit forms of schizophrenia: neuropsychological evaluation. Psychiatry Res 22:319–330, 1987

Watt NJ, Saiz C: Longitudinal studies of premorbid development of adult schizophrenia, in Schizophrenia: A Life-Course Development Perspective. Edited by Walker EF. New York, Academic Press, 1991, 157–192

Weinberger DR: Implications of normal brain development for the pathogenesis of schizophrenia. Arch Gen Psychiatry 44:660–669, 1987

Weiner IB: Child and Adolescent Psychopathology. New York, Wiley, 1982

Wyatt RJ, Alexander RC, Egan MF, et al: Schizophrenia, just the facts. what do we know, how well do we know it? Schizophr Res 1:3–18, 1988

Zigler E, Levine J: Age on first hospitalization of schizophrenics: a developmental approach. J Abnorm Psychol 90:458–467, 1981

Zubin J, Steinhauer SR, Day R, et al: Schizophrenia at the crossroads: a blueprint for the 1980s, in Controversies in Schizophrenia: Changes in Constancies. Edited by Alpert M. New York, Guilford, 1985, pp 48–76

CHAPTER 28

Family Management of Schizophrenia

Julian Leff, M.D.

I n developing countries, families have always been involved with the treatment of patients, whether the illness is physical or psychiatric, and whether the healing approach is biomedical or traditional. However, therapists in the Western world began working with families only in the early 1950s. Because of the development of biomedicine, with its focus on diseased organs, treatment often focused on the individual patient, in isolation from his or her social context. The involvement of family members in therapy in the Western world over the past 40 years represents a return to a traditional approach to healing. This was recognized by Speck and Reuveni (1969), who introduced network therapy for schizophrenia and named it, with a humorous intent, *tribe treatment*.

Initially, family therapy centered on treatment of schizophrenic patients and was shaped by a variety of imaginative theories that linked the origin of the disease to disturbances in family relationships. These theories included the *schizophrenogenic mother* (Fromm-Reichmann 1948), who was postulated to express a combination of overinvolvement and rejection; the *double-bind* (Bateson et al. 1956), an insidious form of emotional blackmail; *communication deviance* (Singer and Wynne 1966a, 1966b); *marital* schism and *marital* skew (Lidz et al.

1957a, 1957b); and *scapegoating* (Laing and Esterson 1964). The therapies developed from these theories inevitably held relatives responsible for the production of schizophrenia in the patient. This led either to the exclusion of relatives from therapeutic activities with the patient or to their inclusion as the target of therapy. Both strategies intensified the feelings of guilt that relatives invariably harbor, and alienated the relatives from the professionals.

A large body of experimental work designed to test the family causation of schizophrenia was built up, but a comprehensive review of this work (Hirsch and Leff 1975) failed to find substantive evidence for any of these theories. Over time, the popularity of these theories waned, although they still have their adherents. The early enthusiasm of family therapists for working with schizophrenia also declined, partly because family therapy seemed to produce little benefit (Rubinstein 1974) and partly because it began to be applied to disorders of childhood and adolescence, in which it often showed a gratifyingly rapid response. Professional interest in working with the families of schizophrenic patients began to revive in the 1970s, at least in part as a response to the emerging research on expressed emotion (EE).

The Implications of Expressed Emotion for Family Work

Relatives' EE is measured from audiotapes of a semistructured interview, the Camberwell Family Interview (Brown and Rutter 1966), which is administered at the first onset or exacerbation of the patient's illness. As used by its originators, it took 4–6 hours to administer. However, Vaughn and Leff (1976a) showed that it could be reduced to about 1½ hours without losing any of its discriminatory value. Four of the five component scales of EE have been shown to be associated with the outcome of schizophrenia. Three components—critical comments, hostility, and overinvolvement—are each significantly linked with relapse of schizophrenia, as measured over a 9-month period following the patient's return to the family home after a hospital admission. On the other hand, one component—high levels of warmth expressed by relatives—is associated with a significantly lower relapse rate (Brown et al. 1972; Vaughn and Leff 1976b). Threshold scores have been established that maximize the difference in patients' outcome between high- and low-scoring relatives. If the relative makes six or more critical comments during the interview, expresses any hostility, or scores three or above on the overinvolvement scale, the relative is categorized as having high EE. If one relative in a household is scored as having high EE, the whole household is classed as being high EE, on the assumption that this relative sets the predominant emotional tone. In practice, it is relatively uncommon to find two household members who rate differently on EE: 10%–15% of households are of this type.

Results from the bulk of published studies support a relationship between relatives' EE and the course of schizophrenia over 9 months (e.g., Brown et al. 1972; Jenkins et al. 1986; Vaughn and Leff 1976b) and over 2 years (e.g., Leff and Vaughn 1980). Only one study (McCreadie 1992) has included a follow-up as long as 5 years; in that study, relapse of patients in high-EE homes was found to be three times as common as that in low-EE homes.

There is less agreement on the importance of social contact between patients and high-EE relatives. This factor was measured from a time budget of a typical week by calculating the number of hours the patient and the high-EE relative spent in the same room, termed *face-to-face contact*. In the two original London studies (Brown et al. 1972; Vaughn and Leff 1976b), patients who spent less than 35 hours per week in face-to-face contact with a high-EE relative had a lower risk of relapse than those with more contact. This finding was not replicated in a number of the succeeding studies, but was substantiated by Vaughan et al. (1992a) in Sydney, Australia.

The data from the two London studies were combined to conduct an analysis of factors possibly mediating between EE and schizophrenic relapse. The results are shown in Table 28–1, where it can be seen that regular maintenance neuroleptics and low face-to-face contact appear to give a similar degree of protection to patients living in high-EE households. Furthermore, the effects seem to be additive, with the consequence that patients who live in high-EE homes but have the benefit of both protective factors have as low a risk of relapse as patients in low-EE homes.

The direction of cause and effect cannot be determined from this type of naturalistic study, which was indeed the impetus for our own decision to mount an experimental study of family intervention. However, one possible interpretation of the figures in Table 28–1 is that if intervention in high-EE homes with patients who have high contact with the high-EE relative is successful in reducing EE, contact, or both, the relapse rate of schizophrenic patients could be substantially reduced. The new generation of studies of intervention with families of schizophrenic patients, which are reviewed here, are all based explicitly or implicitly on these considerations.

Studies of Intervention With Families of Schizophrenic Patients

I review the new generation of controlled trials of family intervention, starting with the first to be published (Goldstein et al. 1978) and encompassing the two studies by my group (Leff et al. 1982, 1989) and the studies by Falloon et al. (1982), Hogarty et al. (1986), and Tarrier et al. (1988). All of these investigators found family intervention to be more effective than control treatments. I also consider three studies conducted within the same period that failed to demonstrate this effect (Dulz and Hand 1986; McCreadie et al. 1991; Vaughan et al. 1992b) because they throw light on those aspects of family intervention that appear to be necessary for its success.

Table 28–1. Relapse rates over 9 months of patients in high–expressed emotion (EE) homes

Regular maintenance neuroleptics	Face-to-face contact	Relapse rate (%)
No	High	92
Yes	High	53
No	Low	42
Yes	Low	15

Source. Brown et al. 1972; Vaughn and Leff 1976b.

In all the above studies, outcome was measured in terms of clinical relapse. Patients with high levels of persisting delusions or hallucinations were excluded because it would be extremely difficult to measure any worsening of their clinical state. For the remainder of patients, relapse was defined as a return of psychotic symptoms in those who were free of them on discharge from the hospital, or an exacerbation of symptoms in those who left the hospital with some persisting symptoms. The most structured definition of relapse was used by Falloon et al. (1982).

In all the trials, the intention was to maintain patients on prophylactic antipsychotic medication, which was usually the main intervention received by the control groups, although some were given additional social treatments that differed in content or intensity from those offered to the experimental groups. In Falloon et al.'s (1982) trial, for example, the control patients received social skills training, whereas in Tarrier et al.'s (1988) study, one control group of relatives was given an education program without the other components of the intervention package.

The relapse rates for patients from all nine studies in the 9–12 months after the beginning of the trial are shown in Table 28–2. The six trials with positive findings used different designs, which require some explanation. Leff et al.'s (1982) study involved a straightforward comparison between an experimental group receiving medication, family intervention, and a relatives' group and a control group receiving routine pharmacological care. In Goldstein et al.'s (1978) study, this type of design was complicated by also introducing a moderate-dosage and a low-dosage medication condition (only the moderate-dosage groups are presented in Table 28–2). In Goldstein et al.'s analysis, crisis family therapy emerged as an independent factor associated with a low relapse rate. Falloon et al.'s (1982) control group received medication plus intensive social skills training, as did one of Hogarty et al.'s (1986) groups. But in Hogarty et al.'s (1986) study, there was also a control group that received pharmacological treatment only, and an additional experimental group that was given medication, family intervention, and social skills training (for the patients). This latter group had the lowest relapse rate at 9-month follow-up. In Tarrier et al.'s (1988) trial, there was an additional experimental group that received only medication plus the education component of the family intervention. This proved to confer no advantage over drugs alone.

Leff et al.'s (1989) trial represented a further stage in the development of this field of research. Having shown that a package of interventions was more effective than routine care, this group then attempted to tease out the contents of the package by comparing education plus family sessions with education plus a relatives' group. Family sessions had produced as low a relapse rate as the combination of family sessions and a relatives' group in the Leff et al. (1982) trial. However, a problem arose in the Leff et al. (1989) trial with regard to compliance when the relatives' group was offered on its own: nearly half the families did not attend the group even once. For those families

Table 28–2. Relapse rates of patients over 9–12 months in family intervention trials

Study	Treatment group	Percentage of relapses
Goldstein et al. (1978)[a]	Drug + crisis family therapy	0
	Drug only	18
Leff et al. (1982)	Drug + family intervention + relatives' group	8
	Drug only	50
Leff et al. (1989)	Drug + family sessions	8
	Drug + relatives' group	17
Falloon et al. (1982)	Drug + family intervention	6
	Drug + social skills training	44
Hogarty et al. (1986)	Drug + family intervention	23
	Drug + family intervention + social skills training	9
	Drug + social skills training	30
	Drug only	49
Tarrier et al. (1988)	Drug + family intervention	12
	Drug + education	43
	Drug only	53
Dulz and Hand (1986)	Drug + relatives' groups + patients' groups	36
	Drug only	54
McCreadie et al. (1991)[b]	Before family intervention	75
	After family intervention	50
Vaughan et al. (1992b)	Drug + relatives' group	41
	Drug only	65

[a]6-month follow-up. [b]18-month follow-up (mirror-image design).

that did attend, the group appeared to be quite efficacious, in that the relapse rate for patients was 17%, compared with 50% for patients in the control (drug only) group in the Leff et al. (1982) trial. But the patients in the noncompliant families had a very poor outcome, with a 60% relapse rate. Tarrier (1991) also found that patients in families that either refused to take up the treatments his group offered or dropped out early had a very high relapse rate (67%). These findings emphasize the importance of engaging families in the treatment programs, an issue that is addressed below.

From the six trials with a positive outcome over 9–12 months, it appears that a variety of interventions have a similar power to reduce the relapse rate in schizophrenia. Consequently, it would be valuable to compare their constituents in detail to bring out common features. Before doing so, however, a longer-term view of outcome is needed.

Outcome Over 2 Years

Schizophrenia persists for years, if not for the sufferer's lifetime, so that a single year of follow-up represents only a fragment of the period of interest. Five of the groups in the above-mentioned studies conducted 2-year follow-ups (Leff et al. 1985, 1990; Falloon et al. 1985; Hogarty et al. 1991; Tarrier et al. 1989). All investigators found a continuing advantage for family interventions in terms of lower relapse rates. However, in Tarrier et al.'s (1989) follow-up, the difference between the experimental and the control groups did not reach significance. In Hogarty et al.'s (1991) follow-up, the superiority of the combination of family intervention and social skills training over family intervention alone, which was evident at 9 months, had disappeared by the 2-year follow-up.

None of these groups has extended the follow-up period beyond 2 years, but this is hardly surprising since it is exceedingly rare for drug studies to incorporate so long a follow-up. The difficulty is ensuring continuing compliance with the treatment to which each group is assigned, obviously a more demanding task when a combination of drug and social treatments is under scrutiny. However, a survival analysis conducted by Leff et al.'s group, using the data from both their 1982 and their 1989 trials, illuminates the longer-term outcome.

As shown in Figure 28–1, patients in the three experimental groups (medication plus family intervention and medication only [control] groups, both from the 1982 trial; and medication plus family sessions and medication plus relatives' groups, both from the 1989 trial), continued to relapse throughout the 2-year follow-up period. The length of time to relapse was longer for the experimental groups, so that fewer of these patients than of the control patients had experienced a relapse by the 2-year follow-up point. There is little doubt that if follow-up were extended by a number of years, virtually all patients in each of the groups would be found to relapse at least once. Indeed, this outcome was found by McCreadie (1992) in his naturalistic 5-year follow-up of patients from high- and low-EE homes. In that study, the proportion of patients relapsing at least once over the follow-up was no different between the high-EE (42%) and the low-EE (56%) groups, but the patients from the high-EE homes had three times as many relapses (mean = 3.4) as those from low-EE homes (mean = 1.1).

Survival curves of patients receiving high-dosage or low-dosage maintenance medication show exactly the same phenomenon, indicating that appropriate pharmacological and social interventions both delay relapse of schizophrenia. The findings of the trials reviewed above show that, when family interventions are added to maintenance medication, the interval between relapses is extended further. There are obvious advantages to patients in this delay, in terms of re-establishing social relationships and improving existing skills or developing new ones. These gains should be measurable, but it is unfortunate that few of the trials of family intervention have attempted to assess them.

Social Performance of Patients

Both Falloon et al.'s and Tarrier's groups used a structured interview to assess the patients' social performance. Falloon et al. (1984) used the Social Behavior Assessment Schedule (Platt et al. 1980), which was completed at baseline and at 9-month and 24-month follow-ups. At 9-month follow-up, the family management group showed significant improvements on household tasks, work or study, and friendship outside the family, compared with the individually treated patients.

Although half of the family management patients continued to show major deficits in one or more areas of social performance, their relatives reported feeling less dissatisfaction with those deficits. No such change was reported by relatives of the control patients. At 2-year follow-up, family management patients performed better on household tasks than did the control patients, and their relatives' dissatisfaction with social performance was further reduced.

Tarrier and Barrowclough (1990) used the Social Functioning Scale (Birchwood et al. 1990), which was designed specifically to assess social functioning in discharged schizophrenic patients. At 9-month follow-up, the patients receiving family intervention showed significant improvements on the withdrawal, interpersonal functioning, and prosocial activities subscales, and on the overall score. The

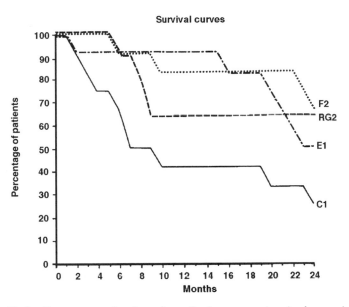

Figure 28–1. Percentage of patients free of relapse over time in the two intervention trials by Leff's group. 0 = beginning date of each trial. C1 = control group (Leff et al. 1982 trial); E1 = experimental group (Leff et al. 1982 trial); FT2 = family sessions (Leff et al. 1989 trial); RG2 = relatives' group (Leff et al. 1989 trial). *Source.* Reprinted by permission from Leff JP, Berkowitz R, Shavit N, et al: "A Trial of Family Therapy Versus a Relatives' Group for Schizophrenia: A Two-Year Follow-Up." *British Journal of Psychiatry* 157:575, 1990.

comparison group showed a significant improvement on interpersonal functioning only. Hence the reduction in social withdrawal by the experimental patients and the increase in their social activities can be attributed to the interventions.

In Leff et al.'s (1989) trial, changes in the patients' social and occupational activity were assessed from a time budget of a typical week. There were modest gains in various aspects of social functioning over 9 months, but none of the changes reached significance. Nevertheless, such gains were of considerable importance for the individual patients (e.g., a small number of patients managed to leave the parental home and live independently).

In summary, improvements in patients' social functioning have been ascertained in those studies in which appropriate measurements were made. These findings indicate that when florid relapses can be delayed by family intervention, it is possible for patients to make gains in their level of activity and to successfully achieve those life transitions that schizophrenia often impedes.

Identifying the Essential Components of Family Intervention

Four of the five groups that have reported positive results from trials of family intervention published books that gave a detailed description of their methods (Anderson et al. 1986; Barrowclough and Tarrier 1992; Falloon et al. 1984; Kuipers et al. 1992). A comparison of these accounts, and consideration of the approaches used in the three studies with negative outcomes (see Table 28–2), enables one to make a reasonably confident identification of those components of family intervention that are essential for its success.

Providing education about schizophrenia.   All of the programs began with the provision of facts about schizophrenia, although the means of presenting the information varied from group to group. Hogarty's group (Anderson et al. 1986) ran multifamily workshops lasting a whole day, whereas Falloon's (Falloon et al. 1984), Leff's

(Kuipers et al. 1992), and Tarrier's (Barrowclough and Tarrier 1992) groups gave the information in two sessions about 1 week apart. Only Falloon's groups (Falloon et al. 1984) included both the patients and the relatives in the education sessions from the beginning; the other groups brought the patients in at a later stage, with or without a separate education program. Falloon's (Falloon et al. 1984) and Leff's (Kuipers et al. 1992) groups imparted the information in the relatives' own homes, based on the reasoning that they would feel less anxious and more receptive, and that there would be fewer refusals to participate. In the studies by Falloon's (Falloon et al. 1984), Leff's (Kuipers et al. 1992), and Tarrier's (Barrowclough and Tarrier 1992) groups, the relatives' knowledge about the illness was assessed just before and after the education program. The results were very similar, suggesting that there was little change in the relatives' understanding of the illness. The main changes recorded were an increase in the proportion of relatives who knew the name of the illness (from half to virtually all) and an increase in relatives' optimism. The latter result indicated that the facts about schizophrenia were less alarming than the relatives' fears and fantasies.

Birchwood et al. (1992) compared information given by therapists in group situations, via written booklet only, and in video presentations. All formats led to gains in knowledge, increased optimism concerning the family's role in treatment, and reductions in relatives' stress symptoms at 6-month follow-up. The limitations of only giving information are underlined by Tarrier et al.'s (1988) trial, in which one group of subjects was randomized to receive education alone without any other components of family intervention. The patients in this group fared no better than those receiving drugs alone.

It is evident from these studies that the imparting of information by itself produces relatively little effect. The educational process continued throughout the therapist's contact with the family, with the same questions and answers being reiterated until the relative was ready to accept the answers. The issue was less one of filling gaps in a relative's knowledge than of negotiating changes in understanding. However, as both Leff's (Kuipers et al. 1992) and Tarrier's (Barrowclough and Tarrier 1992) groups emphasized, the provision of information at the outset of a program of intervention is an effective way of engaging families, as they are eager to hear as much as possible about a condition they often find mysterious and baffling.

Teaching problem solving.   Attempts to teach the families problem-solving techniques were central to all the interventions reviewed, including the pioneering study of Goldstein et al.'s team (Goldstein and Kopeikin 1981). Problem solving was given the greatest emphasis by Falloon's group (Falloon et al. 1984), followed closely by Tarrier's group (Barrowclough and Tarrier 1992), although the latter group reformulated the process as focusing on needs and strengths rather than on problems and deficits. Vaughan et al. (1992b), according to their description of the Sydney study, included a problem-solving approach, which was understandable given that Tarrier was involved in the trial. Leff's group (Kuipers et al. 1992) and Hogarty et al.'s group (Anderson et al. 1986) also emphasized problem-solving techniques, giving them approximately equal weight to attempts to deal with the family's emotional concerns. Only the unsuccessful intervention by Dulz and Hand (1986) gave this approach no mention.

Improving communication.   Communication is not always impaired in families with a schizophrenic member, but in some, particularly those with high-EE relatives, it can be chaotic. Family members talk across each other, the patient tends to be excluded from the conversation, and no one listens to any other person. Falloon's group (Falloon et al. 1984) focused on improving family members' communication skills, particularly the ability to make clear and specific statements, but also emphasized techniques to facilitate active listening. They stressed the importance of members' giving feedback about feelings of appreciation or pleasure. Hogarty's group (Anderson et al. 1986) described similar targets, whereas Leff's group (Kuipers et al. 1992) developed a set of rules for regularizing communications: 1) only one person may speak at a time, 2) everyone should have a fair share of the conversation, and 3) people present should be addressed directly and not talked about in the third person. Hogarty's (Anderson et al. 1986) and Leff's (Kuipers et al. 1992) groups also aimed at improving listening skills and promoting praise and encouragement.

Tarrier's group (Barrowclough and Tarrier 1992) rather downplayed efforts to change communication patterns in the family, whereas Goldstein et al. (1978) did not mention them at all.

Falloon's group (Falloon et al. 1984) placed a unique emphasis on helping families to communicate negative feelings—such as anger, hurt, disappointment, or sadness—in an effective manner. This appeared to run counter to the work on EE, from which the other groups had inferred that patients should be protected from exposure to these negative emotions. Hence, they discouraged family members from expressing such emotions in front of the patient. The resulting problem of how to help relatives deal with these feelings has been tackled by Leff's team (Kuipers et al. 1992) by setting up a relatives' group from which patients are excluded.

Dealing with emotional issues.   Attempts to reduce relatives' critical, hostile, and overinvolved attitudes were central to the interventions developed by Leff's group (Kuipers et al. 1992), but featured equally prominently in the descriptions of interventions by Hogarty's (Anderson et al. 1986) and Tarrier's (Barrowclough and Tarrier 1992) groups. Falloon's group (Falloon et al. 1984) stated that several of their interventions were structured to deal specifically with the EE variable as it presented in each family, but they spent less time elaborating on the techniques than the others. Barrowclough and Tarrier (1992) devoted a lot of space in their book to describing their methods of helping the high-EE relative manage negative emotions, thoughts, and behaviors associated with or triggered by the patient's problems. These methods included more individual-centered techniques (e.g., teaching relaxation exercises, teaching self-calming statements) than the other groups.

Goldstein et al. (1978) specifically mentioned the need for therapists to intervene to prevent conflict from developing, a need that was also stressed by Leff's (Kuipers et al. 1992) and Hogarty's (Anderson et al. 1986) groups. The technique of reframing negative emotional statements in a positive way—derived from strategic family therapy—was mentioned by both Hogarty's (Anderson et al. 1986) and Leff's (Kuipers et al. 1992) groups. The approach to dealing with overinvolvement by gradually achieving physical and emotional separation between the high-EE relative and the patient was described in a very similar way by Hogarty's (Anderson et al. 1986), Leff's (Kuipers et al. 1992), and Tarrier's (Barrowclough and Tarrier 1992) teams. Vaughan et al. (1992a, 1992b) in Sydney also stressed the need to decrease family guilt and anxiety.

Although not a component of EE, relatives' experience of grief and loss is mentioned as an important issue to be dealt with by both Leff's (Kuipers et al. 1992) and Tarrier's (Barrowclough and Tarrier 1992) groups.

Reducing contact.   Strategies to increase the social distance between patient and relatives are described in the accounts of all of the groups with the exception of Falloon et al.'s (1984). A constructive way of achieving this goal is to encourage family members to reengage with or extend their social networks. All the groups, with the exception of Goldstein et al.'s (1978) group, advocated this approach. In parallel with this focus was an emphasis on high-EE relatives' own needs as separate from the patient's. This issue was ascribed importance by Hogarty's (Anderson et al. 1986), Leff's (Kuipers et al. 1992), and Tarrier's (Barrowclough and Tarrier 1992) groups.

It should be noted that although Falloon's group (Falloon et al. 1984) did not specify a diminution in social contact as one of their aims, the attention they paid to improving the patient's social skills was likely to lead to this outcome.

Lowering expectations.   Many relatives hold unrealistic expectations for patients, believing that they will rapidly return to their previous level of functioning after an episode of illness. All the groups stressed the importance of scaling down the relatives' expectations to a level that the patient was capable of attaining. For example, a patient who cannot get up until the afternoon is not going to manage a university course. A more appropriate goal for this person would be to get up half an hour earlier than the day before. All groups emphasized the need for relatives to greet such small achievements with praise and encouragement. As Goldstein and Kopeikin (1981) phrased it, this was "therapists' attempt to lower short-term expectations while holding out hope for the long term" (p. 7). This important function of therapists in sustaining the family's optimism over long periods of time was also mentioned by Leff's group (Kuipers et al. 1992). As was discussed above, education programs contribute to this aim.

The therapist as the family's ombudsperson. Patients with schizophrenia and their caregivers often require a wide variety of services, provided by a number of different agencies. The most common needs are for financial support, sheltered housing, and sheltered occupation, but other requirements specific to individual families also arise. It is very difficult for family members to find their way through the maze of bureaucracy to mobilize these services. Therapists are in a better position to do so, partly because of their professional contacts and their status. The idea that therapists should act in this way on the family's behalf is a radical departure from traditional views of the therapist's role. Nevertheless, this role was advocated by all of the groups except Goldstein et al.'s (1978). Hogarty's group (Anderson et al. 1986) drew a specific parallel between the therapist and the ombudsperson.

Conclusions From Comparison of Approaches

It is evident from this comparison that the programs of the six successful interventions shared the same key components, although there were some differences in emphasis and in the techniques used. This conclusion is of great importance for the design of future intervention studies and for the implementation of family work in clinical practice.

I now turn to the unsuccessful interventions for the lessons that they might teach. The study by Dulz and Hand (1986) clearly used an intervention that differed in kind from those used in any of the six studies that had positive results. They separated patients and relatives into two parallel groups, which were meant to run for 2 years. The researchers had to delay forming each group until sufficient numbers of families entered the study. They reported that it often took months from identification of the first suitable patient to the last to form a group. The aims of their intervention were similar to those of the other workers in the field—namely, to reduce the patient's vulnerability, lower relatives' EE, modify the patient's behaviors that provoked high-EE attitudes, and increase coping skills. However, their approach was an "eclectic-psychodynamic" one, evidently stemming from a different basis than the more behavioral interventions outlined above. Thus, Dulz and Hand's study differed in two key respects from the successful trials: in the delay before engaging with the families and in the content of the intervention. The delay might well have resulted in poorer compliance, but the major factor contributing to their lack of success was the psychodynamic approach of their intervention.

In contrast, the study conducted by Vaughan et al. (1992a, 1992b) in Sydney had a content very similar to the education-behavioral interventions of the six studies considered above. Indeed, the close involvement of Tarrier in the Sydney study after he had completed his successful trial in England ensured a close correspondence in content. Vaughan's intervention differed from most of the others in two main ways: 1) he formed a group of relatives only, from which patients were excluded, with the patients receiving routine care only, and 2) the relatives' group met for no more than 10 weekly sessions. The question of the effectiveness of a relatives' group was addressed in the study by Leff et al. (1989). They found that if relatives were compliant with the group sessions, changes in the family environment and reductions in the patients' relapse rates were as great as with family sessions. Vaughan et al. (1992b) reported that all but 1 of the 18 families in the experimental stream attended the relatives' group regularly. Thus, the most likely factor accounting for their failure was the brevity of the intervention. Goldstein et al.'s (1978) intervention was equally brief, taking place over 6 weeks following discharge, but his patients were easier to deal with, being first- or second-admission patients only. Furthermore, Goldstein et al.'s follow-up period was only for 6 months. By contrast, in the studies by the other teams, sessions were held weekly, extending to fortnightly, over the first 9 months, followed by monthly sessions thereafter for as long as 2 years with some families. Persistence on the part of the therapists and continuity over long time periods appeared to be essential ingredients for a successful outcome.

Finally, there is the study by McCreadie et al. (1991), which was less stringent in its design, being a mirror-image study and not a randomized, controlled trial. Its outcome indicated that simply following written instructions is insufficient to guarantee an effective intervention. These investigators reported that they modeled their intervention on the writings by Leff et al.'s (1982, 1989) groups. At that point, relatively few details were available, as the definitive manual of those studies was published only at the end of 1992 (Kuipers et al. 1992). This experience emphasized the essential requirement for training programs in family work.

From the foregoing comparisons, the content of the intervention can be clearly specified and the duration of the therapists' commitment can be estimated. Despite the long-term nature of this collaborative work with families, it has been demonstrated to be less expensive than routine care, both when direct (Tarrier et al. 1991) and indirect (Cardin et al. 1986) costs are included. As Tarrier et al. (1991) reported, the main financial saving results from reduced hospital admissions.

Given the demonstrable advantages of the family interventions, it is perhaps surprising that they are still a rarity in routine clinical practice 17 years after the publication of the first successful study (Goldstein et al. 1978). One substantial obstacle is the difficulty in obtaining training in the necessary approaches and techniques. Recently, Leff et al.'s and Tarrier et al.'s groups collaborated in setting up a national training network in the United Kingdom, which should make this service accessible to the many thousands of families in need.

References

Anderson CM, Reiss DJ, Hogarty GE: Schizophrenia in the Family: a Practitioner's Guide to Psychoeducation and Management. New York, Guilford, 1986

Barrowclough C, Tarrier N: Families of Schizophrenic Patients: Cognitive Behavioural Intervention. London, Chapman & Hall, 1992

Bateson G, Jackson DD, Haley J, et al: Toward a theory of schizophrenia. Behav Sci 1:251–264, 1956

Birchwood M, Smith J, Cochrane R, et al: The social functioning scale: the development and validation of a scale of social adjustment for use in family intervention programmes with schizophrenic patients. Br J Psychiatry 157:853–859, 1990

Birchwood M, Smith J, Cochrane R: Specific and non-specific effects of educational intervention for families living with schizophrenia: a comparison of three methods. Br J Psychiatry 160:806–814, 1992

Brown GW, Rutter M: The measurement of family activities and relationships: a methodological study. Human Relations 19:241–263, 1966

Brown GW, Birley JLT, Wing JK: Influence of family life on the course of schizophrenic disorders: a replication. Br J Psychiatry 121:241–258, 1972

Cardin VA, McGill CW, Falloon IRH: An economic analysis: costs, benefits and effectiveness, in Family Management of Schizophrenia. Edited by Falloon IRH. Baltimore, MD, Johns Hopkins University Press, 1986, pp 115–124

Dulz B, Hand I: Short-term relapse in young schizophrenics: can it be predicted and affected by family (CFI) patient and treatment variables? in Treatment of Schizophrenia: Family Assessment and Intervention. Edited by Goldstein MJ, Hand I, Hahlweg K. Berlin, Springer-Verlag, 1986, pp 59–75

Falloon IRH, Boyd JL, McGill CW, et al: Family management in the prevention of exacerbations of schizophrenia. N Engl J Med 306:1437–1440, 1982

Falloon IRH, Boyd JL, McGill CW: Family Care of Schizophrenia. New York, Guilford, 1984

Falloon IRH, Boyd JL, McGill CW, et al: Family management in the prevention of morbidity of schizophrenia: clinical outcome of a two-year longitudinal study. Arch Gen Psychiatry 42:887–896, 1985

Fromm-Reichmann F: Notes on the development of treatment of schizophrenics by psychoanalytic psychotherapy. Psychiatry 11:263–273, 1948

Goldstein MJ, Rodnick EH, Evans JR, et al: Drug and family therapy in the aftercare treatment of acute schizophrenia. Arch Gen Psychiatry 35:169–177, 1978

Goldstein MJ, Kopeikin HS: Short- and long-term effects of combining drug and family therapy, in New Developments in Interventions With Families of Schizophrenics. Edited by Goldstein MJ. San Francisco, Jossey-Bass, 1981, pp 5–26

Hirsch SR, Leff JP: Abnormalities in the Parents of Schizophrenics (Maudsley Monograph No 22). Oxford, Oxford University Press, 1975

Hogarty GE, Anderson CM, Reiss DJ, et al: Family psychoeducation, social skills training and maintenance chemotherapy in the aftercare treatment of schizophrenia, I: one-year effects of a controlled study on relapse and expressed emotion. Arch Gen Psychiatry 43:633–642, 1986

Hogarty GE, Anderson CM, Reiss DJ, et al: Family psychoeducation, social skills training and maintenance chemotherapy in the aftercare treatment of schizophrenia, II: two-year effects of a controlled study on relapse and adjustment. Arch Gen Psychiatry 48:340–347, 1991

Jenkins JH, Karno M, De La Selva A, et al: Expressed emotion in cross-cultural context: familial responses to schizophrenic illness among Mexican Americans, in Treatment of Schizophrenia. Edited by Goldstein MJ, Hand I, Hahlweg K. Berlin, Springer-Verlag, 1986, pp 35–49

Kuipers L, Leff J, Lam D: Family Work for Schizophrenia: A Practical Guide. London, Gaskell, 1992

Laing RD, Esterson D: Sanity, Madness and the Family. London, Tavistock, 1964

Leff JP, Vaughn CE: The interaction of life events and relative's expressed emotion in schizophrenia and depressive neurosis. Br J Psychiatry 136:146–153, 1980

Leff JP, Kuipers L, Berkowitz R, et al: A controlled trial of social intervention in schizophrenic families. Br J Psychiatry 141:121–134, 1982

Leff JP, Kuipers L, Berkowitz R, et al: A controlled trial of social intervention in the families of schizophrenic patients: two-year follow-up. Br J Psychiatry 146:594–600, 1985

Leff JP, Berkowitz R, Shavit N, et al: A trial of family therapy versus a relatives' group for schizophrenia. Br J Psychiatry 154:58–66, 1989

Leff JP, Berkowitz R, Shavit N, et al: A trial of family therapy versus a relatives' group for schizophrenia: a two-year follow-up. Br J Psychiatry 157:571–577, 1990

Lidz T, Cornelison AR, Fleck S, et al: The intrafamilial environment of the schizophrenic patient, I: the father. Psychiatry 20:329–342, 1957a

Lidz T, Cornelison AR, Fleck S, et al: The intrafamilial environment of the schizophrenic patient, II: marital schism and marital skew. Am J Psychiatry 114:241–248, 1957b

McCreadie RG: The Nithsdale schizophrenia surveys: an overview. Soc Psychiatry Psychiatr Epidemiol 27:40–45, 1992

McCreadie RG, Phillips K, Harvey JA, et al: The Nithsdale schizophrenia surveys, VIII: do relatives want family intervention—and does it help? Br J Psychiatry 158:110–113, 1991

Platt S, Weyman A, Hirsch S, et al: The Social Behaviour Assessment Schedule (SBAS): rationale, contents, scoring and reliability of a new interview schedule. Soc Psychiatry Psychiatr Epidemiol 15:43–55, 1980

Rubinstein D: Techniques in family psychotherapy of schizophrenia, in Strategic Intervention in Schizophrenia. Edited by Cancro R, Fox N, Shapiro LE. New York, Behavioral Publications, 1974, pp 99–141

Singer MT, Wynne LC: Principles for scoring communication defects and deviances in parents of schizophrenics: Rorschach and T.A.T. Scoring Manuals. Psychiatry 29:260–288, 1966a

Singer MT, Wynne LC: Communication styles in parents of normals, neurotics and schizophrenics. Psychiatry Research Reports 20:25–38, 1966b

Speck RV, Reuvini V: Network therapy: a developing concept. Fam Process 8:182–191, 1969

Tarrier N: Some aspects of family interventions in schizophrenia, I: adherence to intervention programmes. Br J Psychiatry 159:475–480, 1991

Tarrier N, Barrowclough C: Social functioning in schizophrenic patients, I: the effects of expressed emotion and family intervention. Soc Psychiatry Psychiatr Epidemiol 25:125–129, 1990

Tarrier N, Barrowclough C, Vaughn C, et al: The community management of schizophrenia: a controlled trial of a behavioural intervention with families to reduce relapse. Br J Psychiatry 153:532–542, 1988

Tarrier N, Barrowclough C, Vaughn C, et al: Community management of schizophrenia: a two-year follow-up of a behavioural intervention with families. Br J Psychiatry 154:625–628, 1989

Tarrier N, Lowson K, Barrowclough C: Some aspects of family interventions in schizophrenia, II: financial considerations. Br J Psychiatry 159:481–484, 1991

Vaughan K, Doyle M, McConaghy N, et al: The relationship between relative's expressed emotion and schizophrenic relapse: an Australian replication. Soc Psychiatry Psychiatr Epidemiol 27:10–15, 1992a

Vaughan K, Doyle M, McConaghy N, et al: The Sydney intervention trial: a controlled trial of relatives' counselling to reduce schizophrenic relapse. Soc Psychiatry Psychiatr Epidemiol 27:16–21, 1992b

Vaughn CE, Leff JP: The measurement of expressed emotion in the families of psychiatric patients. Br J Clin Psychol 15:157–165, 1976a

Vaughn CE, Leff JP: The influence of family and social factors on the course of psychiatric illness: a comparison of schizophrenic and depressed neurotic patients. Br J Psychiatry 129:125–137, 1976b

CHAPTER 29

Psychiatric Rehabilitation and Case Management in Schizophrenia

Peter J. Prendergast, M.B., M.R.C.Psych., F.R.C.P.C.

The introduction of antipsychotic medication in the 1950s and the movement toward deinstitutionalization in the 1960s changed the nature of the psychiatric treatment of schizophrenia. Custodial care of patients was no longer the norm, and new drugs held out the promise of long-term symptom control, if not absolute cure. That initial optimism has been tempered over the last several decades by the realization that significant numbers of schizophrenic patients have remained seriously disabled despite receiving appropriate pharmacotherapy, and that living conditions in the community may be worse than those in the original institutions. The focus on pharmacological treatments and neuroleptic-induced side effects in Sections III and IV of this book highlights the fact that much work remains to be done to improve the benefit-to-risk ratio for patients taking antipsychotic drugs. There is an emerging consensus that medications are necessary in but not sufficient for the treatment of schizophrenia. Similarly, the overrepresentation of chronic schizophrenic patients among the poor, the unemployed, the homeless, and those who are incarcerated indicates that deinstitutionalization did not always result in an improved quality of life for this population.

Over the last 30 years, various psychosocial treatments have been used in conjunction with medication to optimize the functioning of patients with chronic schizophrenia. These treatments are reviewed in detail in Chapters 27–34 of this book. In this chapter, I review the emergence of psychiatric rehabilitation as a conceptual framework within which to deliver psychosocial treatments and medication, and describe case management as the organizational structure that best meets the needs of individuals with severe psychiatric disabilities. Before reviewing these issues, it is necessary to focus on the concept of continuity of care as a fundamental requirement of any system of health care delivery in this area.

Continuity of Care

Bachrach (1981) defined *continuity of care* as a process that involves the orderly, uninterrupted movement of patients among the diverse elements of the service delivery system. Ten years later, Stein (1992), addressing an American Psychiatric Association symposium on preventing psychotic relapse, referred to the current "nonsystem" of mental health care, which involves interventions and programs that are uncoordinated, noncollaborative, and often in competition with each other. Despite results from studies that have demonstrated the advantages of continuity of care, and descriptions of programs that deliver such continuity (Fuller-Torrey 1986), these programs remain the exception rather than the rule. As a result, as many as two-thirds of psychiatric patients fail to use aftercare services and are readmitted frequently in a process that is referred to as "the revolving door." The results from an aftercare study conducted in Toronto illustrate the problems encountered by this population. Wasylenki et al. (1985) evaluated 747 psychiatric patients at 6-month and 2-year follow-up after discharge from various hospital settings. They found that discharge planning was deficient and that housing, vocational, and social-recreational needs were often neglected, with the result that the readmission rate of those patients had risen to 70% after 2 years.

Harris and Bergman (1988a) described three aspects of continuity of care that are relevant to these "revolving door" patients: *continuity of treatment* refers to the maintenance of specific treatment strategies over time; *continuity of caregivers* refers to the specific relationship between the patient and the treatment providers; and *continuity of caring* refers to the use of that caregiving relationship to provide longitudinal support to vulnerable individuals. Ideally, all three aspects should be provided by continuous treatment teams (Fuller-Torrey 1986) and should be available in inpatient, day care, and outpatient settings so that hospitalization or participation in a day program does not necessitate an interruption in the relationship with regular treatment providers.

Psychiatric Rehabilitation

The terms *psychiatric rehabilitation* and *psychosocial rehabilitation* tend to be used interchangeably in the literature. In a review of the relationship between psychosocial rehabilitation and psychiatry, Bachrach (1992), noting the fact that there is no commonly endorsed definition of psychosocial rehabilitation, provided a summary definition from various sources:

> Psychosocial rehabilitation is a therapeutic approach to the care of mentally ill individuals that encourages each patient to develop his or her fullest capacities through learning procedures and environmental supports. (Bachrach 1992, p. 1456)

Anthony et al. (1990) differentiated treatment—whose aim is to reduce symptoms—from rehabilitation—whose aim is to improve functioning—and emphasized the parallels between psychiatric and physical rehabilitation, both of which aim to develop patients' skills and to maximize environmental supports. These authors outlined the basic principles or essentials of the rehabilitation approach, which can be summarized as follows:

> Psychiatric rehabilitation is an intrinsically positive and hopeful enterprise that seeks to increase the competence of individual patients in the environ-

ment of their choice. It is an eclectic approach that tolerates dependency but encourages independence; that utilizes medication to reduce symptoms but focuses more on vocational, social, and recreational outcomes; and that values patient involvement at an individual and systems level.

There are several models of psychiatric rehabilitation, ranging from the restorative approach of the Fountain House or Club House program (Beard et al. 1982) to the highly systematized Anthony model (Anthony et al. 1990). All of them share the essential features outlined above and use a variety of interventions to effect change in the individual, his or her environment, or both.

Wasylenki et al. (1989) identified the components of care required by schizophrenic patients, components that provide a framework within which specific rehabilitation interventions may be applied:

1. *Medical-psychiatric services,* which include family physicians, a comprehensive biopsychosocial approach to psychiatric care, and a variety of hospitalization options.
2. *Community housing,* a critical and often overlooked environmental component of rehabilitation planning.
3. *A variety of systemized, psychosocial interventions.* These include social skills training, family interventions, social therapeutic clubs, social network therapy, and self-help groups, all of which attempt to address the severe social deficits associated with chronic schizophrenia. In addition, specific attention must be paid to vocational and educational issues and financial services.
4. *Interagency coordination and advocacy,* to ensure that all individuals with long-term mental disabilities receive appropriate treatment and rehabilitation.

Investigators have used differing methodologies and different outcome measures to evaluate the various rehabilitation approaches. This makes it impossible to directly compare these approaches, although Anthony et al. (1990), in reviewing the research in this area, concluded that comparative research is now feasible because of refinements in the description of rehabilitation interventions and in the measurement of outcome variables.

The components of care outlined above offer a comprehensive

rehabilitation approach that incorporates principles developed in some of the more focused interventions such as social skills training (Liberman et al. 1986), family management (Hogarty et al. 1988), and community support systems (Test 1984). The approach also includes a medication strategy that emphasizes the need to focus not just on symptoms, but also on functioning, as stated by Anthony et al. (1990):

> From a rehabilitation perspective, drug therapy is a useful intervention but rarely an entire rehabilitation program. Likewise, practitioners of drug therapy may view rehabilitation as supportive in increasing drug compliance, determining the initial need for drug therapy, and/or decreasing drug dosage. (p. 72)

This treatment approach uses an individual case plan that details patient goals and service plans in five domains:

- Medical-psychiatric
- Housing
- Education
- Work
- Social (including family)

Such case plans can be reviewed periodically by the continuing care team, updated by the case manager in collaboration with the patient, and audited through a peer-reviewed quality assurance process, which would include chart review and interviews with patients.

Case Management

Case managers are the agents of continuity of care and the practitioners of psychiatric rehabilitation. Kanter (1989) defined *case management* as

> a modality of mental health practice that, in coordination with the traditional psychiatric focus on biological and psychological functioning, addresses the overall maintenance of the mentally ill person's physical and social environment with the goals of facilitating his or her physical survival,

personal growth, community participation, and recovery from or adaptation to mental illness. (p. 361)

Harris and Bergman (1988b) identified three therapeutic tasks for case managers: the forging of a relationship with the patient; the modeling of healthy behaviors; and the alteration of the environment in which the patient lives. Hargreaves et al. (1984) described five core case management functions—assessing, planning, linking, monitoring, and advocacy—all of which emphasize the need to help patients navigate a complex array of community programs. Having assessed a patient's strengths and deficits, the case manager works with the patient to develop an individual plan with goals, interventions, and a time frame. Once a patient becomes linked with specific programs or services, the case manager monitors the patient's progress. If programs are unavailable or deficient, the case manager advocates for individual patients and, at a systems level, for mentally ill patients as a group.

Wasylenki et al. (1989) added to the list of core case management functions, suggesting that a direct service provision may be needed and emphasizing the importance of crisis intervention during psychiatric emergencies.

It is clear that there are a range of services that may be considered to be aspects of case management and that there are a large number of models, varying from brokerage services with large case loads to full-support models that emphasize direct service provision and low staff-to-patient ratios.

Robinson (1991) identified four basic models that provide the interventions mentioned above to varying degrees:

1. *Full-support model:* This model is based on the Program for Assertive Community Treatment (PACT) or Training in Community Living model pioneered by Stein and Test (1980) in Wisconsin. The essential features are an interdisciplinary team that provides all the necessary services to all of the target population and an emphasis on continuity of care and 24-hour crisis availability.
2. *Personal-strengths model:* This model, also known as the Developmental Acquisition model, emphasizes individual strengths, self-determination, aggressive outreach, and resource acquisition in the community (Modrcin et al. 1985).

3. *Rehabilitation model:* This model emphasizes the principles of psychiatric rehabilitation and provides case management in the context of an individualized rehabilitation plan (Goering et al. 1988).
4. *Expanded broker model:* In this model, the case manager assesses needs and links the patient to various resources, but does not provide much direct clinical intervention (Johnson and Rubin 1983).

Solomon (1992) reviewed the available studies of these four models and concluded that case management reduces rehospitalization, reduces length of stay, improves quality of life, and increases patient satisfaction. However, she and others emphasized the need for more systematic research to evaluate not just the efficacy but also the degree of intensity of case management, the optimal duration of service, and the case management of subpopulations such as the homeless mentally ill and dually diagnosed patients (Chamberlain and Rapp 1991; Thornicroft 1991).

In the rehabilitation model described above, a multidisciplinary case management team could consist of a psychiatrist, a psychiatric resident, a nurse, an occupational therapist, and a social worker. Case managers would perform the following functions:

- Generic case management functions (e.g., direct skills training)
- Discipline-specific functions (e.g., vocational assessment by an occupational therapist)
- Program functions (e.g., leading a group in the day center)

Thus, case managers have multiple flexible roles, and the case management team functions in a transdisciplinary fashion, meaning that different professions are not just working together but are using clinical skills in a way that crosses traditional professional boundaries.

Using this approach, specific rehabilitation interventions are delivered in the context of a clinical relationship (Goering and Stylianos 1988), which allows for empathic listening and supportive psychotherapy (Wasylenki 1992). In addition to the development of skills and the modification of the environment, patients have the potential to use the relationship with the case manager as a vehicle for modeling, identification, and internalization (Harris and Bergman 1986).

The Role of the Psychiatrist

It is unfortunate that many psychiatrists have avoided working with severely mentally ill patients (Minkoff 1987), and that attitudes of psychiatric residents toward this population have been generally negative (Packer et al. 1994). Meanwhile, funding agencies are targeting these patients, and psychiatric rehabilitation programs and case management services are expanding rapidly throughout Canada and the United States (Goering et al. 1992). There are opportunities for psychiatrists to participate in these developments and to collaborate with an emerging group of professionals who are providing what patients need in a way that is endorsed by the community at large. The involvement of the psychiatrist may vary from consultation and collaboration with case management agencies, to membership in multidisciplinary teams, to administration, planning, and evaluation of programs. Psychiatrists are in a unique position to contribute a biopsychosocial perspective to these endeavors and to facilitate the integration of effective pharmacotherapy and state-of-the-art rehabilitation. To quote Bachrach (1992), "Psychiatry and psychosocial rehabilitation complement each other's contribution to the improvement of long-term patients' life circumstances—and together, these disciplines hold the key to realizing the promise of deinstitutionalization" (p. 1462).

References

Anthony A, Cohen M, Farkas M: Psychiatric Rehabilitation. Boston, MA, Boston University Press, 1990

Bachrach LL: Continuity of care for chronic mental patients: a conceptual analysis. Am J Psychiatry 138:1449–1456, 1981

Bachrach LL: Psychosocial rehabilitation and psychiatry in the care of long-term patients. Am J Psychiatry 149:1455–1463, 1992

Beard JH, Propst R, Malamud TJ: The Fountain House model of psychiatric rehabilitation. Psychosocial Rehabilitation Journal 5:47–53, 1982

Chamberlain R, Rapp CA: A decade of case management: a methodological review of outcome research. Community Ment Health J 27:171–188, 1991

Fuller-Torrey EF: Continuous treatment teams in the care of the chronic mentally ill. Hosp Community Psychiatry 37:1243–1247, 1986

Goering P, Stylianos S: Exploring the helping relationship between the schizophrenic client and the rehabilitation therapist. Am J Orthopsychiatry 58:271–280, 1988

Goering P, Wasylenki D, Farkas M, et al: What difference does case management make? Hosp Community Psychiatry 39:272–276, 1988

Goering P, Wasylenki D, MacNaughton E: Planning mental health services: current Canadian initiatives. Can J Psychiatry 37:259–263, 1992

Hargreaves W, Shaw R, Shadoan R, et al: Measuring case management activity. J Nerv Ment Dis 17:296–300, 1984

Harris M, Bergman HC: Case management with the chronically mentally ill: A clinical perspective. Am J Orthopsychiatry 57:296–302, 1986

Harris M, Bergman HC: Case management and continuity of care for the "revolving door" patient. New Dir Ment Health Serv 40:57–62, 1988a

Harris M, Bergman HC: Clinical case management for the chronically mentally ill: a conceptual analysis. New Dir Ment Health Serv 40:5–13, 1988b

Hogarty GE, McEvoy JP, Munetz M, et al: Dose of fluphenazine, familial expressed emotion, and outcome in schizophrenia: results of a two year controlled study. Arch Gen Psychiatry 45:797–805, 1988

Johnson P, Rubin A: Case management in mental health: a social work domain? Soc Work 28:49–55, 1983

Kanter J: Clinical case management: definitions, principles, components. Hosp Community Psychiatry 40:361–368, 1989

Liberman RP, Mueser KT, Wallace CJ: Social skills training for schizophrenic individuals at risk for relapse. Am J Psychiatry 143:523–526, 1986

Minkoff K: Resistance of mental health professionals to working with the chronic mentally ill. New Dir Ment Health Serv 33:3–20, 1987

Modrcin M, Rapp C, Chamberlain R: Case management with psychiatrically disabled individuals: curriculum and training program. Lawrence, KS, University of Kansas School of Social Welfare, 1985

Packer S, Prendergast P, Wasylenki D, et al: Psychiatric residents' attitudes toward patients with chronic mental illness. Hosp Community Psychiatry 45:1117–1121, 1994

Robinson G: Choices in case management. Community Support Network News 7:11–12, 1991

Solomon P: The efficacy of case management services for severely mentally disabled clients. Community Ment Health J 28:163–179, 1992

Stein LI: A system approach to reducing relapse. Paper presented at Psychotic Relapse: a Multisystems Perspective Symposium at the annual meeting of the American Psychiatric Association, Washington, DC, May 1992

Stein LI, Test MA: An alternative to mental hospital treatment, I: conceptual model, treatment program, and clinical evaluation. Arch Gen Psychiatry 37:392–397, 1980

Test MA: Community support programs, in Schizophrenia Treatment, Management, and Rehabilitation. Edited by Bellack AS. Orlando, FL, Grune & Stratton, 1984, pp 347–373

Thornicroft G: The concept of case management for long-term mental illness. International Review of Psychiatry 3:125–132, 1991

Wasylenki D: Psychotherapy of schizophrenia revisited. Hosp Community Psychiatry 43:123–127, 1992

Wasylenki D, Goering P, Lancee W, et al: Psychiatric aftercare in a metropolitan setting. Can J Psychiatry 30:329–336, 1985

Wasylenki DA, Goering PN, Humphrey BC, et al: Components of care for patients with schizophrenia. J Psychiatry Neurosci 14:287–295, 1989

Psychotherapy, Social Skills Training, and Vocational Rehabilitation in Schizophrenia

J. Steven Lamberti, M.D., and
Marvin I. Herz, M.D.

O ptimal treatment of schizophrenia requires a combination of psychosocial and psychopharmacological
interventions. The importance of psychosocial interventions in the management of schizophrenia is underscored by the
limitations of modern pharmacotherapy. Although antipsychotic medications are generally effective in reducing the psychotic symptoms of
schizophrenia, they have not been demonstrated to be effective in
improving social or vocational functioning.

Psychosocial treatments for schizophrenia encompass a wide variety of therapeutic approaches; the nature and goals of these treatment
approaches vary according to the severity, duration, and phase of the
illness. In this chapter, we focus on three approaches: psychotherapy
(both individual and group), social skills training, and vocational
rehabilitation.

Individual Psychotherapy

Intensive Insight-Oriented Psychotherapy

Following World War II, the predominant psychotherapeutic approach to schizophrenia was psychoanalysis, which flourished in the United States from 1945 to 1965. With the introduction of antipsychotic medications and growing doubts about the efficacy of psychoanalysis, a series of controlled studies during the 1960s examined the efficacy of psychoanalytically oriented treatment of schizophrenia (Bookhammer et al. 1966; Grinspoon et al. 1967, 1968, 1972; Karon and O'Grady 1969; Karon and VandenBos 1970, 1972; May 1968; May and Tuma 1964, 1965). Although results from double-blind placebo-controlled studies demonstrated the efficacy of antipsychotic medications in schizophrenia, most studies of psychoanalytically oriented treatment failed to evidence significant patient improvement.

Questions about the design and methodology of previous psychotherapy studies led to the most rigorously designed psychotherapy study of schizophrenia to date—the Boston Psychotherapy Study (Gunderson et al. 1984; Stanton et al. 1984). In this study, 164 schizophrenic patients were randomly assigned to receive either exploratory insight-oriented (EIO) psychotherapy two to three times per week or reality-adaptive supportive (RAS) psychotherapy conducted weekly to biweekly. All patients in the Boston study were treated over a 2-year period by highly experienced and motivated therapists, and all patients received psychotropic medications. Patients whose illness was either too chronic to be expected to respond to treatment or so acute that it might remit spontaneously were excluded from the study. In general, EIO psychotherapy focused on fostering self-knowledge and self-understanding, and RAS psychotherapy addressed practical issues of daily living. It should be noted that the efficacy of psychotherapy itself was not addressed, as this study did not have a nonpsychotherapy control group.

The principal finding of the study was that the RAS psychotherapy group achieved superior occupational functioning and spent less time in the hospital, whereas the EIO therapy group showed a trend toward better performance on measures of ego functioning. No significant differences were noted between the two types of psychotherapy on other measures, including insight, cognitive functioning, symptomatology, and medication usage. A tendency was noted for patients with acute symptomatology to engage preferentially in RAS psychotherapy, and for patients with more negative symptoms to engage preferentially in EIO psychotherapy (Katz and Gunderson 1990). The fact that only one-third of the patients in each group remained in the study for the entire 2-year period, however, raised questions about the motivation of schizophrenic patients to remain in individual psychotherapy.

The main conclusion to be drawn from the experimental literature is that intensive psychodynamically oriented psychotherapy is not appropriate for most schizophrenic patients (Gomes-Schwartz 1984; Mueser and Berenbaum 1990). This conclusion is especially relevant to current practice, given the growing need for treatments to be cost-effective.

Supportive Psychotherapy

Although the type of psychotherapy should always be determined by the characteristics and needs of the patient, supportive psychotherapy should be regarded as the individual psychotherapy of choice for most schizophrenic patients. Unfortunately, the principles and practice of supportive psychotherapy are not adequately taught at many training centers (Winston et al. 1986). This situation is further complicated by the existence of several different approaches to supportive psychotherapy, which are often difficult to distinguish from one another (Hafez et al. 1990).

In conducting supportive psychotherapy, it is desirable for the therapist to have a comprehensive understanding of the patient and his or her individual needs. Such an understanding may include knowledge of the patient's intrapsychic conflicts and defenses and of his or her coping skills and strengths, in addition to the interpersonal, cultural, and biological factors that affect the patient's life.

The primary goals of supportive psychotherapy are to help the patient manage life stresses, improve social and vocational functioning, and develop a sense of control and increased self-esteem. If interpretations are used with schizophrenic patients, they should be tailored to accommodate the patient's concrete thinking or impaired attention. As noted by Katz and Gunderson (1990), it is generally felt that interpretations should highlight the connections between stressful life events and psychotic symptoms rather than the content of psychotic symptoms. It is clear that some schizophrenic patients can benefit from gaining a better understanding of their reactions to stressful life situations.

The foundation of supportive psychotherapy, as with other types of psychotherapy, is the therapeutic relationship. Continuity of care with one therapist who engages in a collaborative, nonauthoritarian relationship is most beneficial in establishing a therapeutic alliance. Empathy, warmth, and genuineness on the part of the therapist will also enhance development of the relationship. In fact, the role of the therapist in supportive psychotherapy has been compared to that of an effective coach or good parent in terms of being safe, responsible, available, instructive, and encouraging (Adler 1982). However, the therapist differs from those models in that he or she should be trained in psychotherapeutic techniques and be aware of transferential and countertransferential issues.

In addition to facilitating the development of a trusting relationship, the therapist should provide education about schizophrenia, promote medication compliance, facilitate reality testing, help solve problems with the patient, and provide positive reinforcement for adaptive behaviors. The therapist should be prepared to give practical advice and guidance when needed, to set limits on regressive behaviors when necessary, and to collaborate with the patient to help prevent relapse. One promising strategy for preventing relapse involves teaching patients and their family members to monitor for early prodromal signs of relapse and to notify the therapist when those signs occur (Herz 1990).

Flexibility is necessary when conducting psychotherapy with schizophrenic patients. Treatment sessions should not be limited to office visits when there are indications for home visits and other forms of active outreach. Because many schizophrenic patients have deficits in a wide variety of areas of functioning, individual psychotherapy should be integrated into a coordinated treatment plan involving family treatment, case management services, social and residential services, and rehabilitation programs.

Group Psychotherapy

A number of investigators have examined the efficacy of group therapy for schizophrenia (Keith and Matthews 1982; Luborsky et al. 1976; May and Simpson 1980; Mosher and Keith 1980; O'Brien 1975; Parloff and Dies 1977) Review of this literature suggests that group therapy is as effective or more effective than individual psychotherapy for many chronic schizophrenic patients (Kanas 1986; O'Brien 1983).

Several types of group therapy are available for schizophrenic patients, ranging from highly structured behavior therapy groups to less structured social groups. Group therapy is particularly well suited for teaching coping and interpersonal skills and for providing a supportive social network for patients who tend to be socially isolated. In addition, many patients can accept observations about their behavior and symptoms more readily from other group members than from therapists. Group therapy on a weekly basis is also a cost-effective way of monitoring patients for prodromal symptoms (Herz et al. 1991).

In addressing the social and interpersonal deficits of schizophrenia, group therapy should focus on problem solving, goal planning, social interactions, and medication and side effect management, rather than on achieving insight (May and Simpson 1980). Research suggests that, just as in individual therapy, an intensive, insight-oriented group approach is counterproductive for most schizophrenic patients. This finding appears especially applicable to patients receiving psychotherapy in hospital settings or during periods of active psychosis (Kanas 1986). In contrast to the rules governing psychoanalytically oriented groups, flexibility is required in conducting psychotherapy groups for schizophrenic patients. Examples of such flexibility include individualization in attendance contracts, allowance for contact between group members outside of sessions, and less use of confrontation (Group for the Advancement of Psychiatry 1992). In addition, effective group therapy for schizophrenic patients generally requires a high degree of activity and structure by the therapist.

Although no clear consensus exists as to the optimal format for group psychotherapy for schizophrenic patients, Malm (1990) has proposed some useful guidelines:

- The method and goals of the group should be explained clearly to each participant prior to entry into the group.
- The group should consist of up to eight patients with the diagnosis of schizophrenia, including at least two of each gender.
- Patients may be allowed to enter the group during its progress or to reenter the group following relapse.
- All participants should be encouraged to notify the group in advance if unable to attend a session, and the group should always be told why someone is absent.
- Patients should be seated in a circle in a room without a table in the middle, and, if possible, the same room should be used for each session.
- Groups typically meet for 60-minute sessions on a weekly basis.

As with individual psychotherapy, patients receiving group psychotherapy should also be treated with appropriate pharmacotherapy to achieve optimal results. In a well-controlled 2-year study by Malm (1982), schizophrenic patients receiving a combination of communication-oriented group therapy, depot neuroleptics, and living skills instruction demonstrated significantly more improvements in symptomatology and social functioning than those receiving depot neuroleptics and living skills instruction alone. Results from Malm's (1982) study also raised questions about appropriate treatment duration for group psychotherapy. Because the primary purpose of group psychotherapy in schizophrenia is to address social and interpersonal deficits, ongoing, non–time-limited treatment may be the most beneficial. The frequency of group sessions can be decreased (e.g., to biweekly, monthly) in the later stages of treatment. As stated by Keith and Matthews (1984),

> negative symptoms and disordered interpersonal relationships are all pervasive, frequently developmental in origin, and do not spontaneously remit. It becomes less likely, therefore, that a treatment that is time limited . . . or circumscribed . . . can be expected to contribute to reversing this process except in a rather ancillary manner. (p. 341)

When psychotherapy groups are used as the primary treatment mode, individual sessions may be used adjunctively as needed. For many patients, group therapy is at least as clinically effective as individual treatment; furthermore, group therapy is more cost-effective. As in individual therapy, group therapy should be integrated into an overall treatment approach involving a comprehensive system of care.

Social Skills Training

Social skills training is a highly structured behavioral approach to treatment that is usually conducted in groups, although it may be used with individual patients and families. Also called *assertiveness training, personal effectiveness training,* and *structured learning therapy* (Wallace et al. 1980), social skills training is the most thoroughly investigated strategy for treatment of social disabilities in schizophrenia (Bellack and Mueser 1993). The efficacy of social skills training has been documented in more than 50 research studies since the late 1970s (Attkisson et al. 1992). The need for social skills training in schizophrenia is suggested by studies in which a high incidence of social skill deficits in chronic schizophrenic patients has been documented (Sylph et al. 1978), and in which social functioning has been indicated to be a strong predictor of outcome in schizophrenia (Liberman 1982). Despite this evidence, many practitioners have been slow to use social skills training, perhaps because of the nature of the competencies necessary to conduct this mode of treatment (Anthony and Liberman 1986; Backer et al. 1986).

It is important to distinguish between formalized social skills training and social activities, where the acquisition of social skills occurs incidentally (Liberman et al. 1985). According to Bellack and Mueser (1993),

> [social skills training] is a highly structured educational procedure that emphasizes modeling, role playing, and social reinforcement. Complex social repertoires, such as making friends and dating, are broken down into elements such as maintaining eye contact and providing social reinforcers. Patients are first taught to perform the elements and then gradually to smoothly combine them. (p. 321)

In addition to basic conversation and dating skills, social skills training has been used to teach patients skills related to medication management (Eckman et al. 1990), sexual behavior (Lukoff et al. 1986), and job finding (Jacobs et al. 1984; Kramer and Beidel 1982).

Training Models

Social skills training may be broadly grouped into three models: the basic model, the problem-solving model, and the attention-focusing model (Liberman et al. 1985). The choice of a particular model must be determined by the individual needs of the patient. All models use role-playing, modeling, and reinforcement, and often use videotaping to facilitate the delivery of feedback and instruction.

Social skills training more resembles traditional classroom instruction than a therapy session. Patients are required to participate actively in sessions, which can range from 10–15 minutes to 2 hours in length, depending on the patient's level of concentration and attention. Sessions may be conducted several times each week. Social skills training includes an assessment component, during which a variety of modalities—ranging from self-report inventories to direct observation—may be used. Outcome after training is generally assessed by measuring the patient's level of anxiety, number of appropriate behaviors, or successful completion of specific goals (Wallace et al. 1980).

Basic social skills model.   The basic social skills model has been used to teach patients specific verbal and nonverbal social skills, including eye contact, smiling, voice volume, speech duration, asking questions, and giving compliments (Liberman et al. 1985). In a typical basic skills session, a patient and trainer or two patients in a group are asked to role-play a social situation involving a specific goal, such as asking someone for a date. The role-playing is reviewed after completion, often using a videotape, and the patient is given praise and corrective feedback for specific behaviors. Alternative behaviors, such as speaking more quietly or smiling, may be suggested or modeled by the trainer. Training is commonly followed by homework assignments to promote the extension of learned skills to natural settings.

Problem-solving model.   The problem-solving model shares many elements with the basic approach, but also provides strategies to enable patients to manage unrehearsed social situations. Use of this approach is supported by findings that chronic schizophrenic patients often lack problem-solving skills (Liberman et al. 1985; Platt and Spivack 1972).

In the problem-solving approach, the skills necessary for effective interpersonal communication are divided into receiving, processing, and sending. *Receiving skills* are used to accurately perceive verbal, nonverbal, and social cues during interpersonal interactions. *Processing skills* are used to generate alternative responses, to weigh their pros and cons, and to select the most effective response. Once an optimal response is selected, *sending skills* are used to convey the response as a combination of appropriate verbal and nonverbal behaviors.

The problem-solving approach to social skills training has been packaged into a series of training modules that address a variety of social and living skills, including medication management, money management, grooming and self-care, and social problem solving (Roder et al. 1990). Each module contains a patient's workbook, an instructor's guide, and a videotaped skills demonstration, and can be used in small groups during 1-hour sessions. Modules include elements conducted within the treatment setting (e.g., the introduction, videotaped demonstration, role-playing, problem solving) and elements conducted in the natural environment (e.g., in vivo exercises, homework exercises, and "booster sessions"). The purpose of extending social skills training into the patient's natural environment is to promote the transfer of learning to everyday living situations.

Attention-focusing model.   The attention-focusing model was developed for chronic psychiatric patients with severe cognitive, memory, and attentional impairments (Mosk et al. 1983). Such impairments often prevent these patients from participating in standard social skills approaches that require active group participation. The attention-focusing approach is characterized by the use of multiple brief training trials. It is generally used to teach conversational skills; employs role-playing, modeling, and corrective feedback; and often uses food or drink as a reinforcement (Liberman et al. 1985).

Efficacy Studies

The efficacy of social skills training in schizophrenic patients was examined in several large controlled studies during the 1980s. Bellack et al. (1984) found that patients who received a 3-month course of social skills training with day treatment had better social adjustment than those receiving day treatment alone at 6-month follow-up. No differences in relapse rates were noted. Wallace and Liberman (1985) also reported significantly better social adjustment and competence in patients who received a standard treatment plus 9 weeks of social skills training compared with patients who received the standard treatment plus holistic health therapy. The differences were less robust at 24-month follow-up compared with 9-month follow-up, however, and no differences in relapse rates were noted between the groups. Wirshing et al. (1991) compared social skills training, consisting of medication and symptom management modules, with supportive psychotherapy in patients maintained on low-dosage fluphenazine decanoate. The social skills group was found to experience a significantly longer length of time to relapse following the beginning of a prodromal episode than the supportive psychotherapy group.

Perhaps the most rigorously controlled study was that conducted by Hogarty et al. (1991), who compared social skills training with psychoeducational family therapy, a combination of social skills training and psychoeducational family therapy, and a medication-only treatment (as the control condition). All patients in this study resided with relatives rated as having high expressed emotion (which has been implicated in exacerbating relapse in schizophrenic patients [see Chapter 28]). Patients were evaluated during a 2-year follow-up period. Social skills training and family therapy each reduced relapse rates by 50% compared with the control treatment after 1 year, with the combination of social skills training and family treatments resulting in no relapses during that time period. Family therapy alone and in combination with social skills training was effective in reducing relapse at 2 years, but no additive effect was noted for the combination of treatments. The effectiveness of social skills training alone compared with that of the control treatment in reducing relapse rates was lost after 21 months.

Benton and Schroeder (1990) conducted a meta-analytic review of 27 social skills training studies and found this treatment to have a strongly positive impact on behavioral measures of social skills, self-ratings of assertiveness, and hospital discharge rates, and a moderate impact on relapse rates.

A review of the literature raises a number of questions about the extent to which measurable improvement during social skills training is generalized to functional improvement in the community, and about the effectiveness of this treatment in reducing symptomatology. In addition, the effect of patient variables—including level of affiliation motivation, severity and duration of illness, and subtype of schizophrenia—requires further study (Benton and Schroeder 1990).

Another important question concerns the optimal duration of social skills training. Although schizophrenia is known to be a chronic illness, most studies of social skills training have involved brief, time-limited courses of treatment. As noted by Bellack and Mueser (1993), a brief psychosocial intervention is no more likely to be effective at producing sustained improvement in schizophrenia than is a brief course of neuroleptic medication. Offering continued training at lower intensities, the periodic booster sessions over an extended time period, or both strategies combined may help to maximize the long-term effectiveness of social skills training.

Vocational Rehabilitation

The deinstitutionalization of chronically mentally ill patients posed many challenges for community-based treatment programs. This challenge was particularly evident in the field of vocational rehabilitation. In response to increasing numbers of chronically mentally ill patients entering the community, the Rehabilitation Act of 1973, which required state vocational rehabilitation agencies to give priority to psychiatrically disabled individuals, was enacted. In the decade following this legislation, however, employment among individuals with severe physical disabilities rose 19.9%, whereas employment for individuals with psychiatric disabilities declined 3.4% (Andrews et al. 1992). In 1979, the National Institute of Handicapped Research concluded that "although mentally disabled individuals make up the largest number of cases eligible for vocational rehabilitation services, they have the least probability of success before and after rehabilitation" (Ciardiello 1988, p. 264). This situation has been compounded by the fact that mental health professionals typically have had little exposure to vocational rehabilitation during their training and, as a result, often fail to make timely use of vocational interventions (McCrory 1988). As noted by Ciardiello et al. (1988), psychiatry's past failures with vocational rehabilitation highlight the need to understand how schizophrenia impairs vocational functioning and to learn which interventions are most likely to result in vocational success.

There has been a surge of interest in the vocational rehabilitation of schizophrenic patients in recent years. Several approaches currently exist that differ in the degree to which they rely on community placements to achieve vocational outcomes. Vocational rehabilitation services may be viewed as existing on a continuum ranging from hospital-based programs to supported employment and postemployment services (Bond and Boyer 1988; Jacobs 1988).

Hospital-based programs.   Interest in hospital-based vocational rehabilitation programs has declined as lengths of inpatient stays have decreased. Most authors examining the literature in this area have concluded that there is no relationship between involvement in inpatient vocational programs and successful postdischarge employment, and that such programs may actually increase institutional dependency (Bond and Boyer 1988).

Sheltered workshops.   Sheltered workshops, originally designed for individuals with physical and developmental disabilities, have been widely used by psychiatrically disabled individuals. Such programs provide individuals who are not ready for competitive employment with a shortened work day, decreased on-the-job pressures, simplified tasks, and a structured, positive work environment (Jacobs 1988). Review of the literature, however, suggests that psychiatrically disabled individuals earn less income, show poorer workshop attendance, and present more behavioral problems than individuals with other disabilities in these environments (Attkisson et al. 1992). Griffiths (1974) and Weinberg and Lustig (1968), in their controlled studies examining the effects of sheltered workshop programs on competitive employment rates, found no significant differences between the workshop and the control groups. Research has also suggested that work in actual employment settings is better for developing self-esteem and competence among individuals than work in sheltered settings (Conte 1983; Rapp 1979). Although sheltered workshops can be a viable long-term placement for severely disabled patients, they should also be viewed as a step along the rehabilitation continuum for many schizophrenic patients. To function effectively as transitional skill-training environments, sheltered workshops must be embedded in a community support system that includes a full spectrum of rehabilitative services (Jacobs 1988).

Fairweather Lodge model. The Fairweather Lodge model addresses the areas of living, working, and socializing by having the involved individuals reside together in the community and work together in a consumer-owned business (Fairweather et al. 1969). Although more than 100 lodges are currently operating in the United States (Bond and Boyer 1988) and initial studies have demonstrated higher rates of employment among individuals using the Lodge approach than other approaches (Fairweather 1980; Fairweather et al. 1969), further controlled studies of this model are needed.

Consumer-run businesses. Consumer-run businesses range from nonprofit consumer corporations—which contract with community agencies to perform services such as yard work and maintenance—to businesses that are entirely consumer owned and operated. Although these businesses can be demanding on individuals (Salkind 1971), advocates for this approach believe that such demands can have a normalizing and therapeutic impact (Carroll and Levye 1985). Although reports have described experiences with consumer-run businesses (Carroll and Levye 1985), controlled studies are lacking.

Assertive community treatment. Another program that emphasizes vocational rehabilitation of chronically mentally ill patients is Assertive Community Treatment (ACT; Stein and Test 1985). ACT programs involve the use of mobile treatment teams that work to provide ongoing treatment in the community rather than in clinic settings. In addition to psychiatric treatment, these programs provide intensive in vivo training in community living and social support to their patients. For example, patients are taught how to shop on site at their local supermarket. Vocational interventions include assisting patients with job-seeking and maintenance skills, and may involve competitive, volunteer, or sheltered work experiences. The original and best-known ACT program is the Program for Assertive Community Treatment (PACT; Stein and Test 1980). This program emphasizes community-based vocational assessments, employs vocational counselors, and has a large network of job placement sites.

Although a number of studies have demonstrated that ACT programs are effective in reducing the number and length of patient hospitalizations (Group for the Advancement of Psychiatry 1992), their effectiveness compared with that of conventional community treatment programs in achieving vocational outcomes is less certain (Olfson 1990). Many ACT programs do not place primary emphasis on vocational goals, and those that do are often dependent on the availability of community resources to generate job placements.

Psychosocial rehabilitation centers.   Psychosocial rehabilitation centers, as represented by Fountain House in New York City (Beard et al. 1982), are founded on a self-help philosophy. These programs use informal clubhouse settings, call participants "members," and provide residential, social, and vocational services. Members are exposed to a variety of work experiences, ranging from on-site prevocational work to transitional employment. Prevocational activities include clerical work related to clubhouse functioning, tour guide activities, meal preparation, and maintenance work. Although these programs have been shown to reduce hospitalization rates, they have not been demonstrated to be effective in increasing competitive employment (Bond and Boyer 1988)

Transitional employment programs.   Transitional employment programs were originally developed at Fountain House in 1958 (Beard et al. 1982), and they continue to be associated with psychosocial rehabilitation centers. In transitional employment, these centers contract with local businesses to provide community job placements to their members. Placements are usually on a part-time basis, thereby permitting members to spend half days at the clubhouse, and are usually entry-level jobs requiring little experience or training. Staff members begin working at new placement sites to assess the work environments and demands, and are subsequently available at the sites to support members during their initial employment. Placements are transitional or temporary, allowing members to rotate through different placements or to use a placement as an entrance to full-time employment. Transitional employment programs thus provide a bridge to competitive employment, support for clients on the job, and opportunities for community-based vocational assessment of clients. Although transitional employment programs have generally been associated with psychosocial rehabilitation programs, they may also be used with sheltered workshop or day treatment programs. Research has indicated that transitional employment programs are effective in enabling clients to secure employment (Bond 1986) and to hold employment for relatively short periods of time (Cook et al. 1989; Fountain House 1985; I. Rutman and K. Armstrong [Matrix Research Institute, Philadelphia, PA], unpublished manuscript, 1985).

Supported employment programs.   Research has suggested that ongoing job support is necessary for long-term employment of clients with severe mental illness (Cook and Razzano 1992). Supported employment programs differ from transitional employment programs by providing vocational support on an ongoing basis. Such support may range from instruction about hygiene and social skills to providing transportation and on-site job support. Most supported employment programs in the United States are funded to serve mentally retarded clients (Rutman 1986), and outcome studies of schizophrenic patients in supported employment programs are needed.

Job clubs.   Job clubs are structured approaches to job finding that are based on a packaged module originally developed for nonpsychiatric populations from low-income backgrounds (Azrin and Besalel 1980) and later modified for use with psychiatric patients (Jacobs et al.

1984; Kramer and Beidel 1982). Job club programming begins with an intensive, 1-week workshop teaching job-seeking skills, followed by a job-search phase using counselor and peer support to promote daily goal setting, and concluding with weekly aftercare sessions that use problem solving to promote job maintenance. Although research with heterogeneous populations has shown promising results and has suggested that diagnosis does not predict job placement (Jacobs 1988), other work has indicated that this approach may be less effective with schizophrenic patients (Bond, in press).

Boston University model. The Boston University (BU) model of psychiatric rehabilitation is a broad approach that addresses individuals' needs in the areas of living, learning, and working. It is based on principles derived from client-centered therapy and skills training, emphasizes the importance of client choice, and is primarily center based. The BU model of vocational rehabilitation involves extensive assessment of a client's ability to choose, get, and keep a job; development of a rehabilitation plan; and subsequent skills training (Anthony et al. 1984). While evidence to date suggests that such extensive prevocational exploration leads to greater satisfaction with choices, it is unknown whether such exploration also leads to successful employment (Bond 1992).

Dissemination of the BU model has been aided by the existence of an organized training program for mental health workers (Rogers et al. 1986). One study of the BU model by Goering et al. (1988) yielded no significant differences in the rate of paid employment between patients treated by case managers trained in this model and historically matched control subjects. There has been a recent spread of this model, although its efficacy remains to be empirically validated.

Conclusion

In conclusion, psychosocial treatment and rehabilitative programs used in combination with pharmacotherapy can be very beneficial for schizophrenic patients. Interventions should be individualized and modified in a flexible manner according to the changing needs of patients over the course of their lives. Further research is needed to establish the efficacy of many interventions currently in use and to promote the development of new therapeutic techniques.

References

Adler G: Supportive psychotherapy revisited. Hillside Journal of Clinical Psychiatry 4:3–13, 1982

Andrews H, Barker J, Pittman J, et al: National trends in vocational rehabilitation: a comparison of individuals with physical disabilities and individuals with psychiatric disabilities. Journal of Rehabilitation 58:7–16, 1992

Anthony WA, Liberman RP: The practice of psychiatric rehabilitation: historical, conceptual, and research base. Schizophr Bull 12:542–559, 1986

Anthony WA, Howell J, Danley KS: Vocational rehabilitation of the psychiatrically disabled, in The Chronically Mentally Ill: Research and Services. Edited by Mirabi M. New York, Spectrum Publications, 1984, pp 215–237

Attkisson C, Cook J, Karno M, et al: Clinical services research. Schizophr Bull 18:561–626, 1992

Azrin NH, Besalel VB: Job Club Counselor's Manual: A Behavioral Approach to Vocational Counseling. Baltimore, MD, University Park Press, 1980

Backer TE, Liberman RP, Kuehnel TG: Dissemination and adoption of innovative psychosocial interventions. J Consult Clin Psychol 54:111–118, 1986

Beard JH, Propst R, Malamud TJ: The Fountain House model of psychiatric rehabilitation. Psychosocial Rehabilitation Journal 5:47–53, 1982

Bellack AS, Mueser KT: Psychosocial treatment for schizophrenia. Schizophr Bull 19:317–336, 1993

Bellack AS, Turner SM, Hersen M, et al: An examination of the efficacy of social skills training for chronic schizophrenic patients. Hosp Community Psychiatry 35:1023–1028, 1984

Benton MK, Schroeder HE: Social skills training with schizophrenics: a meta-analytic evaluation. J Consult Clin Psychol 58:741–747, 1990

Bond GR: Psychiatric vocational programs: a meta-analysis. Paper presented at the annual meeting of the International Association of Psychosocial Rehabilitation Services, Cleveland, OH, June 1986

Bond GR: Vocational rehabilitation, in Handbook of Psychiatric Rehabilitation. Edited by Liberman RP. Boston, MA, Allyn & Bacon, 1992, pp 244–275

Bond GR: Vocational rehabilitation for persons with severe mental illness: past, present, and future, in Rehabilitation of the Psychiatrically Disabled. Edited by Liberman RP. New York, Plenum (in press)

Bond GR, Boyer SL: Rehabilitation programs and outcomes, in Vocational Rehabilitation of Persons With Prolonged Psychiatric Disorders. Edited by Ciardiello JA, Bell MD. Baltimore, MD, Johns Hopkins University Press, 1988, pp 231–263

Bookhammer RS, Meyer RW, Schober CC, et al: A five year follow-up study of schizophrenics treated by Rosen's "direct analysis" compared with controls. Am J Psychiatry 123:602–604, 1966

Carroll CR, Levye R: Cookie Place and a New Leaf: a profile of two businesses providing supported work for people with psychiatric disabilities. Paper presented at the meeting of the International Association of Psychosocial Rehabilitation Services, Boston, MA, June 1985

Ciardiello JA: Summary and conclusion, in Vocational Rehabilitation of Persons With Prolonged Psychiatric Disorders. Edited by Ciardiello JA, Bell MD. Baltimore, MD, Johns Hopkins University Press, 1988, pp 264–271

Ciardiello JA, Klein ME, Sobkowski S: Ego functioning and vocational rehabilitation, in Vocational Rehabilitation of Persons With Prolonged Psychiatric Disorders. Edited by Ciardiello JA, Bell MD. Baltimore, MD, Johns Hopkins University Press, 1988, pp 196–207

Conte L: Sheltered employment and disabled citizens: an analysis of the work stations in the industry model (abstract). Dissertation Abstracts International 43:2975A, 1983

Cook JA, Razzano L: Natural vocational supports for persons with severe mental illness: thresholds supported competitive employment program. New Dir Ment Health Serv 56:23–41, 1992

Cook JA, Solomon M, Mock L: What happens after the first job placement? Programming for Adolescents With Behavioral Disorders 4:71–93, 1989

Eckman TA, Liberman RP, Phipps CC, et al: Teaching medication management skills to schizophrenic patients. J Clin Psychopharmacol 10:33–38, 1990

Fairweather GW: The prototype Lodge Society: instituting process principles, in The Fairweaather Lodge: A Twenty-Year Retrospective (New Directions for Mental Health Services, No. 7). Edited by Fairweather GW. San Francisco, CA, Jossey-Bass, 1980, pp 13–32

Fairweather GW, Sanders DH, Maynard H, et al: Community Life for the Mentally Ill. Chicago, IL, Aldine, 1969

Fountain House: Evaluation of Clubhouse Model Community-Based Psychiatric Rehabilitation: Final Report to the National Institute of Handicapped Research (Contract No 300-84-0124). Washington, DC, National Institute of Handicapped Research, 1985

Goering P, Wasylenki D, Farkas M, et al: What difference does managed care make? Hosp Community Psychiatry 39:272–276, 1988

Gomes-Schwartz B: Individual psychotherapy of schizophrenia, in Schizophrenia: Treatment, Management, and Rehabilitation. Edited by Bellack AS. New York, Grune & Stratton, 1984, pp 307–335

Griffiths RD: Rehabilitation of chronic psychotic patients. Psychol Med 4:316–325, 1974

Grinspoon L, Ewalt JR, Shader R: Long term treatment of chronic schizophrenia. International Journal of Psychiatry 4:116–128, 1967

Grinspoon L, Ewalt JR, Shader R: Psychotherapy and pharmacotherapy in chronic schizophrenia. Am J Psychiatry 124:1645–1652, 1968

Grinspoon L, Ewalt JR, Shader R: Schizophrenia: Pharmacotherapy and Psychotherapy. Baltimore, MD, Williams & Wilkins, 1972

Group for the Advancement of Psychiatry: Implications for psychosocial interventions in patients with schizophrenia, in Beyond Symptom Suppression (Report No 134). Washington, DC, American Psychiatric Press, 1992, pp 59–78

Gunderson JG, Frank AF, Katz HM, et al: Effects of psychotherapy in schizophrenia, II: comparative outcome of two forms of treatment. Schizophr Bull 10:564–598, 1984

Hafez HM, Frank A, Docherty JP: Individual reality-oriented supportive psychotherapy, in Handbook of Schizophrenia, Vol 4: Psychosocial Treatment of Schizophrenia. Edited by Herz MI, Keith SJ, Docherty JP. New York, Elsevier, 1990, pp 91–105

Herz MI: Early intervention in schizophrenia, in Handbook of Schizophrenia, Vol 4: Psychosocial Treatment of Schizophrenia. Edited by Herz MI, Keith SJ, Docherty JP. New York, Elsevier, 1990, pp 25–44

Herz MI, Glazer WM, Mostert MA, et al: Intermittent versus maintenance medication in schizophrenia. Arch Gen Psychiatry 48:333–339, 1991

Hogarty GE, Anderson CM, Reiss DJ, et al: Family psychoeducation, social skills training, and maintenance chemotherapy in the aftercare treatment of schizophrenia, II: two year effects of a controlled study on relapse and adjustment. Arch Gen Psychiatry 48:340–347, 1991

Jacobs HE: Vocational rehabilitation, in Psychiatric Rehabilitation of Chronic Mental Patients. Edited by Liberman RP. Washington, DC, American Psychiatric Press, 1988, pp 245–284

Jacobs H, Kardashian S, Krienbring R, et al: A skills-oriented model for facilitating employment among psychiatrically disabled persons. Rehabilitation and Counseling Bulletin 28:87–96, 1984

Kanas N: Group therapy with schizophrenics: a review of controlled studies. Int J Group Psychother 36:339–351, 1986

Karon B, O'Grady B: Intellectual test changes in schizophrenic patients in the first six months of treatment. Psychotherapeutic Theory, Research, and Practice 6:88–96, 1969

Karon B, VandenBos GR: Experience, medication, and the effectiveness of psychotherapy with schizophrenics: a note on Drs. May and Tuma's conclusions. Br J Psychiatry 116:427–428, 1970

Karon B, VandenBos GR: The consequences of psychotherapy for schizophrenic patients. Psychotherapeutic Theory, Research, and Practice 9:111–119, 1972

Katz HM, Gunderson JG: Individual psychodynamically oriented psychotherapy for schizophrenic patients, in Handbook of Schizophrenia, Vol 4: Psychosocial Treatment of Schizophrenia. Edited by Herz MI, Keith SJ, Docherty JP. New York, Elsevier, 1990, pp 69–90

Keith SJ, Matthews SM: Group, family, and milieu therapies and psychosocial rehabilitation in the treatment of schizophrenic disorders, in Psychiatry 1982: The American Psychiatric Association Annual Review, Vol 1. Edited by Grinspoon L. Washington, DC, American Psychiatric Press, 1982, pp 166–177

Keith SJ, Matthews SM: Group psychotherapy, in Schizophrenia. Edited by Bellack AS. New York, Grune & Stratton, 1984, pp 337–345

Kramer LW, Beidel DC: Job seeking skill groups: review and application to a chronic psychiatric population. Occupational Therapy and Mental Health 2:37–44, 1982

Liberman RP: Social factors in the etiology of the schizophrenic disorders, in Psychiatry 1982: The American Psychiatric Association Annual Review. Edited by Grinspoon L. Washington, DC, American Psychiatric Press, 1982, pp 97–111

Liberman RP, Massel HK, Mosk MD, et al: Social skills training for chronic mental patients. Hosp Community Psychiatry 36:396–403, 1985

Luborsky L, Singer B, Luborsky L: Comparative studies of psychotherapies: is it true that "everybody has won and all must have prizes"? Proceedings of the American Psychopathological Association 64:3–22, 1976

Lukoff D, Gioia-Hasick D, Sullivan G, et al: Sex education and rehabilitation with schizophrenic male outpatients. Schizophr Bull 12:669–677, 1986

Malm U: The influence of group therapy on schizophrenia. Acta Psychiatr Scand Suppl 297:1–65, 1982

Malm U: Group therapy, in Handbook of Schizophrenia, Vol 4: Psychosocial Treatment of Schizophrenia. Edited by Herz MI, Keith SJ, Docherty JP. New York, Elsevier, 1990, pp 191–211

May PR: Treatment of Schizophrenia: A Comparative Study of Five Treatment Methods. New York, Science House, 1968

May PR, Simpson G: Schizophrenia: evaluation of treatment methods, in Comprehensive Textbook of Psychiatry, 3rd Edition, Vol 2. Edited by Kaplan HI, Freedman AM, Sadock BJ. Baltimore, MD, Williams & Wilkins, 1980, pp 1240–1275

May PR, Tuma AH: The effect of psychotherapy and stelazine on length of hospital stay, release rate and supplemental treatment of schizophrenic patients. J Nerv Ment Dis 139:362–369, 1964

May PR, Tuma AH: Treatment of schizophrenia. Bower J Psychiatry 3:503–510, 1965

McCrory DJ: The human dimension of the vocational rehabilitation process, in Vocational Rehabilitation of Persons With Prolonged Psychiatric Disorders. Edited by Ciardiello JA, Bell MD. Baltimore, MD, Johns Hopkins University Press, 1988, pp 208–218

Mosher LR, Keith SJ: Psychosocial treatment: individual, group, family, and community support approaches. Schizophr Bull 6:10–41, 1980

Mosk MD, Wong SE, Massel HK, et al: Graduated and traditional procedures for teaching social skills to chronic low functioning schizophrenics. Paper presented at the annual meeting of the American Psychological Association, Anaheim, CA, August 1983

Mueser KT, Berenbaum H: Psychodynamic treatment of schizophrenia: is there a future? Psychol Med 20:253–262, 1990

O'Brien CP: Group psychotherapy for schizophrenia: a practical approach. Schizophr Bull 13:119–130, 1975

O'Brien CP: Group psychotherapy with schizophrenia and affective disorders, in Comprehensive Group Psychotherapy, 2nd Edition. Edited by Kaplan HI, Sadock BJ. Baltimore, MD, Williams & Wilkins, 1983, pp 242–249

Olfson M: Assertive community treatment: an evaluation of the experimental evidence. Hosp Community Psychiatry 41:634–641, 1990

Parloff MB, Dies R: Group psychotherapy outcome research. Int J Group Psychother 27:281–319, 1977

Platt JJ, Spivack G: Social competence and effective problem solving thinking in psychiatric patients. J Clin Psychol 28:3–5, 1972

Rapp RE: A normalization approach to the vocational training of mentally retarded adults (abstract). Dissertation Abstracts International 40:1410A, 1979

Roder V, Eckman TA, Brenner HD: Behavior therapy, in Handbook of Schizophrenia, Vol 4: Psychosocial Treatment of Schizophrenia. Edited by Herz MI, Keith SJ, Docherty JP. New York, Elsevier, 1990, pp 107–134

Rogers ES, Cohen BF, Danley KS, et al: Training mental health workers in psychiatric rehabilitation. Schizophr Bull 12:709–719, 1986

Rutman ID: A comprehensive, national evaluation of transitional employment programs for the psychiatrically disabled. Paper presented at the annual meeting of the International Association of Psychosocial Rehabilitation Services, Cleveland, OH, June 1986

Salkind I: Economic problems of workshops, in Rehabilitation in Community Mental Health. Edited by Lamb HR. San Francisco, CA, Jossey-Bass, 1971, pp 71–91

Stanton AH, Gunderson JG, Knapp PH, et al: Effects of psychotherapy in schizophrenia, I: design and implementation of a controlled study. Schizophr Bull 10:520–562, 1984

Stein LI, Test MA: An alternative to mental hospital treatment, I: conceptual model, treatment program, and clinical evaluation. Arch Gen Psychiatry 37:393–397, 1980

Stein LI, Test MA (eds): The Training in Community Living Model: A Decade of Experience (New Directions for Mental Health Services, No. 6). San Francisco, CA, Jossey-Bass, 1985

Sylph JA, Ross HE, Kedward HB: Social disability in chronic psychiatric patients. Am J Psychiatry 134:1391–1394, 1978

Wallace CJ, Liberman RP: Social skills training for patients with schizophrenia: a controlled clinical trial. Psychiatry Res 15:239–247, 1985

Wallace CJ, Nelson CJ, Liberman RP, et al: A review and critique of social skills training with schizophrenic patients. Schizophr Bull 6:42–63, 1980

Weinberg JL, Lustig P: A workshop experience for post-hospitalization schizophrenics, in Rehabilitation Research. Edited by Wright GN, Trotter AB. Madison, WI, University of Wisconsin, 1968, pp 72–78

Winston A, Pinsker H, McCullough L: A review of supportive psychotherapy. Hosp Community Psychiatry 37:1105–1114, 1986

Wirshing WC, Eckman T, Liberman RP, et al: Management of risk of relapse through skills training of chronic schizophrenics, in Advances in Neuropsychiatry and Psychopharmacology, Vol 1: Schizophrenia Research. Edited by Tamminga C, Schulz SC. New York, Raven, 1991, pp 255–267

CHAPTER 31

Quality-of-Life Issues in Medicated Schizophrenic Patients

A. George Awad, M.B., B.Ch., Ph.D., F.R.C.P.C.

O ver the past few years, improving patients' health-related quality of life has become increasingly recognized as an outcome, particularly in patients being treated for chronic and disabling medical conditions (e.g., arthritis, cancer, chronic pulmonary disease). Such increased interest represents a conceptual shift from simply prolonging life to improving the quality of life. A number of factors have contributed to such development: Chronic illnesses have replaced life-threatening conditions of the recent past; with that change in emphasis, the cost of care has become an important concern. Concepts borrowed from the field of economics, such as "cost utility," are increasingly being used in health care evaluations; such concepts involve choices between different health states based on quality of life. Cost-utility studies have also been used in determining the allocation of health care resources at a time when such resources are becoming constrained. In addition, the recent rise in consumerism has forced a redistribution of health care decision-making authority. Families and patients' groups have pressed for more participation in decisions about health care, with clear expectations of better therapies. With the recent scientific and technological advances in medical research, new therapies—frequently expensive—are continuously introduced at a fast rate.

Health-related quality-of-life assessments have become a widely used tool to compare various new therapies. The pharmaceutical industry was quick to seize on the opportunity, motivated by genuine desire to develop better medications as well as eyeing quality of life as an important marketing tool. After all, what matters for the individual patient with a chronic illness is how such an individual feels and functions on long-term drug therapy.

Neuroleptics and Schizophrenia

The introduction in the 1950s of the first neuroleptic, chlorpromazine, and the subsequent development of a long list of other neuroleptics opened an era of therapeutic optimism in the effective management of schizophrenia. Although none of the available neuroleptics offers a cure, these drugs have proven effective in reducing acute psychotic symptoms and preventing relapse in many schizophrenic patients. However, it soon became clear that not all patients benefited equally from medications and that some did not benefit at all (Awad 1989; Rapport et al. 1978). In addition, all neuroleptics can produce a wide array of side effects that may prove disabling to many patients and may offset any improvement, resulting in noncompliance with medications and a less favorable outcome. It is not surprising, then, that schizophrenic patients' functional performance and quality of life can be markedly influenced by factors related to the effects of treatment as well as the severity of emergent side effects.

The Concept of Quality of Life of Schizophrenic Patients on Neuroleptics

Given the extensive use of neuroleptics over the past 40 years, it is surprising that little attention has been devoted to systematic evaluations of the quality of life of schizophrenic patients on neuroleptics.

Only rarely have clinical trials of new neuroleptics included functional performance or issues related to quality of life as an outcome of drug therapy (Awad 1992, 1993a). More frequently, when data are reported about aspects of the functional status of schizophrenic patients on neuroleptics, the impression is that such data are being included as an afterthought. In contrast, there exists an extensive body of literature addressing quality-of-life issues for patients on medications for other chronic medical illnesses (e.g., arthritis, cancer, hypertension). It is paradoxical that the instruments used for assessment of psychosocial performance in these conditions have been borrowed from the behavioral sciences, yet psychiatrists have come relatively late to recognize the importance of using such instruments to evaluate neuroleptic therapy. Although, in clinical practice, psychiatrists may be interested in some global but poorly conceptualized measure of functional performance, rarely do they include systematic and detailed evaluations of functional state. As in clinical trials, physicians are likely to pay more attention to symptomatic change, whether it is improvement or deterioration. As discussed below, a number of factors may have contributed to this relative lack of interest in assessment of quality of life of schizophrenic patients on neuroleptics.

Varying definitions of quality of life. The concept of quality of life is viewed by many as mostly undefinable and, consequently, unmeasurable. However, despite the lack of agreement on a definition of this variable, several investigators have developed operational criteria that can be used in assessments of quality of life. *Quality of life* represents the impact of an illness and its therapy on the functional status of a patient, as perceived by the patient himself or herself (Schipper et al. 1990). It is more than symptomatic improvement or deterioration, and includes assessments of a number of major domains—specifically, illness-related and treatment-related impairments as well as psychosocial performance.

Critical attributes of quality-of-life measures. Any credible quality of life measure has to meet tests for reliability, validity, and sensitivity. The measure has to be reproducible, and it has to satisfy face and construct validity. Unfortunately, criterion validity, which involves testing a measure against some other empirical standard, is very difficult, particularly in assessing psychosocial functioning. The instrument has to be sensitive enough to pick up relatively small changes, such as those that may be expected in drug trials. It is recognized that even the smallest shifts in functional status, although relatively insignificant in the larger picture, may have profound effects on the quality of life of individual patients.

The scarcity of reliable and validated scales that are sensitive enough to pick up small changes has somewhat delayed the interest of both researchers and practicing clinicians in systematic evaluations of quality of life. The few scales available for use in psychiatric populations have been constructed primarily for rehabilitation purposes to measure the impact of psychosocial interventions in chronic schizophrenic patients. Developing a new scale is frequently a demanding process that requires several years as well as extensive efforts. It is surprising that many of the reliable and validated scales that have been extensively used as generic measures of quality of life in other medical conditions frequently include subcategories relevant to assessments of quality of life on neuroleptic therapy. An example of such a useful scale is the Sickness Impact Profile (Bergner et al. 1981), which is a behaviorally based measure of health-related dysfunction. It consists of 12 categories: 1) rest, 2) eating, 3) work, 4) home management, 5) recreation and pastimes, 6) ambulation, 7) mobility, 8) body care and movement, 9) social interaction, 10) alertness behavior, 11) emotional behavior, and 12) communication.

Two years ago, we were searching for a reliable measure of quality of life in the context of a multicenter clinical trial for a new neuroleptic. Since we could not wait for the conclusion of a scale that we had under development, we looked for an available scale or parts of one that could provide us with the information we required. Because the Sickness Impact Profile had been extensively validated in its totality as well as in every one of its 12 categories and could be used on its own, we decided to use preselected categories from this scale in our clinical trial. A summary of the categories chosen as well as a selected sample of the items are presented in Table 31–1.

So far, our experience has shown that such preselected categories are useful in assessing the effects of neuroleptics on aspects of the functional status of schizophrenic patients. As a self-administered scale, it presents no difficulty to patients; most can respond to its 55 items in less than 10 minutes.

Reliability of information from schizophrenic patients about their feelings. Satisfaction and well-being are subjective experiences. Because schizophrenic patients frequently experience disturbed thinking and communication, their reports about their feelings, values, or attitudes toward medications are frequently dismissed as unreliable. Davidhizar (1985) suggested that measurement of feelings and attitudes of schizophrenic patients toward treatment is not only possible but also important. We (Hogan et al. 1983) previously reported on the development of a scale for measuring subjective responses to neuroleptics. In the course of developing such a scale and the necessary test-retest process required over a lengthy period, we were impressed with the consistency of schizophrenic patients in reporting their feelings and attitudes toward their medications.

Table 31–1. Selected categories from the modified Sickness Impact Profile[a]

Category	Sample of selected items
Sleep and rest	• I sit for much of the day. • I sleep or doze most of the time—day or night.
Home management	• I am doing less of the daily household chores that I would usually do. • I am not doing any of the shopping that I would usually do. • I am not doing any of the clothes washing that I would usually do.
Social interaction	• I isolate myself as much as I can from the rest of my family. • I take part in fewer social activities than I used to. • I avoid having visitors.
Recreation and pastimes	• I spend shorter periods of time on my hobbies and recreation. • I am cutting down on some of my usual physical recreation or more active pastimes.
Communication	• I am having trouble writing or typing. • I do not speak clearly when I am under stress.

Note. Patients are also asked to assess globally their own perception of their quality of life.
[a]Bergner et al. 1981.

Lack of integrative conceptual model for quality of life on neuroleptics. A number of the disease-related as well as the treatment-related problems in schizophrenia may be looked on as not different from those of other chronic illnesses with acute exacerbations (e.g., rheumatoid arthritis). A serious problem in assessing schizophrenic patients' quality of life is to define the critical factors that comprise the quality-of-life profile. Any conceptual model of quality of life on neuroleptics has to integrate the factors that may affect the functional status of the individual. Unfortunately, the number of such possible factors is extensive, and their relative contribution to the concept itself is frequently unknown. It is important, then, that only significant factors that make clinical sense or are supported by research evidence be incorporated in conceptual models. Such a model is discussed in the following section.

A Conceptual Model for Measuring Quality of Life

The major determinants of quality of life on neuroleptics are

- Schizophrenic symptoms and their severity
- Side effect profiles
- Psychosocial performance

Other clinically significant factors that may interact with the three major determinants and that are likely to modify outcome of neuroleptic therapy include

- Premorbid characteristics
- Psychosocial adjustment
- Patient's own subjective interpretation of his or her medicated state

In Figure 31–1, all of these factors are integrated in a circular model that underscores the multidimensional aspects of these aspects as well as their interrelatedness. Since these factors are affected to a greater or lesser degree by various interventions, the balance will shift with any change in the patient's regimen. These factors are not merely baseline conceptual factors for judging the quality of life; they are also factors influencing therapeutic outcome.

Symptoms. Schizophrenia is a chronic illness marked with acute psychotic exacerbations. In acute episodes, the picture is dominated by positive symptoms (e.g., delusions, hallucinations, disordered thinking, conceptual disorganization). In the chronic course of the illness, some of these positive symptoms may continue along with a number of negative symptoms (e.g., blunted affect, emotional and social withdrawal, poverty of thought and speech). Focusing on the distinction between positive symptoms and negative symptoms has led to the proposal of two distinct syndromes (Crow 1982). One syndrome is dominated by positive symptoms, responds favorably to neuroleptics, and has a better prognosis than the other syndrome. The other syndrome has negative symptoms as its predominant feature, responds less favorably to neuroleptics, and generally carries a poor prognosis. Such a dichotomy, although proven heuristically valuable in focusing attention on the heterogeneity of schizophrenia, has proven to be at variance with clinical experience.

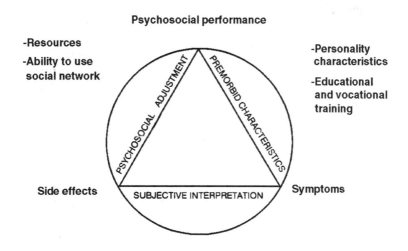

Figure 31–1. Quality-of-life circle on neuroleptics.

Whether schizophrenia is a two-, three-, or even more dimensional illness continues to be an unresolved, but important, issue that needs to be pursued for a number of reasons. Although there is an agreement that certain positive symptoms are sensitive to the effects of neuroleptics, there is no consensus on the degree to which negative symptoms respond to neuroleptic therapy. The debate is confounded by lack of agreement on what constitutes negative symptoms, particularly in light of the fact that neuroleptics themselves can be accompanied by side effects not dissimilar to some negative symptoms (e.g., flattened affect). This debate is relevant to the development of new neuroleptics because the emphasis in such development has shifted to the effectiveness of these medications not only in treating positive symptoms but also in improving negative symptoms. Patients' differential and selective responses to neuroleptics and the ability of the new neuroleptics to treat many symptoms of schizophrenia are central to the level of functional performance of schizophrenic patients on medications.

Side effects.   All available neuroleptics possess a well-known wide range of side effects. The occurrence and severity of such side effects vary markedly among individuals. Neuroleptic side effects not only can affect patients' functional performance but also can prove markedly disabling to many patients and lead to noncompliance with medications and eventually to a less favorable treatment outcome.

Psychosocial performance.   The recent change of emphasis from hospital-based to community-based programs in the management of schizophrenia has focused attention on social and community adjustment of schizophrenic patients. A number of factors have been demonstrated to influence psychosocial adjustment. Good premorbid adjustment is likely to be accompanied by better stability in interpersonal relationships, which in turn contributes to a more favorable outcome. Similarly, educational and vocational characteristics can lead to a better potential for employment. The availability of resources for rehabilitation, housing, and economic support are important components for achieving a reasonable level of functioning for schizophrenic patients in the community. However, symptomatic improvement on neuroleptics, though important for achieving better psychosocial adjustment, by itself may not necessarily allow the patient to become self-sufficient, hold a job, or become socially active. Indeed, other interventions in addition to neuroleptics may influence these functions more effectively than medication alone.

Patients' subjective responses to neuroleptics.   Clinicians have frequently observed that some schizophrenic patients experience a changed subjective state while on neuroleptics. These subjective responses have been invariably labeled as *neuroleptic dysphoria, neuroleptic behavioral toxicity, negative subjective response,* and so on. The construct of subjective response to neuroleptics and its impact on outcome has been neglected in outcome studies as well as in clinical practice. Several investigators have reported a correlation between altered subjective state on neuroleptics and therapeutic outcome (Awad and Hogan 1985; Van Putten et al. 1981), medication compliance (Hogan et al. 1983; Weiden et al. 1991), and aspects of quality of life (Awad and Hogan 1994). Although the nature of these subjective responses to neuroleptics is not clearly understood, such responses are important in any consideration of quality of life (Awad 1993b). The contribution of specific side effects to the genesis of the negative subjective responses to neuroleptics is not clear, although a few reports have implicated the possible contribution of neuroleptic-induced akathisia (Van Putten et al. 1981). In addition to the medications' effects, it is plausible that patients' attitudes and values, their conceptions of health and illness, and their previous experiences on medications contribute to their altered subjective responses to neuroleptics (Awad 1993b).

Whatever the factors that contribute to the genesis of such important and overlooked phenomena, the simple premise is that patients who do not subjectively "feel right" on medications are more likely to discontinue them at the first opportunity. This potential consequence makes it vitally important in clinical practice to recognize and measure the severity of such altered subjective states. Researchers in several successful attempts have managed to develop simplified scales and to apply them to studies of outcome and medication compliance (Hogan and Awad 1992; Hogan et al. 1983; P. J. Weiden, personal communication, September 1992).

Therapeutic and Research Implications of Quality-of-Life Issues

Symptom Improvement Versus Improvement in Functional Status

Recognition of the importance of quality of life of schizophrenic patients on medications will shift the emphasis from symptom improvement to improvement in the functional status of the individual patient. It will serve as an ongoing reminder to clinicians that neuroleptic therapy is an important—but only one—component in the management of schizophrenia. It may also encourage the pharmaceutical industry to pay more attention in their new drug development programs to the impact of neuroleptics on the quality of life of schizophrenic patients. In addition, it may persuade drug regulatory agencies to make quality-of-life assessments a requirement for approval of new neuroleptics for long-term use. As health costs are becoming a major concern, data obtained from quality-of-life evaluations can be used for allocation of resources as well as for comparison of therapies.

Research Implications

As psychiatry is advancing into the field of quality of life relatively late in comparison with other medical disciplines, it is imperative that research interests in this area expand. For that to happen, a number of important conceptual and methodological research issues have to be considered:

1. Future scales for the assessment of quality of life need to be made more specific to a psychiatric population. The scales need to be not only valid and reliable but also sensitive enough to pick up small changes such as are anticipated in a psychiatric population.
2. Quality of life is a multidimensional construct. Accordingly, it has to tap a number of domains, including illness-related and treatment-related issues as well as psychosocial functioning.
3. Better operational criteria are required to define aspects of psychosocial functioning. One example is Thoits' (1982) attempt to define criteria for evaluating social networks. These criteria assess the patient's network in

terms of the quantity of connections (i.e., the number of people in the network) and the quality of those connections (i.e., the degree of trust that the patient invests in such connections). *Utilization* reflects the relative amount of time a patient is prepared to spend with others; *meaning* reflects the importance that the patient attaches to social relationships. *Availability* is an indication of having people when needed.

4. The essential domains that largely contribute to the quality-of-life paradigm need to be identified and some flexibility allowed in choosing quality-of-life parameters. Although certain parameters will be applicable to all populations studied, there must also be specific parameters that suit specific populations in terms of what is realistic and possible to achieve. It is equally important to recognize that quality of life varies over time. For that reason, quality-of-life measurements have to be instituted at regular intervals.

5. Assessment of the quality of life of schizophrenic patients on neuroleptics has to include the patients' own perceptions about their quality of life and their subjective feelings about the medicated state. The unease among researchers about including data on schizophrenic patients' subjective interpretations of their inner feelings has to be tempered with the recognition of the subjective nature of any quality-of-life paradigm. It is paradoxical that clinicians and researchers include patients' self-reports about such personal experiences as delusions or hallucinations as part of their diagnostic formulation, yet are reluctant to accept patients' reports about their inner feelings, their treatment, or their satisfaction with their quality of life.

6. The ideal scale should not only provide separate measures of various dimensions of profiles of quality of life, but also strive to include an index that can be useful for comparisons between treatment groups. Having an index will force the issue of weighing different dimensions of health and their relative significance to the concept of quality of life. In addition, having an index may make it easier to compare data from various studies as well as for use in meta-analyses.

Conclusion

The importance of health-related quality-of-life assessments in schizophrenic patients on neuroleptics and in psychiatric populations in general needs to be recognized. These assessments involve conceptual restructuring of clinical thinking from symptom improvement to improvement in the functional status of the patient. They require a good deal of education among medical students, physicians, and other mental health practitioners about the importance and practical uses of quality-of-life assessments. Such assessments can improve clinical decision making and can assist in making benefit-versus-risk judgments on any therapeutic approach. In addition, they can prove helpful in policy decisions related to resource allocation. Clinical trials of new neuroleptics ought to include measures of quality of life as one outcome, in addition to the traditional symptoms and side effects evaluations. For all of this to be accomplished, there is an identified need for focusing research interests on the development of valid and reliable measures of quality of life suited to the needs of various psychiatric populations.

References

Awad AG: Drug therapy in schizophrenia: variability of outcome and prediction of response. Can J Psychiatry 34:711–720, 1989

Awad AG: Quality of life of schizophrenic patients on medications and implications for new drug trials. Hosp Community Psychiatry 43:262–265, 1992

Awad AG: Methodological and design issues in clinical trials of new neuroleptics: an overview. Br J Psychiatry 163 (suppl 22):51–57, 1993a

Awad AG: Subjective response to neuroleptics in schizophrenia. Schizophr Bull 19:609–618, 1993b

Awad AG, Hogan TP: Early treatment events and prediction of response to neuroleptics in schizophrenia. Prog Neuropsychopharmacol Biol Psychiatry 9:585–588, 1985

Awad AG, Hogan TP: Subjective response to neuroleptics and the quality of life: implications for treatment outcome. Acta Psychiatr Scand 89 (suppl 380):27–32, 1994

Bergner M, Bobbit R, Carter W, et al: The sickness impact profile: development and final revision of health status measure. Med Care 19:787–805, 1981

Crow TJ: Two dimensions of pathology in schizophrenia: dopaminergic and non-dopaminergic. Psychopharmacol Bull 18:22–29, 1982

Davidhizar RE: Can clients with schizophrenia describe feelings and beliefs about taking medication? J Adv Nurs 10:469–473, 1985

Hogan TP, Awad AG: Subjective response to neuroleptics and outcome in schizophrenia: a re-examination comparing two measures. Psychol Med 22:347–352, 1992

Hogan TP, Awad AG, Eastwood MR: A self-report scale predictive of drug compliance in schizophrenic patients: reliability and discriminative ability. Psychol Med 13:177–183, 1983

Rapport M, Hopkins KH, Hall K, et al: Are there schizophrenics for whom drugs may be unnecessary or contraindicated? International Pharmacopsychiatry 13:100–111, 1978

Schipper H, Clinch J, Powell V: Definitions and conceptual issues, in Quality of Life Assessments in Clinical Trials. Edited by Spikler B. New York, Raven, 1990, pp 11–24

Thoits P: Conceptual, methodological and theoretical problems in studying social support as a buffer against life stress. J Health Soc Behav 22:324–336, 1982

Van Putten T, May PRA, Marder SR, et al: Subjective response to antipsychotic drugs. Arch Gen Psychiatry 38:187–190, 1981

Weiden PJ, Dixon L, Frances A, et al: Neuroleptic non-compliance in schizophrenia, in Advances in Neuropsychiatry and Psychopharmacology, Vol 1. Edited by Tamminga C, Schulz C. New York, Raven, 1991, pp 285–296

CHAPTER 32

Psychosocial Treatment of Substance Abuse in Schizophrenic Patients

Lisa Dixon, M.D., and
Thomas A. Rebori, M.D.

C omorbid substance use disorders have emerged as one of the greatest obstacles to the effective treatment of individuals with schizophrenia. The current treatment system often fails patients with these two disorders because of the fragmented and sometimes conflicting approaches of the mental health and substance abuse care systems. Deinstitutionalization, with the subsequent exposure of schizophrenic individuals to drugs within the community and the wider availability of drugs like crack-cocaine, may partially account for the urgency to develop effective treatments for schizophrenic patients who have a comorbid drug or alcohol addiction.

As the extent of the problem has become more severe, clinicians and researchers have begun to develop and test new and integrated clinical interventions to help these dually diagnosed individuals. Although most of the controlled studies are not yet complete, promising treatment programs have some clearly articulated principles. In this chapter, we present background information about the problem and then review psychosocial and psychopharmacological treatments.

Epidemiology

The percentage of schizophrenic patients suffering from a comorbid drug or alcohol use disorder varies tremendously in published studies, ranging from as low as 10% to as high as 70% (Mueser et al. 1990). This wide range is partially attributable to variability in how patients are diagnosed with schizophrenia, to patient characteristics, to the types of populations studied (e.g., inpatient versus outpatient, clinical versus nonclinical), and to the different ways drug and alcohol use disorders are defined (e.g., DSM-III-R diagnosis; evidence of use from urine toxicology screens; other rating scales that assess a variety of issues, including severity of effects of drug and alcohol use and quantitative use) (Mueser et al. 1990). In the Epidemiologic Catchment Area Study patient sample from both community and institutional settings, 47% of all individuals with a lifetime diagnosis of schizophrenia or schizophreniform disorder also met criteria for some form of substance abuse or dependence (33.7% for an alcohol use disorder and 27.5% for another drug use disorder) (Regier et al. 1990). The odds of having a substance abuse diagnosis were found to be 4.6 times higher for schizophrenic individuals than for the rest of the population; their risk for alcohol disorders, over 3 times as high; and their risk for other drug disorders, 6 times as high. Thus, although the comorbidity rate may vary somewhat across different patient samples studied, substance use disorders do seem to occur significantly more frequently in individuals diagnosed with schizophrenia than in the general population and therefore merit special consideration in planning treatment programs.

Characteristics of Substance-Abusing Schizophrenic Patients

The diversity of studies of substance abuse among schizophrenic patients has led to some inconsistencies in characterizing these individuals. Many investigators agree, however, that schizophrenic patients who are young and male are more likely to abuse drugs or alcohol than those who are older and female. Other investigators (Breakey et al. 1974; Tsuang et al. 1982; Weller et al. 1984, 1988) have found that schizophrenic patients with an earlier age at onset of illness and better premorbid characteristics are more likely to have drug or alcohol abuse problems.

Attempts to understand the impact of drug and alcohol abuse on the course of schizophrenia have produced variable results. The overwhelming weight of the evidence points in the direction of substance abuse having adverse short- and long-term effects. Schizophrenic patients who abuse drugs or alcohol have been found to have more psychotic symptoms (Negrete et al. 1986), more psychiatric hospitalizations (Safer 1987), increased utilization of acute services (Goldfinger et al. 1984), increased housing instability and homelessness (Drake et al. 1989), and increased violent and criminal behavior (Abram and Teplin 1991; Safer 1987), including suicide (Caton 1981; Dassori et al. 1990; Drake et al. 1989). These individuals may also cost society more treatment dollars in providing services (Kivlahan et al. 1991). Although these characteristics and possible sequelae have not been found consistently, the existing data paint a picture of the young, chronically ill, often male schizophrenic patient whose course of illness might be significantly improved were his substance abuse problem adequately treated.

Evaluation

Accurate diagnostic evaluation of individuals at risk for comorbid schizophrenic and substance abuse disorders is difficult but essential. A major source of difficulty arises from the fact that the effects of substances may be indistinguishable from the symptoms of schizophrenia. Also, past clinical records often fail to mention a diagnosis of substance abuse or dependence (Ananth et al. 1989). In addition, similar to nonschizophrenic substance abusers, schizophrenic patients often underreport or fail to see the negative consequences of their substance use (Test et al. 1989). Finally, standard assessment tools have not been validated with schizophrenic patients (Drake et al. 1990). Urine and blood toxicology screens can be unreliable, refer only to recent use, and give little information about patterns of use and drug effects.

Most investigators recommend the use of multiple sources of information to diagnose substance use disorders in schizophrenic patients. Such sources include self-reports, collateral reports from significant others, urine and blood screens, and, if possible, longitudinal data from treatment providers who have a long-standing therapeutic relationship with the patient (Mueser et al. 1990). For example, a case manager can assess the interaction between a patient's substance use and his or her functioning in the community (Drake et al. 1990) as well as the patient's subjective view of the positive and negative effects of the substances (Test et al. 1989). Given the tendency of mental health clinicians to overlook the role of substance use, training and supervision are needed to encourage more active investigation of the contribution of substance use to the individual patient's presentation.

Treatment

Integrated Treatment

The most important principle guiding treatment of schizophrenic individuals with comorbid substance use disorders is that both disorders must be treated in an integrated setting in which each diagnosis is treated as primary. Sequential treatment of mental illness and substance abuse may result in a "ping-pong" therapy, in which patients receive conflicting messages about their different diagnoses. This increases the likelihood of poor compliance with both treatment plans. Parallel but separate treatment produces similar results (Osher and Kofoed 1989). Schizophrenic patients may have difficulty attending concurrent programs in separate centers. Also, the cognitive disturbances associated with schizophrenia may make it difficult for patients to integrate the different philosophies of the two treatment systems (Rosenthal et al. 1992).

Patients with a dual diagnosis of schizophrenia and a substance use disorder do not do well in traditional substance abuse treatment centers where confrontational techniques are used, often in group settings with high levels of expressed emotion. This approach may exacerbate symptoms of schizophrenia. Furthermore, most substance abuse treatment centers lack the clinical resources to deal with markedly abnormal behavior, and thus tend to screen out patients with a history of severe mental illness.

On the other hand, patients with a coexisting substance use disorder may not do well in the relatively more permissive traditional psychiatric treatment settings, where substance abuse may not be addressed or even detected (Rosenthal et al. 1992). Thus, "single disability" programs—designed, administered, and financed for one disorder—are not appropriate treatment settings for these dually diagnosed patients. When the dually diagnosed patient attempts to receive treatment at a single-disability setting, the result is often exclusion, dropout, or premature discharge (Ridgely et al. 1990).

Although results of several research trials are still forthcoming, programs with a concurrent dual focus on schizophrenia and substance abuse are reporting improved outcomes. Domains of enhanced outcome include reduced use of services (e.g., decreased days of inpatient hospitalization), decreased need for psychotropic medication, decreased legal involvement, and improvements in housing, physical health, and employment status (Hellerstein and Meehan 1987; Jansen et al. 1992; Kofoed et al. 1986).

Phases of Treatment

Both substance use disorders and other serious mental illnesses are characterized by a high degree of relapse and exacerbation (Minkoff 1989). Patients entering integrated treatment programs are in different stages of their illnesses. Osher and Kofoed (1989) described four phases of treatment based on patients' commitment to substance abuse treatment and the state of their psychiatric disorder. These phases are not necessarily discrete and often overlap, but they help to conceptualize the important steps that these patients need to take to stabilize their illnesses.

First phase: engagement. Engagement is described as the process of convincing patients that the integrated treatment program has something to offer them. Poor treatment retention is characteristic of schizophrenic patients who abuse substances, even in programs specifically designed for them (Lehman et al. 1993). Assistance with food, housing, or clothing, or relief from distressing psychiatric symptoms may be hooks to engage these patients. They often need help with legal difficulties or with negotiating the various state and federal entitlement programs for which they qualify. Homeless or isolated dually diagnosed patients may need assertive outreach services offering help with these problems. Intervention with family or the court system can also include "coercive engagement," by which dually diagnosed patients are required to enter integrated treatment for a variety of reasons. A striking aspect of strategies employed in this phase is that few of them directly highlight the substance abuse problem in itself; instead, they concentrate on other life problems that may be associated with the schizophrenic or substance abuse disorders. This focus has been reported to be helpful in retaining dually diagnosed patients (Osher and Kofoed 1989).

Second phase: persuasion.   The next phase is to persuade patients to accept the concept of treatment aimed at long-term abstinence. Often, schizophrenic patients state that they use substances for the same reasons as other patients with substance use disorders—to escape social pressures or unhappy life circumstances. They may also feel that their substance use is a result of their psychiatric illness and thus does not need specific treatment (Osher and Kofoed 1989). Furthermore, some patients report that some symptoms of their schizophrenia are relieved, at least acutely, by the use of illicit substances (Dixon et al. 1990). Impediments to successfully persuading substance-abusing schizophrenic patients to "buy into" abstinence include defective information processing and the lack of social pressures ordinarily experienced by the nonschizophrenic substance abuser.

The commitment to long-term abstinence for schizophrenic patients must be distinguished from an initial requirement of total abstinence found in many conventional substance abuse treatment programs. A goal of reduced substance use, along with long-term treatment, education, and support, may be better suited to this substance-abusing population. The insistence on total and immediate abstinence that is characteristic of traditional outpatient substance abuse treatment centers—with the exception of methadone clinics—may be unrealistic and may, for many schizophrenic patients who abuse substances, prevent engagement with and participation in treatment (Alfs and McClellan 1992; Hellerstein and Meehan 1987; Polcin 1992; Rosenthal et al. 1992). However, given that schizophrenic patients can experience adverse effects from even small amounts of drug or alcohol use, long-term abstinence should still be an unambiguous treatment goal.

The persuasion process may be achieved by using a variety of individual, group, and family therapies that consistently educate regarding the two diagnoses, their effects on functioning and symptoms, and how they interact. Breathalyzers, toxicology screens, abnormal physical and psychiatric findings, and the legal and social difficulties that can be linked to substance use can all be presented to patients to help reduce their denial that substance abuse is a problem. This process can be particularly effective on an inpatient psychiatric ward, where patients' psychiatric symptoms can be stabilized and their abstinence from substances of abuse facilitated. Furthermore, on an inpatient ward, these individuals are more readily accepting of the patient role and have supportive peers and staff to help them recognize the significance of their substance use. It is imperative that patients who accept the need for treatment of their substance use disorder receive specific assurances of continued support and treatment despite early and repeated relapses (Osher and Kofoed 1989).

Third phase: active treatment. In this phase, emphasis is placed on helping patients acquire the attitudes and skills needed to maintain sobriety. Behavioral, psychosocial, and medical interventions are appropriate for this phase and may be continuations of interventions begun in the engagement and persuasion phases. Having made a commitment to abstinence, patients need ongoing education and support. They may be amenable during this phase to accepting help in restructuring their time and meeting their social needs, which suggests the importance of occupational and recreational approaches. Previously, activities surrounding the use of substances may have filled their time and provided social support.

Fourth phase: relapse prevention. An ongoing relationship between the patient and health care providers is essential in this phase. Providers should acknowledge the patient's successes and monitor for signs of relapse. Both the patient and the treatment team should anticipate some degree of relapse, and this should be discussed before it occurs. Rapid discovery and treatment can help prevent more enduring and serious relapses in the future (Osher and Kofoed 1989).

Patients will not necessarily move unidirectionally from one phase to the next. The complexity of the interaction between schizophrenia and substance use may result in patients making progress but then suffering setbacks. Treatment providers must be prepared to help patients through the various phases many times.

Components of Integrated Treatment

What are the components and structure of an integrated program that can help the substance-abusing schizophrenic patient progress successfully through the phases of treatment? It should be clear from the breadth of services necessary for these patients that the programs likely to be the most effective will offer a wide array of services. As the efficacy of the most comprehensive programs is studied in the near future, it will be important for researchers to assess which specific services or service components are most critical. Given the high cost of comprehensive services, the drive to reduce the cost of care will necessitate an examination and identification of the minimal components that retain treatment effectiveness. Some of the more important components are outlined below.

Appropriate program milieu and philosophy. Substance-abusing schizophrenic patients generally require a supportive environment that is high in structure but low in intensity. To accommodate this population, members of which are difficult to engage and often unpredictable and noncompliant, a philosophy guided by a willingness to perform outreach and a reluctance to discharge is necessary.

Case management with continuous care/crisis intervention. Case managers play a critical role in integrated treatment programs. The preferred case management model involves the "clinical case manager," who provides direct service to patients as well as an appropriate referral when necessary, rather than the "broker case manager," who exclusively refers patients to outside services. As previously mentioned, it is often clinical case managers who provide the best longitudinal data about a patient's functioning, which can aid in the diagnosis of substance use (Drake et al. 1990). Case managers with relatively low case loads (i.e., with a staff-to-patient ratio of 1:10) can provide supportive counseling, assist patients in meeting essential material needs (e.g., for food, clothing, housing), assist patients in obtaining benefits and medical care, and educate patients and their families about potential outcomes and the interaction of substance abuse, psychiatric illness, and psychotropic medication. Attention to social needs may be the critical hook for engaging and retaining patients in treatment. The case manager can provide the continuity so essential to these dually diagnosed patients as they negotiate the myriad of systems necessary for them to meet basic needs and obtain necessary services (Mason and Siris 1992).

Group therapy. Group therapy is a universal mode of treatment in most integrated outpatient treatment programs. Several authors (Alfs and McClellan 1992; Rosenthal et al. 1992; Sciacca 1987a, 1987b) have recommended that groups proceed in a supportive manner when dealing with dually diagnosed schizophrenic patients, as a confrontational exploration of substance use can lead to relapse. Group therapy serves many purposes, including persuasion of dual-diagnosis patients to seek substance use treatment (Kofoed and Keys 1988). The group process can also be used to educate patients about the effects of substance use on their physical and mental health and to provide peer support for the goal of abstinence and use of self-help groups (Hellerstein and Meehan 1987; Jansen et al. 1992; Kofoed and Keys 1988; Rosenthal et al. 1992; Sciacca 1987a).

Toxicologic screening. Random urine toxicology screens and Breathalyzer tests to detect drug use and relapse are necessary procedures. Such measures should be viewed by the staff—and thus communicated to the patients—as devices that are part of the therapy and not for punitive surveillance. They allow the treatment team to assess patterns of substance use and its effects and to prevent a prolonged relapse after abstinence is achieved.

Family involvement. Family education is an important adjunct to the direct treatment of the substance-abusing schizophrenic patient. Families who are already accustomed to coping with schizophrenic family members need education on the separate disease entity of substance abuse, as well as the interaction between the substance abuse and schizophrenia. Persons with mental illness and substance abuse disorders report less satisfaction with family relationships and more need for treatment than do those with severe mental illness only (Dixon et al., in press). Families need help in recognizing substance abuse and in learning how to set limits on the behavior of family members that can be disruptive and dangerous in the household (Hatfield 1991). Families can be referred to self-help groups and advocacy organizations such as Al-Anon and the National Alliance for the Mentally Ill (Osher and Kofoed 1989). Support groups directed specifically toward families with dually diagnosed members have been developed based on the Al-Anon model (Sciacca 1991).

Self-help groups. Self-help groups, such as Alcoholics Anonymous (AA) and Narcotics Anonymous (NA), can be valuable adjuncts to the treatment of the substance-abusing schizophrenic patient. Such groups can provide social support and structure, and the 12-step model may be very helpful in facilitating the patient's acceptance of the need for long-term abstinence. However, not all schizophrenic patients benefit from these groups, and not all NA and AA groups are well suited for schizophrenic patients. Characteristics that may make some schizophrenic patients not suited for AA or NA are their paranoia in groups and their cognitive difficulty in understanding 12-step concepts. Conversely, members of some AA groups may not be educated regarding mental illness and may be averse to the use of medications. The development of dual-diagnosis NA and AA groups as well as staff attendance with the patient at initial AA and NA meetings are strategies that have enhanced the use of self-help groups in the dually diagnosed population (Osher and Kofoed 1989).

Access to detoxification and psychiatric inpatient services. The treatment of substance-abusing schizophrenic patients is characterized by repeated relapse and exacerbation of both their substance use disorder and their schizophrenia. As a result, an outpatient treatment program must have access to an inpatient psychiatric ward that can provide medical detoxification as well as treat severe symptoms of schizophrenia. Traditional community detoxification settings are usually not equipped or willing to treat these patients. There should be frequent communication between the inpatient and outpatient services used, and the treatment of both the substance use disorder and the schizophrenia should be integrated as in the outpatient setting. It should be communicated to patients that despite any relapse in either or both of their disorders, they can have continued access to treatment (Minkoff 1989; Osher and Kofoed 1989).

Vocational, occupational, and recreational therapies. Comprehensive treatment should offer services that help progressing patients develop appropriate structure in their lives in numerous spheres. Assessment and assistance in functioning can help prevent relapse and improve patients' subjective enjoyment of a drug-free existence (Rosenthal et al. 1992). Programs can offer drug-free social events to build group cohesion and promote drug-free leisure activities (Jansen et al. 1992).

Psychopharmacological treatment. Specific psychopharmacological strategies in the treatment of schizophrenic patients who abuse substances have not been well studied. In general, the clinician selecting a psychopharmacological regimen is faced with a double-edged sword: On the one hand, neuroleptics, the mainstay of treatments for schizophrenic patients, are also important in the treatment of the substance-abusing schizophrenic patient. This is especially so because schizophrenic patients may have a preference for abusing drugs that tend to exacerbate psychosis (Schneier and Siris 1987). Neuroleptics would then be a logical choice in preventing drug-induced exacerbations. However, on the other hand, it has been postulated that the side effects of neuroleptics (e.g., the slowed-down, zombielike feeling) may actually enhance the likelihood of drug use to overcome these unwanted effects (Knudsen and Vilmar 1984). Also, the side effects of neuroleptics (e.g., sedation) may be compounded by illicit drug effects. The clinician must therefore consider each patient individually, assessing whether the patient would benefit from aggressive neuroleptic treatment, and, if so, what neuroleptic, dosage range, and route of administration would be best.

Related to the use of neuroleptics is aggressive treatment of neuroleptic side effects with anticholinergic and dopaminergic agents. Aggressive treatment with anticholinergics might minimize the risk of patients self-medicating against neuroleptic side effects with nonprescribed drugs, but anticholinergic drugs are themselves often abused and have street value (Dilsaver 1988). Dopaminergic agents like bromocriptine may serve to reduce side effects, and have themselves been tested in individuals addicted to cocaine to reduce their craving for the drug (Dackis et al. 1987). However, these agents also present the risk of causing psychotic exacerbations of schizophrenia.

Other candidates for pharmacological treatment of schizophrenic patients include antidepressant agents and mood stabilizers. Antidepressants have been used with some success in the treatment of nonschizophrenic individuals addicted to cocaine (Levin and Lehman 1991). The danger with antidepressants is that they may exacerbate psychotic symptoms in unstable patients (Siris 1990). Lithium has also been suggested, but as with antidepressants, there are no clinical trials on its effects in this population, and its use must be evaluated on a case-by-case basis.

The use of benzodiazepines presents the same double-edged sword as neuroleptics and antidepressants. They may be useful for patients who use drugs to self-medicate their anxiety or akathisia, but are themselves agents of abuse. Patients treated with benzodiazepines must be closely monitored.

Other preventive treatments for substance abuse commonly used for nonschizophrenic individuals can be used in schizophrenic patients, but with care. For example, disulfiram can be effective as a deterrent to alcohol use, but has been associated with psychosis and should only be used in patients who are highly motivated and reliable. Methadone may also be useful for patients addicted to opiates and has been reported to have antipsychotic properties (Siris 1990).

The critical aspect of pharmacological treatment of substance-abusing schizophrenic patients is that the pharmacological treatment can only be done successfully in the context of an effective psychosocial program that promotes engagement of patients in treatment, compliance, and monitoring. In that setting, clinicians can prescribe the most appropriate psychopharmacological treatments.

Program Implementation

The way in which health care and service systems have been organized has inhibited the development of integrated programs for the substance-abusing schizophrenic patient. It is only relatively recently that such programs have been developed. In the United States, strategies and the necessary funding and administration for treating mental illness were developed separately from those for treating substance use disorders. This division in resources still exists at the local, state, and federal levels, and thus greatly inhibits the creation of integrated treatment services (Ridgely et al. 1990). The literature on the development of such programs emphasizes the need for creative financing, often combining support from two or more sources (Ridgely et al. 1990). Integrated programs have been created by combining separate service structures or by adding new services to an existing program (Sciacca 1987b).

Another critical issue in program development is staff training. Most professionals are not trained to be experts in treating both disorders. As such, staff education is important, with an emphasis on respecting the knowledge and experience of staff that come to the new system from both areas of expertise (Jansen et al. 1992). Training programs should focus on the unique and special needs this population presents (Ridgely et al. 1990).

Conclusion

Creating treatment programs for patients with both severe, chronic mental illnesses and substance use disorders requires breaking out of the traditional modes of treatment provision, financing, and administration that have excluded these patients from services in the past (Ridgely et al. 1990).

References

Abram KM, Teplin LA: Co-occurring disorders among mentally ill jail detainees. Am Psychol 46:1036–1045, 1991

Alfs D, McClellan T: A day hospital program for dual diagnosis patients in a VA medical center. Hosp Community Psychiatry 43:241–244, 1992

Ananth J, Vandawater S, Kamal M, et al: Missed diagnosis of substance abuse in psychiatric patients. Hosp Community Psychiatry 40:297–299, 1989

Breakey WR, Goodell H, Lorenz PC, et al: Hallucinogenic drugs as precipitants to schizophrenia. Psychol Med 4:255–261, 1974

Caton C: The new chronic patient and the system of community care. Hosp Community Psychiatry 32:475–478, 1981

Dackis CA, Gold MS, Sweeney DR, et al: Single-dose bromocriptine reverses cocaine craving. Psychiatry Res 20:261–264, 1987

Dassori AM, Mezzich JE, Keshavan M: Suicidal indicators in schizophrenia. Acta Psychiatr Scand 81:409–413, 1990

Dilsaver SC: Antimuscarinic agents as substances of abuse: a review. J Clin Psychopharmacol 8:14–22, 1988

Dixon L, Weiden PJ, Haas GH, et al: Acute effects of drug abuse in schizophrenic patients: clinical observations and patient's self-reports. Schizophr Bull 16:69–79, 1990

Dixon L, McNary S, Lehman AF: Substance abuse and family relationships of persons with severe mental illness. Am J Psychiatry (in press)

Drake RE, Osher FC, Wallach MA: Alcohol use and abuse in schizophrenia: a prospective community study. J Nerv Ment Dis 177:408–414, 1989

Drake R, Osher FC, Noordsy DL, et al: Diagnosis of alcohol use disorders in schizophrenia. Schizophr Bull 16:57–67, 1990

Goldfinger SM, Hopkin JT, Surber RW: Treatment resisters or system resisters? toward a better service system for acute care recidivists. New Dir Ment Health Serv 21:17–27, 1984

Hatfield AB: Dual Diagnosis: Substance Abuse and Mental Illness. Arlington, VA, National Alliance for the Mentally Ill, 1991

Hellerstein D, Meehan B: Outpatient group therapy for schizophrenic substance abusers. Am J Psychiatry 144:1337–1339, 1987

Jansen A, Masterton T, Norwood L, et al: Harbinger Team IV: assertive community treatment for people with the dual diagnosis of mental illness and substance abuse. Innovations and Research 1:11–17, 1992

Kivlahan DR, Heiman JR, Wright RC, et al: Treatment cost and rehospitalization rate in schizophrenic outpatients with a history of substance abuse. Hosp Community Psychiatry 42:609–614, 1991

Knudsen P, Vilmar T: Cannabis and neuroleptic agents in schizophrenia. Acta Psychiatr Scand 69:162–174, 1984

Kofoed L, Keys A: Using group therapy to persuade dual diagnosis patients to seek substance abuse treatment. Hosp Community Psychiatry 39:1209–1211, 1988

Kofoed L, Kania J, Walsh T, et al: Outpatient treatment of patients with substance abuse and coexisting psychiatric disorders. Am J Psychiatry 143:867–872, 1986

Lehman AF, Herron JD, Schwartz RP: Rehabilitation for adults with severe mental illnesses and substance use disorders: a clinical trial. J Nerv Ment Dis 181:88–92, 1993

Levin F, Lehman AL: Evaluation of desipramine for the treatment of cocaine addiction. J Clin Psychopharmacol 11:374–378, 1991

Mason S, Siris S: Dual diagnosis: the case for case management. The American Journal on Addictions 1:77–82, 1992

Minkoff K: An integrated treatment model for dual diagnosis of psychosis and addiction. Hosp Community Psychiatry 40:1031–1036, 1989

Mueser KT, Yarnold PR, Levinson DF, et al: Prevalence of substance abuse in schizophrenia: demographic and clinical correlates. Schizophr Bull 16:31–56, 1990

Negrete JC, Werner PK, Doublas DE, et al: Cannabis affects the severity of schizophrenic symptoms: results of a clinical survey. Psychol Med 16:515–520, 1986

Osher F, Kofoed L: Treatment of patients with psychiatric and substance abuse disorders. Hosp Community Psychiatry 40:1025–1030, 1989

Polcin D: Issues in the treatment of dual diagnosis clients who have chronic mental illness. Professional Psychology: Research and Practice 23:30–37, 1992

Regier DA, Farmer ME, Rae DS, et al: Comorbidity of mental disorders with alcohol and other drug abuse: results from the Epidemiologic Catchment Area Study. JAMA 264:2511–2518, 1990

Ridgely MS, Goldman HH, Willenbring M: Barriers to the care of persons with dual diagnoses: organizational and financing issues. Schizophr Bull 16:123–132, 1990

Rosenthal R, Hellerstein DJ, Miner CR: A model of integrated services for outpatient treatment of patients with comorbid schizophrenia and addictive disorders. The American Journal on Addictions 1:339–348, 1992

Safer D: Substance abuse by young adult chronic patients. Hosp Community Psychiatry 38:511–514, 1987

Schneier FR, Siris SG: A review of psychoactive substance use and abuse in schizophrenia: patterns of drug choice. J Nerv Ment Dis 175:641–652, 1987

Sciacca K: New initiatives in the treatment of the chronic patient with alcohol/substance use problems. TIE Lines 4:5–6, 1987a

Sciacca K: Alcohol/substance abuse at the New York State Psychiatric Centers develop and expand. Addictive Intervention With the Disabled (AID) Bulletin 9:1–3, 1987b

Sciacca K: An integrated treatment approach for severely mentally ill individuals with substance disorders. New Dir Ment Health Serv 50:69–83, 1991

Siris SG: Pharmacological treatment of substance-abusing schizophrenic patients. Schizophr Bull 16:111–122, 1990

Test MA, Wallisch LS, Allness DJ, et al: Substance use in young adults with schizophrenic disorders. Schizophr Bull 15:465–476, 1989

Tsuang MT, Simpson JC, Kronfol Z: Subtypes of drug abuse with psychosis. Arch Gen Psychiatry 39:141–147, 1982

Weller MP, Ang PC, Zachary A, et al: Substance abuse in schizophrenia (letter). Lancet 1:573, 1984

Weller MP, Ang PC, Latimer-Sayer DT, et al: Drug abuse and mental illness (letter). Lancet 1:997, 1988

CHAPTER 33

Integrating Pharmacological and Psychosocial Treatments in Schizophrenia

Evan J. Collins, M.D., F.R.C.P.C., and
Heather Munroe-Blum, M.S.W., Ph.D.

S ubstantial evidence exists to support the concept of schizophrenia as a complex, multidetermined illness, the successful treatment of which necessitates a skillful integration of therapeutic modalities over the long-term course. Schizophrenia cannot be fully understood or effectively treated from an exclusively biomedical perspective, although it is recognized as a disorder of genetically predisposed neurophysiologic dysfunction. Incomplete concordance between monozygotic twins from studies suggests that important, nongenetic factors influence the etiology, course, and outcome of schizophrenia. Many of these factors are nonbiological, social, and psychological. For example, social factors were the best predictors of combined clinical and social outcome in the large International Pilot Study of Schizophrenia (Prudo and Munroe-Blum 1987; Strauss and Carpenter 1977). In addition, evidence that 30%–

40% of patients relapse in the first year following hospitalization, even when medication compliance is ensured (Hogarty et al. 1979), indicates that psychological and social factors interact significantly with biological factors in schizophrenia.

If psychological and social factors are critical in the etiology, course, and outcome of schizophrenia, it stands to reason that optimal outcome will be achieved through incorporating these factors into the treatment and management of the disorder. Although there is substantial evidence that psychosocial therapies can be effective in improving outcome in schizophrenia, of concern is the widespread impression that many—and perhaps most—individuals with schizophrenia receive nonintegrated and predominantly biomedical therapies. Usually, treatment draws from a broad array of active antipsychotic pharmacotherapies (with varying degrees of efficacy and a range of side effects) and may, on an ad hoc basis, include nonspecific, supportive individual or family therapies. Although a number of different therapeutic strategies are available, these are often uncoordinated adjuncts to drug therapy with little thought to timing or integration. Furthermore, it has been suggested that the treatment of schizophrenia is often inadequately monitored and revised, ignoring the changing needs of patients as they go through different phases of illness and stages in the life cycle (Dawson et al. 1983; Harding et al. 1987). Consequently, the effects of treatment are uneven, not reaching optimal outcomes in most cases and actually being harmful in the worst-case scenario.

The reasons for this are many, but they rest largely with the ascendancy of the medical model in the face of the failure of psychoanalytic treatments for schizophrenia and the promising early response of schizophrenia to neuroleptic treatments. In addition, a wealthy pharmaceutical industry directs substantial resources into researching the efficacy of pharmacological interventions and promoting medications through advertisements and continuing education programs. There exists no advocate with similar resources to promote research and training in the psychosocial interventions. Finally, many individuals with schizophrenia are cared for by solo practitioners, who are generally untrained in integrated or psychosocial treatments and who operate in resource-strapped contexts without the benefit of psychosocial treatment programs or multidisciplinary teams. Consequently, the benefits of integrated treatment may be unknown to some clinicians, or integrated treatment may seem unrealistic or impractical. Nonetheless, we suggest that much of what is proposed in this chapter can be effected with judicious use of existing community resources and will be best achieved when physicians form a partnership with social workers or public health nurses who can initiate and ensure the stability, timeliness, and effectiveness of linkages with community resources.

In this chapter, we review recent innovations in the pharmacological and psychosocial therapies of schizophrenia and outline ways in which they can be integrated. We propose a framework that clinicians can use in understanding and planning integrated treatment. Finally, we critique current pharmacotherapeutic approaches and suggest ways in which pharmacotherapy can be improved through attention to the psychosocial context.

Framework for Integrated Treatments

World Health Organization Model of Illness

The World Health Organization's (WHO) model of illness is organized along three dimensions: impairment, disability, and handicap (WHO 1980). We have adapted this model for schizophrenia, as illustrated in Table 33–1. In our modified model, *impairment* is the loss of structure and function that results from underlying pathology. As such, impairment includes the core symptoms of the illness—currently typified in positive (productive) and negative (deficit) symptoms—and secondary psychopathological symptoms that might include depression, anxiety, or guilt. As well, we have chosen to recognize the adverse effects of antipsychotic medication as impairment because these are long-term concomitants for a majority of individuals with schizophrenia that become intertwined with the symptoms and phenomenology of the illness, and can be as disabling as core symptoms.

Disability is the restriction of the ability to perform activities that arises from the impairment associated with the disorder; it can include problems in activities of daily living, difficulties in social skills and related social dysfunction, and vocational dysfunction. Dysfunction can also include impaired family relations that may arise secondary to the impairment of the individual with schizophrenia.

Handicap is the disadvantage that follows from the impairment and disability of illness, and includes stigma, discrimination, socioeconomic disadvantage, problems with housing and vocational opportunities, and related disadvantages.

Theoretical Models of Schizophrenia

A range of theoretical models have been proposed to detail the predisposition, onset, treatment, and course of disorder as reflected in the WHO framework. The *biopsychosocial model* provides a conceptual framework relevant for the understanding and treatment of all illnesses, psychiatric and otherwise, even when nonbiological factors are not directly implicated in the etiology of the disorder. Engel (1977) used schizophrenia to illustrate biopsychosocial dynamics in his classic article on the biopsychosocial paradigm.

Consonant with the biopsychosocial model is the *diathesis-stress model,* or the *stress-vulnerability model* (depicted in Figure 33–1), which has been advocated by a number of investigators (Boker et al.

Table 33–1. World Health Organization model of illness (WHO 1980), adapted for schizophrenia

---

Impairment
  Positive symptoms
  Negative symptoms
  Secondary psychopathological symptoms
  Medication side effects
Disability
  Activities of daily living
  Social dysfunction
  Vocational dysfunction
  Family dysfunction
Handicap
  Poverty
  Stigma
  Homelessness
  Discrimination

1989; Liberman 1988; Nuechterlein and Dawson 1984; Zubin and Spring 1977; Zubin et al. 1992) and which describes how these elements interact in schizophrenia. These related paradigms propose a biological diathesis that predisposes an individual to schizophrenia, and a host of biological, psychological, and social factors that affect the individual to determine the expression, course, outcome, and response to treatment of the illness. Currently, the biological diathesis is seen as genetic (Bassett 1991), with the possible addition of alterations of neural development that may arise from obstetrical trauma, infection, or other causes (Murray and Lewis 1987). Once expressed, the vulnerability appears to manifest in deficits in information processing and abnormalities in autonomic arousal (Nuechterlein et al. 1989). In this way, the individual is vulnerable to environmental stressors that can

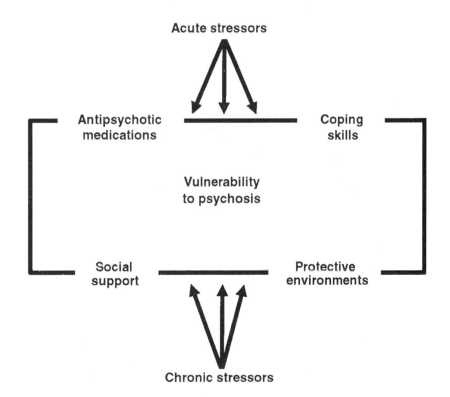

Figure 33–1. The stress-vulnerability model of schizophrenia.

precipitate or perpetuate psychosis. The stressors that affect a vulnerable individual can be acute or acute-on-chronic stressful life events that may be biological (e.g., street drug use, physical illness), psychological (e.g., loss of a significant other), social (e.g., losing one's home or job), or developmental (e.g., completing high school and entering a university). Alternatively, the stressors may be chronic: they may be ambient (i.e., in the family, work, or living environment) or emanate from the conditions of poverty and stigma. Norman and Malla's (1993) review of studies correlating stressful life events and the temporal development of symptoms seems to support this model.

Therapeutic Strategies That Address Key Elements in the Diathesis-Stress Model of Schizophrenia

Strategies for Lessening the Effects of Stressors

In schizophrenia, clinicians aim to lessen the stressors to which the individual is exposed through the utilization of protective environments and family and patient psychoeducation. Strategies for decreasing vulnerability to stress include the use of maintenance antipsychotic medication, the development of social and coping skills, and the enrichment of the patient's social support network. When these mechanisms are overwhelmed, acute antipsychotic pharmacotherapy is used to ameliorate psychotic symptoms. This strategy is analogous to that used with an infectious disease, for which one attempts to decrease exposure to infectious pathogens through sanitation and hygiene, while boosting immunity through nutrition, exercise, and immunization. When prevention fails and an infection takes hold, antibiotics are used to support the body's processes of fighting infection.

Antipsychotic medication appears to both reduce psychotic symptoms and lessen vulnerability through alterations in information processing and an individual's neuropsychological ability to handle stress (Nuechterlein et al. 1989). Maintenance use of medication seems to raise the threshold at which biological and psychosocial stressors exacerbate psychosis.

The protective environments of hospitals and community-based treatment settings (Ciompi et al. 1992; Mosher and Menn 1978) reduce stress by providing support and asylum for those whose routine supportive network has been overwhelmed or rendered unavailable. Other protective environments include sheltered living and working environments and recreational settings where stress is reduced through the modification of performance expectations of community members.

Social support can intervene to protect against social and environmental stressors by cushioning individuals in a manner similar to that described in depression and medical illness (Brown and Harris 1978). Goldstein (1978) demonstrated that individuals with chronic or relapsing courses of schizophrenic illness have weaker social networks than patients with less-severe schizophrenia. Social support can be provided by professionals as well as by family and friends; furthermore, case management and social skills training serve to enrich a person's social network and to increase social support.

Coping skills—the broad range of behaviors that allow individuals to avoid or manage stress, optimize available treatments and supports, and develop social skills that enrich their social network—should also be enhanced.

In addition to therapeutic interventions, it should be noted that an individual's own attempts to lessen stress through social isolation and the development of negative symptoms may in fact be adaptive. Strauss et al. (1989) described how negative symptoms may aid an individual's accommodation to the positive symptoms of psychosis and other aspects of the illness. In the same vein, Rabkin (1980) noted that a stressful circumstance for an individual with schizophrenia may be a normal event for those without the disorder. These factors underscore the importance of administering treatment within the context of a therapeutic alliance that facilitates an accurate assessment of the resources and coping strategies of the patient and his or her current and threatened vulnerabilities and stresses.

Psychosocial Interventions

There are numerous psychosocial interventions that serve to lessen stress in an individual's environment and to decrease his or her vulnerability (see Chapters 27–32 and Chapter 34 of this book). We briefly review the interventions that have been most intensely studied, and identify newer treatments that show promise. These include family psychoeducation, social skills training, case management, vocational rehabilitation, cognitive rehabilitation, and various forms of psychotherapy and coping strategies.

Family psychoeducation.   Family psychoeducation programs arose in response to the many studies indicating that the course of schizophrenia is related to the emotional climate in and communication style of the family (Brown et al. 1972; Doane et al. 1985; Vaughn and Leff 1976). Dysfunctional communication, referred to in the literature as *high expressed emotion (high EE),* includes expressions of criticism and hostility as well as overinvolvement. Investigators in these studies have demonstrated that schizophrenic individuals from high-EE households are three to four times more likely to relapse than those from low-EE families, suggesting that high EE acts as a stressor that can contribute to psychosis.

A number of programs have been developed to provide information about the illness of schizophrenia and to help families develop effective coping strategies for dealing with schizophrenic relatives. Some programs have altered the EE of families, with studies demonstrating that schizophrenic individuals whose families received psychoeducation experience fewer, less frequent, and less severe relapses than those whose families did not (Falloon et al. 1982; Leff et al. 1985; Tarrier et al. 1989). Results from reviews and meta-analyses of the various studies (Lam 1991; Mari 1992) tend to support the effectiveness of these interventions, and suggest that these are some of the most potent interventions (in combination with optimal pharmacotherapy) for influencing the outcome in schizophrenia.

Social skills training.   Social skills training focuses on teaching interpersonal behaviors that address the social deficits commonly documented in individuals with schizophrenia. Behaviors that can be targeted include interpersonal relations, social problem solving, assertiveness, and management of social stress. Social skills training has been viewed as addressing the neuropsychological deficits associated with the social impairments of schizophrenia (Wagman et al. 1987). Although usually conducted in a group format, it can also be conducted one-on-one. Such training relies on the learning principles of goal setting, role-play, behavioral rehearsals, modeling, coaching, reinforcement, and homework. The training is generally offered through modules that may include activities of daily living, medication management, communication skills, stress management, sexuality issues, and vocational preparedness.

The effectiveness of social skills training is the focus of ongoing research. It has been shown that individuals with chronic psychotic disorders can be taught a wide variety of social and living skills. Investigators in five randomized, controlled trials have compared patient-centered social skills training with other therapies (Bellack et al. 1984; Hogarty et al. 1986, 1991; Wallace et al. 1992; Wirshing et al. 1992). It appears that social skills approaches, in combination with optimal pharmacotherapy, have clinical benefits in the short term and can show improvements in quality of life in the long term. Results from a recent meta-analysis of published studies by Benton and Schroeder (1990) demonstrated that skills training can influence behavioral measures of social skills, assertiveness, and discharge from the hospital. In the short term, the greatest benefits appear to occur when social skills training is combined with family psychoeducation (Hogarty et al. 1991; Munroe-Blum et al. 1991), although these effects appear to attenuate over time. Much remains to be learned about the optimal matching of social interventions with specific individual and illness characteristics.

Case management.   Case management attempts to provide psychosocial rehabilitation by linking individuals to needed community resources. It usually contains the elements of functional assessment, patient-directed identification of need, linkages to services, monitoring of progress, and advocacy for the patient. Although, traditionally, case management helped an individual find services, it is now accepted that in many instances the intervention may also be in the form of direct clinical care. Reviews of outcome studies have shown that case management has beneficial effects on social functioning and quality of life and tenure in the community (Goering and Wasylenki, in press; Solomon 1992).

Vocational rehabilitation. There is a broad spectrum of approaches to the assessment and enhancement of vocational and job-readiness skills in schizophrenic individuals. Historically, *vocational rehabilitation* has been a misnomer applied to the institutional provision of low-level, tedious tasks that would challenge the goodwill of the most able. More recently, vocational rehabilitation strategies have taken place in a range of settings, varying from institutions to the community. The key to successful vocational intervention is the combination of effective assessment of the current status of the individual (including cognitive functioning); the development, with the individual, of short-term and longer-term vocational goals; and plans and related activities that facilitate incremental development of skills in the context of realistic incentives and rewards (Jacobs 1988).

Cognitive rehabilitation. Cognitive rehabilitation takes principles from the treatment of individuals with head injuries and related neurocognitive deficits and applies them to schizophrenia. In this rehabilitative model, it is recognized that many individuals with schizophrenia exhibit specific patterns of neurocognitive deficit—especially in the areas of attention, memory, and fine motor skills—that may be addressed with cognitive retraining (Liberman and Green 1992). Given that the vulnerability to psychosis is thought to be related to cognitive information processing, this type of rehabilitation has the potential to address important fundamental components of the disorder (Brenner et al. 1992). Evaluative research on these interventions is just beginning. Preliminary work suggests that cognitive retraining can alter some functions of attention and memory, but it is yet unclear whether these benefits can be sustained.

Other psychosocial interventions. Although traditional, psychodynamic, insight-oriented therapy has been shown to be countertherapeutic in schizophrenia (Drake and Sederer 1986; May 1968), recently there has been a reappraisal of the role of other forms of psychotherapy (Wasylenki 1992). In particular, it has been suggested that individual therapy that is supportive, focuses on stress management, or helps develop coping skills has the potential to be beneficial (Muller et al. 1992).

Other interventions that target coping skills include specific strategies for coping with auditory hallucinations (Romme and Escher 1992), and self-help groups that offer support and encourage sharing of adaptive coping behaviors among group members.

Combined Psychosocial and Pharmacological Treatments

One strategy that is increasingly being advocated as the ideal treatment for schizophrenia is an integration of biological and psychosocial therapies (Carpenter and Keith 1986; Falloon and Liberman 1983). Given that medications are most effective in treating the positive symptoms of schizophrenia (i.e., hallucinations, delusions, and conceptual disorganization) and that psychosocial treatments address functional deficits, behaviors, and possibly negative symptoms, it is evident that the two can be additive. What remains to be seen is the degree to which combined, integrative therapies may be synergistic.

Unfortunately, this area is insufficiently studied, and most of the support for integrated therapy either comes from descriptive case material (Liberman 1988) or is inferred from clinical trials of psychosocial therapies used as adjuncts to pharmacotherapy. Perhaps the best example of a clinical trial of combined treatment is that of the Environmental Personal Indicators in the Course of Schizophrenia Group (Hogarty et al. 1986, 1991), in which the effects of family intervention and social skills training on relapse and social functioning in patients maintained on antipsychotic drugs were studied. At 1-year follow-up, the social treatments used with medication proved to be superior to medication therapy alone, with the strongest effect being in the group receiving both social skills training and family psychoeducation. At 2-year follow-up, some of the effects of social skills training were lost, but the combined treatment was still superior to medication alone. Of the patients receiving psychosocial treatments combined with drug treatment at 2 years, 34% had relapsed, compared with 62% of those receiving medication alone.

Considerably more work needs to be done to evaluate the benefits of integrated therapy. It is not known which combinations of modalities offer the most potential benefit, how they should be timed, and to which subgroup of patients they should be offered. A key question is,

How much do psychosocial treatments work by changing the underlying vulnerability to stress as opposed to sheltering individuals from environmental stress or through targeting medication compliance and other health behaviors?

Pharmacotherapy

Even when pharmacotherapy is the primary or sole treatment, attention to the psychosocial context in which the medication is prescribed can be considered a form of integrated therapy and may optimize drug compliance and enhance the patient's quality of life (Diamond 1985). Consideration of the psychosocial context begins with rational drug prescribing and the avoidance of common mistakes in antipsychotic drug therapy. *Rational drug prescribing* is a concept promoted by pharmacists to motivate prescribers to use drug agents correctly. With antipsychotics, rational use entails choosing an agent with the fewest possible side effects, using the lowest dosage possible, avoiding unnecessary polypharmacy, and prescribing the simplest dose schedule. Unfortunately, pharmacoepidemiological surveys show that antipsychotics are often used in unnecessarily high dosages, that significant polypharmacy occurs, and that unreasonable split-dosage schedules persist (Collins et al. 1992).

In addition to rational drug prescribing, other important elements of pharmacotherapy include collaboration with the patient and significant others, flexibility and appreciation of the longitudinal course of illness on the part of the clinician, a targeting of the patient's quality of life, and clinician empathy.

Collaboration.   Successful pharmacotherapy depends on a consultative, collaborative relationship with the patient. Such a relationship is best effected when both the individual with the illness and his or her significant others are involved in planning therapy, setting treatment goals, and monitoring outcome. This approach can be unfamiliar to clinicians who have excluded families from systems of care or have excluded patients from treatment decisions. Unfortunately, it is easier to infantilize schizophrenic patients and assume control over treatment decisions than to collaborate with them. However, creating a dialogue that allows patients to be informed and to take more control in treatment decisions can be productive, even in the face of poor insight or frank delusions.

Flexibility and appreciation of longitudinal course.   Harding et al. (1987), in their longitudinal studies, demonstrated that individuals with schizophrenia have markedly changing courses of illness over long periods, and that their therapeutic needs vary from one stage of illness to the next. Pharmacotherapy should reflect this symptom fluidity by being flexible in choice of drug, of drug dosages, and even of whether to use medication at all. The tendency to ignore the longitudinal course of schizophrenia and to focus on cross-sectional assessment has been eloquently described by Harding et al. (1992); reliance on cross-sectional assessment has implications for pharmacotherapy as well. Clinicians may ignore the latency period in resolving psychosis and continue to increase medications instead of waiting for resolution. In addition, it is easy to react to fluctuating symptomatology by prescribing more medication, when just riding out the exacerbation may suffice. Greater attention to longitudinal course and a preparedness to ride out behavioral exacerbations without increasing medications are indicated with schizophrenia.

The same short-term bias relates to attempts to lower drug dosages. Drug withdrawal can precipitate cholinergic rebound that is experienced by the patient as agitation and dysphoria. An overemphasis on short-term effects may cause clinicians to misinterpret these withdrawal effects as relapsing psychosis. Patience and attention to longitudinal course will allow patients to ride out any short-term effects.

Quality of life.   Quality of life is an important treatment target of pharmacotherapy (Awad 1992; Collins et al. 1991; Lehman et al. 1982). Traditionally, clinicians have targeted the amelioration of positive symptoms as the key therapeutic end point of antipsychotic pharmacotherapy. Unfortunately, this perspective may ignore negative symptoms of the illness and general issues of quality of life, most notably the impact of adverse effects. Imagine a patient with complete amelioration of hallucinations and delusions but with significant deficits related to sedation, dysphoria, parkinsonism, and akathisia. Then consider a patient on a different drug regimen or dosage who experiences fewer adverse sequelae but persistent hallucinations and delusions. If resolution of positive symptoms is the sole treatment target, then the first scenario would be preferable. If functioning—or quality of life—is key, then the second scenario would be preferred, as long as the positive symptoms did not interfere with functioning.

Clinician empathy.   A final tenet of treatment is the reemphasis on empathy as the cornerstone of drug therapy. Empathy is the ability of the prescriber to communicate an understanding of what the schizophrenic patient is experiencing, especially in relation to the need for medication. Antipsychotic medication is rife with adverse effects, can impair quality of life, and can leave a patient with a distressing, deadened feeling. Its use is recommended only because in most cases the risks and dangers of being psychotic outweigh the risks and dangers of being on medication. However, many schizophrenic individuals struggle with these alternatives and require a psychotherapeutic and psychoeducational process to help them come to terms with the consequences of the illness and its treatments and to make informed and effective decisions. The clinician can help patients in making this transition by communicating an appreciation of the limits of medication and conveying empathy with the patient's situation. All too often a patient's ambivalence to medication and experimentations with self-prescribing are labeled as a denial of illness and met with a clinician's punitive, judgmental admonishments. Prescribers should ask themselves what it would be like to take medication on a regular basis and honestly appraise what their compliance would be. Such an experiment might be facilitated by the knowledge that more patients with hypertension are noncompliant with their prescribed medications than are those with schizophrenia.

Conclusions

The reasoning set forth in this chapter argues for the necessary integration of drug treatments and psychosocial interventions in the therapy of schizophrenia. The stress-vulnerability model, in its various forms, is a template for how biology and environment interact in the expression, course, and outcome of illness, as well as a rationale for the use of both pharmacological and nonpharmacological treatments. Unfortunately, there has been little research into integrative therapies in schizophrenia. If combined treatment approaches are rarely or unsystematically used in clinical practice, it may be because much remains to be clarified about them.

A range of drug and psychosocial interventions have been studied separately, and, in a few cases, together. Still, the rationale for selecting particular strategies in combination remains unclear, and the optimal mix of integrative treatments is unknown. The effects of combined treatments in patients with different clinical, demographic, and prognostic variables are also unknown. The contribution of gender, severity of illness, and other factors may influence the type of treatment mix and its effectiveness. The course of illness is particularly important, as it is expected that treatment needs change significantly throughout different stages of illness.

Although knowledge is lacking, enough information exists to infer the value of integrated treatments in schizophrenia and to make integration a worthy objective in treatment planning. Various psychosocial interventions are possible within an integrated system of care. It is suggested that clinicians who cannot provide psychosocial interventions for their patients because of lack of resources, or because they are in medically oriented systems of care, can still integrate elements of psychosocial therapy into their pharmacotherapy. Such integration provides for a more humane, rational drug therapy, reduces the stress and vulnerability that contribute to schizophrenic symptomatology, and aims to optimize the patient's quality of life.

References

Awad AG: Quality of life of schizophrenic patients on medications and implications for new drug trials. Hosp Community Psychiatry 43:262–265, 1992

Bassett AS: Linkage analysis of schizophrenia: challenges and promise. Soc Biol 38:189–196, 1991

Bellack AS, Turner SM, Hersen M, et al: An examination of the efficacy of social skills training for chronic schizophrenic patients. Hosp Community Psychiatry 35:1023–1028, 1984

Benton MK, Schroeder HE: Social skills training with schizophrenics: a meta-analytic evaluation. J Consult Clin Psychol 58:741–747, 1990

Boker W, Brenner HD, Wurgler S: Vulnerability linked deficiencies, psychopathology and coping behaviour of schizophrenics and their relatives. Br J Psychiatry 155 (suppl 5):128–135, 1989

Brenner HD, Hodel B, Genner R, et al: Biological and cognitive vulnerability factors in schizophrenia: implications for treatment. Br J Psychiatry 161 (suppl 18):154–163, 1992

Brown GW, Harris T: Social Origins of Depression: A Study of Psychiatric Disorders in Women. London, Tavistock, 1978

Brown GW, Birley JLT, Wing JK: Influence of family life on the course of schizophrenic disorders: a replication. Br J Psychiatry 121:241–258, 1972

Carpenter WT, Keith SJ: Integrating treatments in schizophrenia. Psychiatr Clin North Am 9:153–164, 1986

Ciompi L, Dauwalder H-P, Maier C, et al: The pilot project 'Soteria Berne': clinical experiences and results. Br J Psychiatry 161 (suppl 18):145–153, 1992

Collins EJ, Hogan TP, Desai H: Measurement of therapeutic response in schizophrenia: a critical survey. Schizophr Res 5:249–253, 1991

Collins EJ, Hogan TP, Awad AG: Pharmacoepidemiology of treatment refractory schizophrenia. Can J Psychiatry 37:192–195, 1992

Dawson D, Munroe-Blum H, Bartolucci G: Schizophrenia in Focus: Guidelines for Treatment and Rehabilitation. New York, Human Sciences Press, 1983

Diamond R: Drugs and the quality of life: the patient's point of view. J Clin Psychiatry 46:29–35, 1985

Doane JA, Falloon IRH, Goldstein MJ, et al: Parental affective style and the treatment of schizophrenia. Arch Gen Psychiatry 42:34–42, 1985

Drake RE, Sederer LI: Inpatient psychosocial treatment of chronic schizophrenia: negative effects and current guidelines. Hosp Community Psychiatry 37:897–901, 1986

Engel GL: The need for a new medical model: a challenge for biomedicine. Science 196:129–135, 1977

Falloon IRH, Liberman RP: Interactions between drug and psychosocial therapy in schizophrenia. Schizophr Bull 9:543–554, 1983

Falloon IRH, Boyd JL, McGill CW, et al: Family management in the prevention of exacerbations of schizophrenia. N Engl J Med 306:1437–1444, 1982

Goering PN, Wasylenki DA: Case management for the severely mentally ill, in Modern Community Psychiatry. Edited by Breakly W. Oxford, Oxford University Press (in press)

Goldstein MJ: Further data concerning the relation between premorbid adjustment and paranoid symptomatology. Schizophr Bull 4:236–243, 1978

Harding CM, Brooks GW, Ashikaga T, et al: The Vermont longitudinal study, II: long-term outcome of subjects who retrospectively met DSM-III criteria for schizophrenia. Am J Psychiatry 144:727–735, 1987

Harding CM, Zubin J, Strauss JS: Chronicity in schizophrenia: revisited. Br J Psychiatry 161 (suppl 18):27–37, 1992

Hogarty GE, Schooler NR, Ulrich R, et al: Fluphenazine and social therapy in the aftercare of schizophrenic patients: relapse analysis of two year controlled study of fluphenazine decanoate and fluphenazine hydrochloride. Arch Gen Psychiatry 36:1283–1294, 1979

Hogarty GE, Anderson CM, Reiss DJ, et al: Family psychoeducation, social skills training, and maintenance chemotherapy in the aftercare treatment of schizophrenia. Arch Gen Psychiatry 43:633–642, 1986

Hogarty GE, Anderson CM, Reiss DJ, et al: Family psychoeducation, social skills training and maintenance chemotherapy in the aftercare treatment of schizophrenia, II: two-year effects of a controlled study on relapse and adjustment. Arch Gen Psychiatry 48:340–347, 1991

Jacobs HE: Vocational rehabilitation, in Psychiatric Rehabilitation of Chronic Mental Patients. Edited by Liberman RP. Washington, DC, American Psychiatric Press, 1988, pp 245–284

Lam DH: Psychosocial family intervention in schizophrenia: a review of empirical studies. Psychol Med 21:423–441, 1991

Leff J, Kuipers L, Berkowitz R, et al: A controlled trial of social intervention in the families of schizophrenic patients. Br J Psychiatry 146:594–600, 1985

Lehman AF, Ward NC, Linn LS: Chronic mental patients: the quality of life issue. Am J Psychiatry 134:1271–1276, 1982

Liberman RP (ed): Psychiatric Rehabilitation of Chronic Mental Patients. American Psychiatric Press, Washington, DC, 1988

Liberman RP, Green MF: Whither cognitive-behavioral therapy for schizophrenia. Schizophr Bull 18:27–36, 1992

Mari J: A Systematic Overview of Family Interventions and Relapse on Schizophrenia: A Meta-Analysis of Research Findings. M.Sc. thesis, Department of Clinical Epidemiology and Biostatistics, McMaster University, September, 1992

May PRA: Treatment of Schizophrenia: A Comparative Study of Five Treatment Methods. New York, Science House, 1968

Mosher LR, Menn AJ: Community residential treatment for schizophrenia: two-year follow-up data. Hosp Community Psychiatry 29:715–723, 1978

Muller P, Bandelow B, Gaebel W, et al: Intermittent medication, coping, and psychotherapy: interactions in relapse prevention and course modification. Br J Psychiatry 161 (suppl 18):140–144, 1992

Munroe-Blum H, Harris S, Lambert L, et al: A trial of enriched social treatments in schizophrenia: design and outcome. Schizophr Res 6:306–307, 1991

Murray RM, Lewis S: Is schizophrenia a neurodevelopmental disorder? BMJ 295:681–682, 1987

Norman RMG, Malla AK: Stressful life events and schizophrenia, I: a review of the research. Br J Psychiatry 162:161–166, 1993

Nuechterlein KH, Dawson ME: A heuristic vulnerability/stress model of schizophrenic episodes. Schizophr Bull 10:300–312, 1984

Nuechterlein KH, Goldstein MJ, Ventura J, et al: Patient-environment relationships in schizophrenia: information processing, communication deviance, autonomic arousal and stressful life events. Br J Psychiatry 155 (suppl 5):84–89, 1989

Prudo R, Munroe-Blum H: Five-year outcome and prognosis in schizophrenia: a report from the London Field Research Centre of the International Pilot Study of Schizophrenia. Br J Psychiatry 150:345–354, 1987

Rabkin JG: Stressful life events and schizophrenia: a review of the literature. Psychol Bull 87:408–425, 1980

Romme MAJ, Escher ADMAC: Hearing voices. Schizophr Bull 15:209–216, 1992

Solomon P: The efficacy of case management services for severely mentally disabled clients. Community Ment Health J 28:163–180, 1992

Strauss JS, Carpenter WT: The prediction of outcome in schizophrenia, III: five year outcome and its predictors. Arch Gen Psychiatry 34:159–163, 1977

Strauss JS, Rakfeldt J, Harding CM, et al: Psychological and social aspects of negative symptoms. Br J Psychiatry 155 (suppl 7):128–132, 1989

Tarrier N, Barrowclough C, Vaughn CE, et al: The community management of schizophrenia: a controlled trial of a behavioral intervention with families to reduce relapse. Br J Psychiatry 153:532–542, 1989

Vaughn CE, Leff JP: The influence of family and social factors on the course of psychiatric illness. Br J Psychiatry 129:125–137, 1976

Wagman AMI, Heinrichs DW, Carpenter WT: Deficit and nondeficit forms of schizophrenia: neuropsychological evaluation. Psychiatry Res 22:319–330, 1987

Wallace CJ, Liberman RP, Mackain JJ, et al: Effectiveness and replicability of modules for teaching social and instrumental skills to the severely mentally ill. Am J Psychiatry 149:654–658, 1992

Wasylenki DA: Psychotherapy of schizophrenia revisited. Hosp Community Psychiatry 43:123–126, 1992

Wirshing WC, Marder SR, Eckman T et al: Acquisition and retention of skills training methods in chronic schizophrenic outpatients. Psychopharmacol Bull 28:241–245, 1992

World Health Organization: International Classification of Impairments, Disabilities, and Handicaps. Geneva, Switzerland, WHO, 1980

Zubin J, Spring B: Vulnerability—a new view on schizophrenia. J Abnorm Psychol 86:103–126, 1977

Zubin J, Steinhauer SR, Condray R: Vulnerability to relapse in schizophrenia. Br J Psychiatry 161 (suppl 18):13–18, 1992

CHAPTER 34

Individualizing Psychiatric Rehabilitation in Schizophrenia

Pierre Lalonde, M.D., F.R.C.P.C.

Over the last three decades, the treatment and under-standing of schizophrenia have undergone consider-able progress, and future developments in this area appear even more promising. The pessimism of many therapists, pa-tients, and relatives of those with the illness is slowly giving way to optimism in the face of realistic, attainable, and measurable therapeutic goals. The readaptation or development of new skills to compensate for a disability or handicap is the essence of psychiatric rehabilitation in schizophrenia. One definition of *rehabilitate* is "to restore to good repute" (Merriam-Webster 1993, p. 985), something that is import-ant to schizophrenic patients and their families, who often endure the burden of social stigma.

In this chapter, I review general treatment issues that have the potential either to impede or to facilitate the psychiatric rehabilitation of schizophrenic patients. I also discuss the role of the multidiscipli-nary team and that of the clinical psychiatrist.

The Vulnerability-Stress Model of Schizophrenia

The *vulnerability-stress model of schizophrenia*, illustrated in Figure 34–1, integrates various research findings and clinical observations, and demonstrates various biopsychosocial factors involved in schizophrenia and their complex interrelationships.

Recent advances in the genetics of schizophrenia, brain imaging, neurotransmitter function, and receptor physiology, in addition to a better understanding of the mechanisms of action of antipsychotic drugs, provide a strong basis for a biological substrate in schizophrenia in which diverse socioenvironmental factors (e.g., communication patterns such as expressed emotion), life events, and social pressures to "perform" interact and can overload an already vulnerable psyche (Lalonde 1991). Current research is placing less emphasis on pinpointing the exact brain site–specific localization of schizophrenia in favor of a more functional understanding of the illness. The investigation of normal brain function in nonpsychiatric control subjects com-

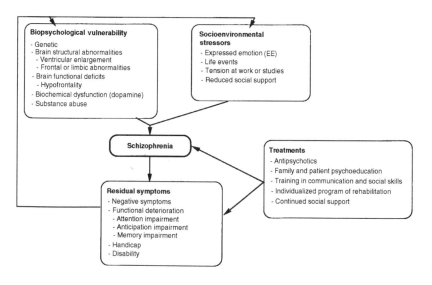

Figure 34–1. Vulnerability-stress model of schizophrenia.

pared with that in schizophrenic individuals is yielding significant contributions (Buchsbaum 1990).

Individualized Treatment Strategies

Schizophrenic patients require an individualized treatment approach whose primary objectives are to reduce disability, improve or control the level of symptomatology, stimulate psychosocial functioning, and decrease patient suffering. Relevant clinical issues presented in this chapter include diagnostic considerations with proper recognition of positive and negative symptoms, helping patients organize their daily living activities, improving patients' social skills, and reducing the impact of cognitive deficits, in addition to providing adequate pharmacotherapy.

Diagnostic considerations and evaluation of positive and negative symptoms.   In North America, a majority of psychiatrists are familiar with DSM-III-R (American Psychiatric Association 1987) diagnostic criteria for schizophrenia and are now becoming familiar with the further changes in these diagnostic criteria in DSM-IV (American Psychiatric Association 1994). Despite the ongoing debate surrounding the use of various diagnostic classifications in psychiatry, the introduction of the DSM classification system has had a lasting impact on general psychiatric practice. With regard to schizophrenic disorders, the DSM classification has undoubtedly improved diagnostic reliability and symptom validity.

The rating scales commonly used for the clinical assessment of schizophrenic disorders include the Brief Psychiatric Rating Scale (Lukoff et al. 1986; Overall and Gorham 1962), the Scale for the Assessment of Negative Symptoms (Andreasen 1982a, 1989), the Scale for the Assessment of Positive Symptoms (Andreasen 1982b; Andreasen et al. 1990), and the Positive and Negative Syndrome Scale (PANSS; Kay et al. 1987). These scales are used to evaluate changes in schizophrenic symptoms and their progression over time, in addition to patients' responses to various pharmacological and psychosocial treatments.

During the last decade, the two-syndrome concept of schizophrenia (Crow 1985) has generated considerable research interest (see discussion in Chapter 5 of this book). Briefly summarized, several research studies have shown that schizophrenic patients with predominantly negative symptoms tend to be unemployed males with poor premorbid social adjustment, an early age at onset of illness, little formal education, impaired cognitive testing, and poor response to neuroleptic treatment (Andreasen et al. 1990). Contrary to earlier findings, these patients do not consistently demonstrate larger ventricle-to-brain ratios (VBRs) than do patients with a mixed or predominantly positive symptom presentation.

Heterogeneity in individual treatment response, family history, age at onset of illness, and symptom presentation are all known to influence the outcome of schizophrenia. In addition, the diagnostic boundaries surrounding schizophrenia-spectrum disorders have even prompted suggestions of the existence of several schizophrenias as opposed to one unique disease process.

Assisting patients in their activities of daily living. Because schizophrenia often appears at a time when a patient's independent living skills are just beginning to mature, it is not surprising that patients with a later age at onset tend to have a better schizophrenic prognosis.

Assisting patients in their various activities of daily living (e.g., budgeting, preparing meals, occupying leisure time, performing work and household tasks) is a major component of psychiatric rehabilitation. Nevertheless, the difficulty experienced in stimulating patients to participate in these programs can be discouraging to any therapist. When negative symptoms (e.g., emotional and passive or apathetic social withdrawal, problem-solving difficulties, poor anticipatory abilities) are not recognized, the therapist or family members can perceive the patient as negligent, lazy, or lacking in motivation.

Diverse interventions—ranging from social skills training to continuity of care throughout inpatient and outpatient services—play an important role in the psychiatric rehabilitation of individuals with schizophrenia (Lalonde 1992). Examples of tasks in which patients frequently require intervention and assistance are managing sleep, acquiring basic motivational skills, training in personal hygiene, developing balanced eating habits, performing housework activities, using public transportation services, conducting errands, managing a budget, planning the day, following up on appointments, scheduling activities and leisure time, and planning for a return to work or school. Results from studies have shown that training patients in these areas increases their ability to cope with the impact of their illness (McCarthy et al. 1986; Waismann and Rowland 1989). Liberman (1992) pioneered the development of psychoeducational modules designed to address the following areas: medication and symptom management, recreation or leisure time management, and conversational skills. Each of these modules has specific training objectives and provides an opportunity for patients to participate in group interactions.

Improving social skills.   Clinicians often encourage patients to participate in group activities. However, schizophrenic withdrawal can be a defense mechanism against an overly stimulating environment. When asked, some schizophrenic patients will link their various interpersonal difficulties with distrust, apathy, or asociality. Patients may also express discomfort with interacting with health care providers and therapists, as well as difficulties in communicating anger or affection to intimate partners, family members, and other individuals. In addition, conceptual disorganization and abstract reasoning difficulties are commonly observed in schizophrenic patients, although they rarely acknowledge having a communication problem (Massel et al. 1991).

Reducing the impact of cognitive deficits.   Neuropsychological function in schizophrenia is the object of much renewed interest (see discussion in Chapter 9 of this book). Several investigators (Andreasen 1982a, 1982b; Reed et al. 1992), using neuropsychological probes such as the Wisconsin Card Sorting Test (Heaton 1985) and the Tower of London test (Krikorian et al. 1994), have demonstrated that attention-span deficits and anticipatory difficulties are components of schizophrenia. We are still unsure of the extent to which neuroleptics and anticholinergic medications contribute to or improve the cognitive functioning of schizophrenic patients. Judgments on the efficacy of cognitive remediation techniques to correct information-processing deficits in schizophrenia await further research (Green 1993).

Individualized Evaluation

The multidisciplinary treatment team often reevaluates the treatment needs of the patient, which often include various degrees of pharmacological, psychotherapeutic, and social treatment interventions. Several investigators (Hogarty et al. 1991; see also Chapters 28 and 33 of this book) have clearly established the value of combining pharmacological treatments with social skills training and family intervention in the prevention of schizophrenic relapse.

Several treatment centers in the United States and Canada have adopted a case management model of care in the treatment of schizophrenic patients in which the role of the case manager is frequently occupied by a nonpsychiatrist mental health professional (see also discussion in Chapter 29 of this book). However, it is often the clinical psychiatrist who coordinates—in a concerted effort with the multidisciplinary treatment team and the patient (Ricci 1990)—the use of complementary resources (see Figure 34–2).

When beginning treatment, many patients do not recognize the importance of rehabilitation. However, once patients are engaged in a rehabilitative effort, they often realize how much "catching up" they have to do. As Bachrach (1992) noted, the credibility of psychiatric treatments resides in their ability to implement effective treatment programs for long-term chronically ill patients.

Evaluation of Needs

A number of scales exist to evaluate a patient's needs and to plan for the level of care required. For example, Brewin et al. (1987) developed the Need for Care Assessment Scale (NFCAS), which measures the patient's level of handicap and physical, psychological, social, and treatment needs. This scale helps to evaluate the patient at the symptom and behavioral levels and to assess his or her daily living skills.

Affleck and McGuire (1984) developed the Morningside Rehabilitation Status Scale, which evaluates four main areas: dependence-independence, activity-inactivity, social integration-isolation, and symptoms and deviant behavior.

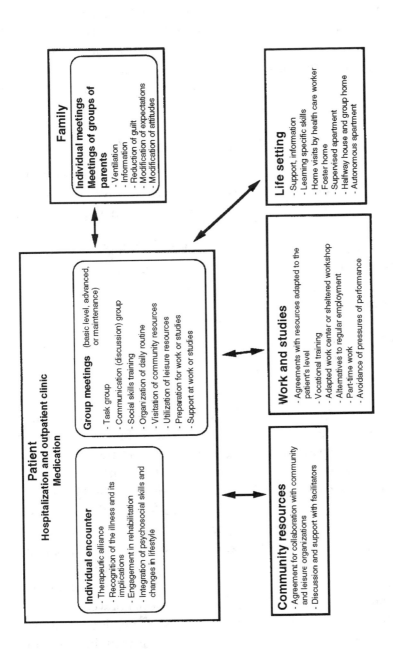

Figure 34–2. Complementary resources for psychiatric rehabilitation.

Wallace (1986) revised several functional evaluation scales that enable the clinician to identify the social skills necessary for community adjustment. Some of these scales evaluate the patient's overall performance in a certain role (e.g., as student, housekeeper, worker), whereas others concentrate on specific skills (e.g., personal hygiene, budgeting).

Quality-of-Life Assessment

Quality-of-life issues in schizophrenic patients are reviewed in Chapter 31 of this book. In recent years, these issues have become increasingly important as studies in this area focus on the assessment of subjective well-being in the patient.

In a 15-point scale, Flanagan (1978) established a series of categories that specify the principal characteristics of quality of life:

- Physical and material well-being
- Relationships with other people
- Social, community, and civic activities
- Personal development and fulfillment
- Recreation

Baker and Intagliata (1982) developed the Satisfaction With Life Domains Scale, using a visual measurement consisting of seven levels, ranging from very satisfied (delighted face with a large upturned smile) to very dissatisfied (terrible face with a deep frown). Lehman (1988) adopted the same visual measurement to develop the Quality of Life Interview, which is but one of a few instruments with known psychometric properties for assessing the quality of life of individuals with chronic mental disorders. This scale is supported by a conceptual base of general quality-of-life theory that integrates access to resources, fulfillment of social roles, satisfaction with life in various domains, and general life satisfaction into a multivariate model of well-being.

When a patient is comfortable in his or her life situation, this comfort can result either from effective treatment interventions or from the patient's lack of ability to deal with or recognize his or her difficulties. For the patient to mobilize himself or herself, overcome apathy, and become involved in the therapeutic process, it is often necessary that the patient perceive something as being unsatisfactory in his or her current life situation. In addition, the patient must believe that the proposed rehabilitation program is within his or her capabilities. Instead of offering a uniform rehabilitation program to all patients, the clinician should make every effort to identify particular areas of dissatisfaction in a patient's life and to suggest appropriate action.

Individualized Intervention

Pharmacological Treatment

With the introduction of antipsychotic medications, clinicians have been able to markedly reduce the anxiety and suffering of the majority of patients with positive symptoms of schizophrenia (see Chapter 12 of this book). Although symptom reduction is a major goal, patients should—as much as is possible—be comfortable with their medication. In this sense, concern over tardive dyskinesia may be exaggerated as patients are often unaware of its presence, and it is primarily family members who notice the grotesque facial expressions that accompany it. On the other hand, patients complain far more frequently of akathisia and drug-induced parkinsonism. To reduce neuroleptic noncompliance, careful attention should be paid to extrapyramidal reactions and other side effects of antipsychotic medications with proper dosage adjustments, use of antiparkinsonian medication, or medication change to another class of antipsychotic agent.

There is increasing evidence that schizophrenic patients who receive early and long-term treatment interventions with neuroleptics have a better prognosis (Ram et al. 1992; see also Chapter 16). In the long term, however, what is important is not so much that patients receive neuroleptics the moment they are hospitalized, but that the experience of taking the medication is sufficiently positive so that patients will agree to continue it over a prolonged period. When positive symptoms are not too anxiety provoking and negative symptoms not too inhibiting, and when patients are comfortable with their medication, it is then that they derive the greatest benefit from a rehabilitation program.

The value of long-acting depot neuroleptic medications in controlling positive symptoms and improving medication compliance has been clearly demonstrated (Hogarty et al. 1991). If symptoms recur, the clinician should always look for psychosocial stresses that can upset the patient's equilibrium (Hogarty 1984).

When a patient insists on interrupting his or her depot neuroleptic injections, the clinician should remind the patient of the risk of relapse and redirect other treatment interventions. Without the biological stabilization afforded by a neuroleptic, the patient is usually not receptive to other psychosocial interventions. Hogarty (1984) demonstrated that the risk of relapse increases markedly following discontinuation of neuroleptics. Nonetheless, many patients will, at some point or another, experience the need to interrupt their neuroleptic medication because of bothersome side effects, pressure from other individuals to interrupt medication, or a desire to see if they can overcome the illness through personal strength. Clearly, it is important to follow the patient even in a period of interrupted neuroleptic medication. In the event of a predicted relapse, it is not uncommon that the patient's confidence in the therapist increases. However, an estimated 20% of patients will not experience a schizophrenic relapse following the withdrawal of neuroleptic medication. For clinicians, the follow-up of such patients who continue to do well off medication is a pleasant experience.

Psychosocial Rehabilitation

The deinstitutionalization movement in psychiatry catapulted thousands of individuals with schizophrenia and other serious mental disorders out of hospitals, often without adequate preparation or suitable resources to successfully integrate them into the community.

The implementation of a rehabilitation program whose aim is the normalization and reintegration of all schizophrenic patients into regular and competitive activities is not a realistic goal. Rather, a rehabilitation program should be tailored to the needs of the individual patient, in a manner that is flexible and gradual and that sets realistic expectations. However, therapists generally do not simply wait for a patient to be motivated for treatment. The ideal rehabilitation intervention should probably be halfway between stressful stimulation and neglectful abandonment.

Clinicians often demonstrate creativity in developing new and effective rehabilitation approaches. Furthermore, a patient will be motivated to participate in a particular activity if he or she recognizes the need for such knowledge. The role of the clinician is to offer a variety of engaging activities adapted to the changing needs of the patient.

Rehabilitation interventions do not oppose or contradict other treatment approaches (e.g., pharmacological, psychodynamic, systemic) but rather interact with other therapeutic factors.

Involvement of the Family

Results from studies of the role of expressed emotion (EE) in schizophrenia (Vaughn and Leff 1981; see also Chapter 28 of this book) have clearly demonstrated the importance of involving families and relatives in the therapeutic process. Patients' families are more often strong allies than nuisances in the rehabilitation process of the schizophrenic patient (Spanoil et al. 1987), and well-informed parents develop attitudes that help prevent relapses (Falloon et al. 1985; Hogarty et al.1991; Mueser et al. 1992). Clinicians generally recognize the importance of family interactions and will often go beyond the familiar dyadic therapist-patient relationship to better understand these issues.

In North America, family support groups have had a considerable impact in improving the quality of care for the mentally ill in addition to promoting and funding new research. These groups—some of which have become important lobbying forces (e.g., the National Alliance for the Mentally Ill)—have greatly contributed to reduce family burden and the social stigma associated with mental illness.

The Biopsychosocial Multidisciplinary Treatment Approach

Multidisciplinary teamwork is indispensable to the treatment process of many schizophrenic patients. More clinical psychiatrists should become actively involved in the coordination of rehabilitation services for the chronically ill schizophrenic patient. If psychiatrists exclude themselves from this process, there is the risk of an unhappy division among the biological, psychological, and social aspects of treatment.

Nevertheless, psychiatry's better understanding of schizophrenia, accomplished through decades of dedicated research, and the prospects of improved psychosocial and pharmacological treatments (as highlighted throughout the course of this book) enable all mental health professionals, patients, and families to be optimistic about the future.

References

Affleck JW, McGuire RJ: The measurement of psychiatric rehabilitation status: a review of the needs of a new scale. Br J Psychiatry 145:517–525, 1984

American Psychiatric Association: Diagnostic and Statistical Manual of Mental Disorders, 3rd Edition, Revised. Washington, DC, American Psychiatric Association, 1987

American Psychiatric Association: Diagnostic and Statistical Manual of Mental Disorders, 4th Edition. Washington, DC, American Psychiatric Association, 1994

Andreasen NC: Negative versus positive schizophrenia: definition and validation. Arch Gen Psychiatry 39:789–794, 1982a

Andreasen NC: Negative symptoms in schizophrenia: definition and reliability. Arch Gen Psychiatry 39:784–788, 1982b

Andreasen NC: The Scale for the Assessment of Negative Symptoms (SANS): conceptual and theoretical foundations. Br J Psychiatry 155:49–52, 1989

Andreasen NC, Flaum M, Swayze VW II, et al: Positive and negative symptoms in schizophrenia: a critical reappraisal. Arch Gen Psychiatry 47:615–621, 1990

Bachrach LL: Psychosocial rehabilitation and psychiatry in the care of long-term patients. Am J Psychiatry 149:1455–1463, 1992

Baker F, Intagliata J: Quality of life in the evaluation of community support systems. Evaluation and Program Planning 5:69–79, 1982

Brewin CR, Wing JK, Mangen SP, et al: Principles and practice of measuring needs in the long-term mentally ill: the MRC needs for care assessment. Psychol Med 17:971–981, 1987

Buchsbaum MS: The frontal lobes, basal ganglia, and temporal lobes as sites for schizophrenia. Schizophr Bull 16:379–389, 1990

Crow TJ: The two-syndrome concept: origins and current status. Schizophr Bull 11:471–486, 1985

Falloon IR, Boyd JL, McGill CW, et al: Family management in the prevention of morbidity of schizophrenia. Arch Gen Psychiatry 42:887–896, 1985

Flanagan JC: A research approach to improving our quality of life. Am Psychol 33:138–147, 1978

Green MF: Cognitive remediation in schizophrenia: is it time yet? Am J Psychiatry 150:178–187, 1993

Heaton R: Wisconsin Card Sorting Test. Odessa, TX, Psychological Assessment Resources, 1985

Hogarty GE: Depot neuroleptics: the relevance of psychosocial factors. J Clin Psychiatry 45:36–42, 1984

Hogarty GE, Anderson CM, Reiss DJ, et al: Family psychoeducation, social skills training, and maintenance chemotherapy in the aftercare treatment of schizophrenia. Arch Gen Psychiatry 48:340–347, 1991

Kay SR, Fiszbein A, Opler LA: The Positive and Negative Syndrome Scale (PANSS) for schizophrenia. Schizophr Bull 13:261–276, 1987

Krikorian R, Bartok J, Gay N: Tower of London procedure: a standard method and developmental data. J Clin Exp Neuropsychol 16:840–850, 1994

Lalonde P: Schizophrénie: vers une nouvelle synthèse. Psychologie Médicale 23:591–593, 1991

Lalonde P: Le programme jeunes adultes. Nervure 4:28–33, 1992

Lehman AF: A quality of life interview for the chronically mentally ill. Evaluation and Program Planning 11:51–62, 1988

Liberman RP (ed): Handbook of Psychiatric Rehabilitation. New York, Macmillan, 1992

Lukoff D, Liberman RP, Nuechterlein KH: Symptom monitoring in the rehabilitation of schizophrenic patients. Schizophr Bull 12:578–602, 1986

McCarthy B, Benson J, Brewin CR: Task motivation and problem appraisal in long-term psychiatric patients. Psychol Med 16:431–438, 1986

Massel HK, Corrigan PW, Liberman RP, et al: Conversation skills training of thought-disordered schizophrenic patients through attention focusing. Psychiatry Res 38:51–61, 1991

Merriam-Webster's Collegiate Dictionary, 10th Edition. Springfield, MA, Merriam-Webster, 1993

Mueser KT, Bellack AS, Wade JH, et al: An assessment of the educational needs of chronic psychiatric patients and their relatives. Br J Psychiatry 160:674–680, 1992

Overall JE, Gorham DR: The Brief Psychiatric Rating Scale. Psychol Rep 10:799–812, 1962

Ram R, Bromet E, Eaton W, et al: The natural course of schizophrenia: a review of first-admission studies. Schizophr Bull 18:185–207, 1992

Reed D, Sullivan ME, Penn DL, et al: Assessment and treatment of cognitive impairment, in Effective Psychiatric Rehabilitation (New Directions for Mental Health Services, No. 53). Edited by Liberman RP. San Francisco, CA, Jossey-Bass, 1992, pp 7–19

Ricci MS: The new after-care clinic: treating individuals rather than masses. J Psychosoc Nurs Ment Health Serv 28:18–21, 1990

Spanoil L, Jung H, Zipple A, et al: Families as a resource in the rehabilitation of the severely psychiatrically disabled, in Families of the Mentally Ill: Coping and Adaptation. Edited by Hatfield AB, Lefley HP. New York, Guilford, 1987, pp 167–190

Vaughn CE, Leff JP: Patterns of emotional response in relatives of schizophrenic patients. Schizophr Bull 7:43–44, 1981

Waismann LC, Rowland LA: Ranking of needs: a new method of assessment for use with chronic psychiatric patients. Acta Psychiatr Scand 80:260–266, 1989

Wallace CJ: Functional assessment in rehabilitation. Schizophr Bull 12:604–630, 1986

Index

Page numbers in **boldface** type refer to figures or tables.